INTRODUCTION TO Neuroscience

1972, To Bill Haney M.D. with great regards – Jeff Minckler

INTRODUCTION TO Neuroscience

Edited by

JEFF MINCKLER, M.D., Ph.D.
Director of Laboratories, Eisenhower Medical Center, Palm Desert, California

With 661 illustrations

Saint Louis

THE C. V. MOSBY COMPANY

1972

Printed in the United States of America

International Standard Book Number 0-8016-3431-8

Library of Congress Catalog Card Number 70-170213

Distributed in Great Britain by Henry Kimpton, London

Contributors

HAROLD B. ANSTALL, M.D.

Professor of Clinical Pathology, University of Utah College of Medicine, Salt Lake City, Utah

THOMAS E. BAUER, B.S.

Programmer-Analyst, Medical Automation, Presbyterian Medical Center, Denver, Colorado

LaVAR G. BEST, Ph.D.

Chief of Speech and Hearing Science, Department of Speech Pathology and Audiology, University of Denver, Denver, Colorado

RONALD COWDEN, Ph.D.

Professor and Chairman, Department of Anatomy, Albany Medical College, Albany, New York

ROBERT LASHER, Ph.D.

Assistant Professor of Anatomy, University of Colorado Medical Center, Denver, Colorado

JEFF MINCKLER, M.D., Ph.D.

Director of Laboratories, Eisenhower Medical Center, Palm Desert, California

TATE M. MINCKLER, M.D.

Associate Professor and Director of Computer Division, Department of Laboratory Medicine, University of Washington, Seattle, Washington

JOHN C. RILEY, M.D.

Radiologist, General Rose Memorial Hospital; Clinical Assistant Professor of Radiology, University of Colorado Medical Center, Denver, Colorado

LUANN M. RINGENBERG, B.A.

Programmer, Medical Automation, Presbyterian Medical Center, Denver, Colorado

DONALD SHEARN, Ph.D.

Associate Professor of Psychology, Colorado College, Colorado Springs, Colorado

To

JOAN

Without whose loving attentions
this book would have been finished long ago

Preface

The multidisciplinary approach to the neurosciences makes sense to most of the pedagogical family oriented about these fields. The only embarrassment associated with this attack arises among the older teachers whose profound interests in one area (say, anatomy) have been permitted to preclude inquiry into the neuroenzyme systems or electrophysiology, for example. Almost everyone agrees that there is enough "business" in each of the splintered disciplines of neurobiology (anatomy, development, physiology, chemistry, psychobiology, communications) to keep an alert teacher or investigator active all his years. Similarly, any one of the more technical approaches (biometrics and quantitative biology, electron microscopy, tissue culture, chemical analysis, electrophysiologic instrumentation, psychologic testing) would appear to be a full-time job. Students in general do not seem to resent the confessed inadequacies of their teachers in highly specialized corners of a subject. Furthermore, they accept with good grace the absolute requirement that they must exceed their mentors' abilities in order to move a subject along. Part of a program in neurosciences to meet these needs is provision at the outset of a broader academic base with depth enough to stay off the "Mickey Mouse" list. This book purports to meet this need.

Fundamental to all the disciplines related to the human nervous system is a solid command of anatomy. The first eleven chapters are directed to this instruction, both in gross and microscopic features. The approach accentuates training in sectional anatomy, which seems to be the most practical means of viewing the various parts of the central nervous system. Basic neuroradiology and growth and biometrics are less usual inclusions but seem to meet a real need in background for neurosciences. Electron microscopy and tissue culture add requisite supporting information relating directly to developmental neurobiology and the review of the histology of neural tissues. Neurochemistry, electrophysiology, and a summary of experimental procedures are added to clarify the functional organization of the nervous system. The classical subdivisions by functional systems are next reviewed. These traditionally provide the knowledge of recognized pathways so important to an assessment of disarray in neural function. Finally, a review of integrative mechanisms is provided to meet the background needs in psychobiology, communications, and a general overview of neural function. The last chapter presents notions of the brain as an engineer might view it in terms of a computer device. It also establishes modeling as a useful tool in exploring the mechanisms of integrated neural function.

The trend in educational circles to provide relevant core curricular material has been kept in mind in formulating this book. An inquiry into the quantitation of peripheral nerves, for example, might be a necessary pursuit for a research student in neurobiology but would be dull indeed for the graduate student in psychology. Similarly, the latter might pry into the integrative sections in detail and omit with profit the sections on electron microscopy and tissue culture. Students in communications might meet a minimal need with the introductory anatomic material, the section on electrophysiology, and the pathway sections covering vestibular and auditory systems together with the motor systems.

The book admits to the occasional need for deferring inquiry in some sections. The core requirement in medical school might well be met with the introductory gross anatomy and the section on pathways. If, however, the student is attracted to pathology as a specialty, a return to background material on microanatomy and basic physiology would be required. If psychiatry became attractive, a return to the sections on integrative physiology would be important.

In providing a source of information for such diversity in the neurosciences, some attention has been directed to reference material. An effort has been made to include principally textual, reference, and review titles at the expense of listing detailed original research. This type of limited bibliography seems more suited to an introductory book. Extended reference material will be found in the cited works.

It is a pleasure to acknowledge the generous participation of the contributors in preparing this book. They have accomplished a proper depth in their sections, which otherwise would not have been possible in a multidisciplinary introductory approach to neuroscience. Nile Root, Sheldon Luper, and Susan Partyka contributed the photographs that distinguish many parts of this work. Sarah Gustafson and Carol Johnson handled the art work with ability and patience. The secretarial load has been carried by Dorothy Nichols. Jeanne Bodson completed the index, a job that always calls for performance above and beyond the call of usual duty.

Jeff Minckler, M.D., Ph.D.

Contents

PART I Gross anatomy

CHAPTER 1

INTRODUCTION

JEFF MINCKLER

BASIC STRUCTURE

The nervous system is an evolutionary product of great complexity. It arises in multicellular animal forms from the necessity to transmit signals from the environment to the organism and from one part of the organism to another. The signal-carrying mechanism is based on at least four interrelated structural neural units. The first of these is the signal receiving unit, the *receptor*. This is a specially designed cell or cellular structure, commonly adapted to respond to only one kind of stimulus. This receptor is responsible for placing the organism, or a part of it, in effective environmental contact. By this means some disturbances in the environment such as changes in temperature, pressure, and chemistry can be "sensed" and translated (transduced) into nervous energy. The second basic strucural unit is the *conductor,* which conveys the signal from the receptor. This nerve cell (neuron), which exists in numerous forms, is adapted to transmit signals as electrochemical "impulses." The impulses are carried to other nerve cells through the third basic structural neural unit, the *synapse,* which is the interrupted union between cells. All neural signals must be transmitted past this synaptic gap in order to provide an effective continuity in the signal from receptor to effector. In general, the synapse is composed of touching or contiguous points of contact, varying in complexity among nerve cells. The fourth and final basic structural unit is the *effector,* which activates the responding part, usually a muscle or a gland. The effector can also be directed to neurons and operate in a manner that will inhibit or augment other neural activities (see Chapter 16). This chain of structures (*receptor* to *conductor* to *synapse* to *conductor* to *effector*) constitutes the simplest expression of a nervous system (Fig. 1-1).[2]

The reflex arc

The primitive nervous system just described can be extended into the prototype of the human nervous system by introducing "connecting" (internuncial) neurons between the receptor and effector.

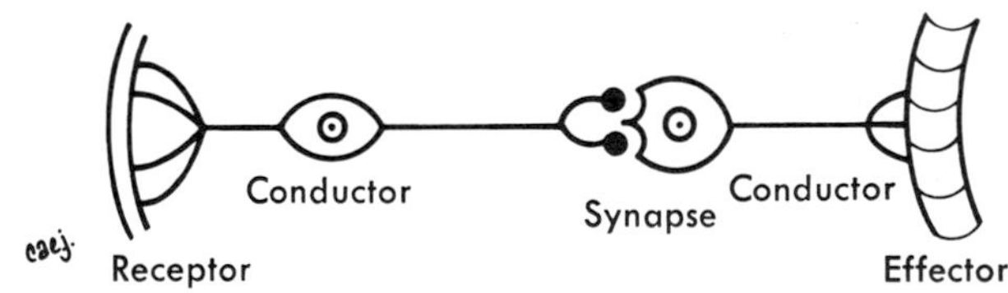

Fig. 1-1. The simplest expression of a nervous system by which a receptor is connected to an effector.

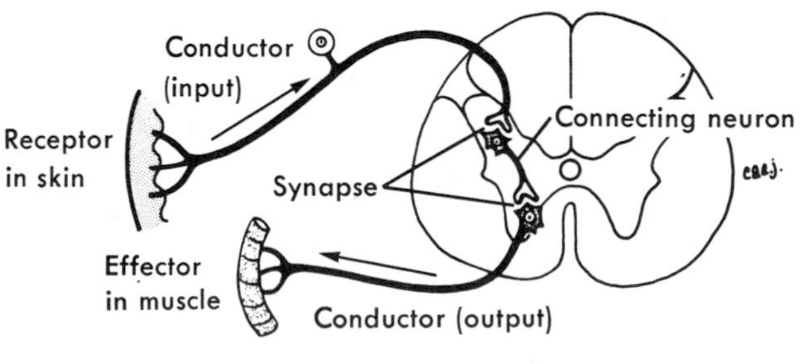

Fig. 1-2. A simple reflex arc with an impulse arising in a peripheral receptor, mediated by a connecting central neuron, and delivered via a peripheral output conductor to an effector.

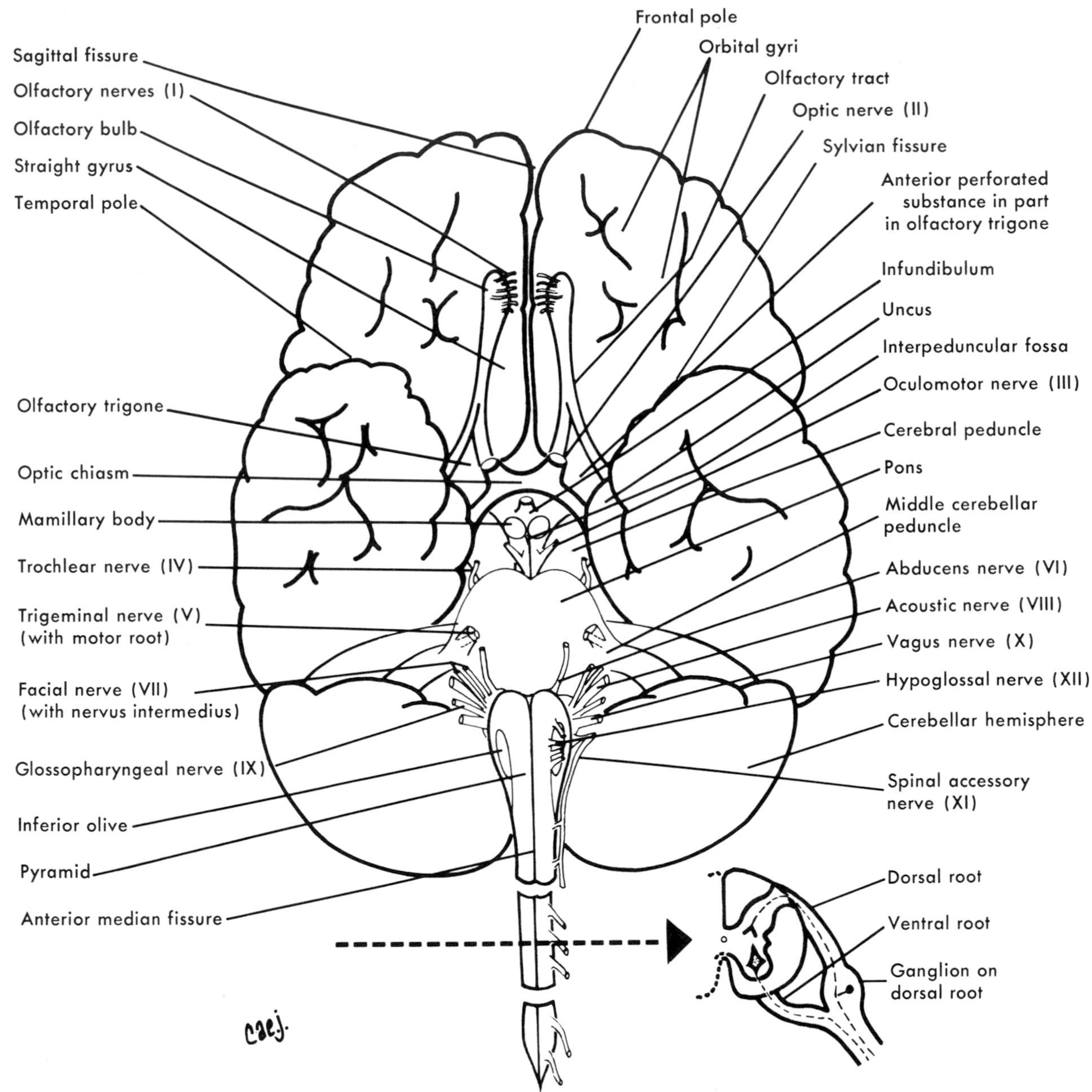

Fig. 1-3. Diagrammatic ventral view of the human CNS; inferior surface of the brain.

This system can now be described as a signal-carrying chain of structural units with the following sequence: *receptor* to *input conductor* to *synapse* to *connecting neuron* to *synapse* to *output conductor* to *effector*. The receptor to effector pathway is realigned (Fig. 1-2) to become the simple *reflex arc* in the human nervous system. A *reflex* traverses this structural arc. This represents a functionally and physiologically primitive response to a stimulus. In the arc displayed in Fig. 1-2, the receptor is a naked nerve ending that can be activated by a painful stimulus to the skin. The input conductor (afferent peripheral nerve) conveys the impulse to the spinal cord (central nervous system), in which a synapse with a connecting or internuncial neuron is located. The impulse is conveyed by this connecting neuron

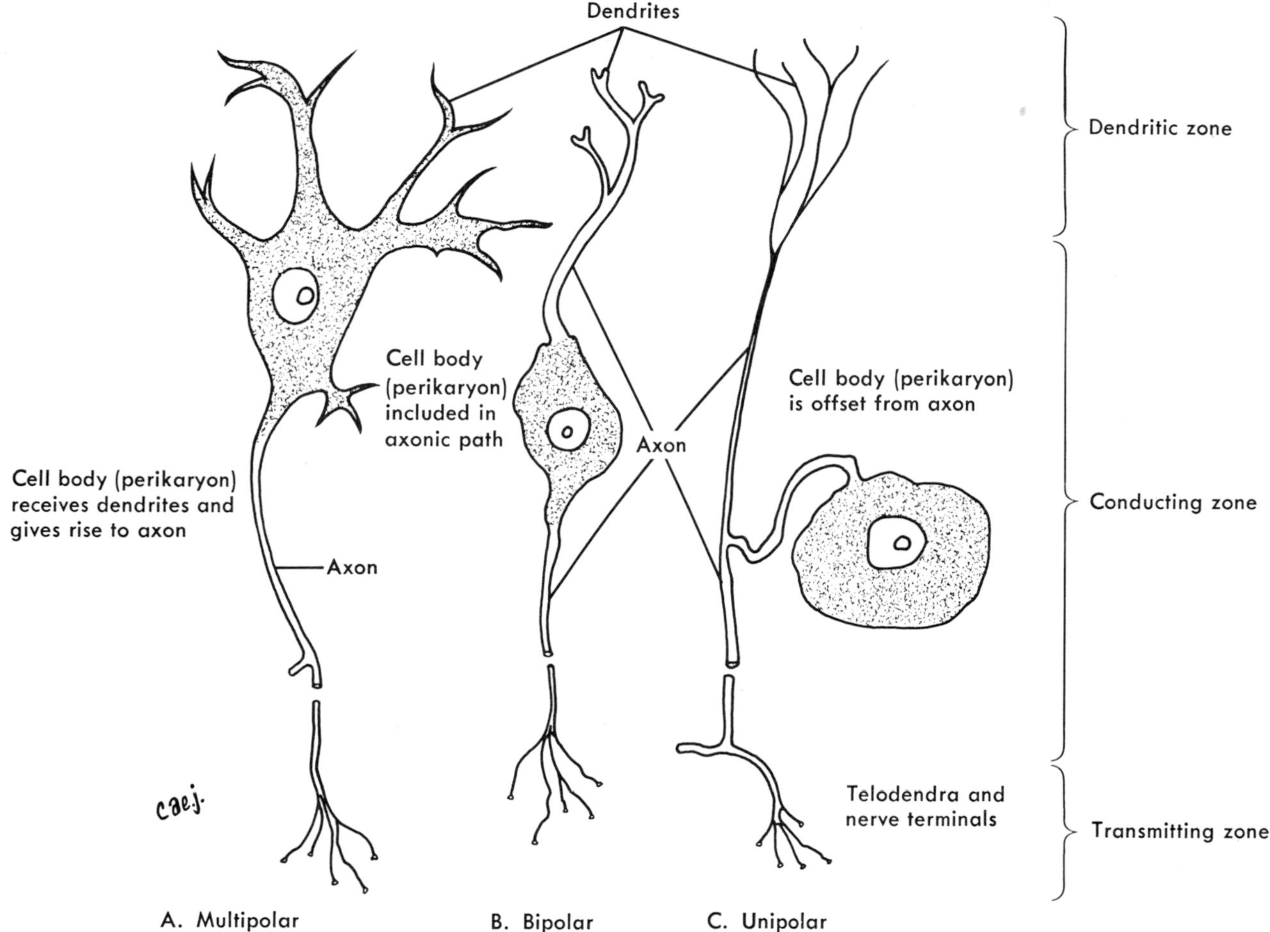

Fig. 1-4. Main types of nerve cells. Perikarya are tracings from photographs.

to the synapse of the output conductor (efferent peripheral nerve), which carries the impulse to the effector in a striated muscle. The usual effect of an impulse carried over this pathway is the reflex withdrawal of the painfully stimulated area. Such reflexes are experienced commonly, in the blinking of a threatened eye, muscle response to a stretched tendon (or tendon reflex), cold sweat from fear, and turning the head in response to noise.

Reflexes vary in the location of the involved structures, in the nature of the receptors, and in the type of the effectors (whether gland, smooth muscle, or striated muscle). Most important, reflex responses vary with the complexity of the connecting neuronal activity in the central nervous system. The connecting neurons possess many alternative routes in the central nervous system, including neural pathways to distant parts of the brain as well as complex activating and inhibiting systems. It is improbable that direct neuronal chains can function without the participation of connecting and activating neurons. Thus, the responses to stimuli in the human organism are probably modified by central neural control. The structural basis for all neural activity, from reflex to complex behavior to thought process, is the interrelationships of neurons. These interrelationships constitute the substance of the study of neuroanatomy.

CENTRAL AND PERIPHERAL SYSTEMS

The nervous system is described, for convenience only, as two principal morphologic units, *central* and *peripheral*. It should be emphasized that these two parts are structurally continuous and cannot function independently. (1) The *central nervous system* (CNS) is comprised of the brain and spinal cord (Fig. 1-3). These structures house the masses of internuncial neurons (probably 15 to 20 billion). The synapses among the CNS cells, with the incoming and outgoing neurons of the peripheral systems, are astronomical in number. The CNS lies within the bony coverings of the cranium and vertebral canal. (2) The *peripheral nervous system* is the aggregate of *afferent neurons* (impulses directed toward the CNS) and their associated receptors, and *efferent neurons* (impulses directed away from the CNS) and their associated effectors (Fig. 1-3). The afferent neurons terminate within the CNS, while the efferent neurons frequently start within the CNS. The peripheral nervous system lies almost wholly outside the cranium and vertebral canal.

The neuron

The *neuron* is the basic cell of both central and peripheral systems.[1,3] (See Chapter 10 for greater detail.) The neuron is made up of (1) a *cell body* or *perikaryon* (the bulky main part), which serves as the trophic center of the entire cell, and (2) a varying number of processes. Those processes, or projections, from the cell body that receive signals from other cells are called dendrites (Fig. 1-4, *A-C*). The dendrites constitute a distinctive functional unit called the *dendritic zone*. In most nerve cells this receptive field includes the nerve cell body as part of the receiving zone, and the dendrites attach to the cell body. In other neurons the dendrites aggregate into a single fiber (axon), and the dendritic zone thus terminates directly in the axon. In these neurons the dendrites are not direct processes of the cell body. This arrangement holds for most general sensory neurons. In both types of neuron, the single process that carries the impulse *away* from the dendritic zone to another neuron or to an effector is called the *axon*. The axon terminates adjacent to other nerve cells in many structural patterns, but most commonly in buttonlike terminals called *boutons*. These terminals make up the afferent limb of the synapse of the neuronal chain. Some axons terminate in special effectors located in muscles or glands. The typical neuron of the CNS possesses many dendrites and a single axon, and is called *multipolar* (Figs. 1-4, *A* and 1-5). The same type of cell also occurs in the peripheral nervous system in the neural units supplying the viscera. Other nerve cell bodies possess only two processes, one conveying the impulse to and the other

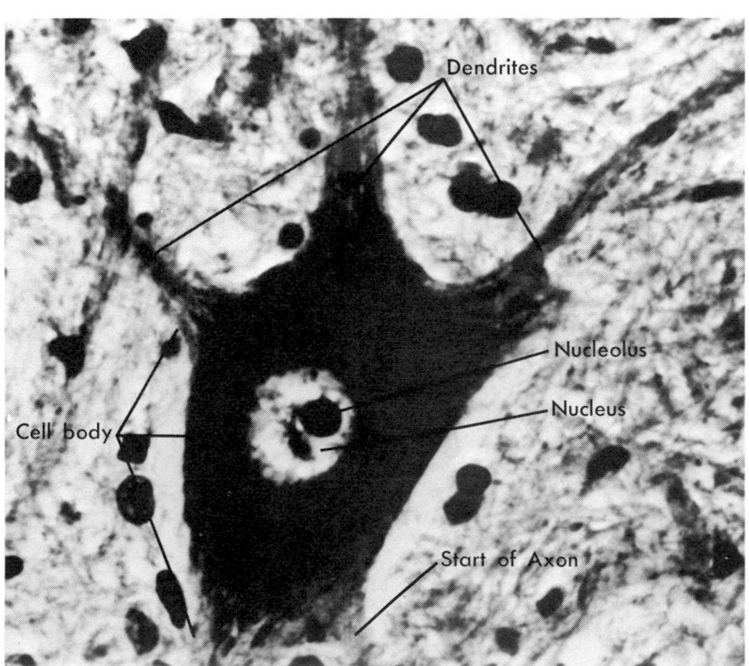

Fig. 1-5. Enlarged neuron from point of arrow in Fig. 1-7.

away from the cell body. In this pattern the cell body is inserted as a swelling along the axon, and the termination of the dendritic zone is some distance away from the cell body. These are *bipolar* nerve cells and are found in afferent nerves serving the special senses (olfaction, vision, hearing, and equilibration) (Fig. 1-4, *B*). Still other neurons have similar cell bodies from which a single process issues. In effect these cell bodies, or trophic centers, are offset from the main conducting stream in the axon. They are *unipolar* and occur in the general sensory nerves of both cranial and spinal origin (Fig. 1-4, *C*). However structured, each neuron possesses a dendritic zone, a conducting zone, a trophic center, and a transmitting zone which arborizes through telodendra into the nerve terminals.

Central nuclei

Within the central nervous system the cell *bodies* of the neurons are located in aggregates called *nuclei* (Fig. 1-6). This term is confusing, as it is also used to designate the vital central structure of individual cells. In some locations (for example, spinal cord) (Fig. 1-7) the nuclei are linear columns of cell bodies. In other places the aggregates are rounded and elliptical (center of brain) or occur in layers, or laminae (cortex of brain) (Fig. 1-6). The axons of these central cells are commonly clustered in bundles that subserve a common function, such as conducting pain, tendon sense, and vision. These bundles are called *tracts* (or *fascicles* when well delineated). They provide the long fiber chains of common conductor systems known as *path-*

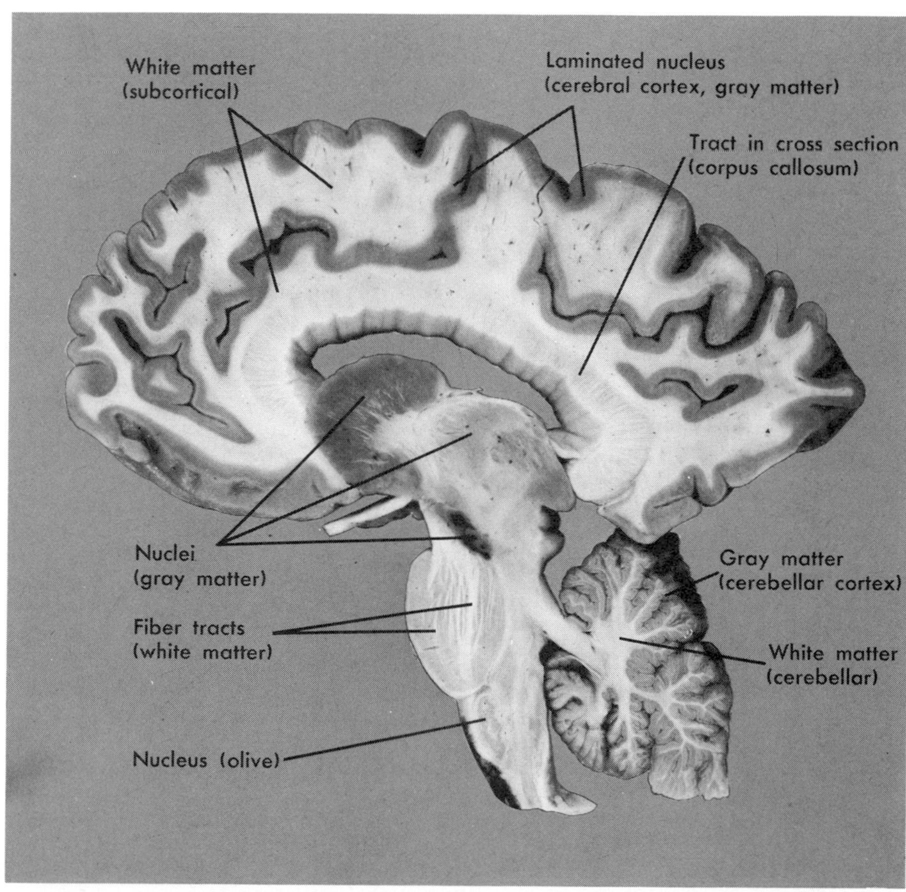

Fig. 1-6. Parasagittal brain section showing nuclei of varying shapes and sizes making up gray matter. Tracts and fascicles show as white matter.

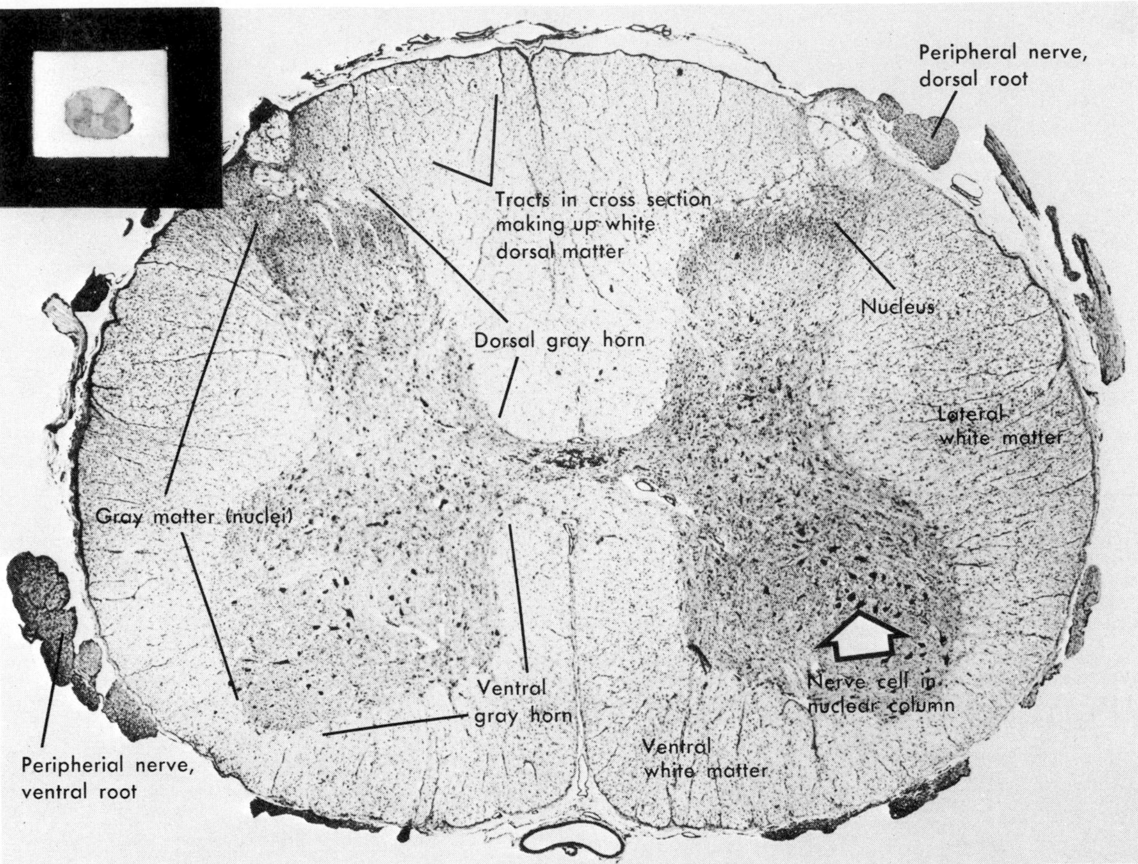

Fig. 1-7. Spinal cord in cross section showing gray matter, made up of nuclei, and white matter, made up of tracts and fascicles. Note dorsal and ventral nerve roots. Inset shows normal size.

ways. Axons of diameters greater than 1.5 μ acquire a fatty sheath of wrapping that is derived from cytoplasmic membrane of adjacent specialized supporting cells. This wrapping is called *myelin*. When fresh it imparts a white appearance to the axons of the brain or spinal cord as well as those peripheral nerves of sufficient size. Masses of myelinated axons thus comprise the *white matter* centrally and make up the "white" nerves peripherally. The nuclei, or cell clusters, of the CNS are devoid of myelin and, in contrast to the white matter, appear gray when fresh *(gray matter)*. Gray and white matter of the CNS are illustrated in Figs. 1-6 and 1-7. The smaller fibers of the peripheral system also do not possess myelin and therefore appear gray rather than white.

Peripheral ganglia and nerves, sensory and motor

The cell bodies of the peripheral system are aggregated in nodular clusters called *ganglia* (singular, ganglion), which correspond to the central nuclei. The axons of these ganglion cells (and frequently the dendrites if elongate) are bound in cable-like structures called *peripheral nerves*. As in the central nervous system, some of these axons attain sufficient size to acquire a myelin sheath *(myelinated nerve)*. Others remain small and *unmyelinated*. Both ganglia and nerves of the peripheral system are to some degree separable into those conducting impulses toward the central nervous system (*afferent* or *sensory*) and those conducting away from the central nervous system (*efferent* or *motor*). It is common to find both sensory and motor *fiber* components in a peripheral nerve (Fig. 1-3). Sensory *ganglia* are, however, usually quite distinct and are isolated from motor nerves throughout the spinal system. Many cranial nerve sensory ganglia, however, are traversed by motor filaments that carry impulses in the efferent direction. The sensory ganglia throughout the spinal nerves are

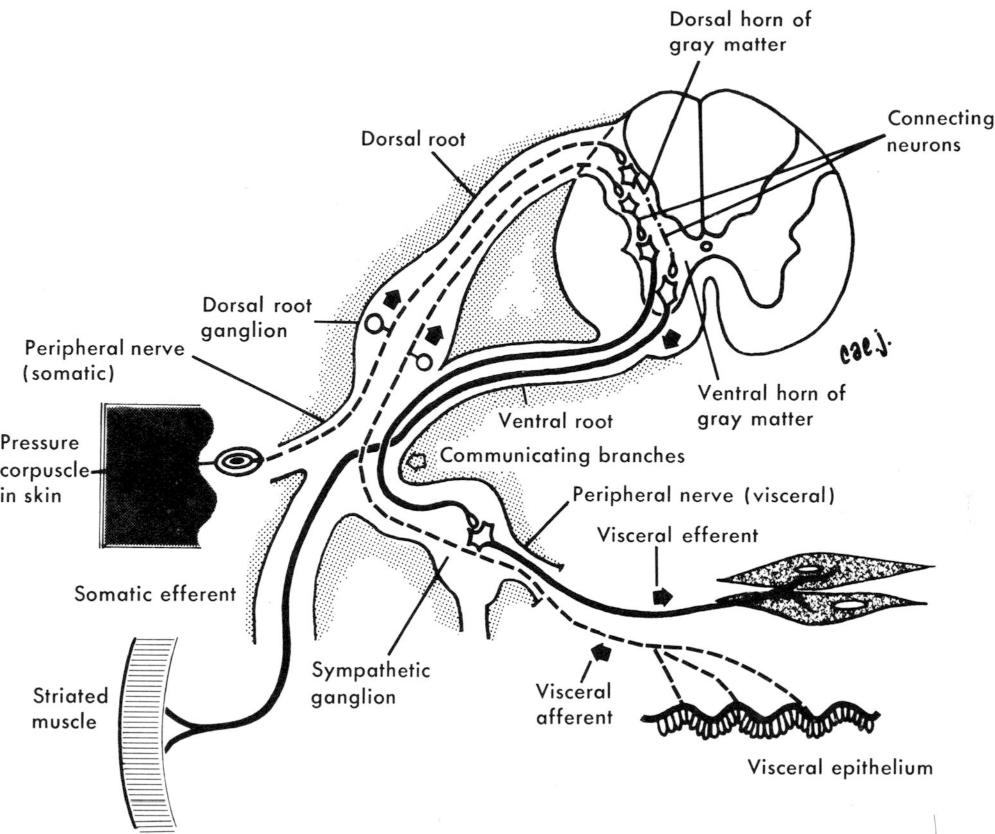

Fig. 1-8. Drawing of somatic and visceral connections in cord.

located on the *dorsal roots,* which are those nerve roots attached to the posterior or dorsal surface of the cord (Fig. 1-8). The ganglia lie immediately proximal to the junction of dorsal and ventral roots. The *ventral roots* are efferent, or motor. Sensory ganglia of *cranial nerves* are commonly placed at a greater distance from the CNS. *Motor ganglia* are traversed by mixed efferent and afferent nerves and are frequently aggregated in plexuses, or network patterns, some distance from the CNS, relatively close to the structures their cells innervate (Fig. 1-8).

Functional divisions of peripheral nerves

The relationship of nerve cell bodies to axons in peripheral nerves is closely tied to function beyond the simple sensory versus motor differential. The function of nerves is frequently related to size or diameter of fibers. This determines to some degree the type of impulse carried and the speed of conduction (large fibers conduct more rapidly). Regardless of function subserved, peripheral sensory neuron cell bodies, with the single exception of those mediating muscle sense from the face, are located in either spinal dorsal root ganglia or in cranial nerve ganglia. This situation obtains whether the impulse arises from a *somatic* or from a *visceral* source (Fig. 1-8). "Somatic" refers to the general body substance. *Somatic afferent impulses* therefore arise in skin, muscle, bone, or in special receptors in contact with the external environment (eye and ear). Thus areas in the nervous system from which sensory signals normally reach conscious levels constitute the *somatic* system. It is common to classify somatic afferent nerves as *general somatic afferent* (those pertaining to cutaneous and deep sense) and *special somatic afferent* (those functionally related to equilibration, audition, and vision). "Visceral," on the other hand, refers to body substance that normally is not in contact with the external environment, and *visceral afferent impulses* are those which arise in blood vessels, bowel walls, and cavity membranes. All of these areas are classed as "general" viscera, from which sensory signals seldom reach conscious levels. They therefore constitute the *general visceral afferent system.* By contrast, the olfactory and gustatory systems are viscera-related, but their impulses reach conscious levels. Therefore, they are called *special visceral afferent* systems.

General body structures (voluntary striated muscles) are supplied by *somatic efferent nerves.* Visceral structures (glands, vessels, smooth muscles, cardiac muscle) are supplied by nerves that are called *visceral efferent. Somatic efferent nerve* cell bodies lie within the central nervous system, and their fibers pass to the effector end-organs via the somatic efferent nerves. In the somatic efferent group no "special" category is definable. *General visceral efferent* (also called *autonomic)* fibers also arise from cell bodies in the CNS but terminate abjacent to cells in outlying motor ganglia or paraganglia (Fig. 1-8). These ganglion cells are interposed between the CNS and the end-organs. They supply the effector terminals in glands and smooth or cardiac muscles. In the visceral efferent system the components are subdivided into *general* and *special* functional units. The general visceral efferent, or *autonomic,* system operates, as the name implies, almost wholly without volitional control. On the visceral motor side, the term "special" is applied to the visceral efferent nerves supplying the striated muscles of the upper digestive and respiratory tracts, including the larynx. These muscles are striated and are at least partially volitionally controlled, but are derived from visceral sources (branchial) in the embryo. Hence the nerve cells are called *special visceral efferent.* In contrast to the general visceral efferent (autonomic) system, the cells of the special visceral efferent system do not have an autonomic ganglion interposed between the CNS and the effectors.

• • •

To summarize, the functional divisions of the peripheral nervous system are outlined below.

- I. *Somatic afferent*
  - A. *General*
    1. Cutaneous sense (pain, temperature, light touch)
    2. Deep sensibility (pressure; muscle sense; vibratory sense; bone, joint, tendon, and ligament sense; spatial and tactile discrimination)
  - B. *Special*
    1. Vestibular (equilibration)
    2. Auditory
    3. Visual
- II. *Visceral afferent*
  - A. *General* (unconscious reflexes from bowel, vessels, glands; complex visceral sensations of thirst, hunger, etc.; visceral pain, temperature)
  - B. *Special*
    1. Olfactory
    2. Gustatory
- III. *Somatic efferent* (nerves to striated muscles of the general body)
- IV. *Visceral efferent*
  - A. *General* or *autonomic* (to glands, smooth muscles, vessels, heart)
  - B. *Special* (to striated muscles of visceral origin)

REFERENCES

1. Bodian, D.: The generalized vertebrate neuron, Science **137**:323, 1962.
2. Bullock, T. H., and Horridge, G. A.: Structure and function in the nervous systems of invertebrates, San Francisco, 1965, W. H. Freeman & Co., publisher.
3. Luse, S.: The neuron. In Minckler, J., editor: Pathology of the nervous system, vol. I, New York, 1968, McGraw-Hill Book Co.
4. Richins, C. A., and Saccomanno, G.: Anatomy of the peripheral nervous system. In Minckler, J., editor: Pathology of the nervous system, vol. 1, New York, 1968, McGraw-Hill Book Co.

CHAPTER 2

THE CENTRAL NERVOUS SYSTEM

JEFF MINCKLER

STRUCTURAL DIVISIONS

Structure and function are so closely interrelated in nervous tissue that both must be studied simultaneously. In Chapter 1 it was stated that nervous tissue is divisible into units that are distinctive in function (such as sensory or motor). This is the basis for studying neuroanatomy in its functional systems, such as pain, vision, muscle sense, and motor acts. These systems will be discussed in Chapters 16 through 22. The systems are commonly defined in specific anatomic units, or *pathways,* which are oriented with the long axis of the nervous system. In addition to these longitudinally oriented functional divisions the CNS also displays structural subdivisions that are segmentally or transversely defined. These segments differentiate very early in the embryo and lose their definable segmental character above the level of the midbrain (see Chapter 9). They also carry some measure of functional distinction, as each higher segment adds greater and greater complexity in its neural activity. This culminates in the cerebral cortex as the "highest" neural center. On developmental, gross anatomic, and physiologic grounds, the CNS is hierarchically divisible into: (1) *telencephalon,* or end-brain (cerebrum); (2) *diencephalon,* or thalamus; (3) *mesencephalon,* or midbrain; (4) *metencephalon,* or pons and cerebellum; (5) *myelencephalon,* or medulla oblongata; and (6) *medulla spinalis,* or spinal cord. The terms *prosencephalon* (forebrain) for the combined cerebrum and thalamus, and *rhombencephalon* (hindbrain) for the parts related to the rhomboid fossa (pons and medulla) are seldom used in human neuroanatomy. The *isthmus rhombencephali* in the human brain is reduced to a junction plane between midbrain and pons (origin of cranial nerve IV) and is seldom used as a term for a point of reference.

The subdivisions can best be grossly visualized by studying the CNS from several angles, such as superior view, medial view of a sagittal section, lateral view, and basal view. Frequently, the gross inspection of the subdivisions is aided by dissections to remove overlying or obscuring parts. This technique is employed to uncover the *brainstem,* which is arbitrarily employed in this text to include the diencephalon, mesencephalon, metencephalon without the cerebellum, and medulla oblongata (Fig. 2-1). The medulla is often referred to as the *bulb,* and nuclei or diseases related to them are *bulbar.* Because so many parts are deeply buried, they frequently can be discerned only by extensive dissection or by viewing sections in various planes, as presented in Chapter 4. Coronal, transverse, and sagittal planes as well as dissections are employed in displaying the attachments of nerves (Chapter 6) and the tracts (Chapters 16 to 22).

Telencephalon

Superior view (Fig. 2-2). The bulky cerebrum, when viewed from above with the membranes removed, displays the complex irregularities of the surface. The projecting coarse ridges form the *convolutions,* or *gyri,* and the depressed valleys between them form the *sulci.* Each side represents a *cerebral hemisphere* that is wrapped around the nuclei of the diencephalon (Fig. 2-3). The hemispheres are separated by the large midline cleft, the *median sagittal fissure.* In the depths of this cleft is a massive transversely oriented bundle of nerve fibers, the *corpus callosum,* which interconnects the two hemispheres. This is the largest of the side-to-side inter-

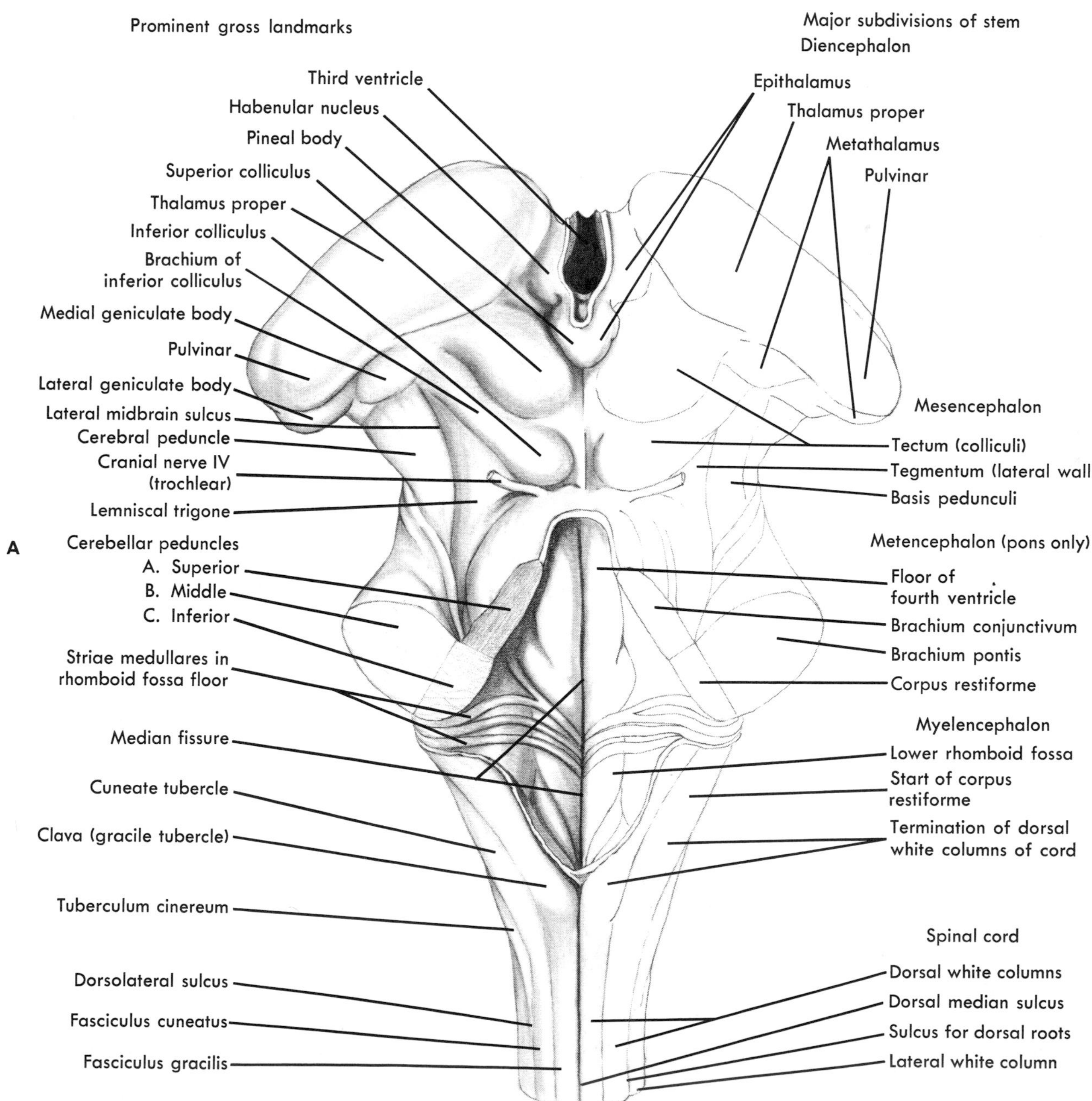
Prominent gross landmarks
Major subdivisions of stem
Diencephalon
Third ventricle
Habenular nucleus
Pineal body
Superior colliculus
Thalamus proper
Inferior colliculus
Brachium of inferior colliculus
Medial geniculate body
Pulvinar
Lateral geniculate body
Lateral midbrain sulcus
Cerebral peduncle
Cranial nerve IV (trochlear)
Lemniscal trigone
A
Cerebellar peduncles
A. Superior
B. Middle
C. Inferior
Striae medullares in rhomboid fossa floor
Median fissure
Cuneate tubercle
Clava (gracile tubercle)
Tuberculum cinereum
Dorsolateral sulcus
Fasciculus cuneatus
Fasciculus gracilis
Epithalamus
Thalamus proper
Metathalamus
Pulvinar
Mesencephalon
Tectum (colliculi)
Tegmentum (lateral wall)
Basis pedunculi
Metencephalon (pons only)
Floor of fourth ventricle
Brachium conjunctivum
Brachium pontis
Corpus restiforme
Myelencephalon
Lower rhomboid fossa
Start of corpus restiforme
Termination of dorsal white columns of cord
Spinal cord
Dorsal white columns
Dorsal median sulcus
Sulcus for dorsal roots
Lateral white column

Fig. 2-1. Diagram of brainstem: **A,** posterior view; **B,** lateral view; **C,** sagittal view.

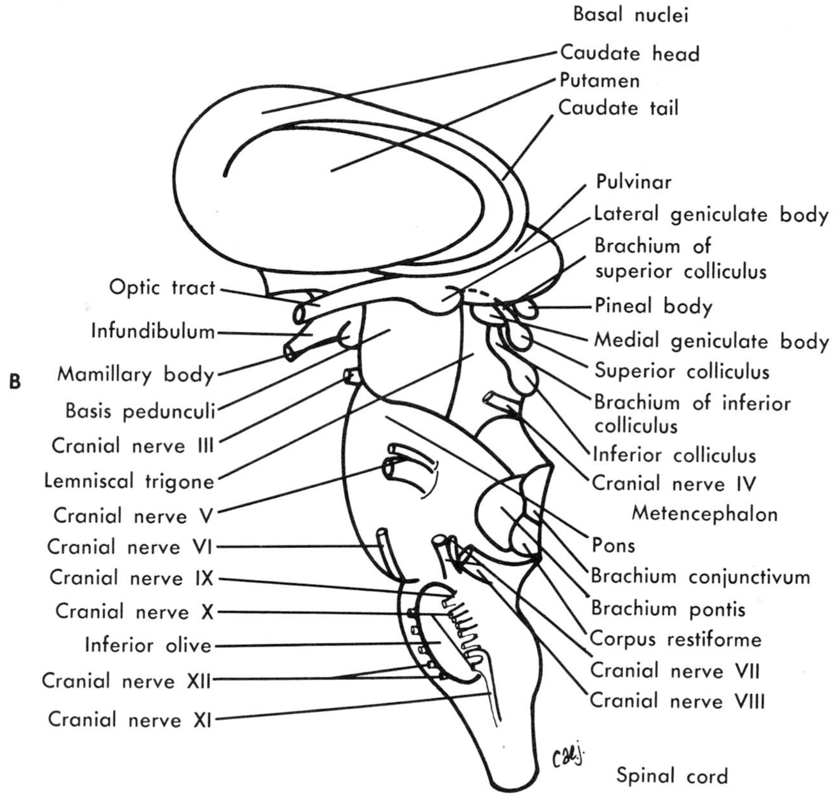
Basal nuclei
Caudate head
Putamen
Caudate tail
Pulvinar
Lateral geniculate body
Brachium of superior colliculus
Pineal body
Medial geniculate body
Superior colliculus
Brachium of inferior colliculus
Inferior colliculus
Cranial nerve IV
Metencephalon
Pons
Brachium conjunctivum
Brachium pontis
Corpus restiforme
Cranial nerve VII
Cranial nerve VIII
Spinal cord
Optic tract
Infundibulum
B
Mamillary body
Basis pedunculi
Cranial nerve III
Lemniscal trigone
Cranial nerve V
Cranial nerve VI
Cranial nerve IX
Cranial nerve X
Inferior olive
Cranial nerve XII
Cranial nerve XI

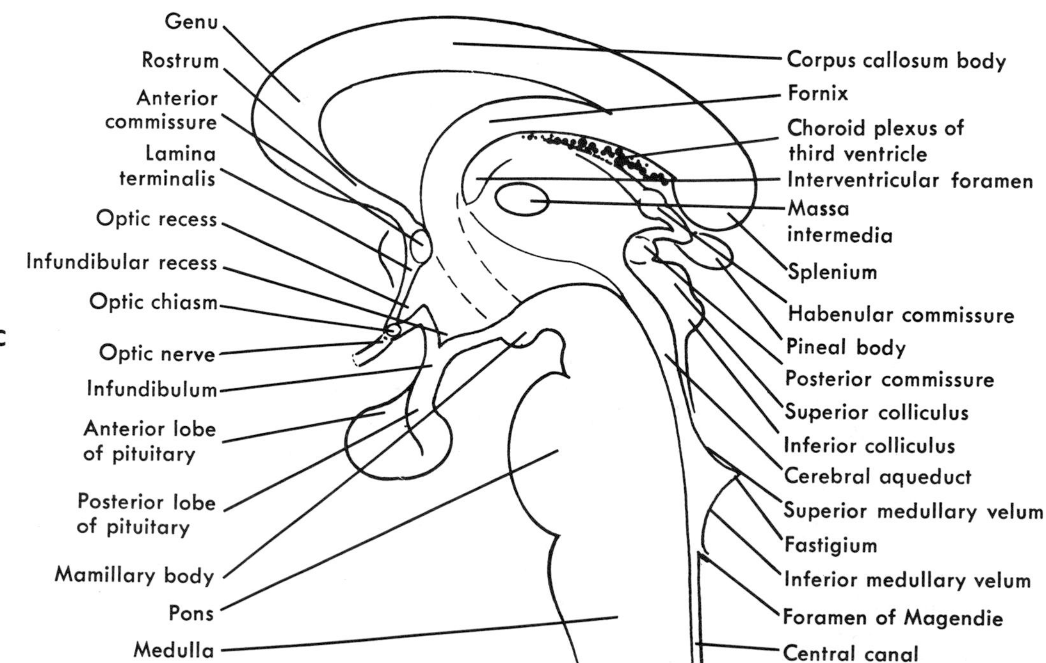
Genu
Rostrum
Anterior commissure
Lamina terminalis
Optic recess
Infundibular recess
Optic chiasm
C
Optic nerve
Infundibulum
Anterior lobe of pituitary
Posterior lobe of pituitary
Mamillary body
Pons
Medulla
Corpus callosum body
Fornix
Choroid plexus of third ventricle
Interventricular foramen
Massa intermedia
Splenium
Habenular commissure
Pineal body
Posterior commissure
Superior colliculus
Inferior colliculus
Cerebral aqueduct
Superior medullary velum
Fastigium
Inferior medullary velum
Foramen of Magendie
Central canal

Fig. 2-1, cont'd. For legend see opposite page.

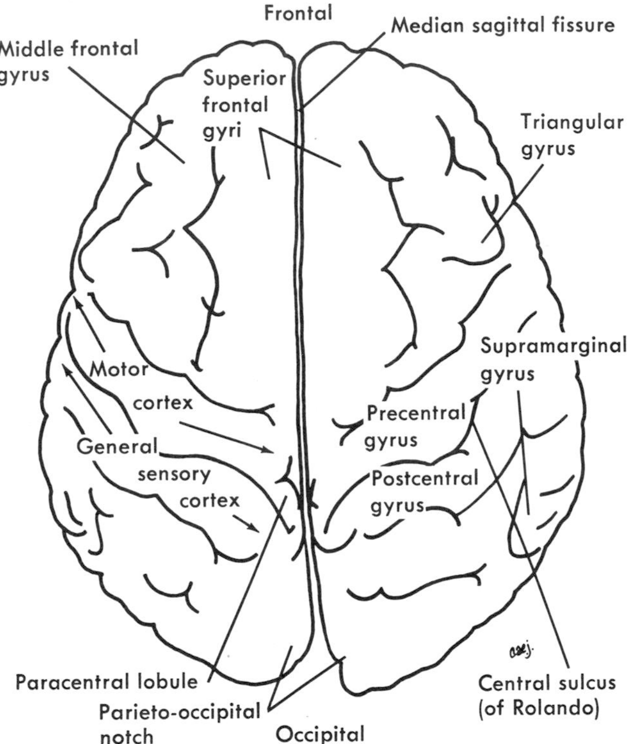

Fig. 2-2. Diagram of cerebrum, superior view.

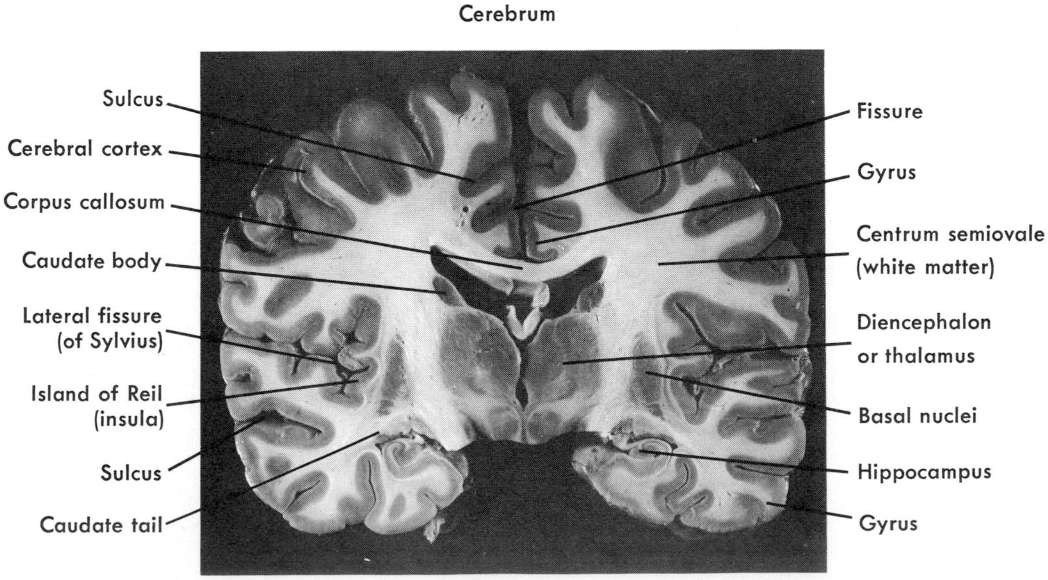

Cerebrum

Sulcus
Cerebral cortex
Corpus callosum
Caudate body
Lateral fissure (of Sylvius)
Island of Reil (insula)
Sulcus
Caudate tail
Fissure
Gyrus
Centrum semiovale (white matter)
Diencephalon or thalamus
Basal nuclei
Hippocampus
Gyrus

Fig. 2-3. Coronal section through level of thalamus. Photograph of unstained gross section.

connections that are known as *commissures.* The corpus callosum is displayed better in the sagittal section of Fig. 2-4. In the superior view (Fig. 2-2) it is possible to delineate some fairly constant gyral and sulcal patterns. The *superior frontal gyrus* is oriented anteroposteriorly near the vertex in the frontal part. The *central sulcus* can be seen as a particularly deep cleft running obliquely from the vertex, roughly at the beginning of the posterior third, downward and forward. At the vertex, the *central sulcus* ends as the cleft in the *paracentral lobule,* which extends somewhat over the medial surface of the hemisphere. Bordering the central sulcus are two gyri that parallel it, the *precentral gyrus* (motor area) in front, and the *postcentral gyrus* (general sensory area) in back. The central sulcus is the arbitrary dividing structure between the *frontal lobe* anterior and the *parietal lobe* posterior to the sulcus. In this view the superior part of the parietal lobe is illustrated as the *superior parietal lobule.* There is a distinct notch in the vertex of the hemisphere (Fig. 2-4) that is the arbitrary posterior terminus of the parietal lobe. This is the *occipitoparietal notch.* The part of the hemisphere posterior to this is the *occipital lobe.*

Medial view (Fig. 2-4). Viewing a sagittal section of the brain from the medial aspect reveals two distinctive patterns of tissue: (1) a cerebriform, or convoluted, portion disposed in a circumferential pattern around the smoother brain substance, and (2) a smoother brain substance with a complex anatomy that principally represents diencephalon and the extending brainstem. Some of this central substance belongs, embryologically, to the cerebrum. This part is called the *telencephalon medium* and includes the midline structures at the anterior border of the third ventricle, as shown in Fig. 2-4. The dividing line between cerebrum and thalamus extends from the lower border of the optic chiasm to the interventricular foramen. Anterior to this

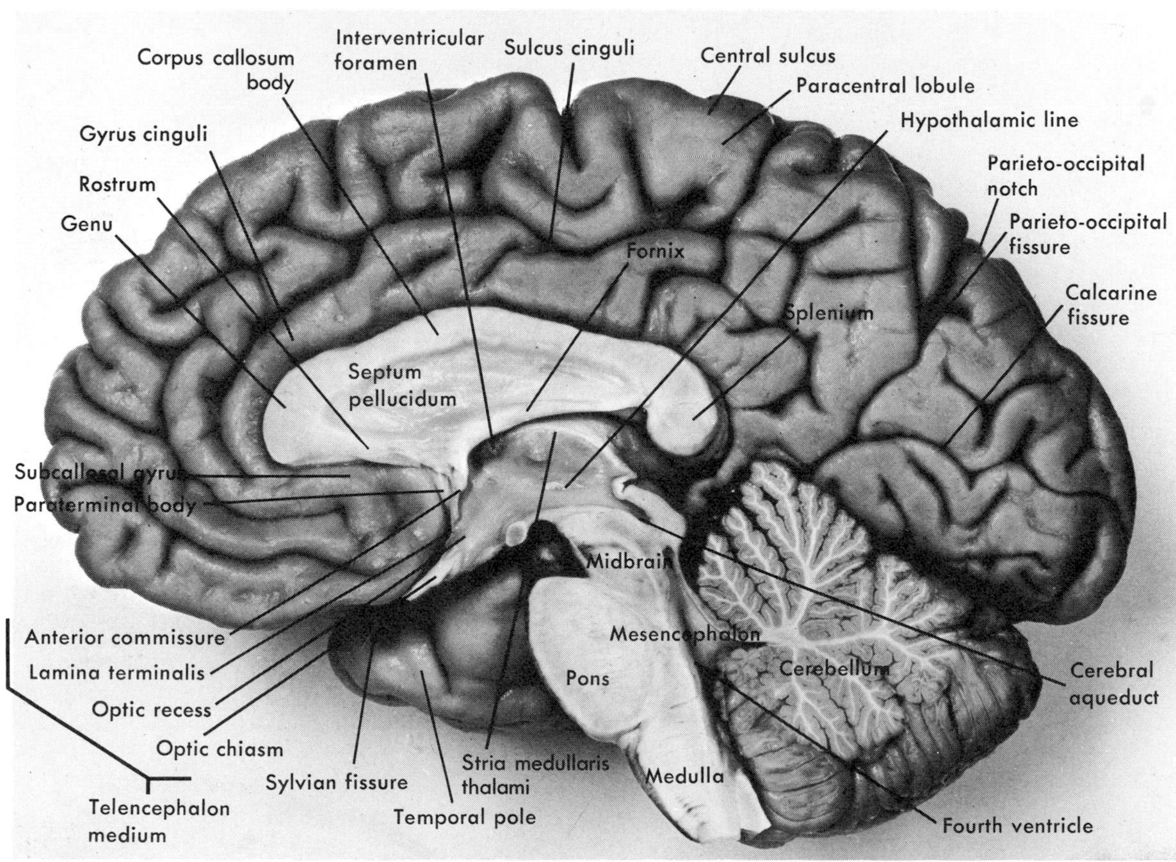

Fig. 2-4. Medial view of sagittal section of normal brain.

line are the cerebral parts: (1) the *optic chiasm;* (2) the projecting *optic recess* of the third ventricle above the chiasm; (3) the *lamina terminalis,* which is the thin membrane limiting the third ventricle anteriorly; (4) the *anterior commissure,* which interconnects the temporal parts of the two hemispheres; (5) the *triangular recess* which projects anteriorly above the commissure as a recess of the third ventricle; and (6) the *paraphysis,* a transitory embryonic structure that occurs near the junction of telencephalon and diencephalon in the roof of the third ventricle, between the interventricular foramina. While the paraphysis normally disappears, it sometimes persists as a possible source of cystic tumors (colloid cysts of the third ventricle).

The *corpus callosum* is also a part of the cerebrum and is continuous with the telencephalon medium through its beak-like extension, the *rostrum* (Fig. 2-4). The anterior end of the corpus callosum is the *genu,* or knee. At the genu it bends downward and posteriorly to form the rostrum. The bulky central part of the corpus callosum is the *body,* which terminates posteriorly as the slightly expanded *splenium.* The *fornix* (plural, fornices) is the longitudinal compact tract that curves anteriorly, medially, and downward from the inferior surface of the area of the splenium along the posterior two-thirds of the undersurface of the corpus callosum. The fornices extend by columns over the roof and anterior borders of the bilateral interventricular foramina, disappearing into thalamic substance just behind the anterior commissure. The *septum pellucidum* is the thin membrane bridging the fornix to the corpus callosum in midline (Fig. 2-6). This separates the two lateral ventricles as a septum. Sometimes it is split by a cavity, the *cavum* of the septum pellucidum, or "fifth" ventricle (Fig. 2-5).

The convoluted parts of the cerebrum exhibit fairly constant patterns that establish accurate reference points (Fig. 2-6). The *subcallosal body* is the small gyrus inferior to the rostrum. It continues into the *gyrus cinguli,* which goes around the genu and body of the corpus callosum. The *paraterminal* body is the narrow gyrus applied vertically along the side of the lamina terminalis. While the gyral pattern of the medial surface of the hemispheral cortex is confused and variable, certain major sulci are consistent enough in their appearance to assist in subdividing the forebrain into lobes. At the junction of the anterior two-thirds and the posterior third of the corpus callosum, the *sulcus cinguli* (above the gyrus) turns toward the vertex. Immediately anterior to this is a deep sulcus projecting over the vertex to the medial surface. This is the upper extremity of the *central sulcus,* as seen in the superior view (Fig. 2-2). This structure defines the *paracentral lobule* with the surrounding gyri. The central sulcus separates the anterior lobe from the parietal lobe on the medial surface, as it does in the superior view. Approximately half the distance from the central sulcus to the occipital pole is a deep notch (*parieto-occipital*) that marks the dividing point between *parietal* and *occipital* lobes. On the anteroinferior medial view below the thalamus, a deep cleft in the convolutional pattern, the *lateral* or *Sylvian* fissure, separates the *frontal lobe* above from the *temporal lobe* below.

After elevating or removing part of the brainstem by transecting at the midbrain, the medial surface of the temporal lobe comes to view. The uppermost gyrus on the medial aspects is the *hippocampal,* which has an upward and forward projecting bulge, the *uncus* (Fig. 2-6). At the posterior third mark of the inferior border of the temporal lobe is the *temporo-occipital notch,* which marks the division between *temporal* and *occipital* lobes. The *calcarine fissure* (visual area) appears as the prominent cleft along the medial aspect of the occipital lobe. This separates the *lingular gyrus* below from the *cuneus* above. The *parieto-occipital* fissure extends from the calcarine fissure to the parieto-occipital notch (Fig. 2-6). In this medial view with the brainstem removed, it is apparent that an arch-like pattern of cortex surrounds the nonconvoluted central part. This almost circular arch is formed by the subcallosal gyrus, gyrus cinguli, isthmus, hippocampal gyrus, and uncus. Together they form *fornicate* or *limbic* lobe. Sometimes the limbic lobes together with the olfactory structures, including the amygdaloid nuclei, are termed *rhinencephalon,* but this representation is more helpful in comparative studies than in human neuroanatomy.

Lateral view (Fig. 2-7). Viewed laterally, the telencephalon presents two principal landmarks that aid in defining lobes: (1) the *lateral* (Sylvian) fissure, which is the prominent separation between frontal and temporal lobes; and (2) the *central sulcus* (Rolando), which is the conspicuous diagonal crevice extending from the middle of the Sylvian fissure to the paracentral lobule. The central sulcus separates *frontal* (anterior) and *parietal* lobes. The anterior boundary of the *occipital lobe* is defined in this view by a line from the parieto-occipial notch to the temporo-occipital notch. The dividing line between parietal and temporal lobes is a projected line extending posteriorly from the Sylvian fissure

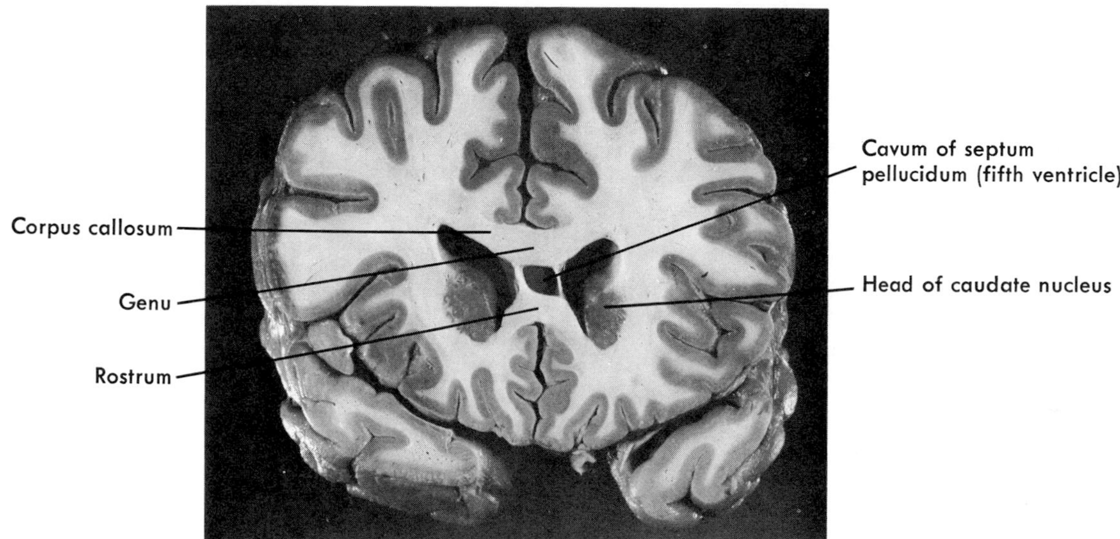

Fig. 2-5. Coronal section showing cavum of septum pellucidum (fifth ventricle).

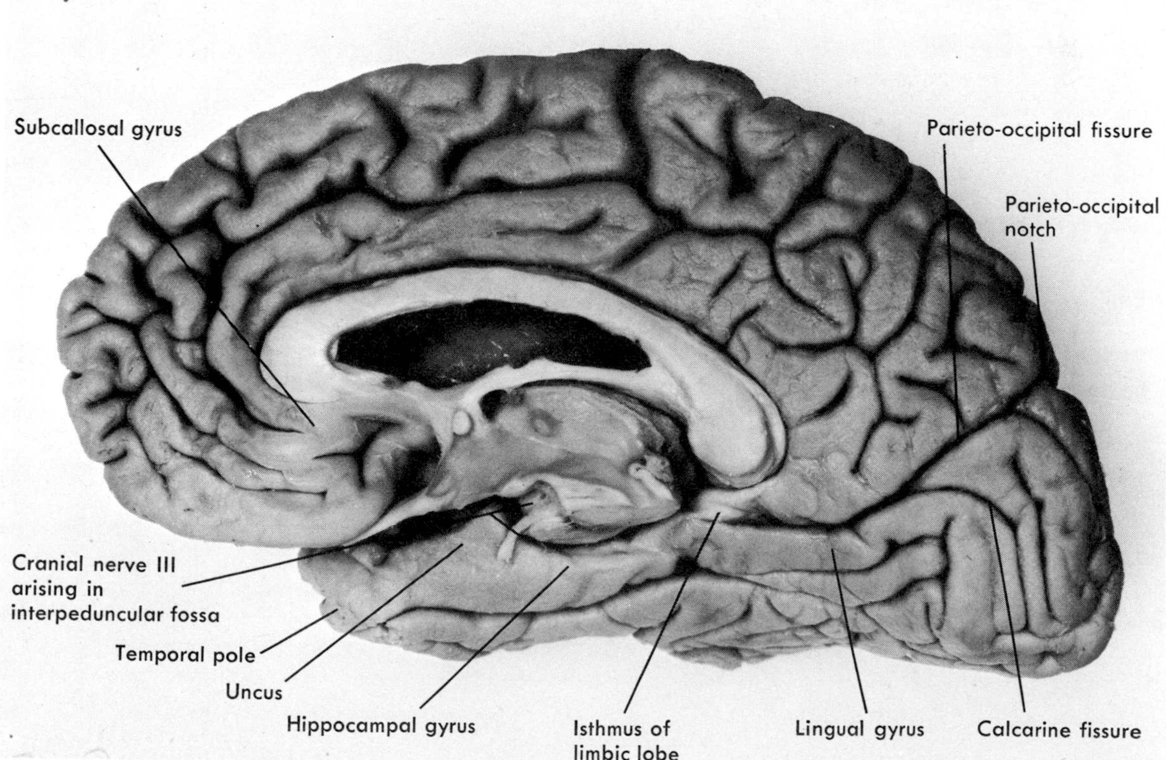

Fig. 2-6. Medial view of brain with the stem removed at the level of the midbrain.

to the midpoint of the anterior boundary of the occipital lobe. On the *anterior* or *frontal lobe,* a *precentral gyrus* can be discerned in front of the central sulcus. This runs parallel to the central sulcus and represents the motor area. *Superior, middle, and inferior frontal gyri* are delineated in longitudinal pattern and are discernible toward the frontal pole. The inferior frontal gyrus contains an *orbital* part lying adjacent to the underlying orbit, a *triangular* part that is named by its shape, and an *opercular* part that overlies the Sylvian fissure (Fig. 2-7). The *parietal lobe* can be divided into a *postcentral* gyrus immmediately behind and parallel to the central sulcus (general sensory area), and a *superior* and *inferior parietal lobule.* The inferior parietal lobule is distinguished by a *supramarginal gyrus* that extends around the posterior extremity of the Sylvian fissure, and by an *angular gyrus* that passes around the posterior extremity of the superior temporal sulcus. The occipital lobe can be further distinguished on lateral view only by the vertical character of the convolutions. The temporal lobe exhibits *superior, middle,* and *inferior* gyri. By retracting or removing the temporal lobe and the overhanging frontal and parietal lobes to widen the Sylvian fissure, the *insula* (*island of Reil*) is exposed. This presents a transverse *central fissure of the island* with two *long gyri* posterior and variable *short gyri* anterior to it (Fig. 2-8). At the posterior extremity of the upper surface of the temporal lobe are the *transverse gyri of Heschl* (auditory area) (Fig. 2-8). These gyri are buried in the depths of the Sylvian fissure posteriorly, and are related externally to the superior temporal gyrus and anteromedially to the long gyri of the island of Reil.

Basal view (Fig. 2-9). The *orbital gyri* in a basal view lie lateral to the *straight gyri* (recti). The former are separated from the latter by the line of the *olfactory bulb* in the anterior and the *olfactory tract* extending to the posterior. This is commonly but improperly designated cranial or olfactory nerve I. The *first cranial nerves* are actually the filaments passing from the bulbs to the nasal mu-

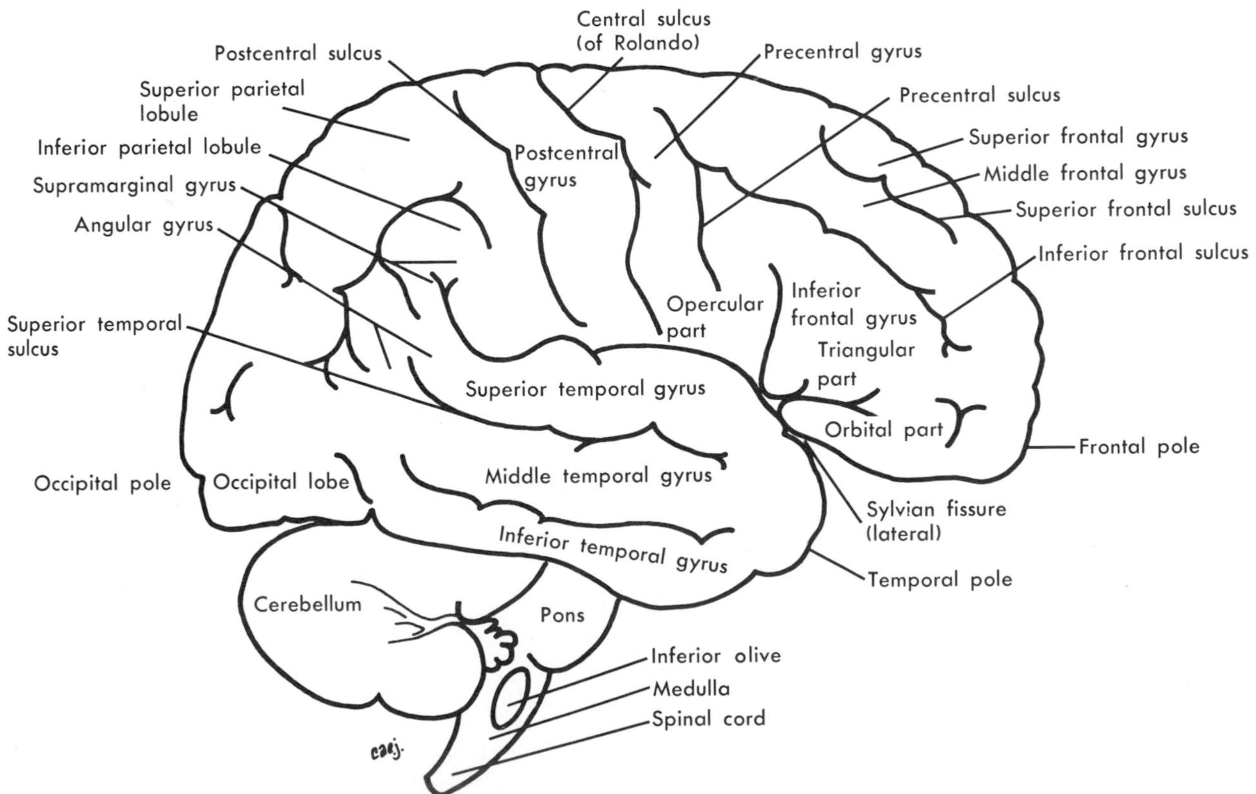

Fig. 2-7. Diagram of the lateral view of the cerebrum.

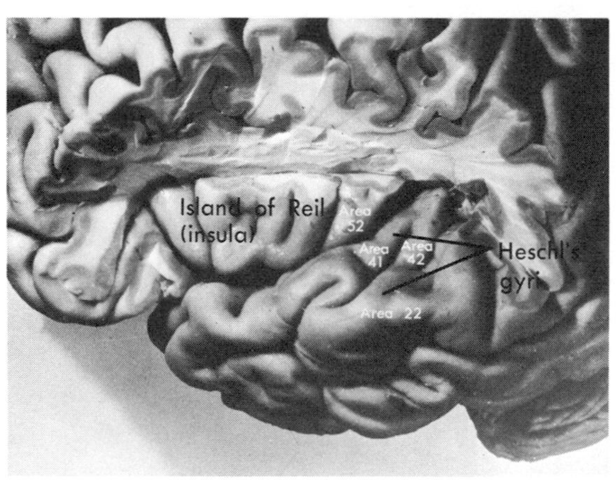

Fig. 2-8. The Island of Reil (insula) and the transverse gyri of Heschl exposed by removing overlying forebrain.

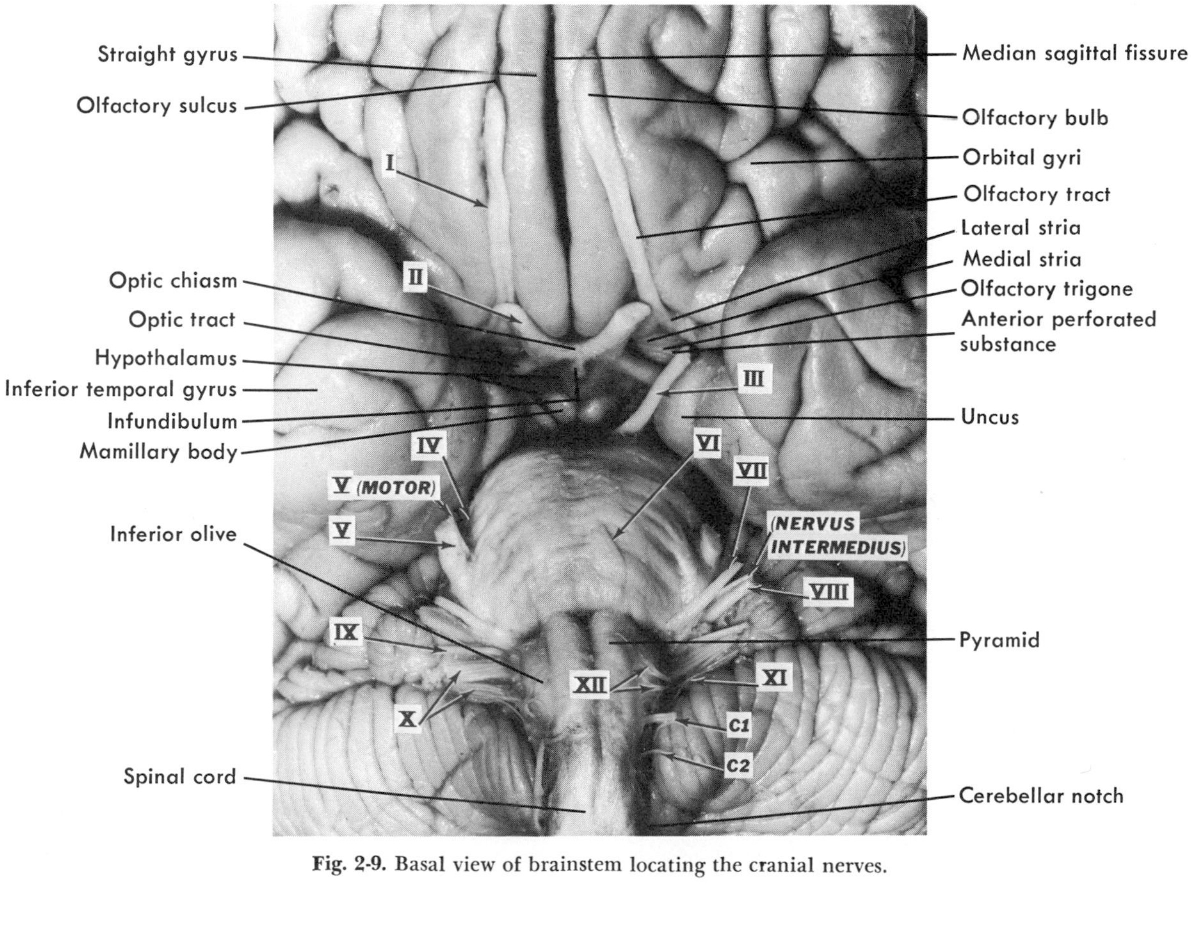

cous membrane (Chapter 18). The tracts occupy the *olfactory sulcus*. The olfactory tracts divide posteriorly to form *medial* and *lateral striae,* which define the *olfactory trigone*. The *central stria* is faintly outlined and projects posteriorly into the trigone. Immediately posterior to the trigone is the *anterior perforated substance,* named for the holes produced by penetrating small vessels. The *optic nerves* (cranial II), *chiasm,* and *optic tracts* (the parts posterior to the chiasm) are telencephalic units that define the lower boundary of the endbrain and mark the junction of the telencephalon with the diencephalon. Diencephalic parts (*hypothalamus*) are framed by the optic components in this basal view. Laterally the temporal lobes exhibit a medially projecting *uncus* as well as *the hippocampal* gyrus and the *inferior temporal gyrus* on either side. The *lateral* (*Sylvian*) *fissure* marks the division between frontal and temporal lobes. Much basal surface of the occipital lobes is covered by the

Fig. 2-9. Basal view of brainstem locating the cranial nerves.

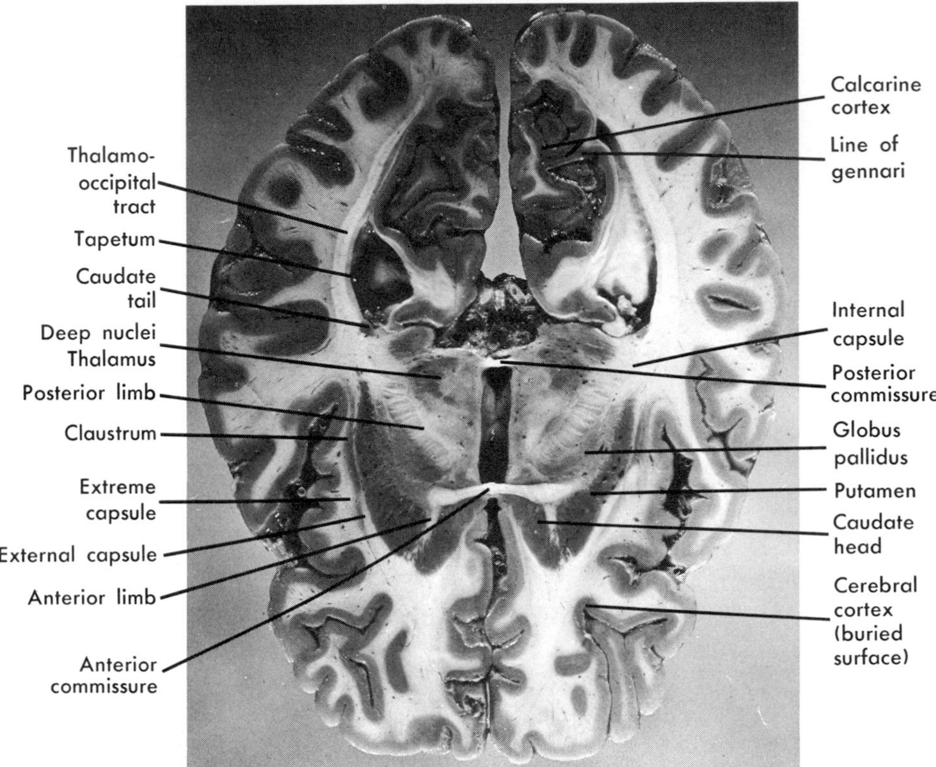

Fig. 2-10. Transverse section of brain through the anterior and posterior commissures.

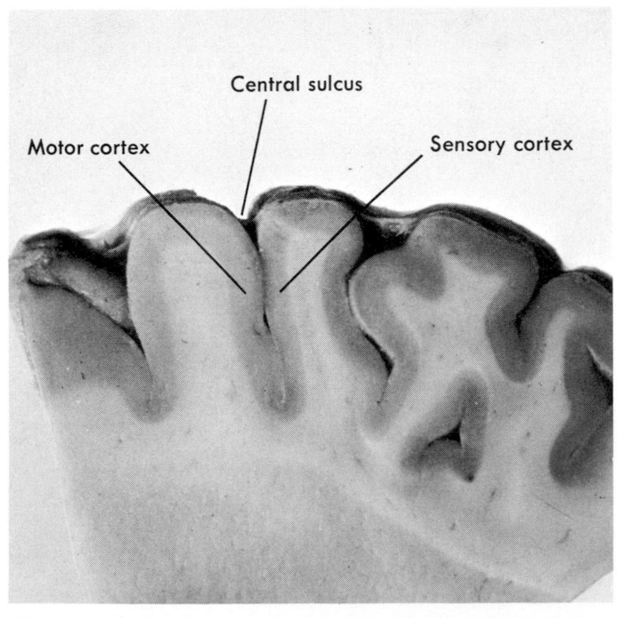

Fig. 2-11. Unstained photo showing varying width in the cortical areas adjacent to the central sulcus.

brainstem and the expanding cerebellar hemispheres. By removing the brainstem below the midbrain the features of the medial aspect of the posterior part of the temporal lobes and the occipital lobes are brought to view in the walls of the *cerebellar notch* (Fig. 2-6).

Nuclei of the telencephalon. The gray matter of the endbrain occupies two major nuclear masses, the *cerebral cortex* and the *basal nuclei*. The latter are frequently called *basal ganglia* and, despite the inconsistency with the definition, this last term is well established by use. The *cerebral cortex* provides a rind of gray nuclear structures following the cortical gyral pattern superficially to varying depths. This can be viewed to best advantage in coronal and transverse sections of the brain (Figs. 2-3 and 2-10). The cortex presents to the cerebral surfaces in all fields of the convolutions. Most of the cortex is buried in the depths of the sulci. The remarkable enhancement of surface area through convolutional patterns is evident in the sections. Several cortical gray areas merit special consideration here by virtue of their distinguishing gross

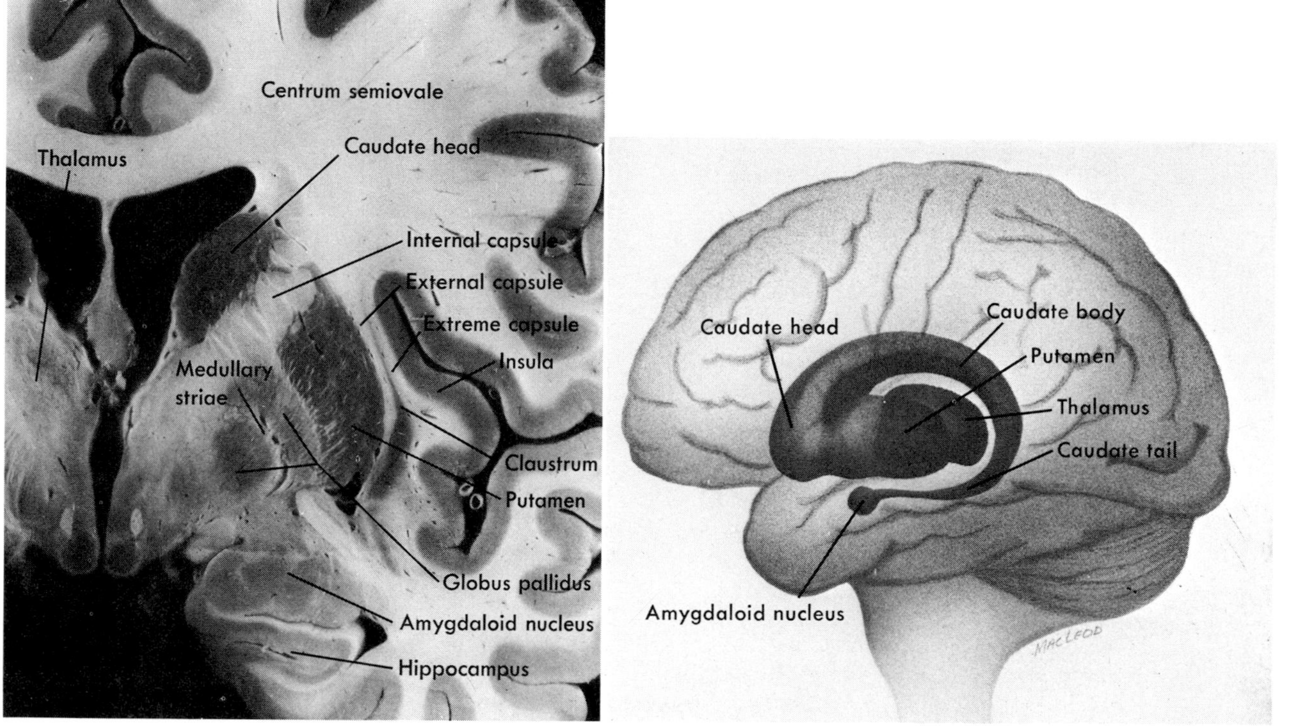

Fig. 2-12. A, The basal nuclei in coronal section; **B,** reconstruction of the basal nuclei.

characteristics. The *central sulcus* area (Fig. 2-7) presents a junction at its deep point between the thick-walled cortex of the motor (precentral) area and the much thinner cortex of the sensory (postcentral) area (Fig. 2-11). No other juncture in the cortical gray matter has this striking change in thickness, and this feature is helpful in identifying the central sulcus in gross sections. The *calcarine cortical* gray matter possesses a distinctive line paralleling the gyral surface (line of Gennari) that identifies the visual cortex (Fig. 2-10). The *hippocampus* presents a distinctive outline by which it can be identified (Figs. 2-3 and 2-12). The remaining cortical gray matter possesses few distinctive gross features, and the areas are dependent upon tagging for identification after gross section.

The second massive group of nuclei that represents telencephalic cell clusters is embodied in the *basal nuclei* (ganglia), which lie between the *centrum semiovale,* or central white matter, of the telencephalon and the nuclei of the diencephalon, or *thalamus.* They are separated from the thalamus by the *internal capsule* (Figs. 2-1 and 2-10). These basal nuclei include: (1) *corpus striatum* (the head of the *caudate* nucleus and adjoining anterior part of the *putamen,* with the intervening *internal capsule*); (2) the *lentiform nucleus* (*putamen* and *globus pallidus*); (3) the *claustrum,* which is separated from the lentiform nuclei by the *external capsule;* and (4) the *amygdaloid nucleus* in the temporal pole (Figs. 2-3 and 2-12, *A*). These nuclei (ganglia) are also viewed to best advantage in coronal, transverse, and parasagittal sections of the brain or by dissection (Chapter 4). Their general outline in reconstructed and combined gross pattern is presented in Fig. 2-12, *B*. The gross structure of each of the nuclei is discussed in the following paragraphs.

The *caudate nucleus* forms at its anterior extremity a bulky expansion, the *head,* which is partially in contact with the putamen of the lentiform nucleus. These two nuclei are separated superiorly by the anterior limb of the internal capsule (Fig. 2-10). This limb is crossed by numerous transverse fibers that pass between the head of the caudate nucleus and the putamen. The striated nature of these crossing fibers accounts for the term *corpus striatum,* which applies to all three parts (caudate head, anterior limb of internal capsule, and putamen). The head of the caudate tapers posteriorly into a narrower *body* (Fig. 2-12). Eventually this extends into the narrow *tail,* which follows the line of the isthmus and hippocampal gyrus into the temporal lobe. The tail of the caudate terminates anteriorly by blending with the amygdaloid nucleus in the tip of the temporal lobe (Fig. 2-12, *B*). The *putamen* is the bulky, densely gray, and cellular outer part of the *lenticular nucleus* (Fig. 2-12). This cone-shaped nuclear mass continues medially as the whiter (pallid) *globus pallidus.* The lenticular nucleus, particularly the pallidum, is subdivided by white strands of fibers called *medullary striae.* The lenticular nucleus borders the *internal capsule* on its medial surface and the *external capsule* on its lateral surface. The *claustrum,* the basal nucleus lateral to the external capsule, lies between the external capsule and the *extreme capsule,* which underlies the cortex of the island of Reil. The *amygdaloid nuclei* occupy the tips of the temporal lobes beneath the uncus of either side. The nucleus on each side fuses posteriorly with the tail of the caudate and is superiorly in apposition with the putamen (Figs. 2-3 and 2-12). These basal nuclei are reviewed further in connection with motor regulation in Chapter 22.

The basal nuclei give rise to fibers from cells lodged within them to the internal capsule; the fibers interconnect thalamic nuclei, cortex, and other basal nuclei. They also receive fibers from the internal capsule and other white areas. The main efferent bundle leaves the lentiform nuclei via the apex of the globus pallidus. This is the *ansa lenticularis,* which delivers fibers from the lentiform nuclei to the thalamus and to the lower nuclei of the brainstem, especially midbrain.

White matter of the telencephalon. Named for the half-oval shape of the cerebral white matter in transverse sections above the corpus callosum, this fiber mass is called *centrum semiovale* (Fig. 2-2). The masses of fibers in the centrum are derived from four sources. Those passing from the cortex to lower nuclei are called *projections.* This term is also arbitrarily used to describe the extension of fibers from any nuclear mass to another. The fibers arising from cells in the thalamus and passing to the cortex are called *radiations.* Fibers interconnecting parts of the same cerebral hemisphere are called *associations.* Those that pass from side to side, connecting right and left hemispheres, comprise the *commissures.* All are commingled in parts of the centrum. Many form definitive bundles with known relationships.

The *internal capsule* (Fig. 2-3) contains both projections and radiations, with the fibers aggregating in two *limbs* (*anterior and posterior*) and a *genu,* as seen in transverse section (Fig. 2-10). The anterior limb of the internal capsule carries fibers to and from the frontal lobe cortex, relating this to the nuclei of the thalamus as well as to the caudate nucleus and putamen. The *genu* is related to both the precentral (motor area) and part of the premotor (anterior to the motor) area of the cortex. It relates these cortical fields primarily to bulbar nuclei. The posterior limb carries fibers in its anterior part to and from the precentral gyrus (motor area) to the spinal cord. These are located close to the genu and run with other fibers from premotor fields to brainstem nuclei. Adjacent to these fibers in the posterior limb are the projections and radiations from thalamic and basal nuclei to parietal cortex. Next in the posterior limb are the *general sensory radiations,* which pass from the thalamus to the postcentral gyrus. The *special sensory radiations* (auditory and visual) pass from their thalamic nuclei via the *sublenticular* and *postlenticular* parts of the internal capsule to their respective cortical areas in the temporal lobe (Heschl's gyri) and occipital lobe (calcarine fissure) (Fig. 2-10). Both projections and radiations interdigitate within the centrum semiovale with the transversely oriented fibers of the corpus callosum. This forms a radiating crown (corona radiata) of fiber bundles projecting from the internal capsule upward past the commissural fibers. Some projections and radiations travel via the external capsule.

The *commissures* of the telencephalon include the *corpus callosum,* the *anterior commissure,* and the *hippocampal commissure.* The *corpus callosum* is the largest of the commissures and interconnects the cerebral cortices of frontal, parietal, occipital, and parts of limbic and temporal lobes. Its fibers radiate through the centrum on either side and interdigitate with those of the internal capsule. Some fibers pass between the upper parts of the temporal lobes via both the external and extreme capsules (Fig. 2-12). In transverse sections of the brain the extensions of the corpus callosum form anterior and posterior pincer-like patterns called *anterior* and *posterior forceps,* respectively. The part of the corpus callosum that passes over the posterior part of the lateral ventricles is the tapetum (Fig. 2-10). The *anterior commissure* (Fig. 2-10) principally interconnects the temporal lobes and amygdaloid nuclei. It also conveys crossing fibers from olfactory centers on one side to temporal lobe on the contralateral side. The *hippocampal commissure* interrelates the hippocampus and hippocampal gyrus of one side with the other through bundles of fibers. The fibers cross deep to the splenium of the corpus callosum between the converging crura of the fornix. The fiber pattern produces the harp-like *psalterium* of the classic anatomies.

Association bundles interconnect parts of the same hemisphere in short chains and long bundles. The short association fibers (*arcuate*) pass between gyri and, if myelinated, hug the gray matter of the cortex. Some are unmyelinated and are located within the cortical layers. A short association bundle of prominence is the *stratum calcarinum,* which interconnects visual cortical areas from cuneus to lingula around the calcarine fissure. Long association bundles include: (1) *uncinate fasciculus,* connecting frontal and temporal lobes; (2) *inferior occipitofrontal fasciculus,* interconnecting occipital and frontal cortices and running ventrolateral to the lentiform nuclei; (3) *inferior longitudinal fasciculus,* interconnecting temporal pole and occipital cortex and running in the inferior temporal white matter inferior and lateral to the lateral ventricle; (4) *superior longitudinal fasciculus,* running from frontal to temporal and occipital cortices and placed lateral to the corona radiata; (5) *superior occipitofrontal fasciculus,* running from frontal to occipital cortex and occupying the area of interdigitation of the corpus callosum and internal capsule dorsolateral to the caudate nucleus; (6) *cingulum,* running from parieto-occipital and temporal cortex to frontal lobe by relays within the gyrus cinguli; and (7) *vertical occipital* bundle, connecting upper and lower lateral occipital cortices (Fig. 2-13). The association bundles are reviewed in Chapter 21.

The cavities of the telencephalon are the bilateral *lateral ventricles,* which continue into the cavity

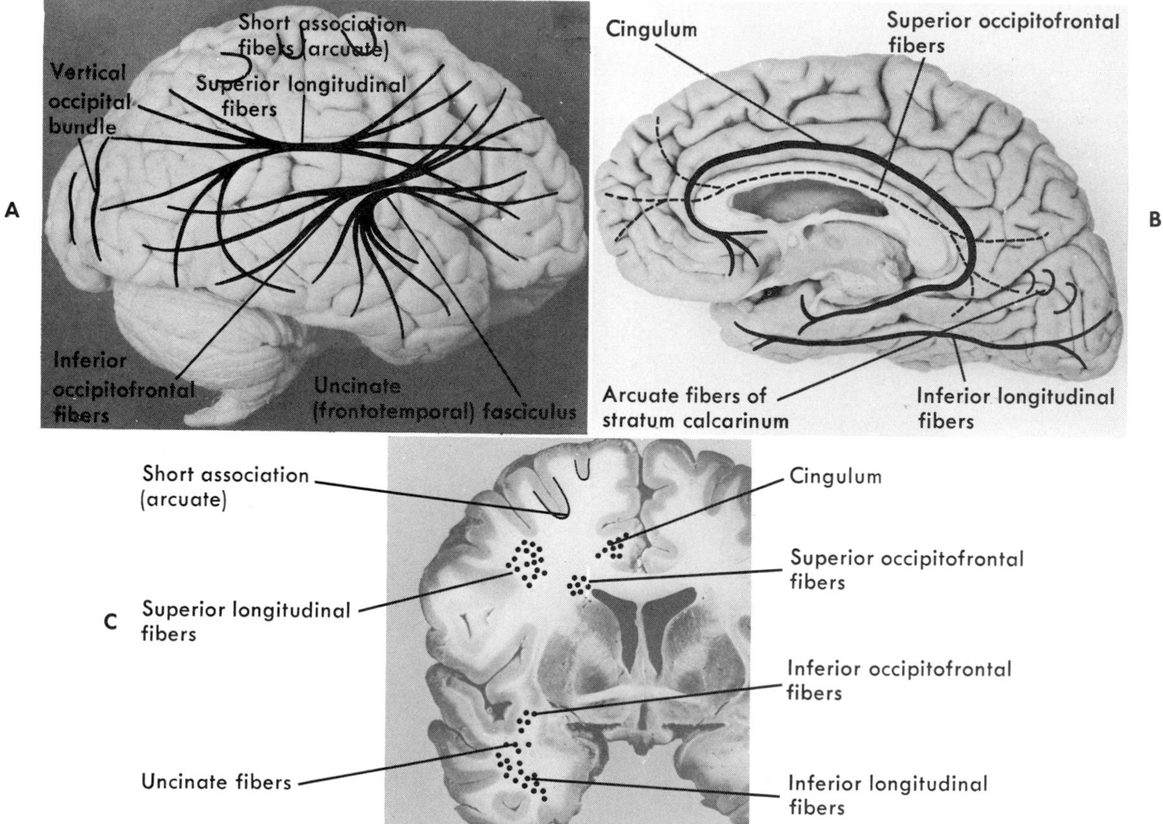

Fig. 2-13. Association bundles: **A,** in lateral projection; **B,** in medial projection; **C,** marked on coronal section.

of the *third ventricle* through the *interventricular* foramina on either side (Fig. 2-4) (see Chapter 3).

Diencephalon

Division of the diencephalon or thalamus. The thalamus is represented in superficial presentation as the lateral walls of the third ventricle in sagittal sections (Fig. 2-4). The best illustrations are in the coronal and transverse sections (Chapter 5). The diencephalon includes *thalamus proper, metathalamus, epithalamus, subthalamus,* and *hypothalamus;* each part possesses distinct anatomic and functional characteristics.[3,4]

The *thalamus proper* (dorsal thalamus proper) is the diencephalic structure comprising the bulk of the wall of the third ventricle and extending posteriorly as the pulvinar (Figs. 2-1, *A,* 2-3, and 2-10). The opposing structures on either side connect across the third ventricle through the constricted massa intermedia. Cell groups in the massa intermedia and adjacent periventricular structures comprise an ill-defined nucleus called *midline.* The major parts of the thalamus proper are divided by a narrow band, the *internal medullary lamina.* This contains cells that form the *intralaminar nucleus.* The *anterior* nucleus separates anteriorly and dorsally (Figs. 2-3 and 2-15). A *medial nucleus* forms the bulky mass to the side of the midline group. The *lateral nucleus* of the thalamus proper lies against the *external medullary lamina,* which is separated from the posterior limb of the internal capsule by the narrow *reticular nucleus.* The *ventral nuclear group* of the thalamus proper is divided into an anterior ventral nucleus, a lateral ventral nucleus (ventral posterolateral), and a medial ventral nucleus (ventral posteromedial). The lateral nucleus carries posteriorly into the *pulvinar,* which overhangs the midbrain (Figs. 2-1, *A* and 2-10). The thalamus proper connects to the insula and temporal lobe by a ventral stalk or peduncle (ansa peduncularis), which curves around the anterior boundary of the internal capsule. The functional relationships of the thalamic nuclei are reviewed in Chapter 21.

The *metathalamus* includes the bilateral *geniculate bodies, medial* and *lateral.* The medial geniculate body is an oval tubercle between pulvinar and midbrain, adjacent to the cerebral peduncle (Figs. 2-1, *A* and 2-14). It connects with the *inferior colliculus* of the midbrain through the brachium of the latter and is a relay station for auditory impulses from the colliculus and lower centers to the auditory cortex in the temporal lobe. The *lateral geniculate body* is a similar oval tubercle at the posterior

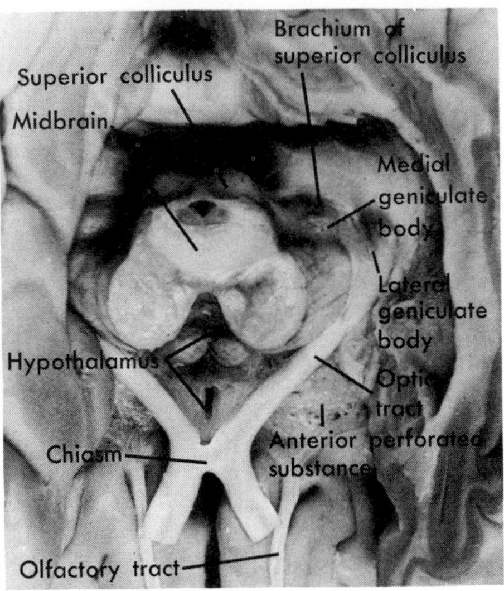

Fig. 2-14. Optic tract and lateral geniculate body.

extremity of the thalamus anterolateral to the medial geniculate body. It represents the thalamic terminus of the optic tract, which can be traced to it (Fig. 2-14). The lateral geniculate body connects to the *superior colliculus* of the midbrain through the *brachium* of the latter (Fig. 2-1). This part of the thalamus mediates visual impulses as a relay station projecting to the visual cortex.

The *epithalamus* includes the *pineal body,* the *habenular nuclei* and their *commissure,* and the *posterior commissure* (Figs. 2-1, *A,* 2-4, and 2-10). The pineal is an organ of uncertain function that projects posteriorly from the roof of the third ventricle. Recently the pineal has been shown to store serotonin and a derivative, melatonin, which may influence gonadal function.[10] *Habenular nuclei* occupy the posterior, superior, and lateral areas of the third ventricle roof adjacent to the pineal stalk and interconnect through the stalk as the habenular commissure. The *posterior commissure* lies in the inferior part of the stalk of the pineal, and through it some of the fibers interconnect the bilateral superior colliculi (Figs. 2-1, *A* and 2-4).

The *subthalamus* is the diencephalic area at the junction of the thalamus proper and the midbrain (Fig. 2-15). Its principal structure is the *subthalamic body* (of Luys), which receives fibers from the globus pallidus and cerebral peduncle and functions in extrapyramidal regulation of motor control. The *ansa lenticularis* is the interconnecting group of subthalamic fibers passing from the lenticular nuclei of the telencephalon to the nuclei of the midbrain and subthalamus. This peduncle is well

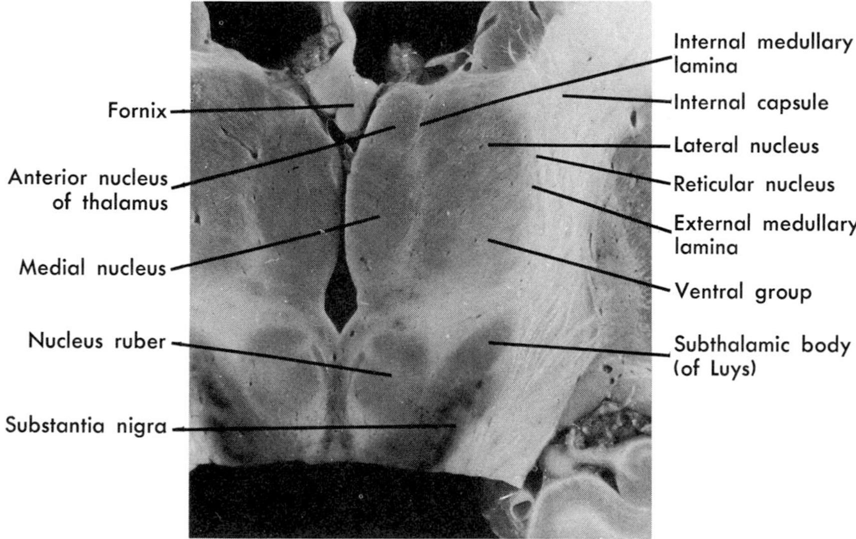

Fig. 2-15. Thalamic and subthalamic nuclei.

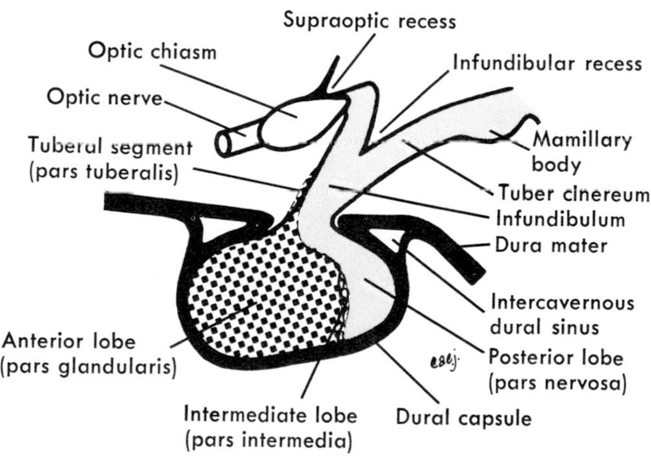

Fig. 2-16. Diagram of pituitary body and coverings.

displayed in coronal and parasagittal sections (Chapter 4).

The *hypothalamus,* on the medial view of a sagittal section, is that part of the brain adjacent to the third ventricle and below a line connecting the interventricular foramen with the aqueduct of Sylvius (hypothalamic line) (Fig. 2-4). It includes all the structures below this line except the parts of the telencephalon medium. The *tuber cinereum* is the funnel-like floor of the third ventricle leading into the *infundibulum,* or stalk, of the pituitary gland (hypophysis). The *neural lobe* of the hypophysis is part of this complex, although it is usually discussed with the gland. The *mamillary bodies* are the breast-like projections from the posterior part of the third ventricle floor (Figs. 2-4 and 2-9). These hypothalamic structures enter into control of vegetative functions (metabolism, temperature regulation), interrelate brain and neurohypophysis in the *neuroendocrine system,* and provide many thalamic interconnections having to do with viscera-related activities (see Chapter 22).[3,6]

Pituitary (hypophysis). The pituitary gland is closely related to the hypothalamus both anatomically and functionally (see p. 383). Its *posterior lobe* (pars nervosa) is an extension of the infundibulum. Besides the pars nervosa, the gross subdivisions of the gland (Fig. 2-16) include the *anterior lobe* (pars glandularis), the *intermediate lobe* (pars intermedia), and the *tuberal segment,* which extends up the stalk (pars tuberalis). The role of the pituitary in the neuroendocrine system is reviewed in Chapter 22.[6]

The *third ventricle* is the cavity related to the diencephalon. It is continuous with the lateral ventricles through the *interventricular foramina of Monro* and with the *cerebral aqueduct* of the midbrain (see Chapter 3).

Mesencephalon

The *mesencephalon,* or midbrain, is the short constricted segment of the brainstem that connects the diencephalon with the metencephalon. It is best seen by detaching the brainstem from the overhanging cerebrum and by dorsally removing the cerebellum (Fig. 2-1). In posterior view the four *colliculi* stand out prominently as the *corpora quadrigemina.* The two *superior colliculi* are related to the visual system. These connect with the *lateral geniculate bodies* through the *brachium of the superior colliculus* on either side (Fig. 2-1). The two inferior colliculi are auditory way stations and connect to the *medial geniculate bodies* on either side by means of the brachium of the *inferior colliculus.* At the inferior border of the inferior colliculi, the *trochlear nerves* (cranial IV) originate on either side and pass around the midbrain to approach the orbit. In side view the bulge of the longitudinally oriented *basis pedunculi* produces a shallow valley called the *lateral midbrain sulcus.* Dorsal to the sulcus is the *lemniscal trigone* which terminates superiorly at the line of the brachium of the inferior colliculus (Fig. 2-1, *B* and *C*). In anterior view the bulges of the *cerebral peduncles* are the longitudinal fiber masses on each side. These are continuous above with the internal capsule. Between them is the *interpeduncular fossa,* with the *posterior perforated substance* at its depths. The *oculomotor nerves* (cranial III) issue on either wall of the interpeduncular fossa (Fig. 2-9).

In cross section (Figs. 2-17 and 2-18) the midbrain presents three definable layers anteroposteriorly: the *basis pedunculi,* the *tegmentum,* and the *tectum.* The basis pedunculi represents the cerebral peduncles, which are fibrous continuations of the internal capsule. The fibers of the anterior limb of the internal capsule (frontal cortex relationships) pass into the medial fifth of the basis en route to the pons. The fibers from the genu of the internal capsule pass lateral to these and occupy the next fifth of the cross sectional area. These pass to bulbar nuclei from the motor cortex. The next two-fifths of the cross sectional area of the basis is occupied by the fibers from the medial part of the posterior limb of the internal capsule. These are en route to nuclei in the spinal cord from the motor cortex. The lateral fifth of the basis includes fibers from the posterior limb of the internal capsule that originate in parietal, occipital, and temporal cortex. These are en route to the pons (Fig. 2-19). The *tegmentum* of the midbrain represents the structures intervening between the basis pedunculi and the transverse line of the aqueduct, as displayed in cross section. The principal gross anatomic units are the *substantia nigra,* the *nucleus ruber,* and the *decussation of the brachium conjunctivum.* The substantia nigra is the black pigmented field lying immediately dorsal to the basis pedunculi on either side. The nucleus ruber (red nucleus) is the massive central nucleus of the midbrain on either side of midline. It represents an important relay station for fibers entering the midbrain from the basal nuclei and for fibers from the cerebellum reaching the red nucleus via the brachium conjunctivum, or superior cerebellar peduncle. The latter fibers cross at midline (decussate), producing a conspicuous midbrain structural entity (decussation of the brachium conjunctivum) immediately below the red nuclei. Dorsal to a line roughly drawn transversely across the cerebral aqueduct of the midbrain is the *tectum.* This part of the midbrain contains the four *colliculi,* the *cerebral aqueduct* of Sylvius, and the surrounding periaqueductal *gray matter* (Figs. 2-1, *A,* 2-17, and 2-18).

The ependyma-lined channel of the midbrain is the aqueduct of Sylvius (Fig. 2-17).

Metencephalon

The metencephalon includes the *pons* and *cerebellum,* which as a unit is the part of the brain continuous with the midbrain above and with the medulla below. The pons is the ventral swelling that continues dorsally on either side of the stem into the cerebellum. Each extension becomes a *middle cerebellar peduncle,* or *brachium pontis.* On cross section (Figs. 2-19 to 2-21) the pons presents a dorsal *tegmentum* that is continuous with the tegmentum of the midbrain and a ventral *basilar* portion, or *basis pontis.* Note that no tectum exists in the pontine structure. The roots of the *trigeminal nerve* (cranial nerve V), with both motor and sensory components, issue from the sides at the base of the middle cerebellar peduncle. The *abducens* (cranial VI), *facial* (cranial VII), and *acoustic*

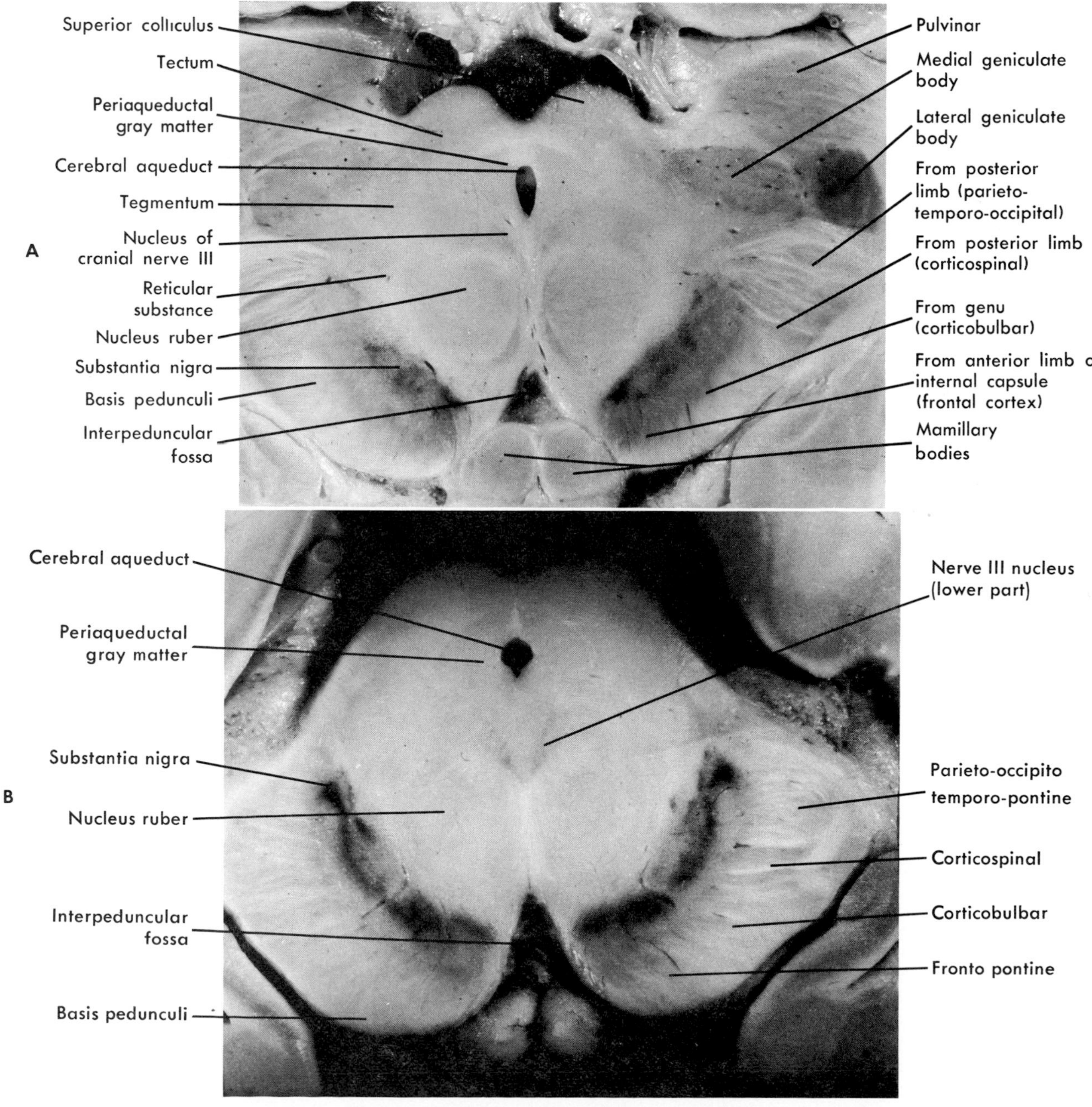
A
Superior colliculus
Tectum
Periaqueductal gray matter
Cerebral aqueduct
Tegmentum
Nucleus of cranial nerve III
Reticular substance
Nucleus ruber
Substantia nigra
Basis pedunculi
Interpeduncular fossa
Pulvinar
Medial geniculate body
Lateral geniculate body
From posterior limb (parieto-temporo-occipital)
From posterior limb (corticospinal)
From genu (corticobulbar)
From anterior limb of internal capsule (frontal cortex)
Mamillary bodies
B
Cerebral aqueduct
Periaqueductal gray matter
Substantia nigra
Nucleus ruber
Interpeduncular fossa
Basis pedunculi
Nerve III nucleus (lower part)
Parieto-occipito temporo-pontine
Corticospinal
Corticobulbar
Fronto pontine

Fig. 2-17. A, Upper midbrain; **B,** lower midbrain.

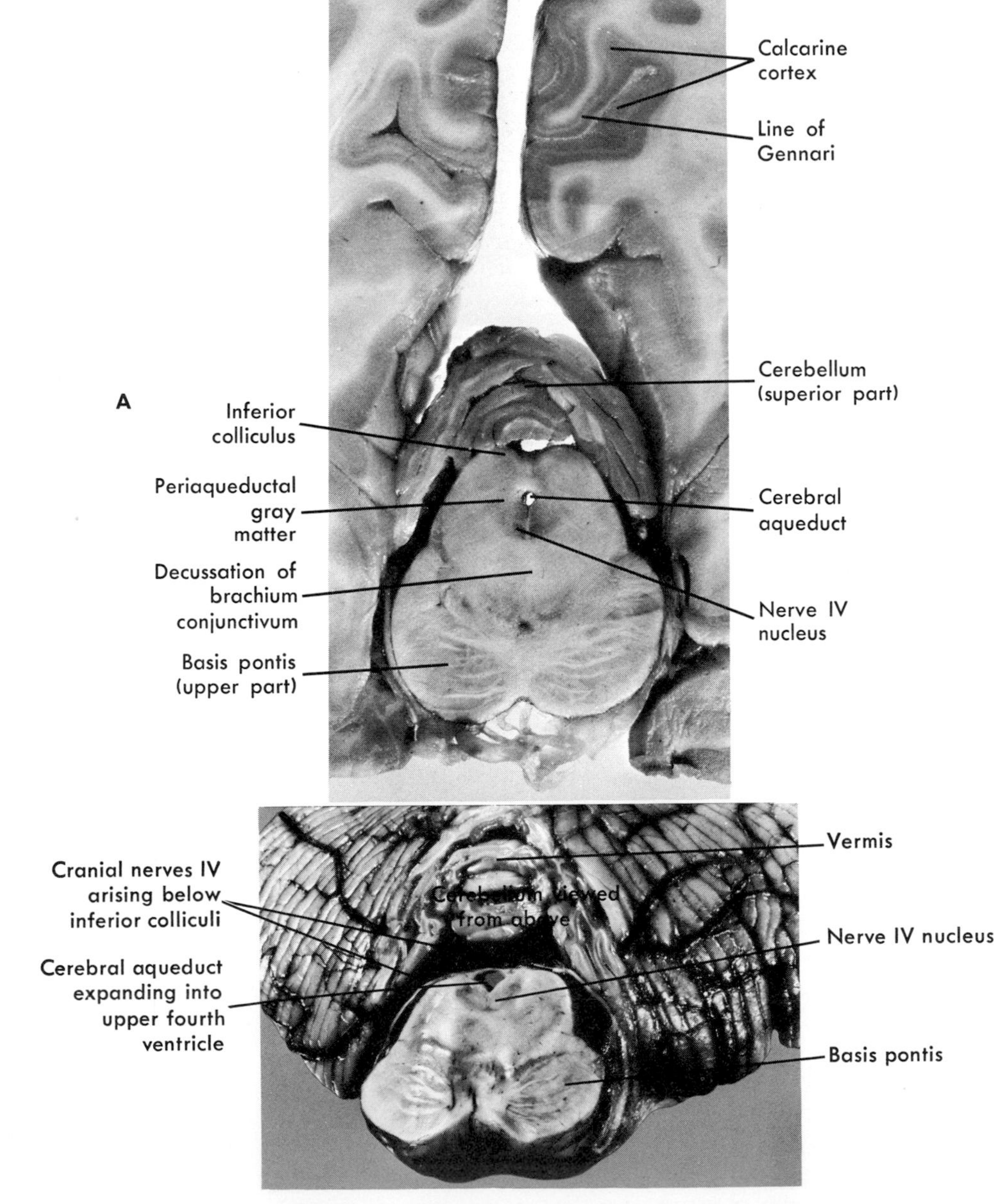

Fig. 2-18. Low midbrain: **A,** with upper pontine base; **B,** with cranial nerve IV.

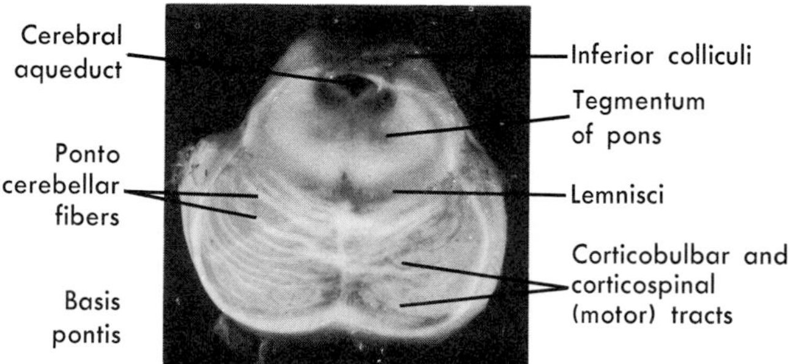

Fig. 2-19. Upper pons.

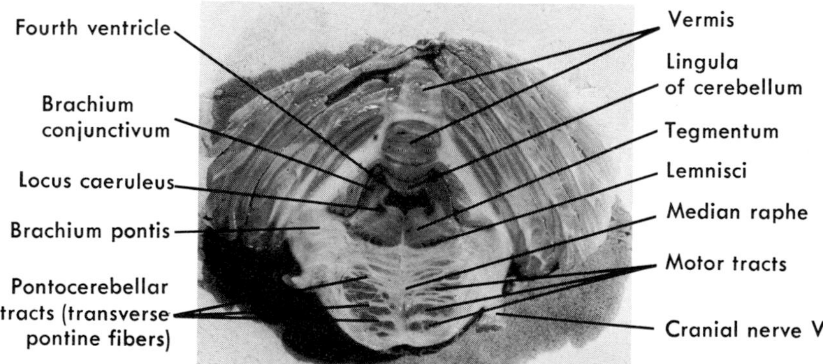

Fig. 2-20. Pons at level of nerve V.

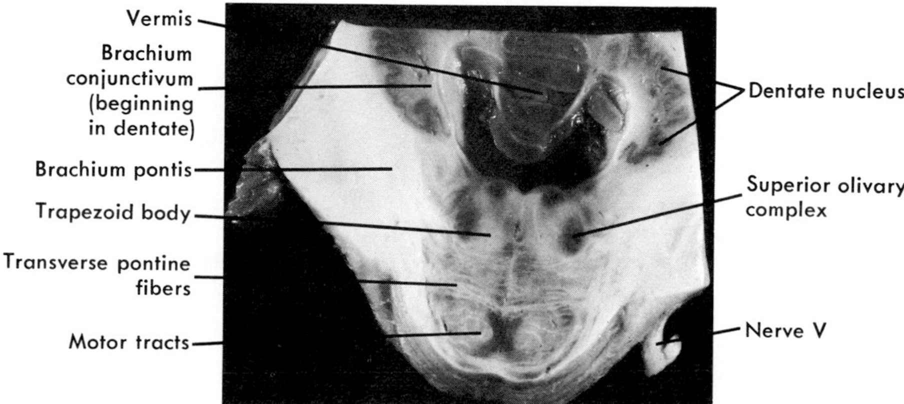

Fig. 2-21. Lower pons viewed from below.

(cranial VIII) nerves issue around the lower borders (Fig. 2-9). On gross examination, the *basis pontis* displays transverse fibers that arise in pontine nuclear cells. These fibers cross their counterparts from the other side in midline, producing the *median raphe* of the pons. The fibers in the basis pontis in cross section are the continuing projections from the cerebral cortex that have reached this position by traversing the internal capsule and the basis pedunculi. As stated previously, those fibers running in the medial fifth (frontopontile) and lateral fifth (parieto-occipito-temporo-pontile) of the basis pedunculi terminate in the pons. The fibers of the central three-fifths of the cerebral peduncle for the most part traverse the pons longitudinally to reach the bulbar and spinal nuclei. The *tegmentum* contains tracts and nuclei that are somewhat difficult to delineate grossly. The *brachium conjunctivum,* or superior cerebellar peduncle however stands out clearly on either side of the fourth ventricle (Fig. 2-1, *A*).

The cerebellum is the "small brain" lying dorsal to the pons. It is distinguished by the small straight gyri called *folia,* which are separated by compressed *sulci* and larger *fissures.* The largest of the fissures, designated *great horizontal,* is most conspicuous on the ventral surface. On this surface it splits over the middle cerebellar peduncle. This fissure extends laterally around the projecting hemispheres to a cleft inferior to a deeply buried *folium vermis* in dorsal midline (Fig. 2-4). At this midplane position the fissure roughly marks the midpoint of the cerebellum in the superoinferior axis. A second major structural subdivision is the *vermis,* which is a sagittally-placed, worm-like mass of short transverse folia vertically oriented side-to-side and separating the right and left *hemispheres* (Fig. 2-22). Note that a cleft, the *posterior incisure,* is formed inferiorly between the hemispheres. Further subdivisions of cerebellar structure are best introduced in sagittal section (Fig. 2-22).

Viewed medially, the sagittal section of the vermis of the cerebellum presents folia, sulci, and fissures disposed in a radiating pattern. The thin, branching white matter resembles a branching tree (*arbor vitae*), with gray cortex capping each folium. The white matter is continuous superiorly with a thin lamina overlying the fourth ventricle, the *anterior (superior) medullary velum.* A similar membrane extends inferiorly over the roof of the ventricle as the *posterior (inferior) medullary velum.* Viewed from above, the lobular pattern is separated, as in Figs. 2-4 and 2-22. The superiormost lobule is the *lingula,* which usually takes the form of two small folia attached at their bases to the superior medullary velum. The lingula is limited from behind by the *precentral fissure.* This fissure and the *postcentral fissure* define the *central lobule.* A massive lobule, the *culmen,* extends from the postcentral fissure to the deep *preclival fissure.* This fissure extends around the hemispheres and separates *anterior lobe* from the more bulky *posterior lobe.* The *declive* is the next subdivision of vermis and lies between the *preclival* and *postclival* fissures. The deep-seated *folium vermis* lies between the postclival and *great horizontal* fissures and is the smallest of the lobules of the vermis. The *tuber vermis* is located between the horizontal fissure and the *postpyramidal fissure.* Next is the *pyramidal lobule,* which is limited anteriorly by the *prepyramidal fissure.* The bulky *uvula* extends from this fissure to the *postnodular* fissure, and the nodule lies adjacent to the posterior medullary velum. The postnodular fissure separates the posterior lobe from the *flocculonodular lobe.* Three lobes are thus defined by fissures that involve hemispheres as well as vermis (*anterior, posterior,* and *flocculonodular*).[3,6]

By extending the principal fissures laterally the hemispheres are divided into units that are lateral continuations of the vermal lobules (Figs. 2-4 and 2-22, *B*). The *lingula* possesses no significant extension. The *central lobule* becomes the *ala (wings) centralis.* The culmen is continuous with the *anterior crescentic (semilunar) lobules* of the hemispheres. These structures comprise the *anterior lobe.* The *declive* extends to become the *posterior crescentic (semilunar) lobules.* The *folium vermis* expands greatly into the hemispheres as the *posterior superior* lobules. The *tuber* extends into the *posterior inferior lobules.* The pyramid expands into the *biventer* lobules. The *uvula* expands bilaterally into the *tonsils,* which project downward as bulky rounded nodular masses located medially on either side near the more anterior brainstem. The parts from declive and its hemispheral extensions to the uvula and its tonsillar extensions constitute the *posterior lobe.* The remaining *nodule* extends laterally via a narrow *peduncle* to the *flocculus.* This combination makes up the *flocculonodular* lobe (Fig. 2-9). The flocculus can be isolated as a bilaterally projecting nodule on the ventral surface, closely related to the nerves at the inferior border of the pons and near the start of the great horizontal fissure.

The *gray matter* of the cerebellum includes the narrow cortex covering the folia and deeper nuclei in the central white matter, called *dentate, emboliform, globose,* and *fastigial.* These nuclei are well

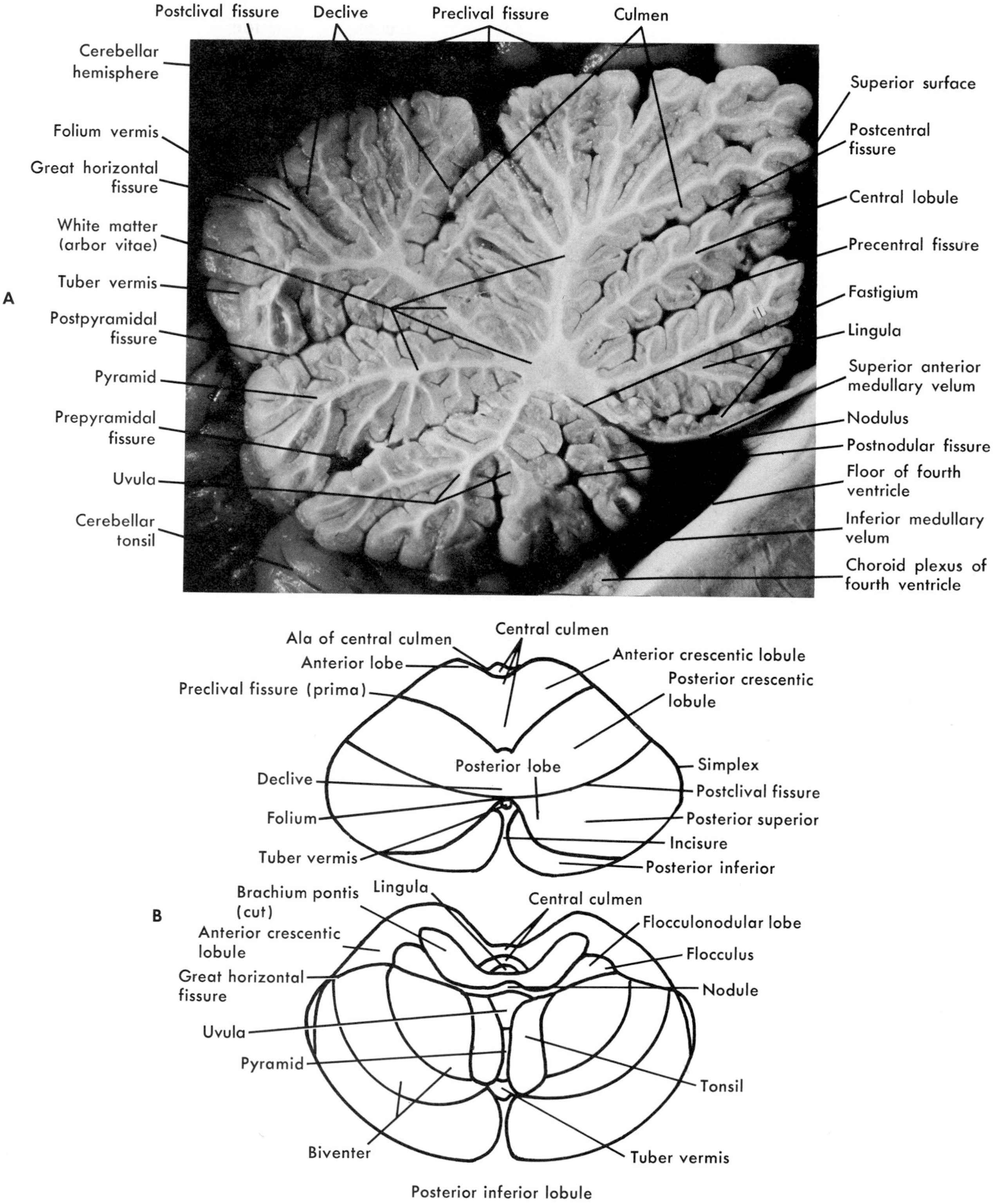

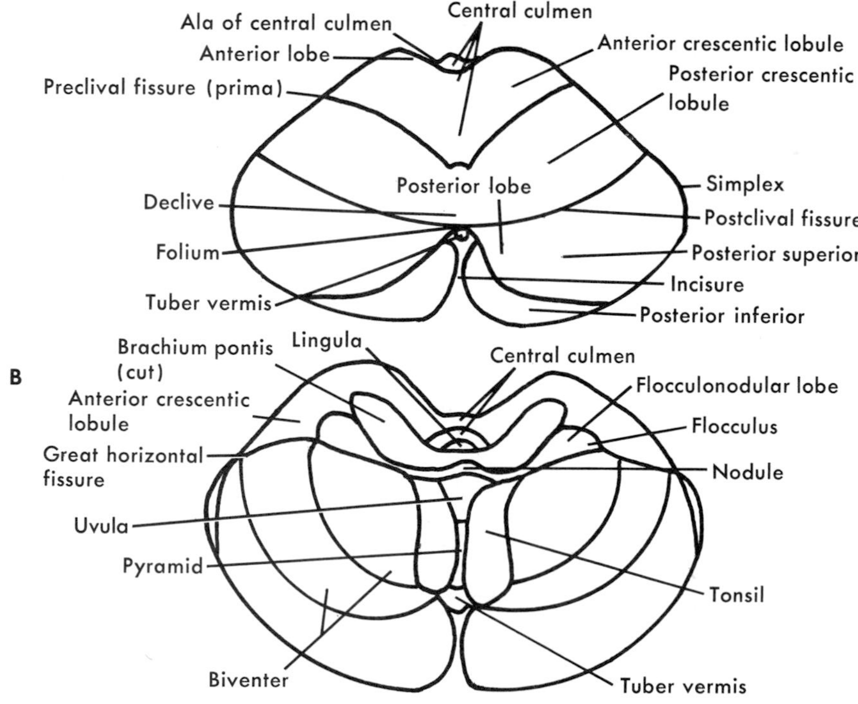

Fig. 2-22. A, Medial view of cerebellar vermis; **B,** cerebellar surfaces.

displayed by a transverse section through the peak, or fastigium, of the fourth ventricle (Fig. 2-23). These nuclei receive the fibers originating in the cerebellar cortex, and cells within them provide the axons that carry efferent signals from the cerebellum. The *white matter* of the cerebellum has previously been called *arbor vitae* in the distal branching patterns related to the centers of the folia. The axons passing both to and from the cerebellum travel via three cerebellar peduncles: (1) *brachium conjunctivum* (superior cerebellar peduncle), (2) *brachium pontis* (middle cerebellar peduncle), and (3) *corpus restiforme* (inferior cerebellar peduncle) (Fig. 2-1, *A*). The superior cerebellar peduncle originates principally in the dentate nucleus. It passes to midbrain and higher centers (especially nucleus ruber) after decussating where the pathway enters the midbrain *(decussation of the brachium conjunctivum)*. The middle cerebellar peduncle is principally comprised of fibers arising in pontine nuclei and passing across the median raphe of the pons *(pontocerebellar)* to the brachium pontis. The inferior cerebellar peduncle is more complex in structure and includes fibers from many nuclei in the medulla and spinal cord. Some fibers extend from the cerebellar nuclei (especially fastigial) to bulbar nuclei via paths closely related to the inferior peduncle. (For details concerning cerebellar connections in the motor system see Chapter 23.)

The cavity of the metencephalon is the *fourth ventricle,* which connects with the cerebral aqueduct above and with the spinal canal below. This cavity is also related to the myelencephalon. It opens into the meningeal spaces related to the medulla via apertures of Luschka and Magendie (see Chapter 3).

Myelencephalon

The *medulla,* or bulb, is the part of the brainstem that connects the metencephalon to the spinal cord. It forms the terminal segment of the brain-

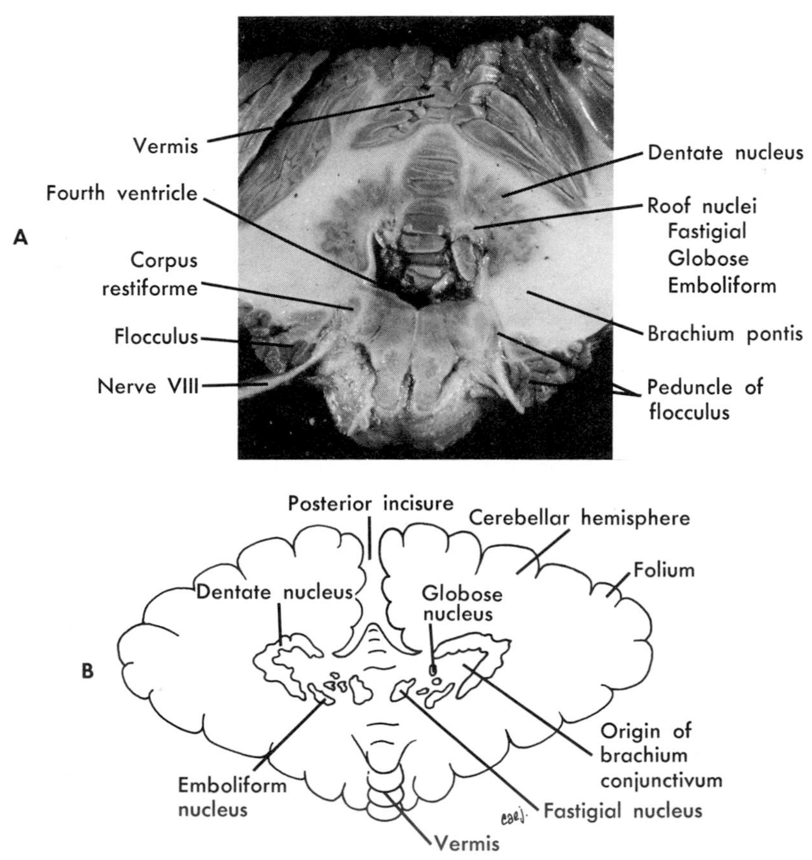

Fig. 2-23. A, Transverse section through cerebellar nuclei; **B,** diagram of cerebellar nuclei.

stem and arbitrarily ends at the foramen magnum. The anterior surface (Fig. 2-9) is distinguished by two prominent longitudinal ridges that issue below the belly of the pons. These are the *pyramids,* which are the continuation of the corticobulbar and corticospinal fibers, previously identified in the internal capsule, basis pedunculi, and basis pontis in downward succession. The pyramids are separated by the *anterior median fissure* in midline. This fissure is bridged throughout the medulla by the bulky crossing fibers of the pyramids (*decussation of the pyramids*); however, the bridge is most prominent in the deeper part of the fissure. Immediately lateral to the pyramids are the projecting oval prominences, the *inferior olives.* The sulci anterior and posterior to the olives are called *preolivary* and *postolivary* respectively (Fig. 2-9). The longitudinal ridge dorsal to the postolivary sulcus that continues inferiorly throughout the length of the medulla is the *tuberculum cinereum* (related to the tracts of the trigeminal cranial nerve V). On the dorsal surface of the medulla adjacent to the tuberculum cinereum is the slightly nodular projection, the *cuneate tubercle,* which overlies the *nucleus cuneatus* (Fig. 2-1, *A*). This tubercle continues downward as the *fasciculus cuneatus* through the length of the medulla and into the upper spinal cord. The sulcus between the tuberculum cinereum and the cuneate fasciculus becomes the *dorsolateral sulcus* of the spinal cord, by which the *dorsal roots* of spinal nerves enter the cord (beginning at cervical segment 2). Immediately adjacent to the cuneate system and separated from it by the *dorsal intermediate sulcus* is the *gracile* prominence. This structure also is oriented longitudinally and exhibits a nodular prominence, the *clava,* in its superior part (overlying *nucleus gracilis*), and a continuing ridge, the *fasciculus gracilis,* which parallels inferiorly the fasciculus cuneatus. The two gracile fasciculi are separted in midline by the *dorsal median sulcus,* which continues into the cord.

Related to the medullary and pontine contours on the ventral surfaces are the cranial nerves VI through XII, which will be discussed in detail later. The abducens (VI) is identified between pyramid and pons, and curves over the latter. Lateral to the abducens is the facial (VII) with its small branch, *nervus intermedius.* Closely related to the lateral side of nerve VII is the acoustic nerve (VIII), which is bulkier. The seventh and eighth cranial nerves are immediately superior to, and partly covered by, the flocculus of the cerebellum. In the postolivary sulcus the glossopharyngeal (IX), vagus (X), and spinal accessory (XI) nerves appear in successions downward from above. The hypoglossal nerve (XII) arises as several filaments in the preolivary sulcus. Nearer the spinal cord on the ventral aspect of the medulla, nerve XI (spinal accessory) runs slightly dorsal to the line of *ventral roots* of spinal nerves, which begin at the first segment of the cord. The ventral roots occupy the slight *anterolateral sulcus,* which marks the exit line of the motor filaments of the cord (Fig. 2-9).

The floor of the fourth ventricle (rhomboid fossa)

The *rhomboid fossa* is exposed by removing the cerebellum from the brainstem. As viewed posteriorly, it represents the contours of the dorsal parts of both the pons and medulla. The area is thus both metencephalic and myelencephalic. At the juncture of pons and medulla in the dorsolateral areas, prominent ridges rise from the medulla and extend into the cerebellum. These ridges are called the *inferior cerebellar peduncles* (corpora restiforme) (Figs. 2-1, *A* and 2-24).

The transected parts of all three cerebellar peduncles are evident in the lateral boundaries of the fossa. The superior boundary is formed by the narrow, transected superior medullary velum and its overlying cerebellar lingula. The inferior border is defined by the broader inferior medullary velum, which terminates inferiorly as a slight nodule, the *obex.* This nodule is the pointed terminus of the fossa. The fourth ventricle extends on both sides into its *lateral canals* and *apertures* (of *Luschka*), putting the cavity of the fourth ventricle into communication with the meningeal spaces. A similar *midline aperture* (of *Magendie*) penetrates the inferior medullary velum overlying the obex.

The floor exhibits a somewhat complex contour pattern that provides important landmarks to underlying nuclei of the pons and medulla (Fig. 2-24). In the upper third of Fig. 2-24, a longitudinal ridge, the *medial eminence,* runs on either side of the *median fissure* of the floor. At the approximate midpoint of the fossa, the median eminence expands into bilateral projecting nodules called the *facial colliculi.* These overly the nuclei of the VIth nerves and parts of the nerves VII as they extend dorsally to the nuclei of the nerves VI within the brainstem substance. The sulcus lateral to the median eminence and the facial colliculus on each side is the embryonic *sulcus limitans,* which separates sensory from motor primordial sites. A depressed fossa above the facial colliculus in this sulcus is called the *superior fovea.* Below the colliculus is a similar fossa, the *inferior fovea,* which represents the lowest grossly rec-

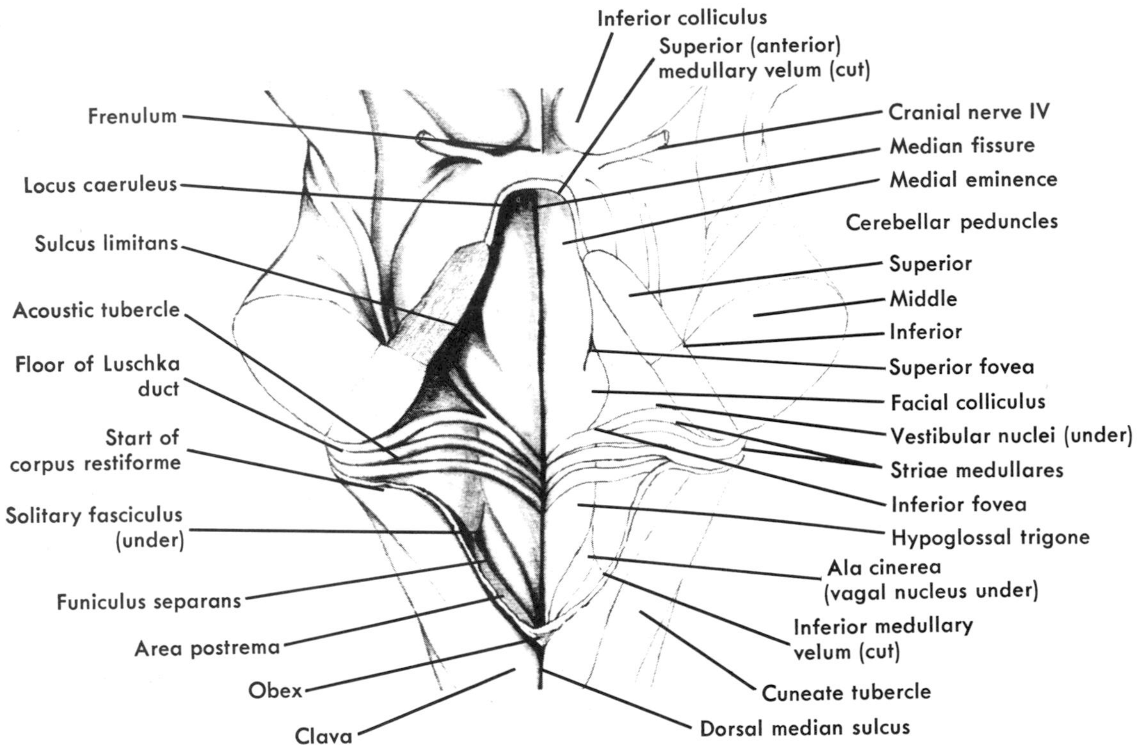

Fig. 2-24. Diagram of floor of fourth ventricle (rhomboid fossa).

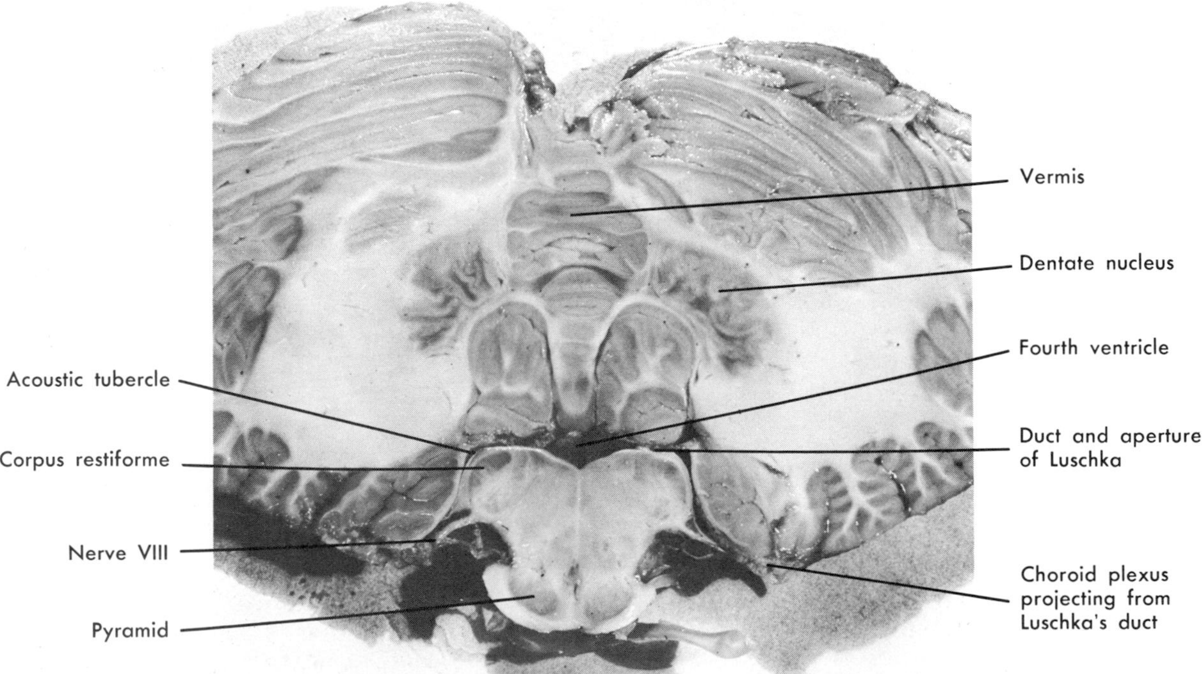

Fig. 2-25. Upper medulla at the level of the cochlear nuclei.

ognizable sulcus limitans. The *locus caeruleus,* a bilateral pigmented nucleus, is located in the upper pontine levels. It underlies the superior medullary velum at the lateral extremities of the narrowed part of the fourth ventricle. This is variable in length and can best be viewed by laterally retracting the superior cerebellar peduncles (Fig. 2-24). Immediately below the facial colliculi are fiber bundles of variable size that elevate the floor in a transverse pattern and disappear into the central fissure. These are the *striae medullares,* which pass from nuclei on the ventral surface of the medulla (arcuate nuclei) to the cerebellum. Lateral and inferior to the facial colliculus and covered variously by the striae medullares are the bilateral elevations, the *acoustic tubercles.* These overlie the dorsal cochlear nuclei of the auditory system. Lateral to the acoustic tubercle and bending inferiorly, the duct-like extension of the fourth ventricle continues to the *aperture of Luschka* on each side. A tringular eminence with the point toward the obex located near midline below the striae defines the *hypoglossal trigone.* This overlies the hypoglossal nucleus and is separated by a fine sulcus from the *ala cinerea,* which lies lateral to the trigone. The ala cinerea terminates at the inferior fovea above, and its boundaries define the underlying dorsal *vagal nucleus* (vagal trigone) on either side. The lateral border of the ala cinerea is also a landmark to the *solitary fasciculus,* a longitudinally-oriented bundle of incoming fibers related to cranial nerves VII, IX, and X (see Chapter 6). The narrow lateral border of the ala cinerea is the *funiculus separans,* which also defines the upper medial border of the *area postrema.* The area postrema is the last differentiable structure of the floor of the fourth ventricle. A combination of triangles points to the obex and ressembles a pen point. Because of its shape, this area is called *calamus scriptorus.*

The *medulla* oblongata is generally too small and

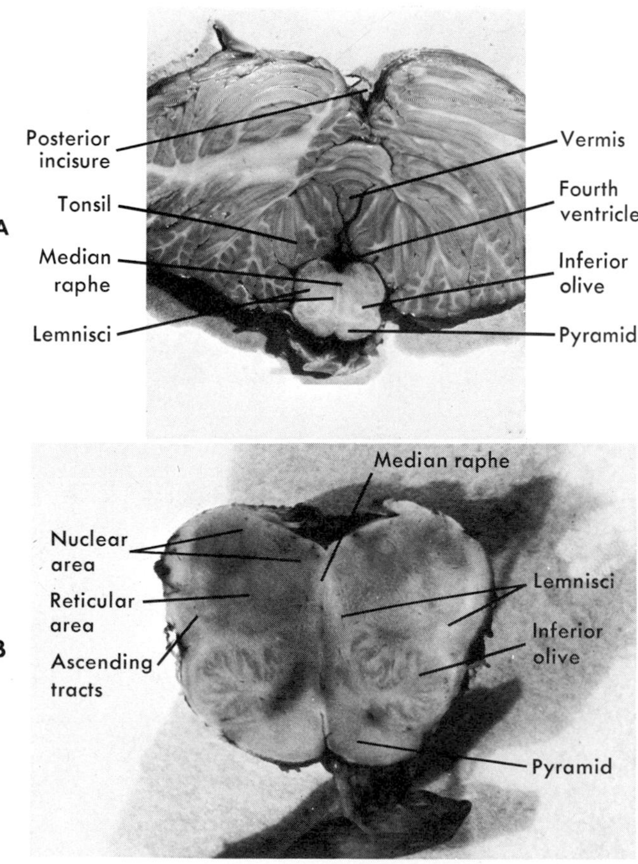

Fig. 2-26. A, Mid medulla through inferior olives; **B,** isolated medulla through olives.

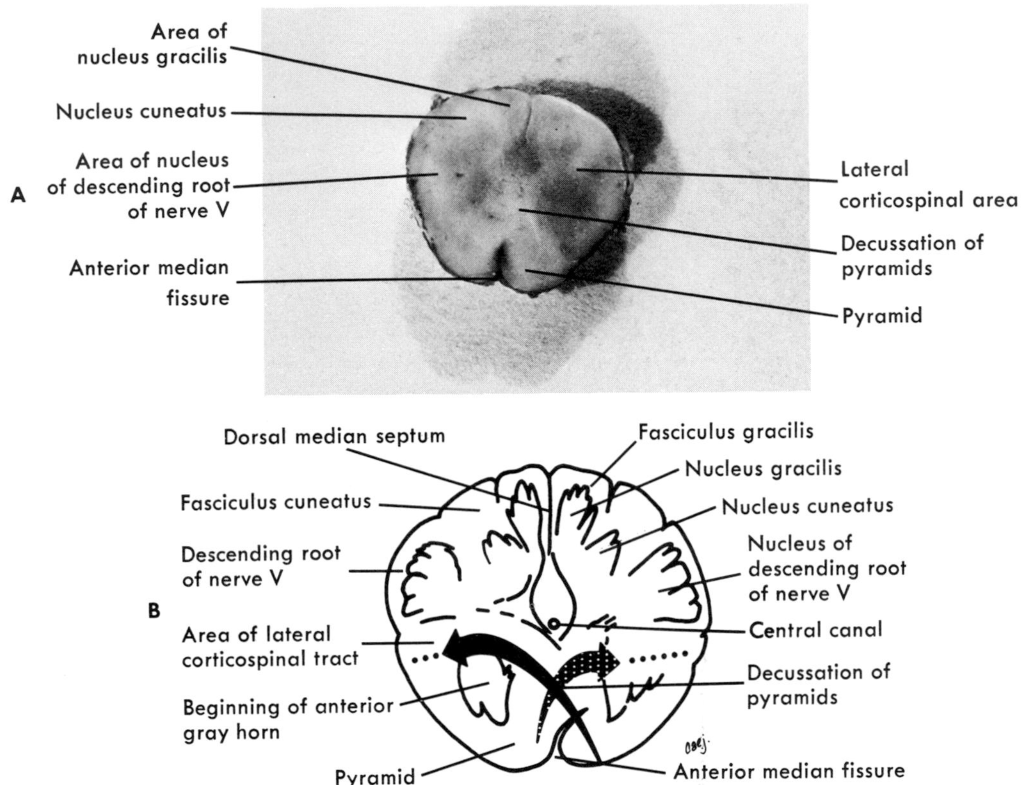

Fig. 2-27. A, Lower medulla at level of decussation of pyramids; **B,** diagram of medulla at decussation of pyramids.

complex for gross study of its cross sections. The following anatomic areas can be defined, however grossly alone or with a hand lens (Figs. 2-1 and 2-27 to 2-30). The *pyramids* stand out prominently along the ventral part in the upper segments and disappear as prominent gross landmarks in the lower medulla. In Fig. 2-27 they are shown to decussate and assume a central and lateral position, continuing into the cord as the lateral corticospinal tracts. The *inferior olives* are located dorsal to the pyramids and produce the bilateral prominences on either side of the medulla (Figs. 2-1, *B* and 2-25). Dorsal to the olives are the mixtures of tracts and nuclei that are obscure in gross inspection but that come to light by staining. These are the extremely important *pathways,* to be reviewed later (Chapters 16 to 19), and the *nuclei* associated with the cranial nerves (Chapter 6). At the dorsolateral extremities of the medulla are the bilateral fiber bundles that comprise the *inferior cerebellar peduncles* or *corpora restiforme.* The bundles are most conspicuous in the upper part. They stand out prominently in gross view (Figs. 2-24 and 2-25).

Spinal Cord

The *spinal cord* is the extracranial continuation of the medulla through the foramen magnum into the vertebral canal. It terminates inferiorly in a cone-like, tapering extremity called the *conus medullaris,* which is located at the low part of lumbar vertebra 1 (Fig. 2-28). Its connective tissues aggregate at the tip of the conus to form a filamentous strand, *filum terminale,* which continues caudally to attach to the sacrum. The spinal cord exhibits a striking segmentation, with each segment identified by a corresponding spinal nerve. There are eight cervical segments, twelve thoracic segments, five lumbar segments, five sacral segments, and one coccygeal segment. The segments are unequal in length and volume and, with the spinal cord terminating at lumbar 1 of the vertebral levels, are frequently distantly related to their corresponding vertebrae. These topographic relationships are displayed in Fig. 2-28. The segments of the lower cord become increasingly distant from their vertebrae. Note that the nerves of the cervical segments pass *over* the related vertebrae (cervical nerve 8 passing *under*

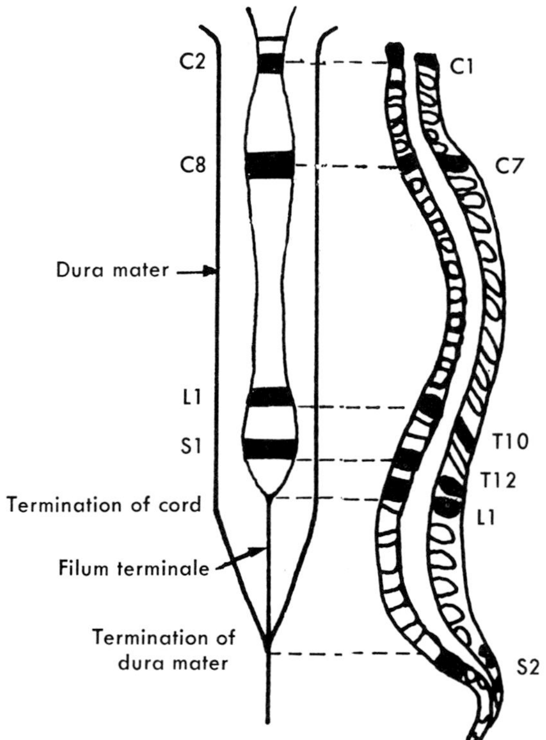

Fig. 2-28. Spinal cord segment levels and corresponding vertebral levels.

cervical vertebrae 7 and *over* thoracic vertebra 1) while the nerves from other segments pass *under* the vertebra with the same number. As the vertebral canal descends it becomes filled with nerves that are oriented longitudinally in relating cord segment to vertebral level. This produces an aggregate of nerves reminiscent of a horse's tail, the *cauda equina* (Fig. 2-29), below the lumbar vertebra 2.

Enlargements. The spinal cord is somewhat flattened anteroposteriorly, especially in the cervical part. It contains two enlargements, *cervical* and *lumbar*. These are the segments of the cord related to the upper and lower extremities respectively. The cervical enlargement occurs with some variability in segments from cervical 4 to thoracic 2, reaching maximum dimensions at cervical 6. The enlargement is topographically related to cervical vertebrae 3 to 7 and thoracic vertebrae 1 and 2 (Fig. 2-28). The nerves issuing from these segments supply the upper extremity, related trunk segments, and the diaphragm (see Chapter 5). The lumbar enlargement involves spinal cord segments from thoracic 12 down to sacral 4. It is compressed into a relatively short section corresponding to vertebral levels from the thoracic 9 to 12. Below this level, the spinal cord tapers into the conus, which extends approximately one disk and vertebral length further (to lumbar 1 or the upper part of lumbar 2). The

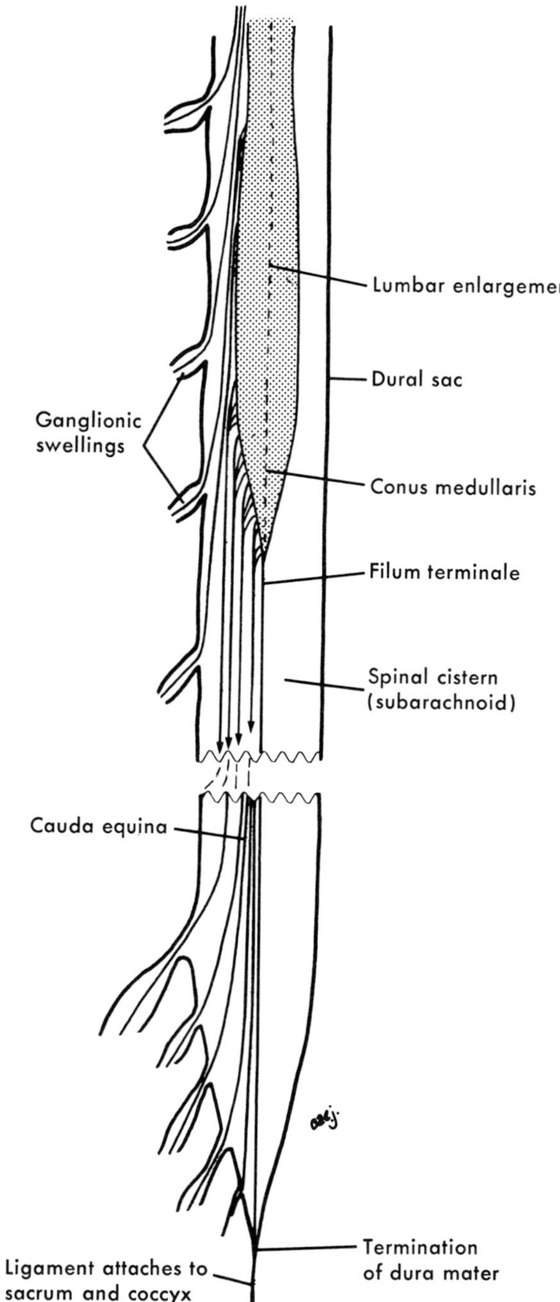

Fig. 2-29. Cauda equina and spinal cistern.

lumbar enlargement (lumbosacral) distributes its nerves principally to the lower extremity. The thoracic segments intervene between, and gradually blend with, the cervical and lumbar enlargements. These segments correspond to the level of thoracic 2 to thoracic 9 (Fig. 2-28). Above the cervical enlargement the upper cervical segments are uniform in dimension and extend upward to blend with the medulla at the foramen magnum. The position of these upper cervical segments corresponds to the levels of the first three cervical vertebrae (Fig. 2-28).

Surface markings. The spinal cord is divided into symmetrical halves by a deep fissure anteriorly (*ventral median fissure*) and a less conspicuous sulcus (*dorsal median sulcus*) posteriorly. These are continuous with the markings on the medulla. On the ventral surface, the spinal cord is joined by a row of nerve filaments that represent the *ventral roots* (motor). These form a shallow *ventral lateral sulcus* (Fig. 2-29). The posterior attachments of dorsal nerve roots (sensory) form a more prominent *dorsal lateral sulcus.* These two principal sulci (ventral lateral and dorsal lateral) on either side provide the external limits of the three major white columns, or *funiculi,* of the spinal cord: (1) *dorsal funiculus,* between the dorsal median sulcus and the dorsal lateral sulcus; (2) *lateral funiculus,* between the dorsal lateral sulcus and the ventral lateral sulcus; and (3) *ventral funiculus,* between the ventral lateral sulcus and the ventral median fissure (Fig. 2-29). The dorsal surface of the spinal cord in the cervical and upper thoracic segments is also marked by a narrow sulcus, the *dorsal intermediate sulcus.* It divides the dorsal funiculus into a medial *fasciculus gracilis* and a lateral *fasciculus cuneatus.* These are continuous with the same fascicles of the medulla above but disappear as separate tracts below the cervical enlargement.

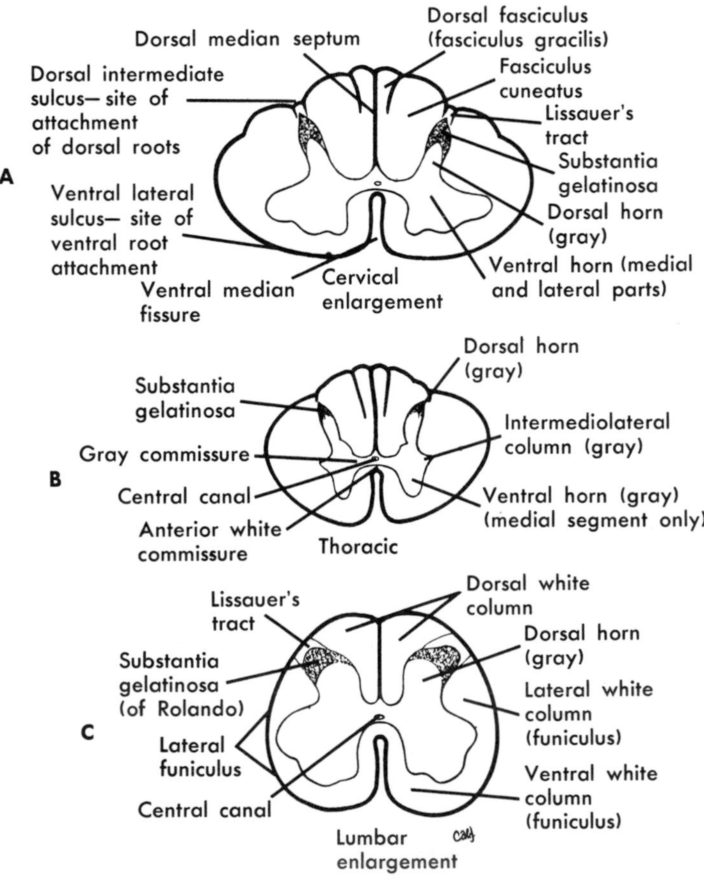

Fig. 2-30. Diagrams of cord levels: **A,** cervical; **B,** thoracic; **C,** lumbar.

The dorsal funiculus of the thoracic and lower cord is directly continuous with the fasciculus gracilis. This fascicle is compressed medially by incoming fibers in the levels of the cervical enlargement. These fibers, arising from the upper extremity, ascend as the fasciculus cuneatus and remain distinct to their termination in the medulla.

Gray and white matter. The nuclei of the spinal cord are lodged in columns of cell bodies located centrally in patterns that are best viewed in cross section. A hand lens is usually required to examine these gross features. The gray matter is disposed in an H shaped pattern that varies from level to level. The central bar of the H is called the *gray commissure.* It is oriented around the *central canal,* which is the part of the ventricular cavity in the spinal cord. The *anterior white commissure* passes transversely ventral to the gray commissure. The gray commissure is called *dorsal* or *ventral,* dependent upon its position relative to the canal. The posterior limbs of the H extend to the dorsal surface of the cord at the dorsal lateral fissure, where the dorsal roots enter. This limb on either side forms the *dorsal horn* and provides the lateral limits of the dorsal funiculus (Fig. 2-29). The anterior limb of the H forms the *ventral horn* on each side, which extends nearly to the surface at the attachment of the ventral roots in the ventral lateral fissure. The horns thus define the funiculi of white matter in the cross-sectional views. These are the dorsal, lateral, and ventral funiculi that are marked on the surface by the sulcal divisions (Fig. 2-29). The horns of gray matter are also referred to as gray columns, since their pattern persists in longitudinal columns of cells (see Chapter 6). The outlines of gray matter in sections of the cord differ from level to level, as displayed in Fig. 2-29. The dorsal horns are elongate, and the ventral horns narrow in the upper cervical segments. The cervical enlargement is distinguished by large expansions of the ventral horns (to house the cells supplying the upper extremity). Thoracic levels are characterized both dorsally and ventrally by narrow horns and by a slight lateral projection on either side at the level of the gray commissure, called the *intermediolateral gray column* or lateral horn. This column contains cells of the visceral efferent system. The lumbosacral enlargement is unique in the relative bulk of both gray horns and the relative small size of the white funiculi (Fig. 2-29). The nuclear groups are reviewed in Chapter 6, and the organization of the tracts in the funiculi are discussed in Chapters 16 to 22.

REFERENCES

1. Crosby, E. C., Humphrey, T., and Lauer, E. W.: Correlative anatomy of the nervous system, New York, 1962, The Macmillan Co.
2. Dow, R. S., and Moruzzi, G.: The physiology and pathology of the cerebellum, Minneapolis, 1958, University of Minnesota Press.
3. Haymaker, W., Anderson, E., and Nauta, W. J. H.: The hypothalamus, Springfield, Illinois, 1969, Charles C Thomas, Publisher.
4. Riley, H. A., An atlas of the basal ganglia, brain stem and spinal cord, New York, 1960, Hafner Publishing Co., Inc.
5. Russell, W. O., and Bowerman, D. L.: Pineal body. In Minckler, J., editor: Pathology of the nervous system, vol. I, New York, 1968, McGraw-Hill Book Co.
6. Scharrer, E., and Scharrer, B.: Neuroendocrinology, New York, 1963, Columbia University Press.

CHAPTER 3

VENTRICULOMENINGEAL SYSTEM AND VASCULATURE

JEFF MINCKLER

The fluid transport systems of the brain and spinal cord are unique among the tissues of the body. The most distinguishing feature of the neural tissues is the absence of a lympatic system. Fluid exchanges are made without a special means of intercellular drainage. A second distinguishing feature is the development of a series of cavities (ventricles) within the CNS that contain fluid. In this system *cerebrospinal fluid* (CSF) is elaborated and transported outside of the main nervous tissue mass. The ventricular system thus becomes a dynamic pathway in the fluid transport activities of the brain. Enroute, this CSF provides a universal incompressible, but movable fluid cushion within and around the structures of the CNS to protect them mechanically. In accomplishing these functions, the CSF is channeled through spaces in the membranous coverings of the brain, the *meninges,* and in the ventricular cavities. The meningeal and ventricular spaces are continuous. Like other tissues of the body the CNS is provided with a blood supply in the arterial system and a drainage mechanism in the venous system. This vasculature is closely related to the ventriculomeningeal system and is discussed with it. This section concerns the gross anatomy of the ventricular system, the meninges, and the vasculature of the brain and spinal cord. The histology of these tissues and the details of functional anatomy are presented in Chapter 10 and neuroradiology in Chapter 5.

VENTRICULAR SYSTEM

Each major segment of the CNS is oriented around a cavity (ventricle) or duct that serves to convey CSF from its origin in the choroid plexus to the meningeal spaces (Fig. 3-1). Each cerebral hemisphere of the telencephalon possesses a *lateral ventricle.* The diencephalon is disposed around a centrally located *third ventricle.* The third ventricle connects with the lateral ventricles on each side through an *interventricular foramen of Monro.* The mesencephalon has a dorsal *cerebral aqueduct (aqueduct of Sylvius)* that is continuous above with the third ventricle. The cerebral aqueduct expands in the metencephalon into the upper part of the *fourth ventricle.* This ventricle also represents the cavity of the myelencephalon. The fourth ventricle is continuous below with the central canal of the spinal cord. The fourth ventricle possesses two lateral extensions, the *foramina of Luschka,* which open into the subarachnoid meningeal spaces on either side of the pontomedullary junction. A central *foramen of Magendie,* of controversial existence, opens in midline into meningeal spaces between medulla and overlying cerebellum in the area of the posterior medullary velum (Fig. 3-1). The entire ventricular system is lined with an epithelium called *ependyma.* A secreting organ, the *choroid plexus,* is found in part of the walls of the lateral ventricles, in the roof of the third ventricle, and in the posterior medullary velum and lateral apertures of the fourth ventricle. The CSF arises in the choroid plexus and flows from lateral ventricles through the interventricular foramina to the third ventricle. From the third ventricle it travels through the cerebral aqueduct into the fourth ventricle and from there into the meningeal spaces through the foramina of Luschka and Magendie. A small amount of CSF passes into the central canal of the spinal cord.[3,5,10]

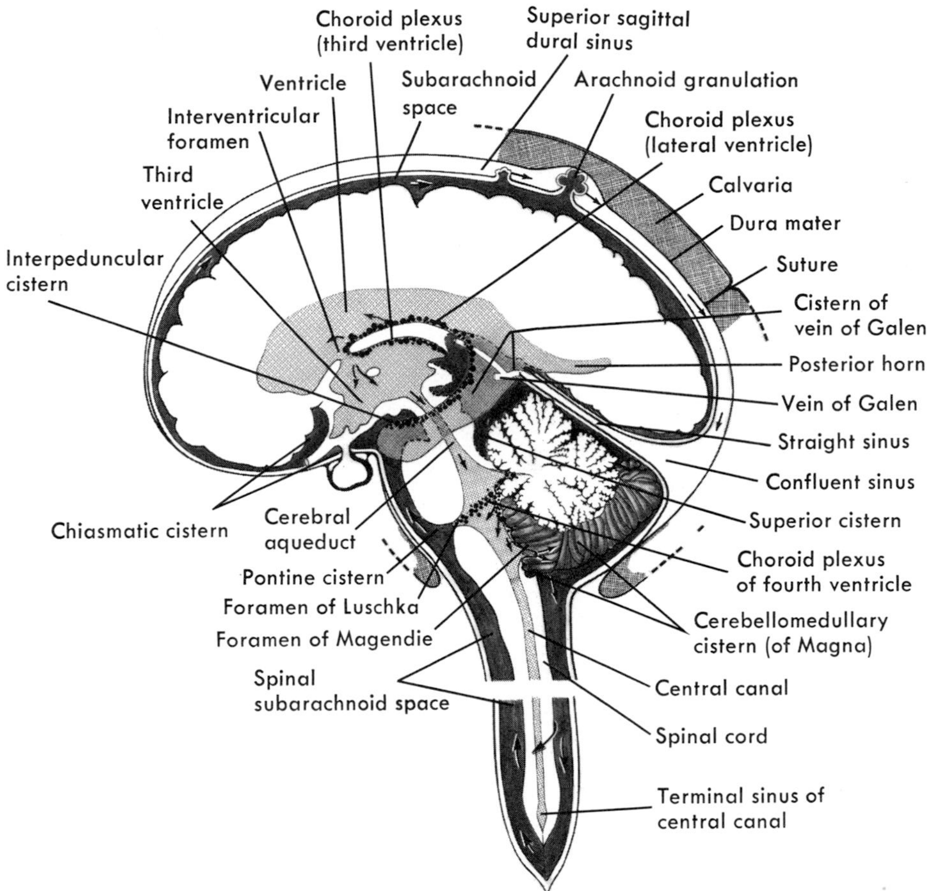

Fig. 3-1. CSF pathway.

Lateral ventricle

This cavity of the cerebral hemisphere is remarkably irregular in shape. It is best totally viewed as a casting (Fig. 3-2, *B*). The lateral ventricles communicate with the third ventricle by bilateral channels, the interventricular foramina of Monro, which pass under the arches of the fornices on either side. Anterior to the foramen, each ventricle projects into the frontal lobe as the *anterior horn* (Fig. 3-2, *A*). The head of the caudate nucleus forms the lateral wall of the anterior horn. This is well displayed in coronal section (Fig. 2-12, *A*), although the extent of the relationship is more apparent in transverse section (Fig. 3-3). The medial wall is mainly formed by the septum pellucidum and slightly formed, where the anterior horn terminates posteriorly, by the walls of the fornices. The medial aspect, anterior extremity, and roof of the horn are more anteriorly walled by the corpus callosum and its genu. In coronal sections the normal configuration of the anterior horn is the "hockey-stick" outline (Fig. 4-4). The anterior divergence of the anterior horns is well displayed in transverse section (Fig. 3-3). The *body* of each ventricle extends posteriorly from the interventricular foramen to the more expanded, vertically-oriented *confluent part*. The body of the ventricle is related laterally to the body of the caudate nucleus and medially to the short septum pellucidum and its attached fornix. The roof is the corpus callosum, and the floor is made up of thalamic nuclei. The ventricular cavity through the area of the body is superoinferiorly flattened and is similar in coronal section to an inverted boot with the toe pointing to the upper outer reflection of the wall. Deep to this reflection is the superior *occipitofrontal association fasciculus* (Fig. 2-13, *C*). It is also an area of prominent vascularity. Ependyma commonly be-

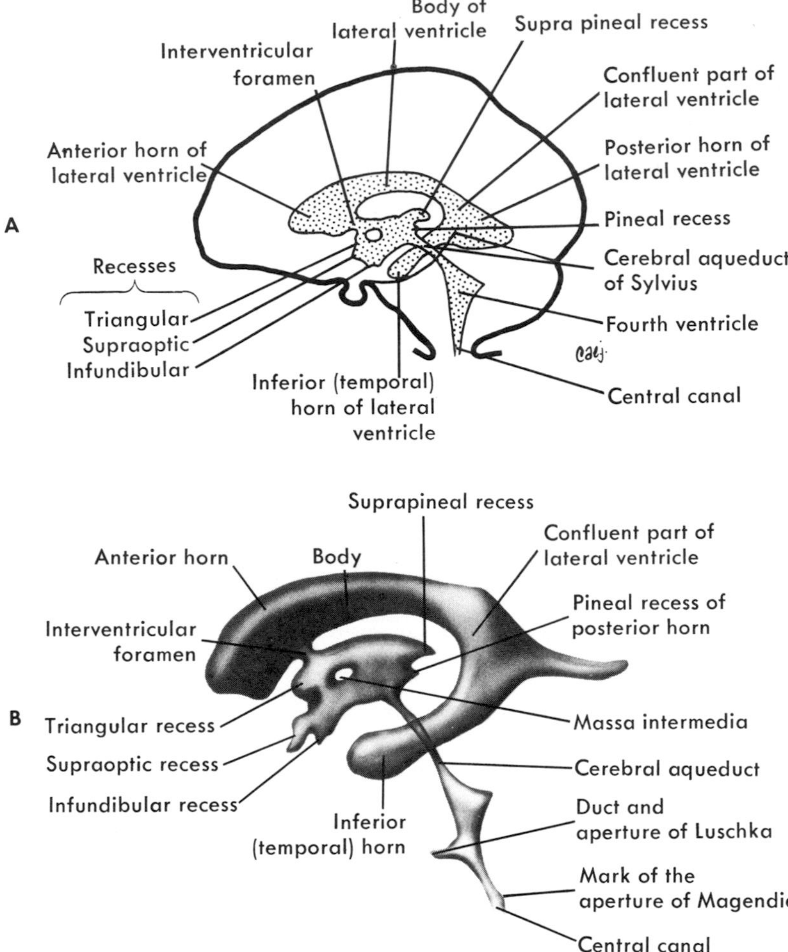

Fig. 3-2. A, Silhouette of ventricles showing topography; **B,** ventricular cast.

comes isolated as inclusions within the brain substance in the area of the occipitofrontal association fasciculus.

The *confluent* part of the lateral ventricle is formed by the expanded meeting point of body, inferior horn, and posterior horn. The anterior aspect of this part of the ventricle is limited by thalamic and retrolenticular internal capsule structures (Fig. 3-3). The confluent ventricle is bordered medially by the posterior *pillars (crura)* of the fornices and their continuing fimbriae. The *tapetum* continues laterally from the corpus callosum to become a roof and lateral wall for this segment of the ventricle. The layers of deeper contiguous laminae are better seen along the *posterior horn* of the lateral ventricle. This extends posteriorly into the occipital lobe from the confluent part of the ventricle. The horn tapers to a point and is narrow in cross section (Fig. 3-3). The outer wall and roof include the grossly visible thin line of the tapetum, which is bordered by the *thalamo-occipital radiations.* The outer part of this last stratum is visibly enhanced by the density of the fibers of the *inferior longitudinal* and *inferior occipitofrontal association* fascicles (Fig. 2-16). The medial wall of the posterior horn is distinguished by two elongate ridges, the *bulb* and the *calcar avis.* The bulb of the posterior horn is the intraventricular projection of the posterior forceps of the corpus callosum (Fig. 3-4). The calcar avis (bird's beak) arises irregularly as the prominence from the infolding of the deep calcarine fissure (Fig. 3-4). It is not unusual for the medial and lateral walls of the posterior horns to be partly fused. The *inferior horn* of the lateral ventricle projects downward, laterally, and anteriorly from the confluent part into the temporal lobe (Fig. 3-5). It curves medially and terminates, abutted against the amygdaloid nucleus, deep to the uncus. The lat-

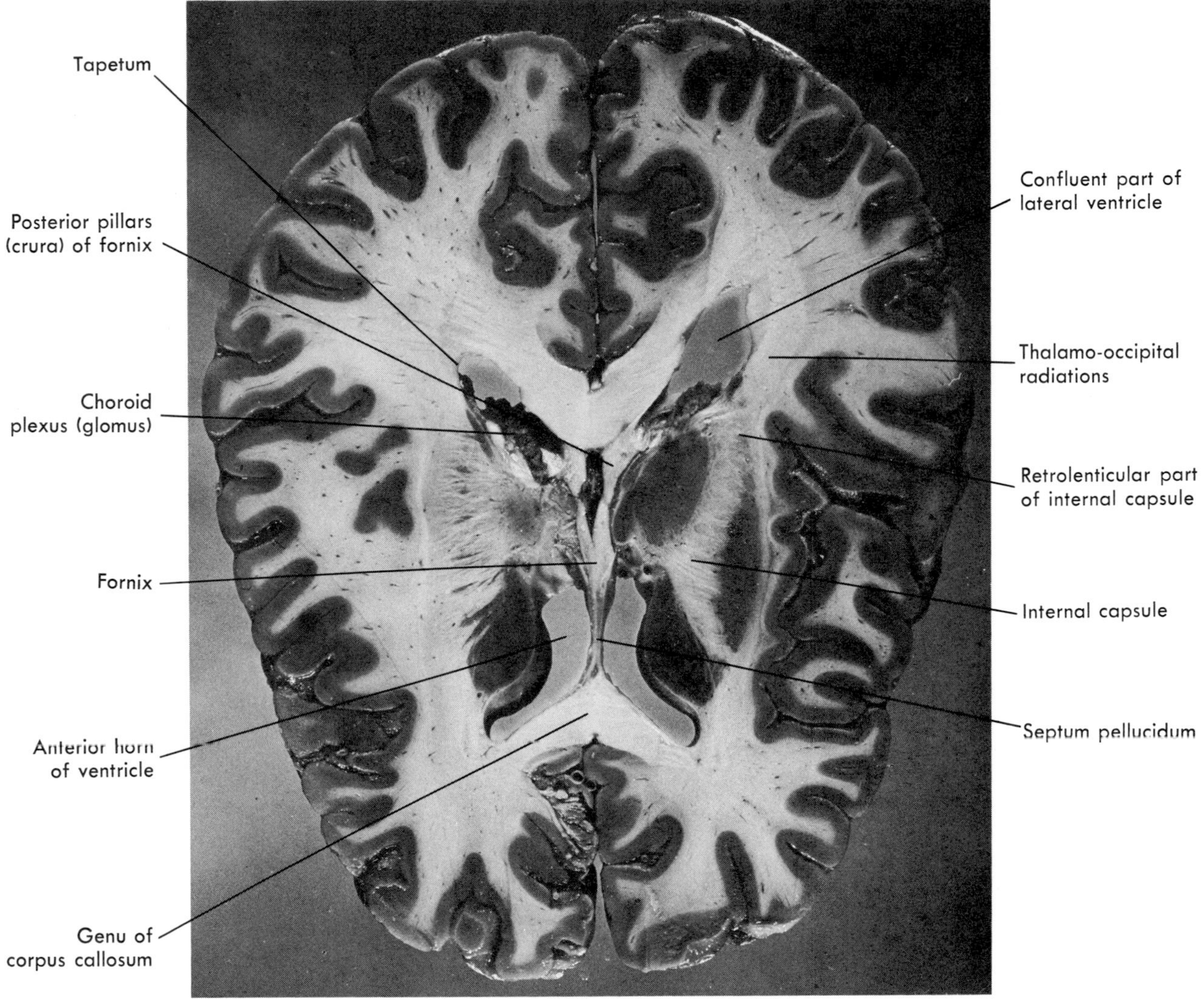

Fig. 3-3. Transverse section of brain showing ventricular contour and choroid plexus.

eral wall of the inferior, or temporal, horn is covered by tapetum. The tail of the caudate nucleus follows the line of the roof of this part of the ventricle and continues to the amygdala. Located anteriorly along the medial wall of the inferior horn are the fimbria, the alveus of the hippocampus and the infolded choroid plexus, and finally the amygdaloid nucleus near the tip of the ventricle (Fig. 3-5). The separation in the confluent ventricle, where the calcar avis projects posteriorly and the hippocampus projects anteriorly, forms a triangular field on the floor of the ventricle. This is the *collateral trigone,* which bulges slightly into the ventricle.

The *choroid plexus* of the lateral ventricle is the multitufted vascular organ that arises essentially as a layer of ependyma infolded by meninges and vessels and adapted to a structure that elaborates CSF (see Chapter 10). It overlies the hippocampus in the inferior horn of the lateral ventricle and follows the hippocampus posteriorly to the fimbria and crus of the fornix in the confluent part. The choroid plexus then rounds the posterior bulge of the thalamus and continues through the interventricular foramen to extend along the roof of the third ventricle (Figs. 3-3 and 3-6). It receives choroidal vessels in the choroid fissue of the temporal lobe. Formation of choroid plexus by the ependymal layer

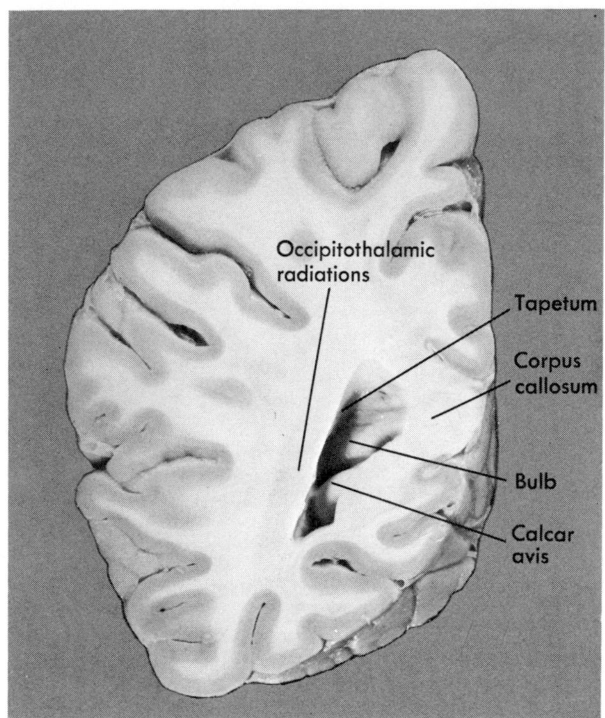

Fig. 3-4. Contour of posterior horn showing bulb and calcar avis.

is diagrammed in Fig. 3-7. This relationship obtains throughout its course, and an ependymal layer separates the structure from the ventricular lumen in all areas. The linear, raised ribbons of ependyma that are elevated for covering the choroid plexus are called *taeniae*. Each taenia is named by its structure of origin (such as taenia of the fornix and taenia of the fimbria). In the confluent part of the ventricle the choroid plexus is invariably enlarged and distended *(glomus)*. Frequently it forms cysts in this location. For histologic details of choroid plexus, see Chapter 10. The *stria terminalis* and *vena terminalis* are respectively important as a land mark and a major vessel. They comprise the fiber tract and associated vein running in the valley between the caudate nucleus (telencephalon) and thalamus (diencephalon) (Figs. 3-3 and 3-7). These structures follow the caudate tail from the temporal horn around the ventricular surface to the area of the anterior commissure. The vein joins the internal cerebral vein near the interventricular foramen.

Third ventricle

This represents the cavity of the diencephalon and is continuous with the lateral ventricles on each side through the bilateral interventricular foramina. These foramina are bounded posteriorly by the anterior prominence of the thalamic nuclei and

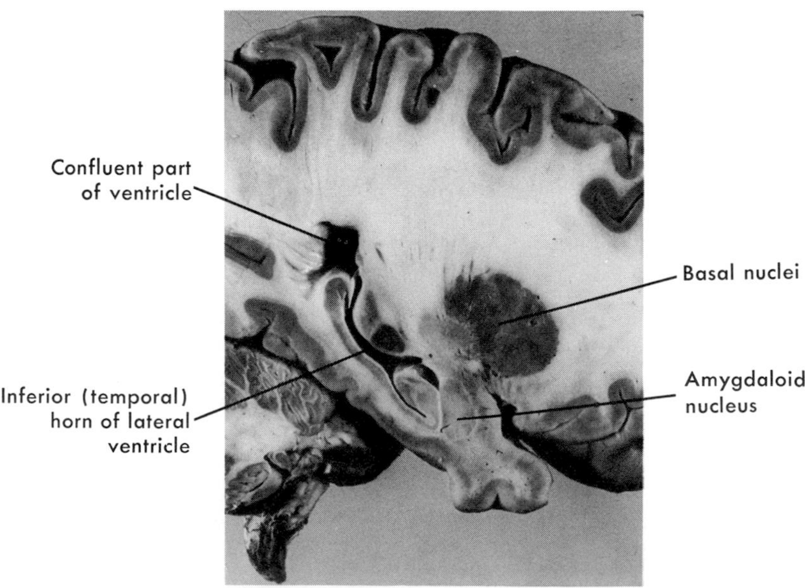

Fig. 3-5. Oblique parasagittal cut through the inferior horn of the lateral ventricle.

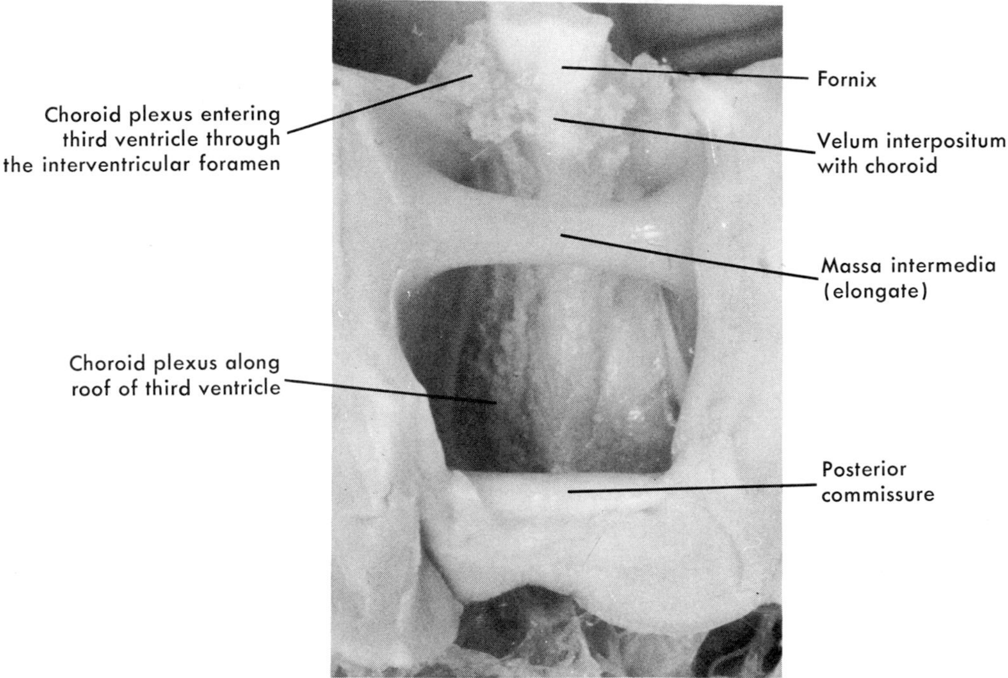

Fig. 3-6. Inferior view of roof of dilated third ventricle showing choroid along roof (hydrocephalus).

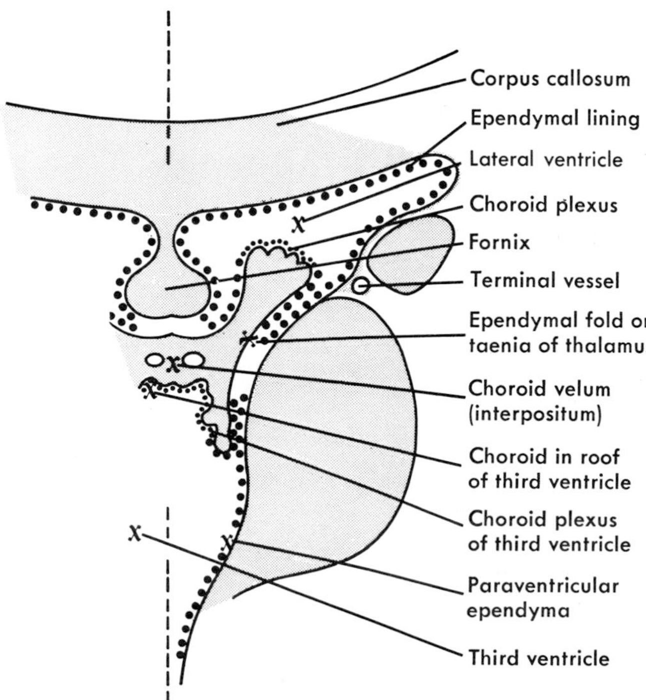

Fig. 3-7. Diagram of choroid projections; inset, plane through interventricular foramina.

are limited above and anteriorly by the arching columns (anterior pillars) of the fornix (Fig. 2-4). The choroid plexus from the lateral ventricle continues through the foramen in its upper posterior part and joins the plexus of the third ventricle (Fig. 3-3). The roof of this ventricle is the inferior ependymal cover of the *tela choroidae,* or *velum interpositum.* This membrane possesses an ependymal bridge that passes on its undersurface from side to side between the taeniae of the thalamus. Each taenia overlies the medial ridge of the thalamus, the *stria medullaris thalami,* which runs from the area of the interventricular foramen in front and curves posteriorly and medially to the root of the pineal body (Figs. 2-4 and 3-7). This stria becomes related to the *habenular trigone* and *habenular commissure* in this manner. As stated previously, the choroid plexus of the third ventricle is continuous on either side with that of the lateral ventricles through the interventricular foramina. This plexus continues posteriorly along the roof of the third ventricle in two parallel, down-folding linear tufts that project from the velum interpositum (Fig. 3-6). They invaginate the ependymal membrane in the same manner that the choroid invaginates the ependyma in the choroidal sulcus where

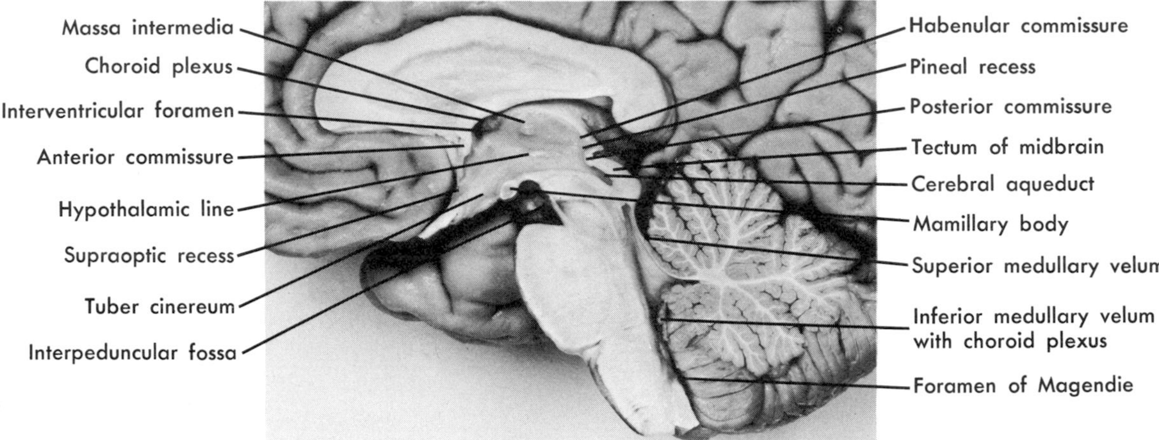

Fig. 3-8. Sagittal section of brain and stem.

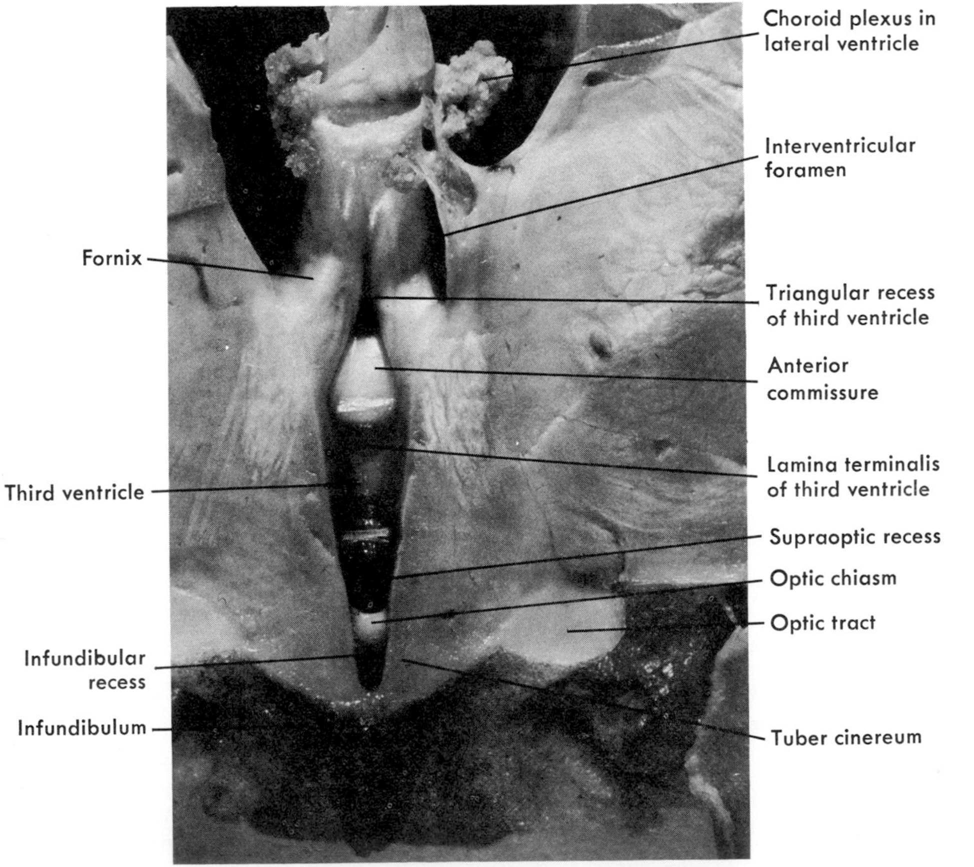

Fig. 3-9. Triangular recess viewed posteriorly.

the plexus projects into the lateral ventricle and its inferior horn (Fig. 3-7). Further details of choroidal gross structure are presented in the succeeding discussion.

The contours of the third ventricle are shown in some detail in a medial view of a sagittal section (Fig. 3-8). The roof is slightly arched posteriorly from the interventricular foramen. The cavity, the *suprapineal recess,* projects a varying distance above the pineal body. The *habenular* and *posterior commissures* form the upper and lower margins of the *pineal recess,* which projects into the pineal body. Below the posterior commissure the third ventricle continues into the *cerebral aqueduct.* A shallow groove on the walls of the ventricle extends from the cerebral aqueduct in a slightly curved line to the interventricular foramen. This is the *hypothalamic* line, which marks the upper border of the hypothalamus. Above the line is the thalamus proper. The two sides of the thalamus are usually joined across the ventricular cavity by the *massa intermedia* (Figs. 3-6 and 3-8). The third ventricle arches over the midbrain in the region behind the mamillary bodies, It projects downward and forward as the cavity of the *tuber cinereum,* terminating as the *infundibular recess.* This projects into the pituitary stalk. Above and anterior to this stalk are the parts of the telencephalon medium (Fig. 3-8). The contours of this structure include the *supraoptic recess* above the optic chiasm, the anterior extremity of the ventricle carrying to the thin *lamina terminalis,* and the *triangular recess* projecting into the depression formed by the anterior commissure and the two columns of the fornix (Fig. 3-9). Two special areas of the third ventricle are: (1) the *paraphyseal area* at the junction of telecephalon and diencephalon in the roof near the columns of the fornix, and (2) the *subcommissural organ,* which is a specialized area underlying the posterior commissure and extending into the cerebral aqueduct. The paraphysis is an embryonic vestige that is important as a rare source of cystic tumors. The function of the sub-

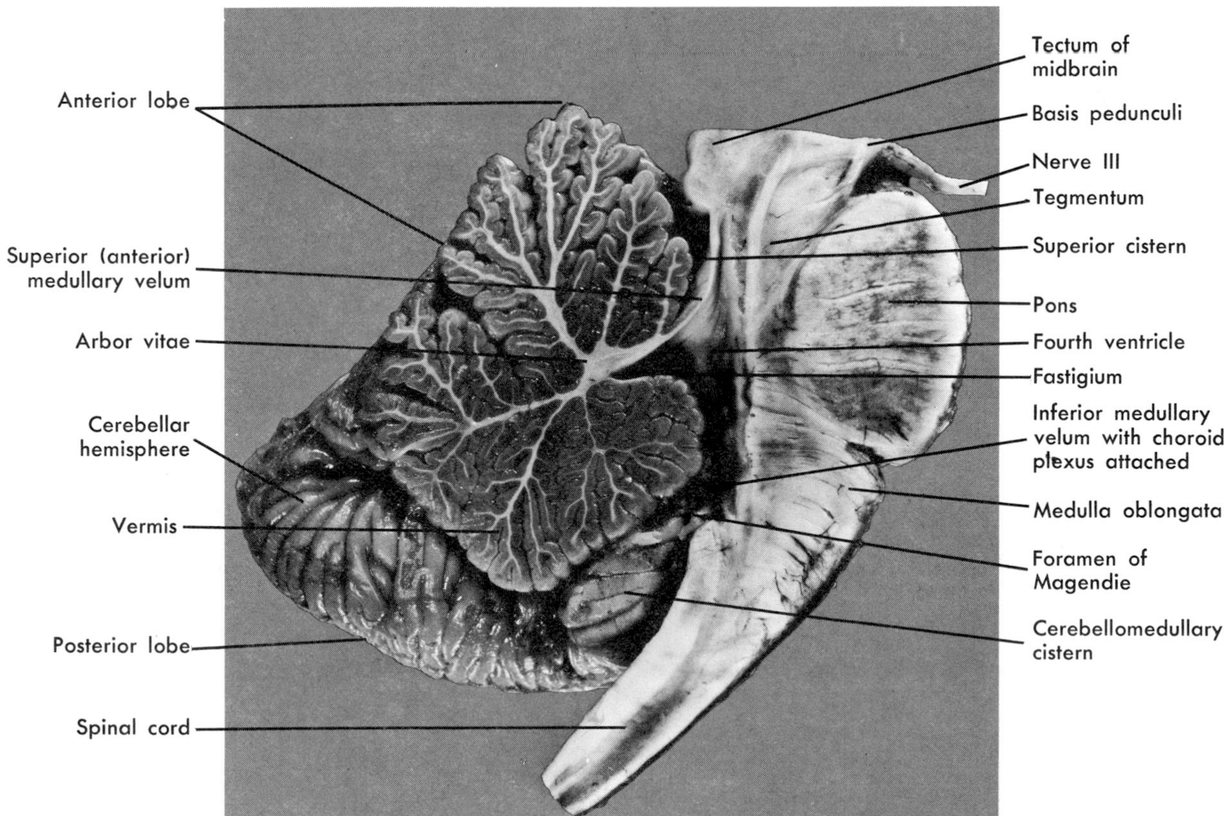

Fig. 3-10. Sagittal plain of brainstem and cerebellum.

commissural organ is uncertain, but it may be related to control of water metabolism.[9]

The *cerebral aqueduct* is the ependyma-lined channel of the midbrain (mesencephalon) that is continuous above with the third ventricle and below with the fourth ventricle. It is well displayed in a sagittal plane (Fig. 3-8) and in cross sections of the upper brainstem (see Chapter 4). Dorsal to the cerebral aqueduct is the quadrigeminal body, and ventral is the tegmentum of the midbrain.

Fourth ventricle

This is the cavity of both the metencephalon and the myelencephalon. Hence it is related in its floor to both the pons and the medulla. The roof is related to the cerebellum. The floor was described in some detail as topographic areas of the related parts of the brainstem (p. 33). In its superior part, the ventricle narrows into the aqueduct. It is dorsally covered in by this area by the anterior (superior) medullary velum and at the sides by the superior cerebellar peduncles. The pons underlies the floor. The pattern of the roof is best seen in sagittal view (Fig. 3-10). The anterior medullary velum rises to a peak *(fastigium)* where it meets the posterior medullary velum. This slopes back toward the floor and attaches along the velum margin, which defines the inferior margin of the rhomboid fossa. At the expanded portion, approximately at the junction of the posterior and middle thirds of the fossa, the ventricle extends laterally and inferiorly into the *lateral recesses.* These extend over the acoustic tubercle in a tubular fashion and open into meningeal spaces through the *foramina of Luschka* (Fig. 4-40). The actual foramina represent apertures in both ependyma and the inner meningeal layer, which is applied closely to the brain substance. The posterior medullary velum also possesses an aperture, the *foramen of Magendie,* which penetrates the ependyma and meningeal membrane as a single opening immediately over the obex (Fig. 3-1). A choroid plexus also invaginates the fourth ventricle. The line of invagination runs through the posterior medullary velum beginning above the foramen of Magendie on both sides. The lines curve to follow the lateral aperatures. Choroid

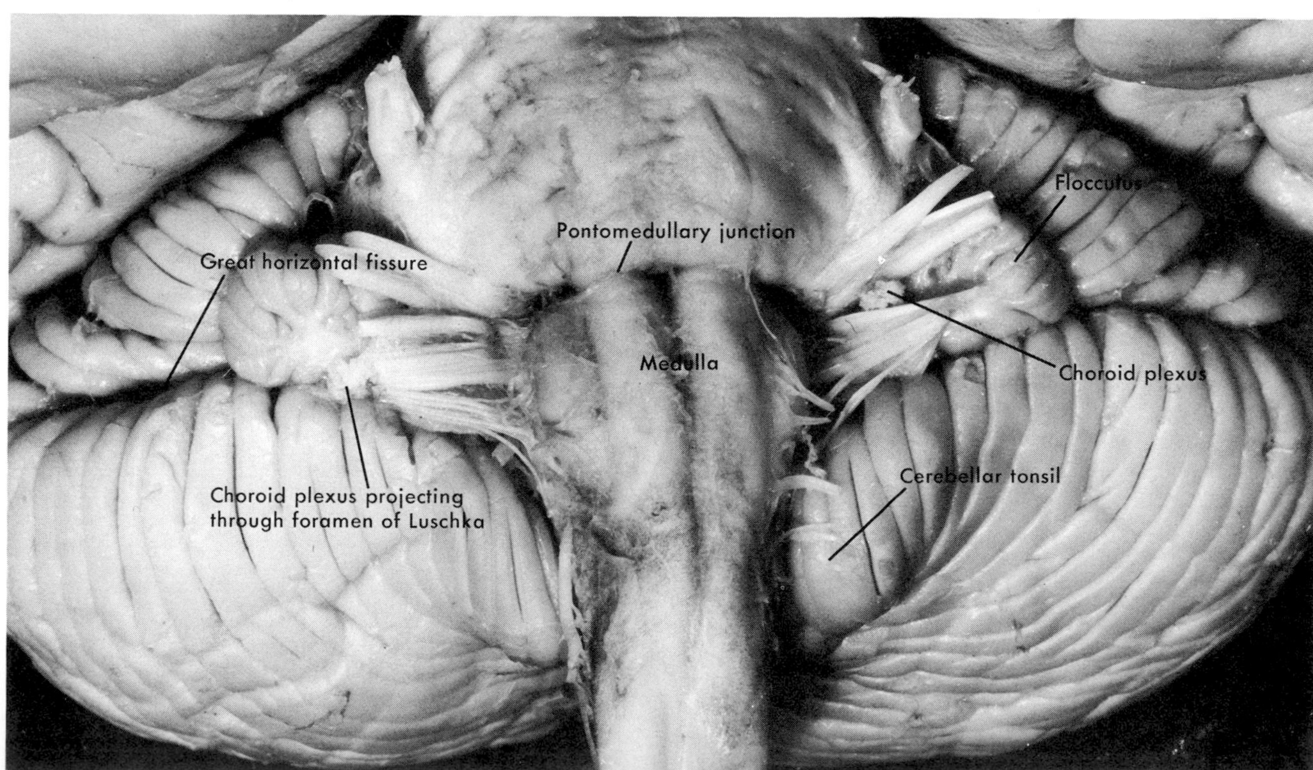

Fig. 3-11. Basal view of choroid and flocculus.

plexus protrudes from the foramina of Luschka into the meningeal spaces on either side of the medulla below the pons. This segment of choroid lies adjacent to the flocculus, deep to cranial nerves VIII and IX (Fig. 3-11).

Central canal

This canal represents the cavity of the spinal cord and continues throughout the length of this organ. Probably very little CSF circulates through the canal, since it normally obliterates in part during early adulthood. Ependyma lines the canal and commonly appears as "inclusions" marginal to the main canal, especially in areas of obliteration. The central canal dilates slightly in the conus and extends for varying distances into the filum terminale. This cavity is the *terminal sinus* (terminal ventricle), which sometimes appears as a grossly visible thin-walled saccule of variable shape (Fig. 3-1). Ventricle outlines as seen in radiographs contribute enormously to an understanding of structure and function (see Chapter 5).

MENINGES

The membranous coverings of the brain and spinal cord intervene between bone and nervous tissue in two soft tissue layers and a fluid cushion. These layers are: (1) an outer *pachymeninx,* or dura mater, and (2) an inner *leptomeninx.* The dura mater is a thick, tough, fibrous membrane. The leptomeninx is a sponge-like, fluid-filled mass comprised of an outer *arachnoid* membrane that is applied to the deep surface of the dura mater and an inner *pia* mater that is applied to the surface of the brain and cord. The arachnoid membrane and pia mater are interconnected by thin filaments called *arachnoid trabeculae,* which subdivide and sustain the space between these layers, the *subarachnoid space* (Fig. 3-12).

Pachymeninx or dura mater

In the cranial cavity the dura mater possesses two somewhat indistinct and almost inseparable layers, an outer (periosteal) layer and an inner (meningeal) layer (Fig. 3-14, *A*). The outer layer is the same as the inner periosteum of the cranial bones and is attached to them by many fibers that pull away on traction as hair-like extensions of the membrane. The outer dura mater continues around the lips of cranial foramina and is tightly applied at the sutures between cranial bones. The potential cleft between dura and bone is *epidural space,* which is compartmentalized by the limits of bony outlines. The inner layer of the cranial dura mater is closely applied to the outer layer, but the junction is usually apparent by a vascular zone of the inner layer. The two layers separate in specific patterns to form the *dural sinuses,* which become part of the venous system and contribute to the drainage mechanism for CSF. The layers also separate to form the periosteal lining of the sella turcica and the covering of the pituitary fossa. The leaflet of meningeal dura mater overlying the fossa is called the *diaphragma sellae* (Fig. 3-14, *B*). It is perforated by a central opening that accommodates the infundibulum, or pituitary stalk. Second pockets are formed on either side in the middle cranial fossae by layers of dura mater that encase the fifth cranial nerves and ganglia *(Meckel's cave)* (Fig. 3-14, *D*).

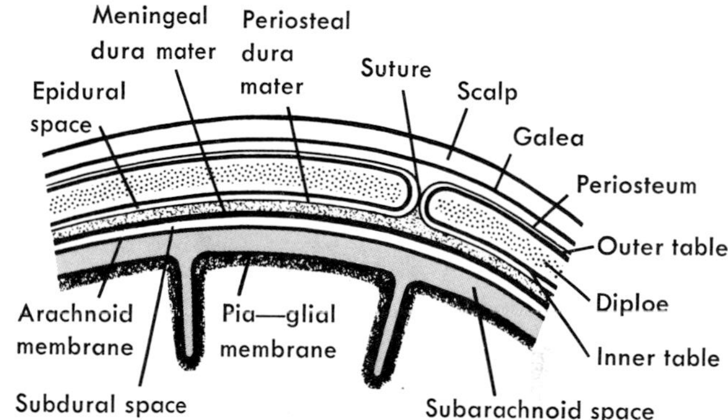

Fig. 3-12. Diagram of meningeal layers.

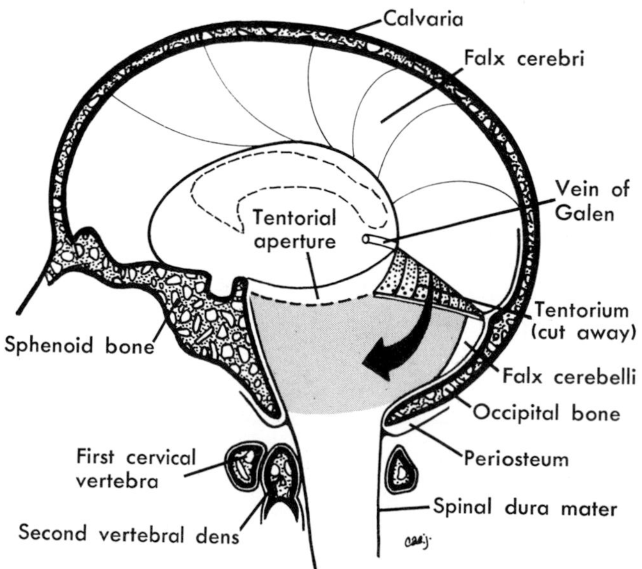

Fig. 3-13. Dural folds and intracranial compartments.

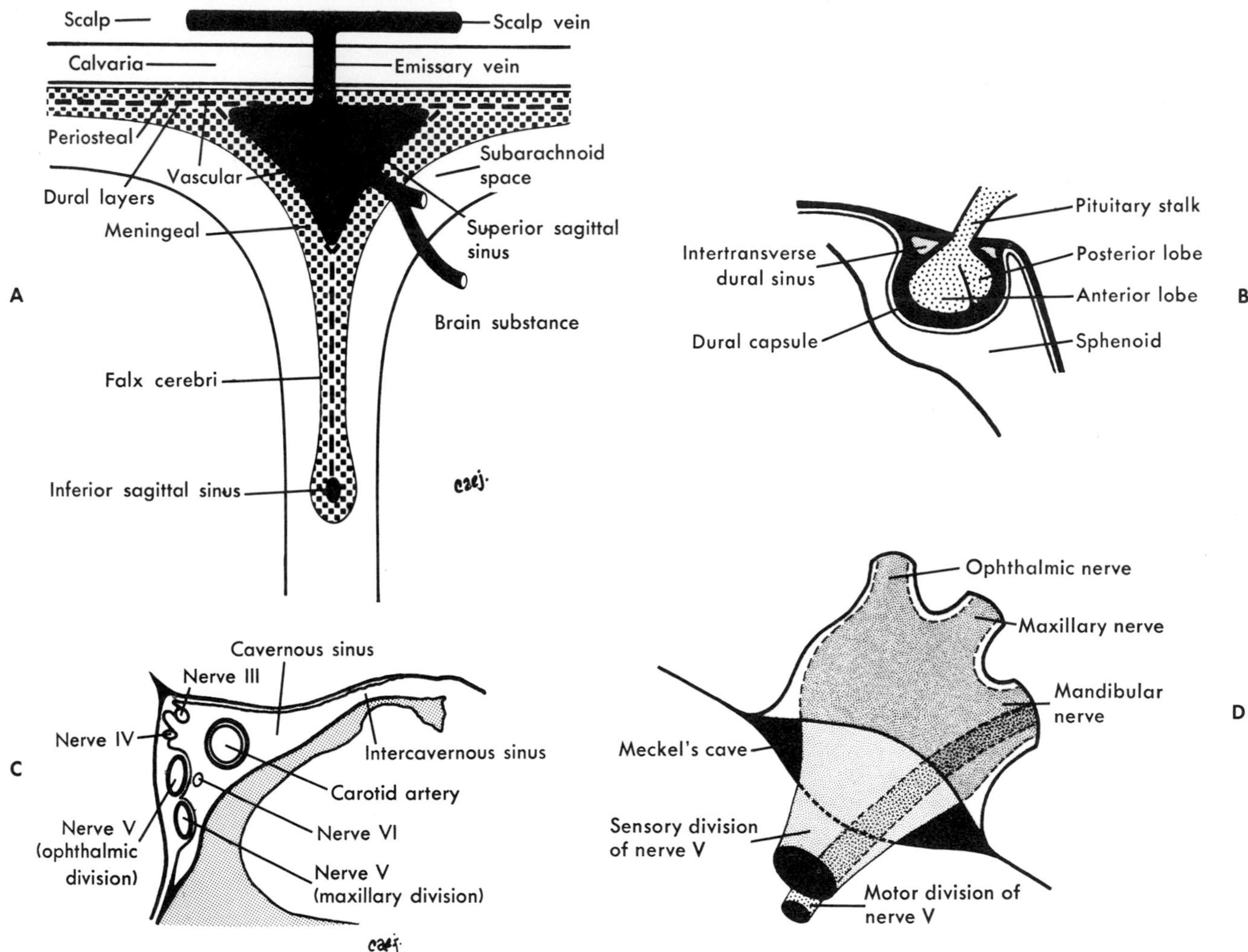

Fig. 3-14. Special dural complexes: **A,** sagittal sinuses and falx; **B,** diaphragma sellae; **C,** cavernous sinus; **D,** Meckel's cave; **E,** olfactory nerves; **F,** optic nerve; **G,** auditory nerve; **H,** spinal root.

The cranial dura mater has complex folds and attachments that serve to subdivide the cranial cavity and fix the brain in place. The *falx cerebri* is a sickle-shaped sagittal leaf that extends into the median sagittal fissure between the hemispheres (Fig. 3-14, *A*). It stretches from the crista galli to the internal occipital protuberance (Fig. 3-13). At the inferior margin, near the junction of its posterior and middle thirds, the falx cerebri is joined on its sides by tent-like wings. These extend to it from the petrous ridges and occipital bone in a circular pattern that follows the course of the transverse sinuses in the posterior cranial fossa. This is the *tentorium cerebelli,* which separates the cerebellum from the occipital lobes above. The tentorium extends anteriorly in its bony attachment only to the posterior clinoid processes. This leaves a semicircular opening, the *tentorial aperture,* which has free margins surrounding the midbrain at the waist of the brainstem (Fig. 3-13). A shallow midline projection of dura mater, the *falx cerebelli,* also separates the cerebellar hemispheres

The spinal dura mater duplicates the intracranial arrangement only in the levels of the first three cervical veretbrae. Below this, the outer layer becomes independent periosteum for the vertebrae

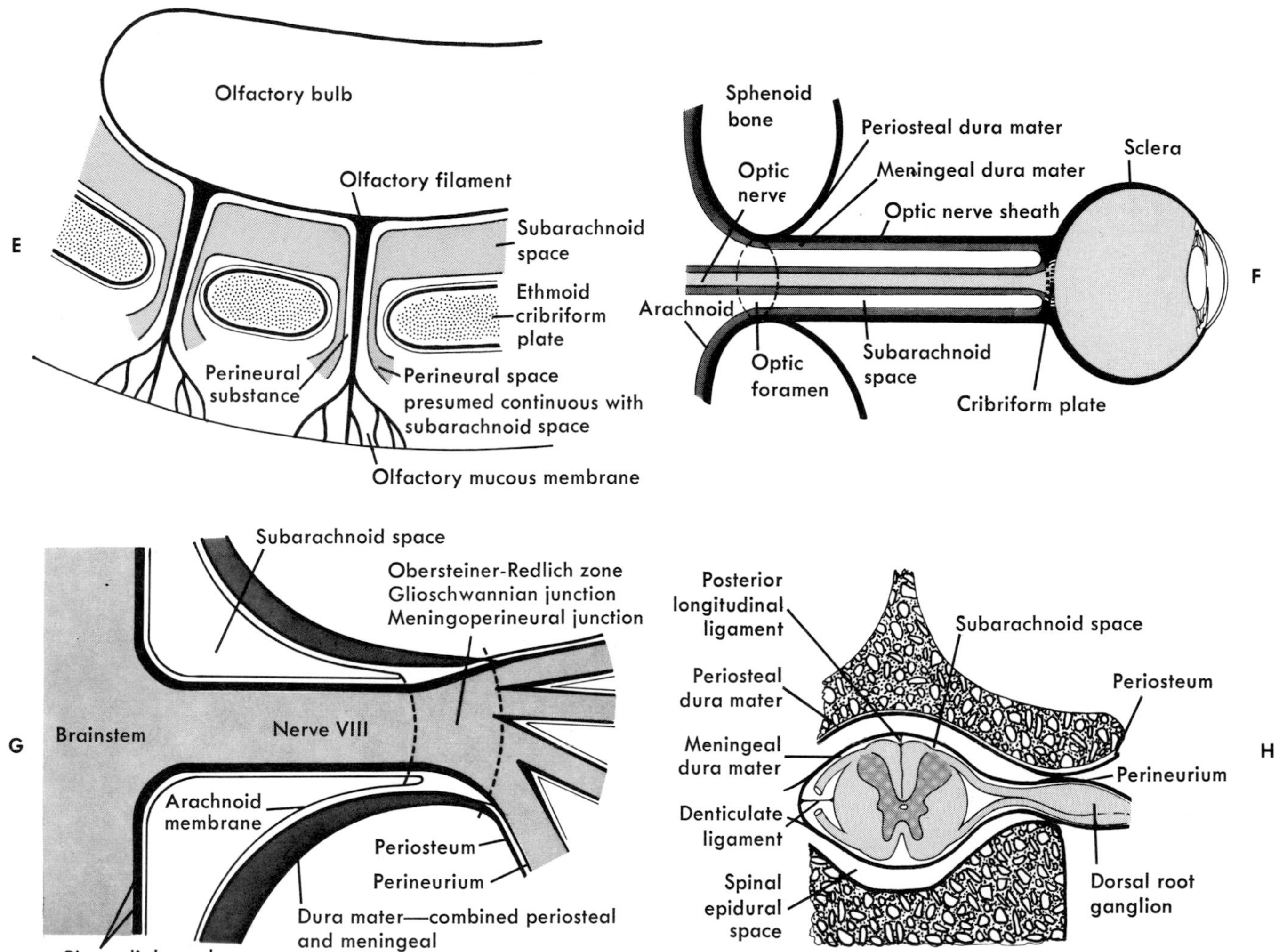

Fig. 3-14, cont'd. For legend see opposite page.

and liner for the supporting ligaments of the vertebral canal (Fig. 3-14). The inner layer of dura mater becomes widely separated from the outer layer by a fat-filled spinal *epidural space*. The dural layer continues as a sac to the second sacral piece, where it terminates in a ligament that joins the filum terminale to attach to the sacral and coccygeal pieces. The dural pattern at the exit of nerves of both cranial (Fig. 3-14, *C* and *E* to *G*) and spinal origin is essentially the same and is illustrated for spinal nerves in Figs. 3-14 and 3-15. The *subdural space* extends deep to the dural inner layer and contains a thin layer of fluid that separates the dura mater from the apposed, underlying arachnoid membrane (Fig. 3-12).

Leptomeninx

The arachnoid membrane is the outer layer of the leptomeninx and follows the dural folds and contours. The pia mater, on the other hand, is applied to the cerebral and spinal surfaces and follows the convolutional patterns to the depths of the sulci and folds (Fig. 3-12). The space between the pia mater and arachnoid membrane (subarachnoid space) varies greatly in shape and depth, depending upon the contours of the brain surface. This ir-

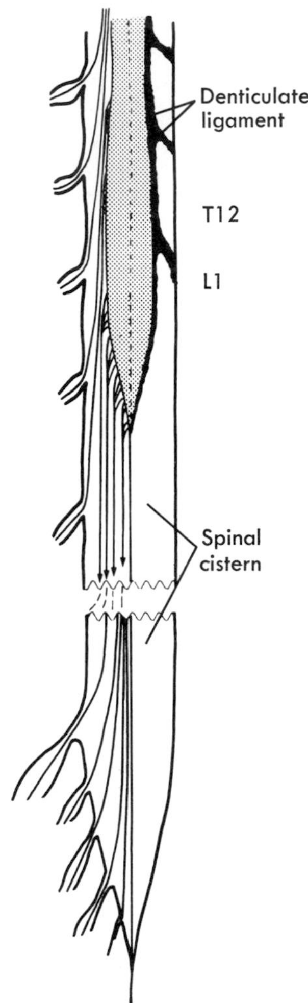

Fig. 3-15. Dural and arachnoid terminations and denticulate ligaments (heavy black).

regularity in contour produces several large subarachnoid spaces known as *cisterns.* These play some role in the flow pattern of the CSF that occupies the subarachnoid space. As previously stated, this space is continuous with the ventricular cavities and receives CSF from the fourth ventricle through the apertures of Luschka and Magendie. The following cisterns merit special mention. (1) The great cistern *(cistern magna),* or cerebellomedullaris, is the massive subarachnoid space between the undersurface of the cerebellum and the dorsal surface of the medulla (Fig. 3-1). (2) The foramen of Magendie opens into the great cistern in midline through the posterior medullary velum. (3) The *pontine cistern (cisterna pontis)* lies ventrally and laterally over the bulge of the pons, between it and the medulla. (4) The foramina of Luschka open into the lateral parts of the pontine cistern. (5) The *interpeduncular cistern* lies between the cerebral peduncles of the midbrain. This cistern is anteriorly continuous with the *chiasmatic cistern,* which surrounds the optic chiasm. These two, together with the large space underlying the hypothalamus and surrounding the infundibulum, constitute the *basal cistern.* (6) The *superior cistern* lies between the quadrigeminal bodies of the midbrain and the overlying cerebellum. (7) The *cistern of the vein of Galen* surrounds the vascular area near the pineal body and projects between the pial layers following the corpus callosum and the roof of the third ventricle. (8) The *Sylvian cistern* lies in the depths of the Sylvian or lateral fissure.

Leptomeningeal spaces seem to be lacking in the sella turcica that surrounds the pituitary. This arises apparently by close application of dural membrane to the body of the gland as its capsule (Fig. 3-14, *B*).

The spinal subarachnoid membrane follows the dura mater to the second sacral piece, while the pia mater terminates at the second lumbar level with the conus. A particularly large reservoir of CSF occupies this space (Fig. 3-15). This space is used as an elected site for subarachnoid puncture to obtain CSF. The leptomeninges of the spinal cord are the same as those of the brain, except for two added ligaments, the *longitudinal septum* and the *denticulate ligaments.* The longitudinal septum is a midline dorsal leptomeningeal density extending from the posterior median septum of the cord to the overlying arachnoid membrane and dura mater. While it is discontinuous, it tends to separate the left and right posterior subarachnoid channels (Fig. 3-14, *H*). The denticulate ligaments on either side of the cord are tooth-like projections that connect pia mater through arachnoid membrane to dura mater, with the line of attachment occurring between the exit points of nerve roots. The denticulate projections meet the root intervals to the level between thoracic 12 and lumbar 1. The last ligament thus serves as a reliable landmark to determine nerve levels at their exists (Fig. 3-15).

Arachnoid granulations

These villous structures (*Pacchionian bodies*) project into venous sinuses of the dura mater, particularly along the superior sagittal sinus (Fig. 3-16). They represent arachnoid projections into the venous stream that permit drainage of the subarachnoid fluid into the blood (p. 182). Similar arachnoid-to-vein mechanisms exist in the spinal canal. The flow of CSF from the foramina of the

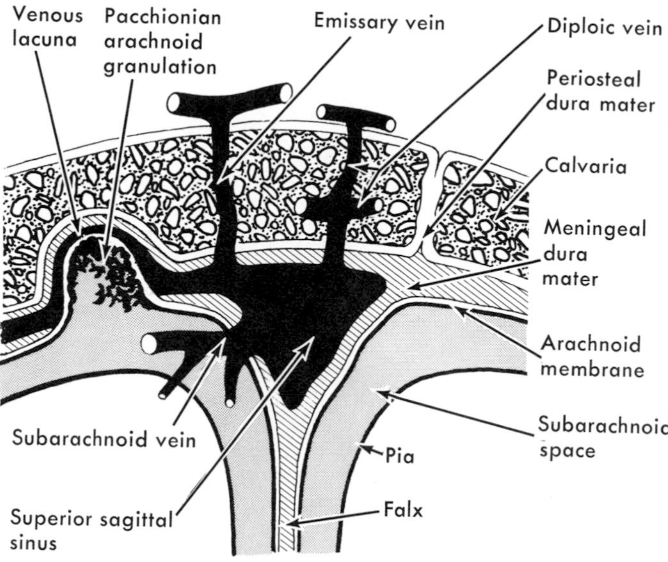

Fig. 3-16. Arachnoid granultaion (Pacchionian body).

fourth ventricle principally occurs in the following sequence: cisternae pontis and magna upward through the cisterns and sulci of the brain to the arachnoid granulations along the vertex. Here the CSF is emptied into the dural venous sinuses. A small exchange undoubtedly takes place in the spinal subarachnoid spaces (Figs. 3-14, *H,* and 3-15).[1,8] The meningeal spaces are radiographically represented in Chapter 5.

VASCULATURE

The importance of the vascular supply and drainage of the central nervous system can hardly be overemphasized because of the frequency of serious disease involving the system. Because of the acute metabolic demands of nervous structures, the human organism has cultivated ways of preserving the integrity of the blood supply through *anastomoses* that permit alternate routes of both supply and drainage (see p. 60). Because of supply demands, failure in arterial integrity commonly causes death of neural tissue in a very short time after cessation of circulation. In this way the vessels function as terminal arteries, although their distribution beds possess alternate supplies. The distribution of vessels thus becomes an anatomic process of great interest. The vasculature is classified as *extracranial arterial supply, intrinsic arterial supply, venous drainage, dural sinuses, emissary vessels, vessels of peripheral nerves,* and *major anastomoses.*

Extracranial arterial supply

The main arterial supply to the brain follows one of two principal pathways, the *carotid artery system,* or the *vertebral artery system.* The carotid system arises in bilateral *common carotid arteries,* which take off from the innominate artery on the right and from the arch of the aorta on the left. The common carotid arteries ascend to the level of the upper border of the thyroid cartilage and divide on either side into *internal carotid* and *external carotid* branches. At or near this dividing point is a slight distention, the *carotid sinus,* which plays a part in the neuroregulation of arterial pressure. The external carotid supplies the superficial parts of the scalp and skull and the deep and superficial parts of the face. In the latter distribution a major branch, the external maxillary, continues via orbital vessels to anastomose with the ophthalmic artery. This is a terminal branch of the internal carotid complex. The *ophthalmic anastomosis* is thus formed. It becomes important in supplying the brain in the event of obstructive disease of the internal carotid complex (Fig. 3-17). In the deeper distribution of the external carotid complex, the internal maxillary division gives off the main supply to the meninges, the *middle meningeal artery.* This artery enters the skull through the foramen rotundum and spreads over the dura mater from the floor of the middle cranial fossa in a broad fan-shaped distribution (Fig. 3-18). The middle meningeal artery anastomoses with the anterior menin-

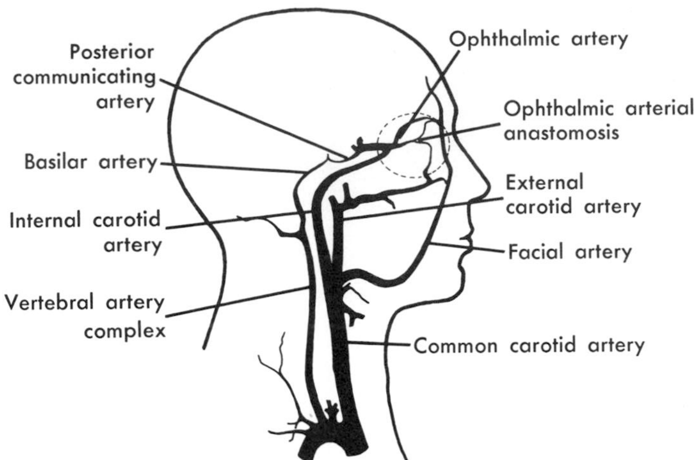

Fig. 3-17. Ophthalmic anastomosis.

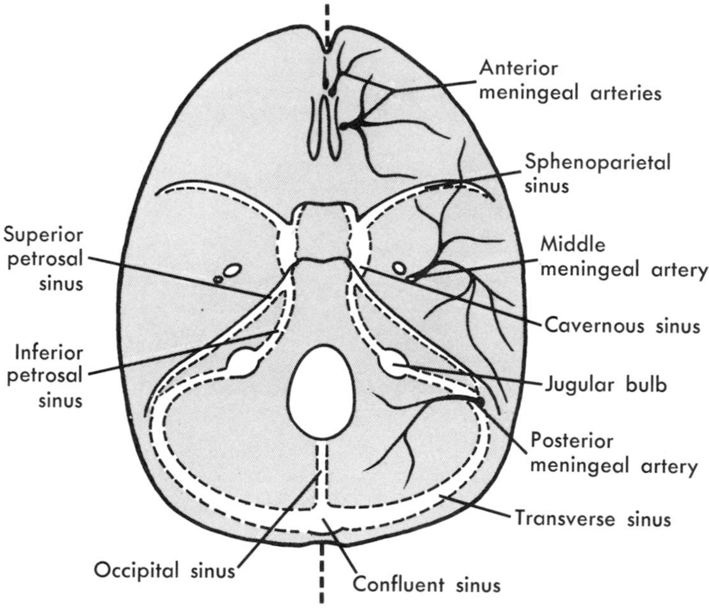

Fig. 3-18. Base of skull with meningeal vessels and dural sinuses.

geal artery from the internal carotid complex and with the posterior meningeal artery from the pharyngeal branch of the external complex.[7,12]

The internal carotid artery ascends deep in the neck to the carotid foramen and through the carotid canal to enter the cranium. It crosses the cartilage plate in the foramen lacerum. It then lies along the medial wall of and projects into the cavernous sinus (Fig. 3-14). Through the intracranial, subdural position, the artery has a sigmoid contour that is believed to account for its resilience. It penetrates the dura mater medial to the anterior clinoid process and at this point gives off the ophthalmic branch that goes to the orbit. The ophthalmic branch provides the anastomosis with the external carotid complex. The internal carotid penetrates the arachnoid membrane in the area of the anterior perforated substance and divides into its terminal branches, the middle and anterior cerebral arteries. Before dividing, it gives off the following arteries:

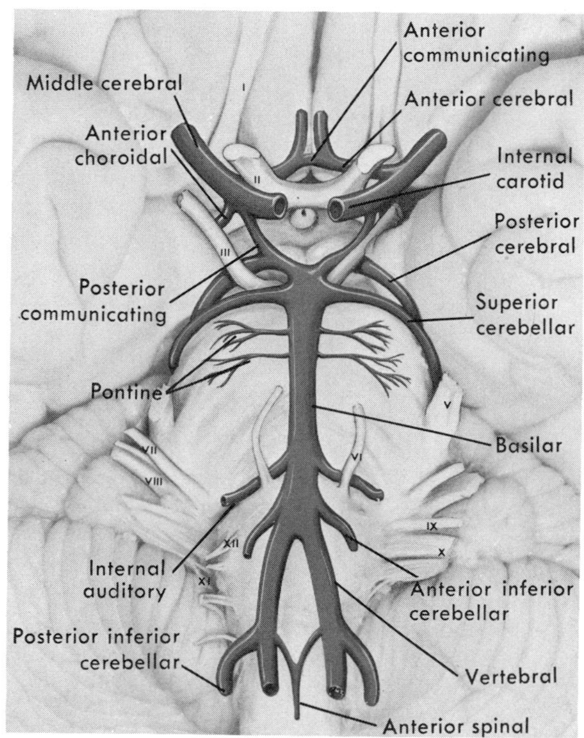

Fig. 3-19. Basal vessels and circle of Willis.

(1) the posterior communicating artery, which anastomoses with the vertebral complex, and (2) the anterior choroidal artery, which runs to the choroidal fissure to supply the choroid plexus (Fig. 3-19).

The vertebral arteries arise bilaterally from the subclavian arteries and ascend through the transverse foramina on each side of the sixth through second cervical vertebrae. Here the arteries turn laterally, pass through the transverse foramen of the atlas, and continue through the atlanto-occipital ligament. There they enter the cranium via the foramen magnum. The arteries terminate by anastomosing side-to-side and becoming the basilar artery. The extracranial branches of the vertebral arteries include *spinal branches,* which follow the spinal nerve roots into the canal. A small *posterior meningeal branch* supplies the meninges of the posterior fossa and anastomoses with meningeal branches from the external carotid complex. Within the cavity, the vertebral arteries give off *posterior spinal arteries* that descend behind the spinal nerves and join the direct spinal arteries from the cervical portion of the vertebral arteries (Fig. 3-19). The *posterior inferior cerebellar arteries* arise directly from the vertebral arteries, pass around the medulla, and supply the medial and posterior parts of the cerebellar hemispheres and the vermis. Enroute, they supply blood to the medulla and provide a choroidal artery to the choroid plexus of the fourth ventricle. Direct *medullary branches* also arise from the vertebral vessels themselves. The *anterior spinal artery* arises from the union of two vessels that pass anteriorly from their bilateral origins in the vertebral arteries just before the latter combine to become the basilar artery (Fig. 3-19). The anterior spinal artery passes down the medulla and cord in the anterior median fissure. Another major arterial source for the spinal cord arises as segmental vessels along the aorta that accompany nerve roots into the vertebral canal. The intrinsic distribution pattern of spinal arteries is discussed in the following section. Of the root vessels *(radicular arteries),* the largest is usually one of the lumbars (p. 61).[4]

Intrinsic arterial supply

The carotid and the vertebral complexes deliver major arteries to the base of the brain to form the anastomotic *circle of Willis.* The *basilar* artery, formed from the fusion of the two vertebral arteries, divides into two *posterior cerebral arteries* near the upper border of the pons. Each posterior cerebral artery gives off a *posterior communicating* artery that runs forward to join the *internal carotid* artery on either side of the tuber cinereum, underlying the anterior perforated substance. The internal carotids give rise on either side to *anterior cerebral arteries,* which pass deep to the optic nerves and reach anterior sufaces of the splenium. There they turn superiorly into the median sagittal fissure. Anterior to the optic chiasm the two anterior cerebral arteries are bridged by an *anterior communicating artery.* This completes the arterial circle of Willis of the base of the brain (Fig. 3-19). All the significant direct arterial supply to the brain is derived from this basal arterial complex. The arterial branches of the vertebral vessels to the cord have already been reviewed.

The *basilar artery,* en route to its bifurcation into posterior cerebral arteries, gives off small *pontine arteries,* which arise at right angles and penetrate the pons. Near the middle of the basilar artery, the small *internal auditory artery* arises to join the nerve VIII and passes with the nerve into the internal auditory meatus to be distributed to the internal ear. The *anterior inferior cerebellar artery* leaves the basilar on either side near its lower part and continues to the anterior inferior surface of the cerebellum. It anastomoses with the posterior inferior cerebellar artery below and with the superior cerebellar artery above. The *superior cerebellar arteries* arise on either side of the basilar artery, immediately below the terminal posterior cerebral arteries. These vessels pass around the cerebral peduncles and are distributed over the superior cerebellar surface. They anastomose with the inferior cerebellar arteries. Important branches supply the anterior medullary velum, the pineal, and project into the transverse fissure overlying the third ventricle. These branches contribute to the choroid plexus in the roof of this ventricle (Fig. 3-19).

The *posterior cerebral artery* on either side is a dichotomous branch of the basilar artery. Each extends laterally and is joined by the posterior communicating branch of the internal carotid artery as part of the arterial circle. Occasionally this anastomotic branch provides the major blood supply to one or both posterior cerebral vessels. The course of the posterior cerebral artery runs over the lip of the tentorial aperture to the tentorial surface of the temporal and occipital lobes. This topography makes the vessel subject to compression from any excursion of cerebral substance over the tentorial lip. The artery gives off branches to the interpeduncular posterior perforated substance; these branches spread to the third ventricular wall and medial thalamus. The posterior cerebral artery also contributes posterior choroidal vessels to the choroidal fissure in the lateral aspect of the transverse fissure and to the tela choroidea overlying the third ventricle. Lateral branches supply the posterior thalamus. The distal branches are distributed to the medial side of the temporal and occipital lobe, as shown in Fig. 3-20. Radiographic silhouettes in both lateral and anteroposterior views clarify this relationship (see Chapter 5).

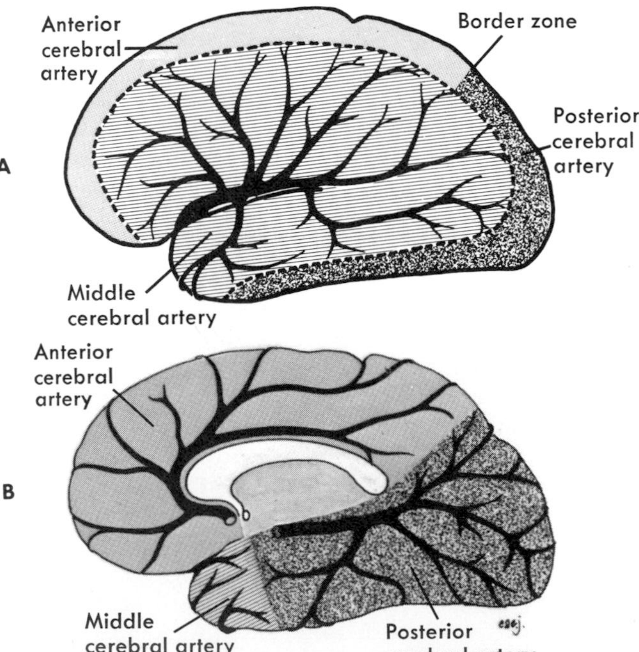

Fig. 3-20. Cerebral arteries. **A,** Lateral view of distribution; **B,** medial view of distribution.

The *basal vessels* include small but important penetrating branches from the posterior communicating and carotid arteries. Branches of the posterior communicating vessels reach the infundibulum, optic tract, part of the genu of the corpus callosum, and part of the posterior limb of the internal capsule. Branches also share with the posterior cerebral arteries the blood supply to the walls of the third ventricle. The *anterior choroidal* artery arises from the internal carotid and follows the course of the optic tract around the midbrain. It provides the main arterial supply to the choroid plexus of the inferior horn and gives branches to the base of the brain, optic tract, cerebral peduncle, lateral geniculate body, caudate tail, posterior limb, and sublenticular and retrolenticular parts of the internal capsule (Fig. 3-19).

The *middle cerebral artery* is the most direct continuation of the internal carotid. It runs laterally into the depths of the Sylvian fissure and is divided into many branches that serve the insular cortex and the cortex of the lateral surface of the brain (Figs. 3-20 and 3-21). The artery also supplies blood to the lateral orbital and lateral inferior frontal parts of the frontal lobe and the medial aspect of the temporal pole. In its transverse course, the middle cerebral artery gives off lateral striate arteries that supply the basal nuclei, including the putamen, head and body of the caudate nucleus, the lateral globus pallidus, and the upper part of the internal capsule. The middle cerebral artery extends only to the anterior and lateral parts of the thalamus. The distribution is displayed in Figs. 3-20 and 3-21. In coronal sections the middle cerebral arteries associate with the Sylvian fissure (Fig. 3-21).

The *anterior cerebral artery* crosses the anterior perforated substance en route to the genu. It supplies the lamina terminalis, rostrum, and septum pellucidum in this course and gives off a lateral, recurrent (medial striate) branch that penetrates to the basal nuclei (lower putamen, globus pallidus,

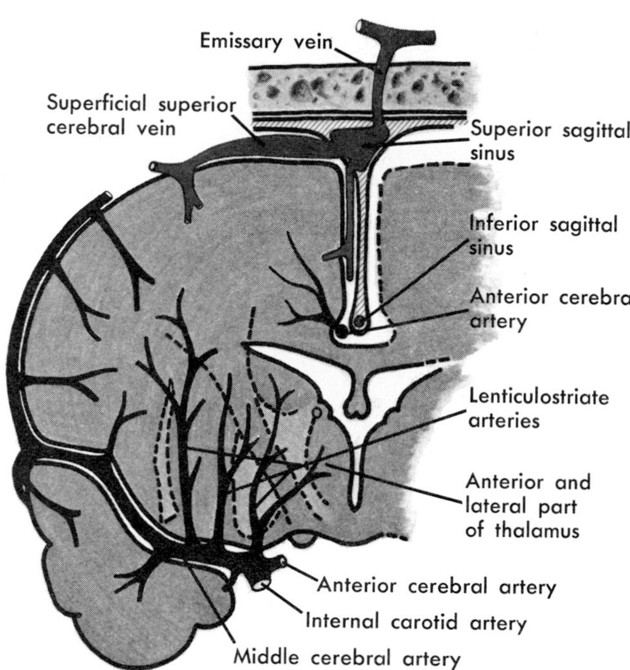

Fig. 3-21. Coronal diagram of arterial distribution. (After Rasmussen.)

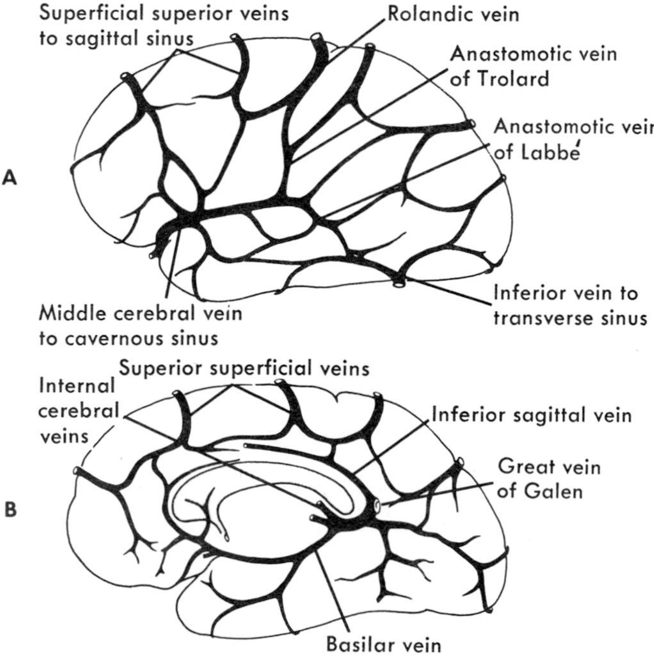

Fig. 3-22. Superficial cerebral veins. **A,** Laterial view; **B,** medial view.

internal capsule, and caudate head) (Fig. 3-20). The cortical distribution is reviewed in Fig. 3-21. The extremities of the supply areas anastomose with terminal branches of the middle and posterior vessels. In coronal sections the anterior cerebral branches are associated with the median sagittal fissure. The arteriograms are discussed in Chapter. 5.

Venous drainage

The veins of the brain can be separated descriptively into *superficial* and *deep* sets. The superficial veins drain the cortical fields and run in the subarachnoid space applied closely to the arachnoid membrane. The deep veins are within the cerebral substance or related to ventricular walls. The superficial veins aggregate into three drainage systems, *superior, middle,* and *inferior.* The *superior group* drains principally to the superior sagittal dural sinus along the vertex (Fig. 3-22, *A*). The vessels enter the sinus at right angles or slanted anteriorly against the flow of the blood in the dural vessel. The *middle group* drains toward the temporal pole, where veins enter the sphenoparietal and cavernous sinuses. The *inferior group* drains from the lateral posterior surfaces into the transverse sinuses on either side. The three systems are interconnected by anastomotic veins. Two of these veins are particularly prominent. The *anastomotic vein of Trolard* connects the superior and middle groups, and the *anastomotic vein of Labbé* connects the middle and inferior groups (Fig. 3-22, *A*).

The deep veins include the systems leading to the great vein of Galen. The *basal vein* crosses the perforated substance and receives vessels from the corpus striatum, interpeduncular fossa, midbrain, inferior horn, and temporal lobe. This reception is made as the vessel passes posteriorly in the lateral cerebral fissure around the cerebral peduncle to join the internal cerebral veins near their fusion into the vein of Galen. In the distal frontal part the basal vein is joined by drainage vessels from the cortical fields of both the frontal and Sylvian areas (Fig. 3-22, *B*). The paired *internal cerebral veins* are formed near the interventricular foramina by the junction of the septal veins, the vena terminalis, and choroidal veins of both sides. The two vessels run posteriorly parallel over the roof of the third ventricle and join the basal veins of each side near the pineal body. The two vessels then fuse to form the *great cerebral vein* (of Galen), which almost immediately joins the straight sinus (Fig. 3-22, *B*). The cerebellar veins and the veins of the brainstem aggregate into two sets, one joining the great vein of Galen over the superior vermis and the

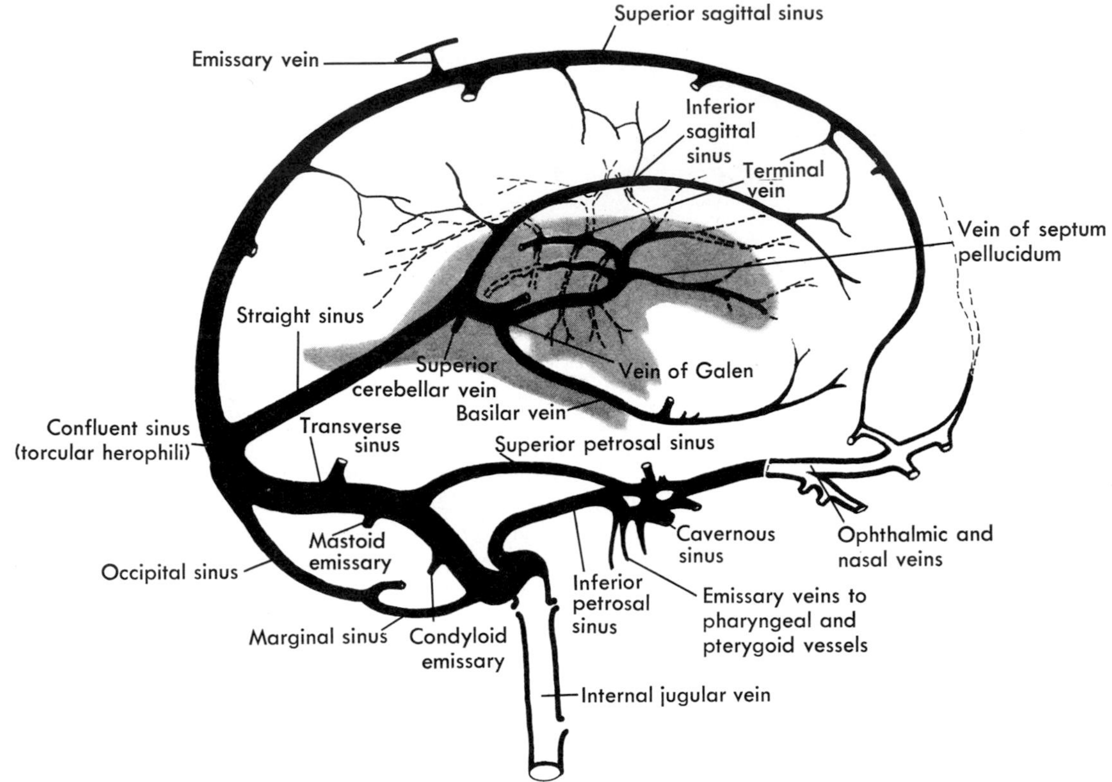

Fig. 3-23. Diagram of dural sinuses, lateral projection.

other directly joining the petrosal, transverse, or occipital sinuses of the dura mater (Fig. 3-23).

Dural sinuses

The folds and reflections of the dura mater form between its two layers a series of venous vascular channels that are continuous with the jugular system. As stated previously, the cerebral veins join these sinuses, and the CSF is emptied into the special arachnoid granulations that project into the sinus wall. The *superior sagittal* sinus follows the vaulted line of the superior aspect of the falx cerebri. It is in most cases continuous posteriorly with the right transverse sinus, although occasionally it joins the left. The junction of the two sinuses is at the internal occipital protuberance via the *confluent sinus* (torcular Herophili). The superior sagittal sinus is joined by the superior superficial cerebral veins and by emissary and diploic veins (Fig. 3-23). Lateral extensions of the sinus called *lacunae* are found throughout the course of the sinus, concentrated posteriorly. These receive most of the arachnoid granulations and many of the large superficial veins. The confluent sinus represents the common meeting point of the superior sagittal sinus, the straight sinus, and the occipital sinus as tributaries to the two *transverse sinuses*. The *inferior sagittal sinus* is located along the free edge (inferior) of the falx cerebri. It joins the *straight sinus* at the tentorium, which has already received blood from the great cerebral vein of Galen. The straight sinus continues posteriorly along the line of junction between falx and tentorium and empties into the confluent sinus. It usually is primarily continuous with the left transverse sinus. The *occipital sinus* is a small dural vessel, running in the free margin of the falx cerebelli from the margin of the foramen magnum to the confluent sinus. It anastomoses laterally with the transverse sinus, and through the foramen magnum with the vertebral venous plexus. The *transverse sinuses* continue around the occipital part of the skull at the attachment of the tentorium to the wall. They turn downward to follow the line of the base of the petrous ridges along irregular grooves *(sigmoid sinuses)* and become continuous through the jugular foramina with the jugular veins on each side (Figs. 3-18 and 3-23).

Several sinuses are concentrated in the antero-inferior parts of the cranial cavity (Fig. 3-18). An inferior petrosal sinus extends anteriorly from the jugular foramen to the cavernous sinus on either side of the sella turcica. The inferior petrosal sinuses on either side interconnect across the midline via the *basilar venous plexus*. This lies on the basilar part of the occipital bone and anastomoses with the vertebral venous plexus. A *superior petrosal sinus* connects an area from the transverse sinus, along the petrous ridge, to the cavernous sinus on each side. The *cavernous sinuses* lie on either side of the sphenoid body next to the sella turcica. They connect posteriorly with the petrosal sinuses. Anteriorly, they are joined by the sphenoparietal sinuses, which follow the sphenoparietal ridges. *Intercavernous sinuses* (Fig. 3-14), anterior and posterior to the pituitary, interconnect the two cavernous sinuses. This union forms the circular venous sinus surrounding the gland. The cavernous sinuses are joined anteriorly by the ophthalmic veins (superior and inferior), which drain the orbit. The dura mater has a venous outflow that follows the incoming arteries. In the vertebral canal, the venous drainage is organized into anterior and posterior internal venous plexuses that anastomose freely through venous rings. The drainage to extravertebral areas is principally through intervertebral veins, via the intervertebral foramina. The intrinsic veins of the spinal cord join the internal venous plexuses via veins in the fissures. They also join directly to the intervertebral veins (Fig. 3-24).

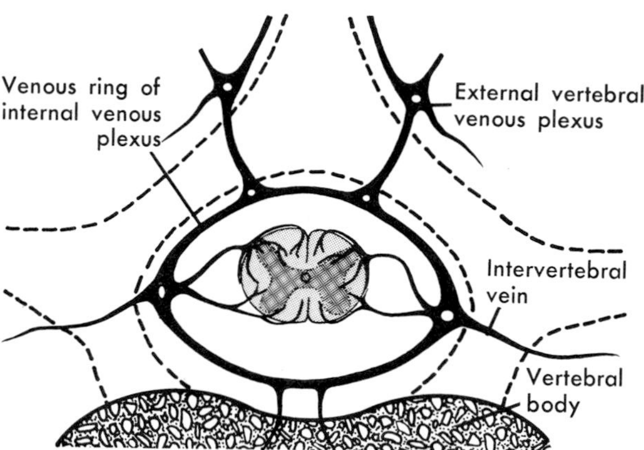

Fig. 3-24. Spinal veins and vertebral venous plexus; main longitudinal channels clear.

Table 3-1. Emissary veins

Vein	Connections formed
1. Frontal	Nasal mucous membrane to superior sagittal sinus
2. Ethmoidal	Nasal mucous membrane to superior sagittal sinus
3. Mastoid	Postauricular and occipital regions to transverse sinus
4. Parietal	Scalp to superior sagittal sinus
5. Condyloid	Deep veins of neck to transverse sinus
6. Hypoglossal	Deep veins of neck to occipital sinus
7. Ophthalmic	Face to orbit to cavernous sinus
8. Pharyngeal	Pharyngeal and pterygoid plexuses to cavernous sinus
9. Diploic	Numerous connections between intracranial venous sinuses and supraorbital, deep temporal, posterior temporal, and occipital veins

Emissary veins

The emissary vessels directly connect the extracranial tissues to the dural sinuses by a system of veins. Some are quite constant, and all serve in prospective transport (infection) from extracranial to intracranial positions. The principal emissary vessels are listed in Table 3-1. The veins that interconnect diploë to the dural sinuses are similar, as they also connect to veins of the scalp. Diploic veins open directly into the superior sagittal sinus from the frontal bones, into the sphenoparietal sinus from the frontal bone and greater wing of the sphenoid, into the transverse sinus from the parietal bone, and into the transverse sinus complex from the occipital bone (Figs. 3-14, *A* and 3-16).

Vessels of peripheral nerves

Arteries for the largest nerves arise by short trunks from major arteries and are directed exclusively to the nerves near their roots. Smaller neural branches from distal muscular arteries enter more distal nerve branches. In this way a succession of anastomosing vessels will enter a single long nerve. The anastomotic chain lies superficially within epineurium and may anastomose further by transverse or oblique branches with similar linear chains on the opposite side of the long nerve. Penetrating arterioles enter the perineurial connective tissue and those with capillaries provide a dense vascular plexus that reaches into the depths of the nerve along the fine filaments. An intraneural plexus of veins drains blood from the nerves into adjacent muscular veins or into subcutaneous vessels that accompany superficial cutaneous nerves.

In contrast to CNS tissues, which are devoid of lymphatics, peripheral nerves possess lymph vessels that drain fluid from superficial interstices into the regional node systems. The possible relationship of neural lymphatics to CSF drainage is still controversial. Experimentally, diffusable substances injected into spinal CSF can be recovered in intraneural spaces. Conversely, diffusable materials within peripheral nerve tissue will reach CSF within the subarachnoid space. There is however some uncertainty regarding the relationship of CSF drainage to lymphatic pickup in peripheral nerve tissue. Possibly the uptake is directly into venous channels, paralleling the circumstances occurring in cerebral CSF exchanges.

Major anastomoses

Equally important in the vasculature of the CNS are the interrelationships of the principal vessel systems in providing alternate anastomotic routes of blood supply. Frequently these anastomotic systems are critical in securing continuing blood flow to the CNS and operate in normal circumstances. In conditions of vascular insufficiency they sometimes become vital. The major systems to be reviewed include: (1) the spinal anastomotic tracts, (2) extracranial carotid systems, (3) the vertebral complex, (4) the circle of Willis, and (5) meningeal anastomoses.

Spinal anastomotic tracts. As stated previously, the arterial supply to the spinal cord arises from two major sources: (1) the *vertebral complex,* which provides the anterior and posterior spinal arteries, and (2) the *radicular arteries,* which are segmentally supplied. The anterior and posterior spinal arteries are better represented as *anterior* and *posterior anastomotic tracts.* The anterior spinal artery is formed from fusion of branches from each vertebral artery (sometimes from each posterior inferior cerebellar). These branches of the vertebral arteries arise close to the fusion of the vertebrals into the basilar vessel (Fig. 3-19). The posterior spinal arteries also arise from the vertebral arteries, but they do not fuse. Instead they form the upper extremity of the posterior anastomotic tract on each side. This posterior tract divides near the first cervical segment into a lateral anasto-

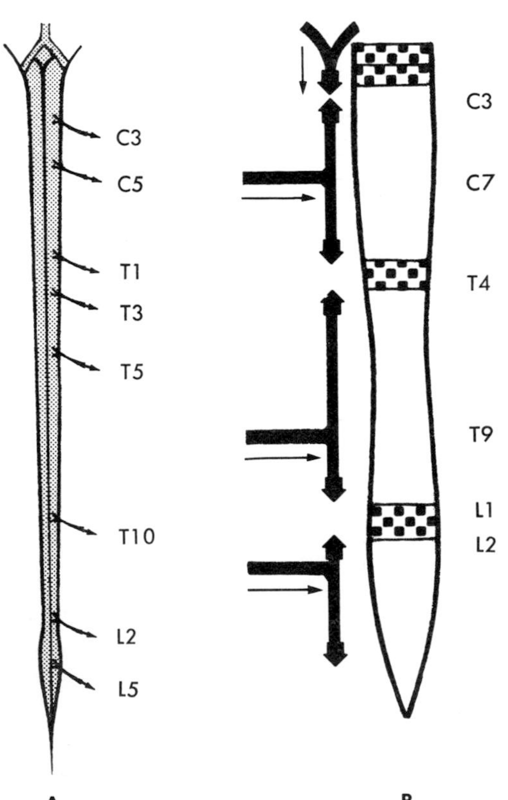

Fig. 3-25. A, Main radicular vessels by segmental source; **B,** relatively bare anastomotic zones in areas of supply by longitudinal anastomotic tracts.

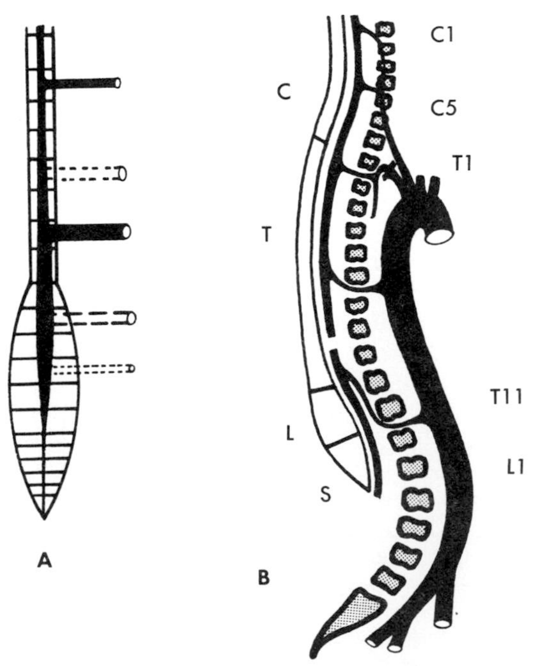

Fig. 3-26. A, Adamkiewicz artery and accessory vessels in black; alternate supply pattern dotted; **B,** manner of spinal supply and overlap with principal levels of radicular vessel sources.

motic tract and the continuing posterior tract (Fig. 3-25). Functionally these anastomotic tracts that carry blood from the vertebral arteries serve only the first few spinal segments. The remaining segments are supplied blood by radicular arteries.

The radicular vessels represent the terminal branches of vertebromedullary arteries, which arise segmentally downward in vertebral, intercostal, abdominal, iliac, and sacral arteries. While these arteries distribute by both anterior and posterior rootlets in the embryo (four per spinal segment), they disappear with age until only a few are significant contributors to the adult longitudinal anastomotic tracts. Approximately five to ten anterior radicular vessels usually persist in functional size, and about fifteen to twenty-two posterior radicular vessels remain. The latter are smaller than the anterior radicular vessels and contribute to the posterior longitudinal anastomotic tracts. The major anterior radicular vessels are variable and include: two or three cervical arteries below level C2, with a principal vessel usually occurring at C6; one or two small vessels in the upper thoracic segments, usually T4 or T5; and one to three vessels in the lower thoracic and lumbosacral region. One of the last group (Adamkiewicz's, or great radicular, artery) characteristically stands out prominently on one side (usually the left) at the lumbar enlargement and provides most of the blood for the lower thoracic and lumbosacral cord. The artery arises at varying levels. If located high (from T8 to T10), it usually is the only artery for the region; if low (from T11 to L2), it is accompanied by a small vessel appearing at T7 to T9, (Fig. 3-26). The irregu-

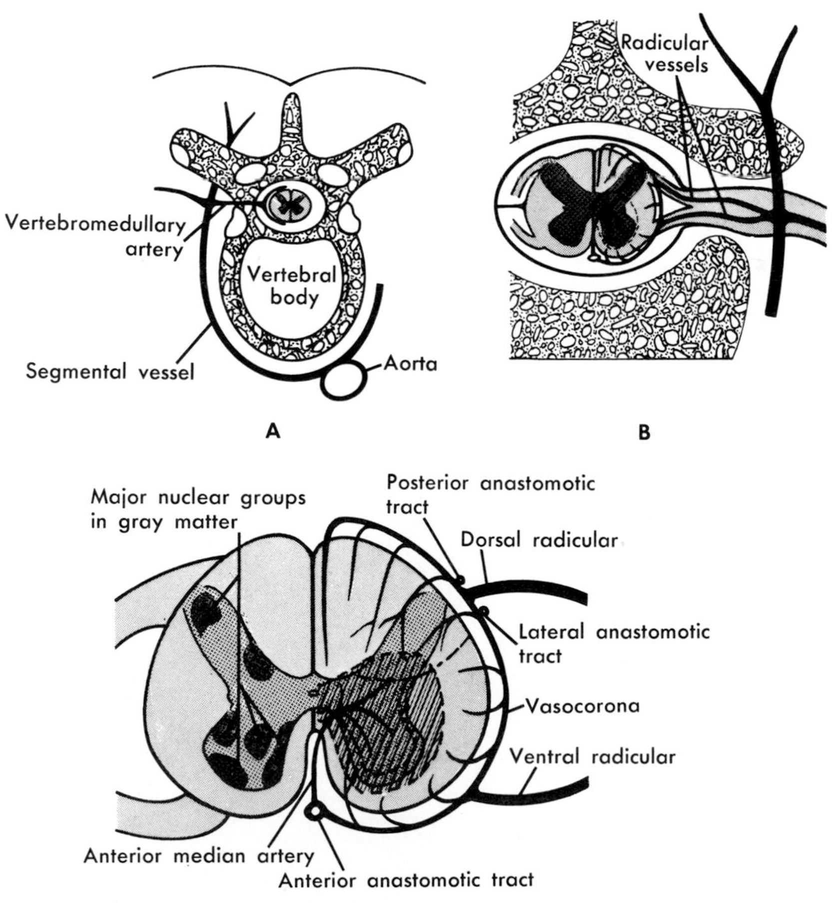

Fig. 3-27. A, Spinal arterial source; **B,** pattern of radicular supply; **C,** arterial distribution within cord. Note main nuclei on left, **C,** and relationship to radicular and vasocoronal supply.

larity of the contributing vessels produces marked variation in the size of the longitudinal anastomotic tract. Its largest dimension is at the entry of the great radicular artery.[4]

Intraspinal arteries. The peripheral arteries of the spinal cord anastomose freely in a network overlying the cord substance. This produces the *vasocorona,* from which penetrating vessels arise as part of the intraspinal vascular system. The surface vessels aggregate into poorly defined and inconstant groups longitudinally aligned as anterior (related to anterior roots), lateral (related to lateral columns), posterior (near posterior roots), and intrafunicular (penetrating the glial septa) (Fig. 3-27). The *anterior median arteries* arise as branches at right angle to the anterior anastomotic tract. They pass anteroposteriorly into the anterior median sulcus (Fig. 3-27). The vessels number from 180 to 260, but their distribution is uneven (from one to five per segment), with the greatest density of these vessels in the enlargements.

Extracranial carotid systems. The extracranial interconnections between the external and internal carotid complexes are numerous and well understood.[12] Of particular importance to CNS vascular supply is the interconnection via the ophthalmic artery (Fig. 3-17). The main link is from the external carotid through the ethmoidal to the ophthalmic artery. Accessory connections occur between the nasal and frontal vessels. It is known that an entire hemispheral blood supply can be accomplished through the ophthalmic anastomosis in the event of occlusion of an internal carotid artery.

Vertebral anastomosis. The muscle branches of the vertebral arteries anastomose with the external carotid branches. The two vertebral arteries also interanastomose via the anterior spinal vessels. It is possible for these connections to produce retrograde filling in many related vessels. The physiologic significance is subject to question. Both the carotid complex and the vertebral arteries function with the intracranial anastomoses.

Circle of Willis. The classic contributing vessels to the circle of Willis are reviewed on p. 55. (Fig. 3-19). It should be noted that the "classic" arrangement occurs in only twenty percent of the brains examined routinely.

The circle's functional capabilities as an anastomotic channel are frequently compromised by structural variations in its make-up. The right vertebral artery is commonly hypoplastic. About one-fifth of brains examined display the origin of posterior cerebral vessels in the carotids. Hypoplasia, or absence of one limb of the circle, is very common.

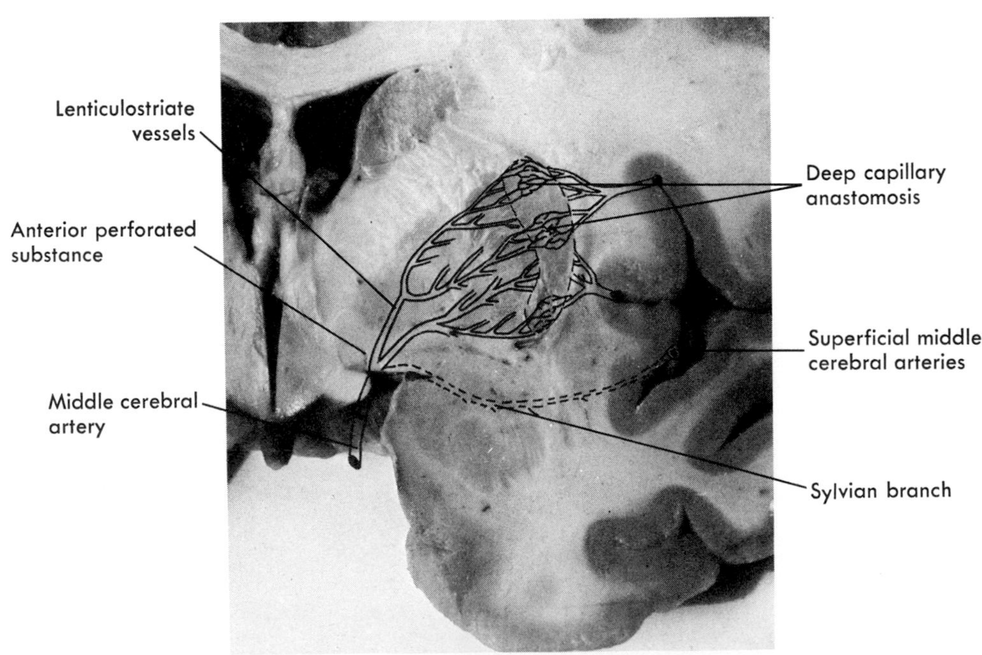

Fig. 3-28. Deep capillary anastomosis in outer basal nucleus (putamen).

Both anterior cerebral arteries may arise from one carotid.[6,12] Hemisphere-to-hemisphere anastomosis is accomplished by routes other than the circle of Willis, notably via the anterior cerebral vessels through the midportion of the corpus callosum.[2]

Meningeal anastomoses. Late in the nineteenth century Heubner developed the idea that any of the major vessels (the two carotids and the vertebral arteries) could supply any cerebral cortical area by anastomoses through their meningeal branches. This hypothetical model remained controversial as a functioning anastomosis and stimulated the cultivation of the opposing "end-artery" notions regarding cerebral blood supply, at least in regard to physiologic behavior. The outcome of the investigations may be summarized briefly as follows. (1) Several *meningeal anastomoses* do, in fact, exist.[11] These relate to each of the major cerebral supply vessels and to the cerebellar supply. Such an anastomosis, for example, is known to bridge around a basilar vessel occlusion. (2) The arachnoidal vessels anastomose freely as *arachnoidal rings.* (3) After penetrating the cortical substance, the superficial vessels interconnect by *transverse* anastomoses that are capillary links. It appears that these various meningeal connections serve as functional as well as structural interconnections and contribute to cortical integrity as part of the normal blood flow system. In addition to the cortical supply, those vessels that penetrate deeply to supply the lenticulostriate area also form their anastomotic links via capillary beds (Fig. 3-28). In circumstances of partial deprivation of blood supply, those areas with collateral feeding through capillary systems are most likely to fail. This concept of the special effects on the "last meadow" when the main pipeline is impaired has contributed greatly to theories of cerebral circulatory mechanics.

Radiographic demonstrations of anastomoses are given in Chapter 5.

REFERENCES

1. Austin, G.: The spinal cord, Springfield, Illinois, 1961, Charles C Thomas, Publisher.
2. Baptista, A. G.: Studies on the arteries of the brain, II. The anterior cerebral artery: some anatomic features and their clinical implications, Neurology **13**:825, 1963.
3. Davson, H.: Physiology of the ocular and cerebrospinal fluids, Boston, 1956, Little, Brown and Co.
4. Fazio, C.: Vascular pathology of the spinal cord. In Minckler, J., editor: Pathology of the nervous system, vol. II, New York, 1970, McGraw-Hill Book Co.
5. Mettler, F. A.: Fluid exchanges. In Minckler, J., editor: Pathology of the nervous system, vol. I, New York, 1968, McGraw-Hill Book Co.
6. Meyer, J. S., and others: New technics for recording cerebral blood flow and metabolism in subjects with cerebrovascular disease. In Millikan, C. H., editor: Cerebral vascular disease, New York, 1966, Grune & Stratton, Inc.
7. Moossy, J.: Cerebral atherosclerosis, intracranial and extracranial lesions, In Minckler, J., editor: Pathology of the nervous system, vol. II, New York, 1970, McGraw-Hill Book Co.
8. Slager, U. T.: The meninges. In Minckler, J., editor: Pathology of the nervous system, vol. I, New York, 1968, McGraw-Hill Book Co.
9. Tennyson, V. M., and Pappas, G. D.: Ependyma. In Minckler, J., editor: Pathology of the nervous system, vol. I, New York, 1968, McGraw-Hill Book Co.
10. Tourtellotte, W. W.: Cerebrospinal fluid and its reactions in disease. In Minckler, J., editor: Pathology of the nervous system, vol. I, New York, 1968, McGraw-Hill Book Co.
11. Vander Ecken, H. M., and Adams, R. D.: The anatomy and functional significance of the meningeal arterial anastomoses of the human brain, J. Neuropath. Exp. Neurol. **12**:132, 1953.
12. Zülch, K. J.: Thrombosis, hemorrhage, embolism. In Minckler, J., editor: Pathology of the nervous system, vol. II, New York, 1970, McGraw-Hill Book Co.

CHAPTER 4

SECTIONAL ANATOMY

JEFF MINCKLER

Advantageous views of most of the structures of the central nervous system can be obtained by serial coronal, transverse, or parasagittal sections. Usage has established a standard pattern of cutting that is nicely adapted both to anatomic review and to sighting pathologic changes. The brainstem is transected at the midbrain through the cerebral peduncles, between the inferior and the superior colliculi. The knife passes inferior to the mamillary bodies, leaving thalamic parts intact. The forebrain is then cut coronally while resting on its vertex through the landmarks as indicated in Fig. 4-1. It is helpful to hold the brain against a firm plane while cutting. These levels include the following eight standard cuts that provide pieces for histologic study of critical locations, as well as gross display of major anatomy: (1) through the frontal lobes and tips of the temporal lobes; (2) through the optic chiasm; (3) through the tuber cinereum; (4) through the mamillary bodies; (5) through the middle of the cerebral peduncles; (6) through the lateral midbrain sulcus; (7) through the superior colliculi dorsal to the cerebral aqueduct; and (8) through the occipital lobes. The plane of sectioning is perpendicular to the base plane of the temporal lobes. It is common to standardize the viewing to the attiude as if the viewer were looking at the subject. This method is utilized in all of the following photographs, unless otherwise mentioned in the caption. This places the subject's left side to the viewer's right, with vertex up. In viewing the transverse sections of the brain and spinal cord, it is customary to view the pieces as if the subject were cut transversely and tipped toward the viewer. This places the posterior or dorsal aspect up and the subject's left side to the viewer's right. The midsagittal plane is equally valuable and has been utilized in previous illustrations (Fig. 4-31). Parasagittal sections will often be particularly useful (for example, in outlining the length of a tract) and will be utilized in this book when helpful. The following gross photographs are of unstained material. Atlases of stained sectional pieces are available in Villiger[5] (brainstem), Riley[3] (central brain), Matzke and Roofe[1] (coronal), and Singer and Yakovlev[4] (sagittal). Stained sections through many of these levels will also be included in this book. Each cut will vary considerably from all others in the same plane, however meticulous the start. Some of the structures to be sought are barely visible without aid and are frequently missed in the sections. These important structures will be displayed by gross magnification photography. Special sections will be displayed to identify structures that are missing in the major photos of the routine sections. In reviewing these pictures, it will be necessary to refer frequently to the surface topography in the various views of the brain shown in Chapter 2 and in following chapters. One of the greatest difficulties in the actual cutting is preservation of gyral identity. This is accomplished by tagging the principal convolutions by markers (such as pins, tags, and coloring) before doing the coronal sections. The accessory views will be discussed principally in the captions.

CORONAL SECTIONS OF FOREBRAIN

Plane through frontal lobes and anterior poles of temporal lobes (Fig. 4-2)

In the central focal field is the *genu of the corpus callosum*. The lower part becomes the *rostrum*, and the upper part continues into the body as the cuts are continued posteriorly (Figs. 4-4 and following). At this level the anterior horn of the ventricle is round or triangular and, viewing the end cut from

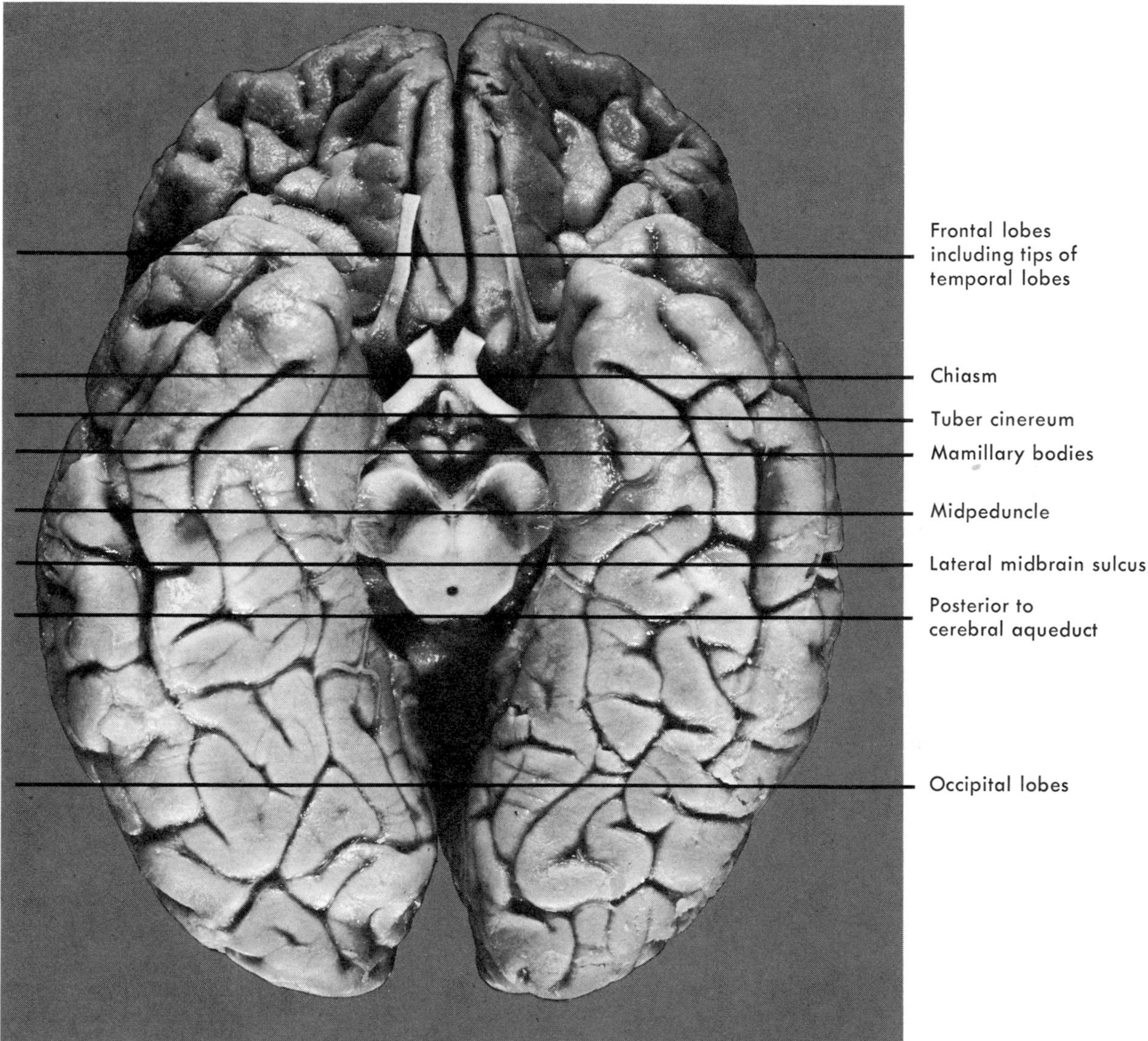

Fig. 4-1. Basal view of brain with major planes of section.

the posterior aspect or in transverse section (Fig. 4-19), the poles of the horns diverge. This broadens the genu anteriorly, with the extremities continuing forward into either frontal pole as limbs of the *anterior forceps*. This is seen to advantage in a transverse section (Fig. 4-19). Note in the depths of the median sagittal fissure the cut ends of the anterior cerebral arteries as they pass around the genu. The cortical fields and gyral patterns are markedly irregular and are even more difficult to define in coronal section than in surface view (Fig. 4-3). At this level however the superior, middle, and inferior gyral clusters stand out well. The deep unnamed sulcus that separates the inferior frontal gyral configuration and the orbital gyri establishes the overlying (or opercular) character of the frontal group. This overhang gradually meets the opercular parts that overlie the insula (Fig. 4-5). The *subcallosal area* is well shown in this level, and its relationship to parolfactory area, anterior perforated substance, and amygdala can be traced posteriorly in the next three levels. The *gyrus* and *sulcus cinguli* form a continuing convolution and overlying crevice that can be seen passing around the genu from the subcallosal area. The *olfactory tracts* occupy the *olfactory sulcus,*

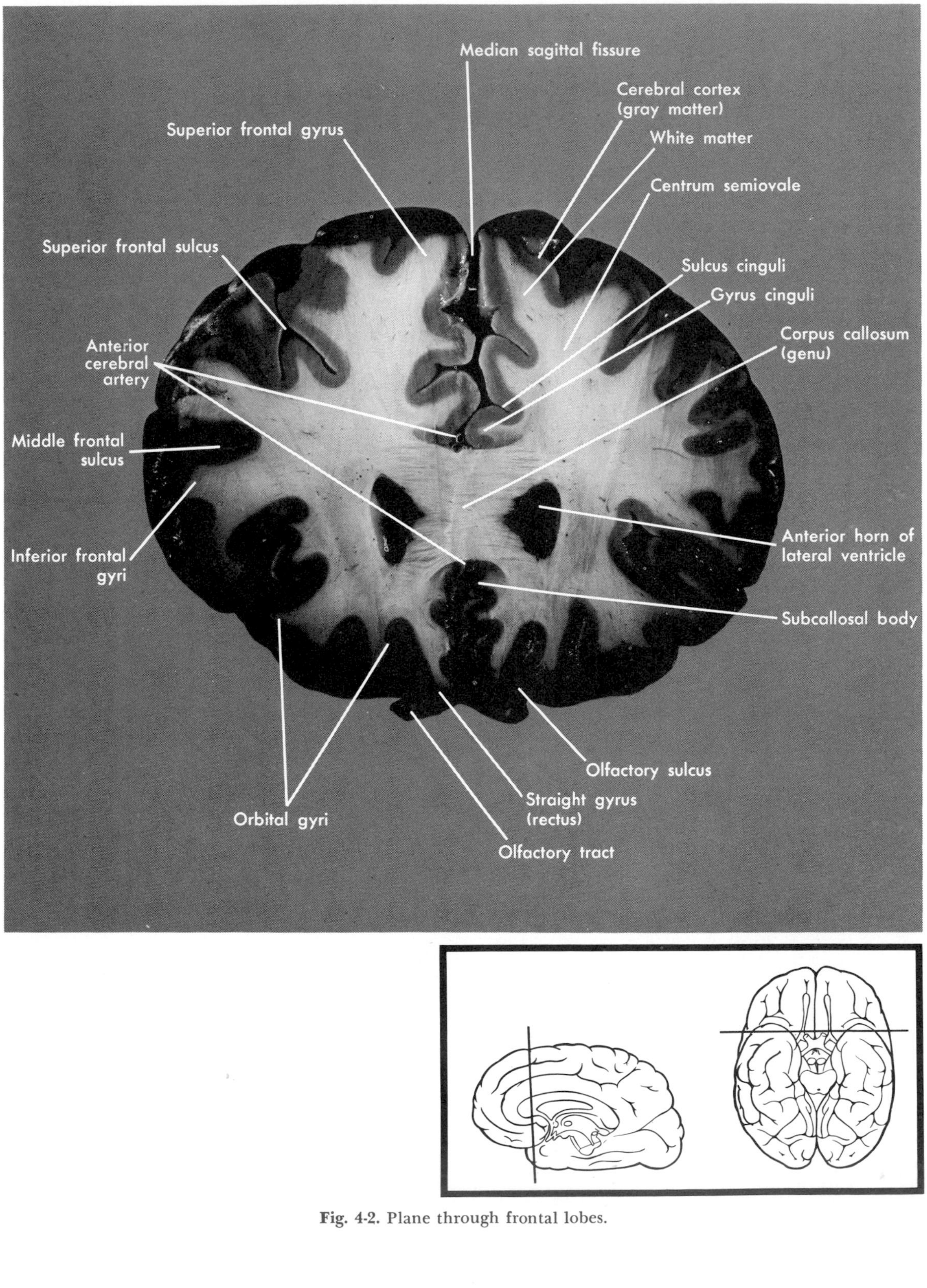

Median sagittal fissure
Cerebral cortex (gray matter)
Superior frontal gyrus
White matter
Centrum semiovale
Superior frontal sulcus
Sulcus cinguli
Gyrus cinguli
Anterior cerebral artery
Corpus callosum (genu)
Middle frontal sulcus
Anterior horn of lateral ventricle
Inferior frontal gyri
Subcallosal body
Olfactory sulcus
Straight gyrus (rectus)
Orbital gyri
Olfactory tract

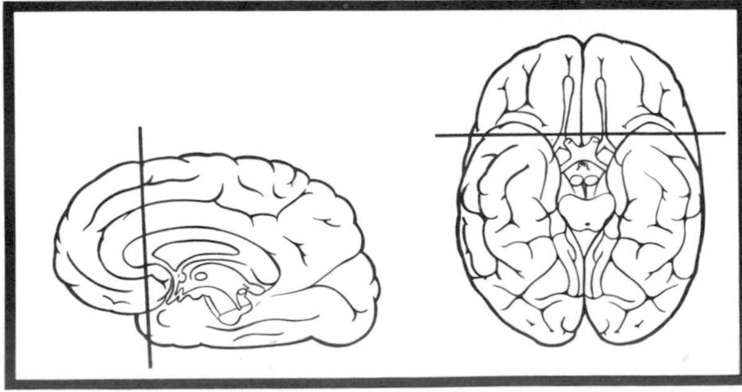

Fig. 4-2. Plane through frontal lobes.

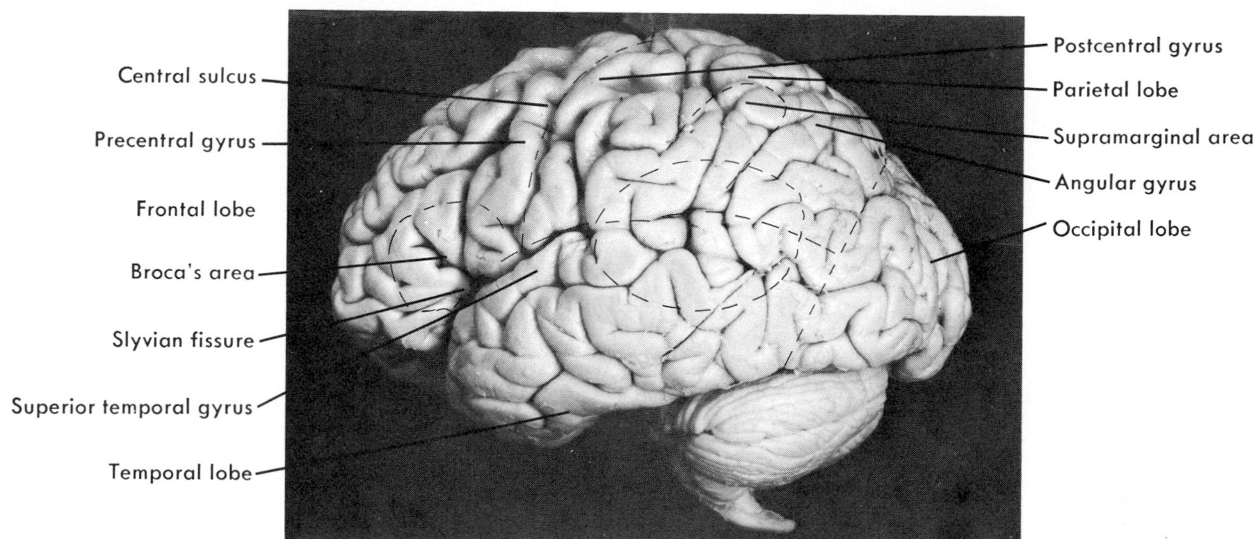

Fig. 4-3. Lateral view of brain with arachnoid removed; major landmarks and areas identified. Variations should be compared with idealized areas in Fig. 2-7. The central dotted circle is Wernicke's area.

and medial to this is the *straight gyrus*. Tips of temporal lobes frequently occur in this section.

Plane through the level of the optic chiasm (Fig. 4-4)

The lateral ventricular cavities at this level have a typical "hockey-stick" outline in cross section and are separated by the thin *septum pellucidum*. Here this membrane bridges the area between the rostrum and the central part of the genu and body. This membrane is sometimes divided by the *cavum septi pellucidi* (fifth ventricle) and has two limbs bridging the space between rostrum and genu (Fig. 2-6). When the septum is single, it can be traced posteriorly where it joins the fused *fornices* at the body of the corpus callosum (Fig. 4-18). When the cavum septi pellucidi exists, each limb of the septum continues posteriorly to bridge the space between each individual fornix and the overlying *body of the corpus callosum*. The bulge projecting into the lateral ventricle is the head of the *caudate nucleus*, which lies medial to the anterior limb of the internal capsule. Anterior and inferior to the capsule, the caudate head blends with the *putamen*, which expands laterally to the internal capsule. The combination of head of caudate, anterior limb of internal capsule, and putamen constitutes the *corpus striatum*. Note that the *subcallosal body* expands into a *parolfactory gray area*, which is continuous with the *anterior perforated substance* and laterally approaches the *amygdala* (Fig. 4-7). These primary olfactory receptive areas have appeared in the path of the olfactory tract, which has disappeared into them via the olfactory striae (Fig. 4-1). Lateral to the putamen are the white *external capsule*, the faintly defined gray *claustrum*, and the thin extreme *capsule* immediately deep to the cortex. The Sylvian fissure has come into view at this level, accentuating the opercular, or overhanging, character of the inferior frontal lobe and superior temporal gyrus. Note that the inferior frontal gyrus is continuous with the precentral gyrus. This establishes a motor relationship of interest (see Chapters 21 and 22). The *optic chiasm* can be seen dividing posteriorly into the two *optic tracts*. The subdivisions of the gyri in the temporal lobe can be seen, and the vascular complex of the middle cerebral vessels is evident in the depths of the Sylvian fissure. The sulcal pattern of the frontal area is irregularly divided into its three tiers. The *gyrus cinguli* continues along the superior surface of the corpus callosum.

Plane through the level of the tuber cinereum (Fig. 4-5)

The lateral ventricles at this level are slightly larger but retain the general shape, as in Fig. 4-4. The base of the septum is broadened by the appearance of the *columns of the fornices*. These split over the *anterior commissure* into a precommissural and postcommissural pillar. The pos-

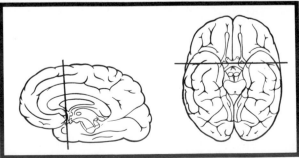

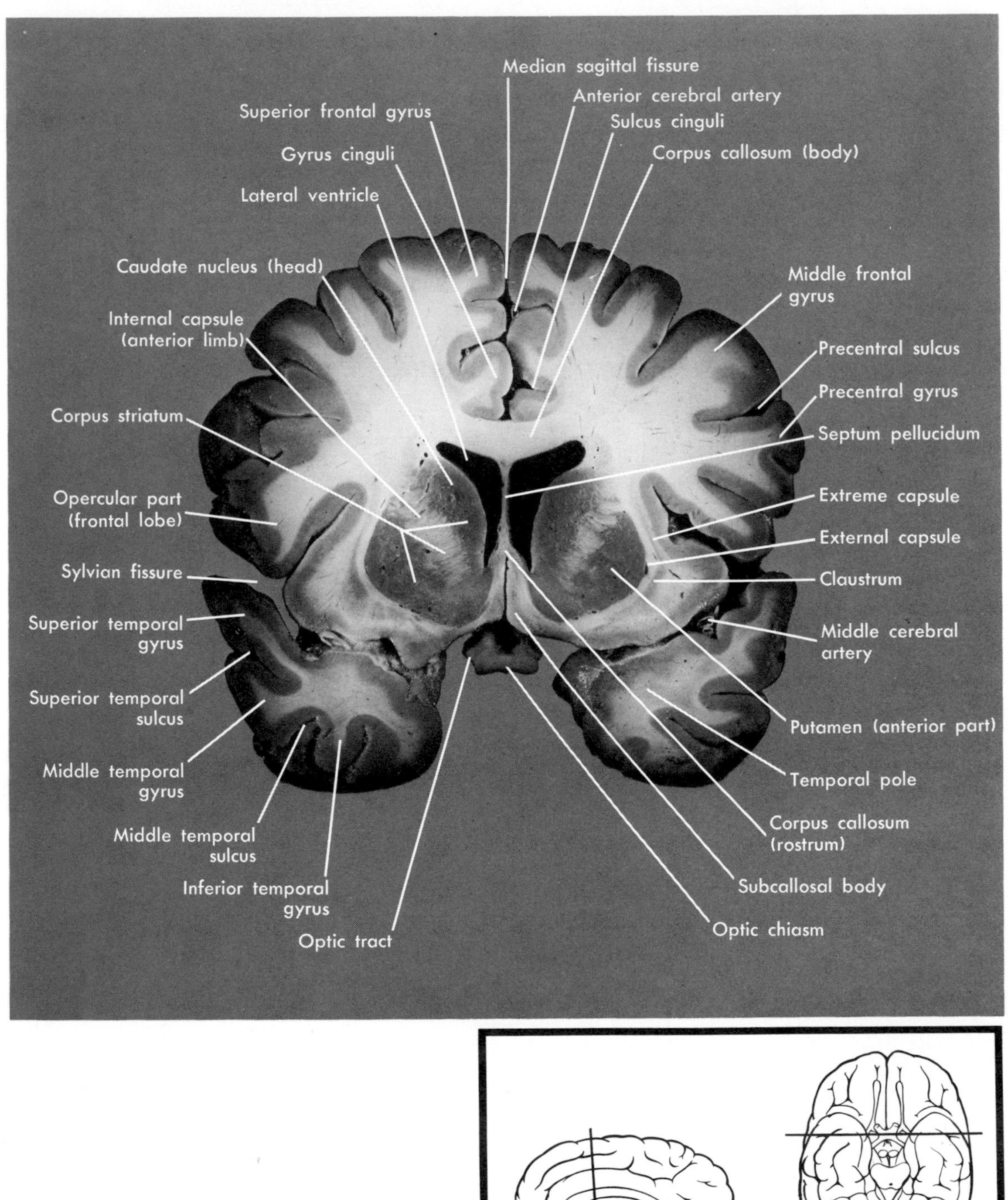
Median sagittal fissure
Anterior cerebral artery
Superior frontal gyrus
Sulcus cinguli
Gyrus cinguli
Corpus callosum (body)
Lateral ventricle
Caudate nucleus (head)
Middle frontal gyrus
Internal capsule (anterior limb)
Precentral sulcus
Precentral gyrus
Corpus striatum
Septum pellucidum
Opercular part (frontal lobe)
Extreme capsule
External capsule
Sylvian fissure
Claustrum
Superior temporal gyrus
Middle cerebral artery
Superior temporal sulcus
Putamen (anterior part)
Middle temporal gyrus
Temporal pole
Corpus callosum (rostrum)
Middle temporal sulcus
Subcallosal body
Inferior temporal gyrus
Optic chiasm
Optic tract

Fig. 4-4. Plane through optic chiasm.

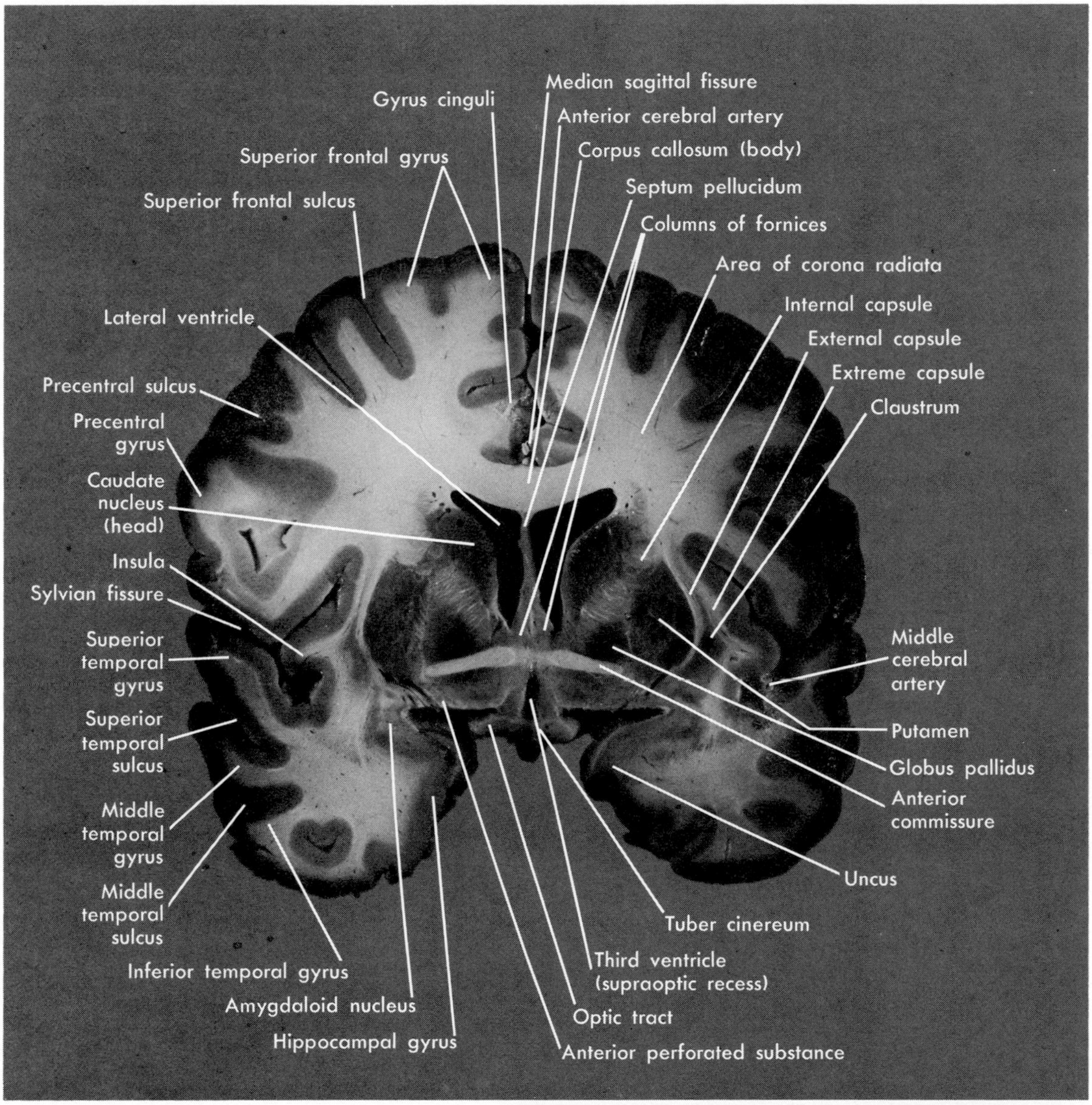

Gyrus cinguli
Median sagittal fissure
Anterior cerebral artery
Corpus callosum (body)
Superior frontal gyrus
Septum pellucidum
Superior frontal sulcus
Columns of fornices
Area of corona radiata
Internal capsule
Lateral ventricle
External capsule
Extreme capsule
Precentral sulcus
Claustrum
Precentral gyrus
Caudate nucleus (head)
Insula
Sylvian fissure
Superior temporal gyrus
Middle cerebral artery
Superior temporal sulcus
Putamen
Globus pallidus
Middle temporal gyrus
Anterior commissure
Uncus
Middle temporal sulcus
Tuber cinereum
Third ventricle (supraoptic recess)
Inferior temporal gyrus
Amygdaloid nucleus
Optic tract
Hippocampal gyrus
Anterior perforated substance

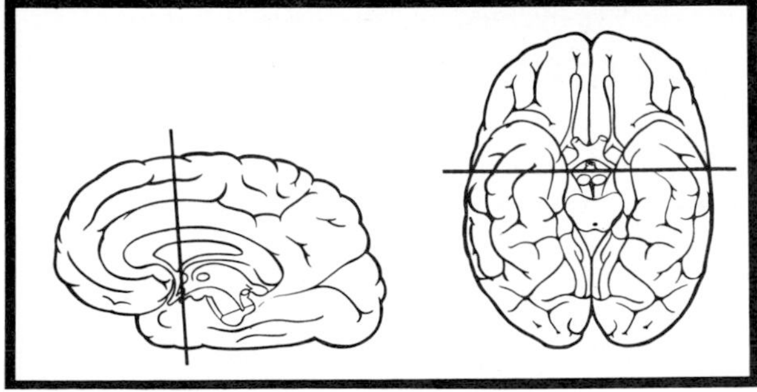

Fig. 4-5. Plane through tuber cinereum.

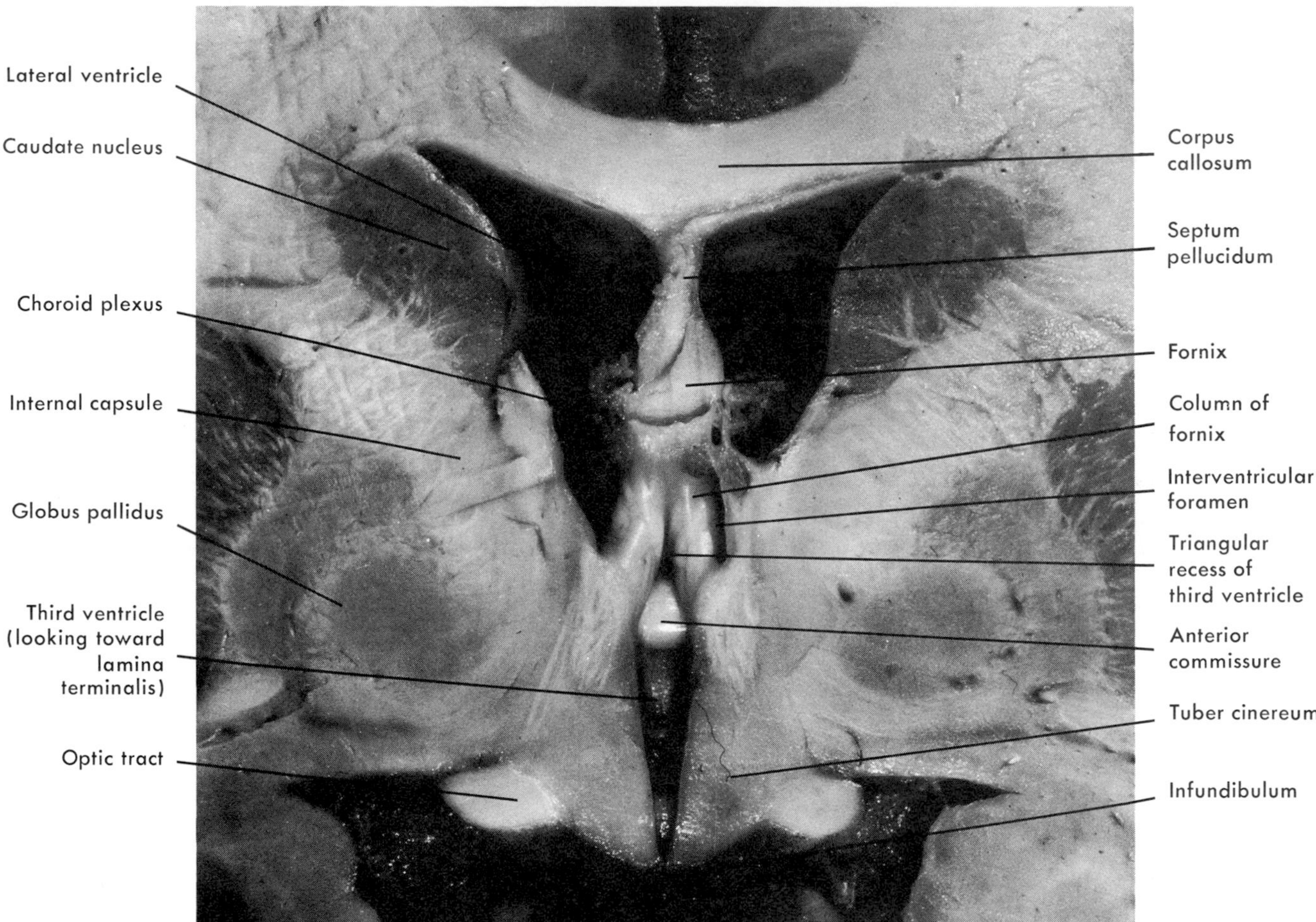

Fig. 4-6. Fornices and anterior commissure viewed from behind.

terior is largest and passes behind the central area of the anterior commissure, which is barely shaved away in the central part of Fig. 4-5. A posterior view of this area showing this relationship is displayed in Fig. 4-6. The *triangular recess* of the third ventricle is formed by the two columns of the fornix and the crossing anterior commissure. In this third level the *supraoptic recess* has been opened. This projection of the third ventricle cavity in posterior view also appears in Fig. 4-5. The *tuber cinereum* is the funnel-shaped, downward extension of the hypothalamus that is embraced laterally by the optic tracts. The expanded anterior perforated substance and amygdala extend laterally. Note the posterolateral extension of the anterior commissure in the next level (Fig. 4-7), which shows fibers joining the commissure from the temporal lobe and amygdaloid nucleus. The basal nuclei are somewhat more complex in this level, with the anterior limb of the capsule completely separating the head of the caudate and the putamen. Note the appearance of the *globus pallidus* medial to the *putamen*. The *insula* (*island of Reil*) is a definitive cortical field deeply buried in the Sylvian fissure. The anterior extremity of the *hippocampal gyrus* (better seen in the next level) is expanded into the projecting uncus, which overlies the amygdala. Only the anterior part of this nucleus is evident here. The gyral configurations retain their general relationships over frontal and temporal lobes. The white centrum semiovale shows the interdigitations of the transverse fibers of the corpus callosum with the nearly vertical fibers of the internal capsule. The re-

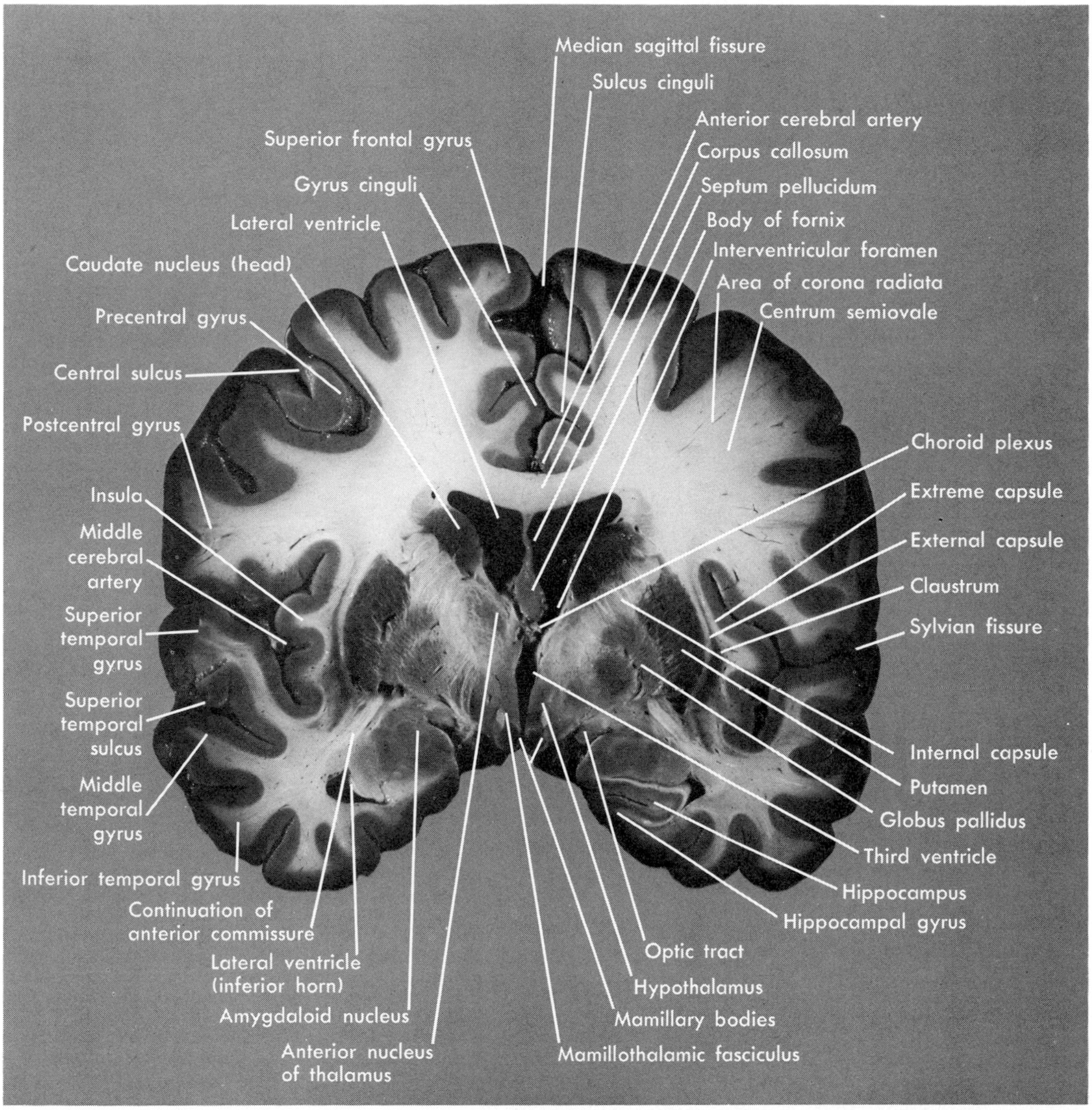

Median sagittal fissure
Sulcus cinguli
Anterior cerebral artery
Corpus callosum
Septum pellucidum
Body of fornix
Interventricular foramen
Area of corona radiata
Centrum semiovale
Superior frontal gyrus
Gyrus cinguli
Lateral ventricle
Caudate nucleus (head)
Precentral gyrus
Central sulcus
Postcentral gyrus
Insula
Middle cerebral artery
Superior temporal gyrus
Superior temporal sulcus
Middle temporal gyrus
Inferior temporal gyrus
Continuation of anterior commissure
Lateral ventricle (inferior horn)
Amygdaloid nucleus
Anterior nucleus of thalamus
Choroid plexus
Extreme capsule
External capsule
Claustrum
Sylvian fissure
Internal capsule
Putamen
Globus pallidus
Third ventricle
Hippocampus
Hippocampal gyrus
Optic tract
Hypothalamus
Mamillary bodies
Mamillothalamic fasciculus

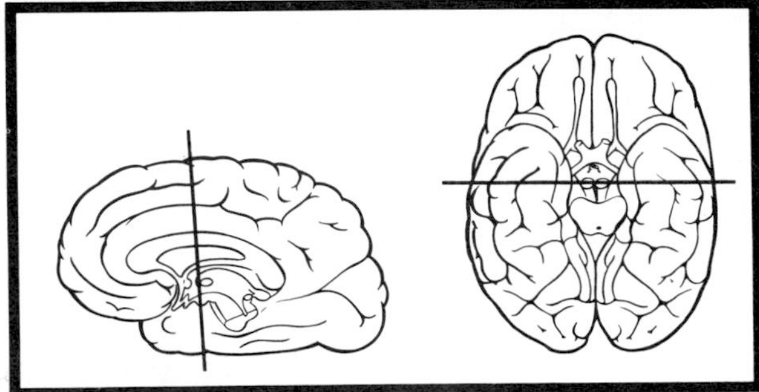

Fig. 4-7. Plane through mamillary bodies.

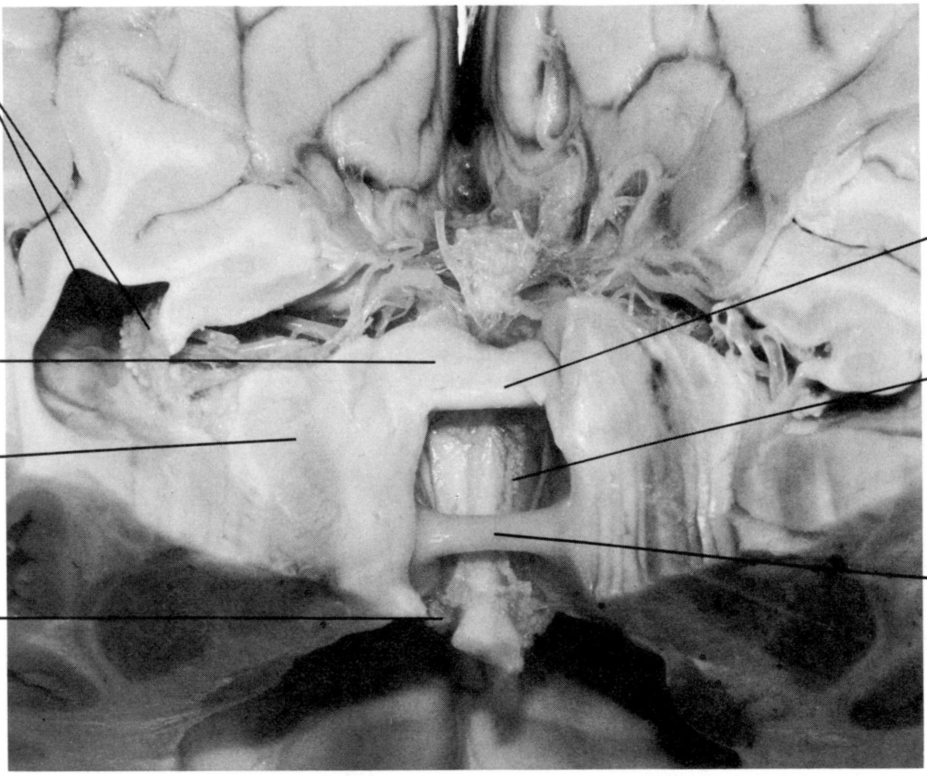

Confluent part of lateral ventricle with choroid plexus
Tectum of midbrain
Basis pedunculi
Choroid plexus passing through interventricular foramen
Posterior commissure
Third ventricle with strips of choroid along roof
Massa intermedia (thinned and elongated from hydrocephalus)

Fig. 4-8. Roof of third ventricle viewed from below (case of hydrocephalus with ventricle distended).

Choroid plexus
Anterior commissure
Amygdaloid nucleus
Mamillothalamic fasciculus (Vicq d'Azyr)
Interventricular foramen
Globus pallidus
Third ventricle
Optic tract
Mamillary body

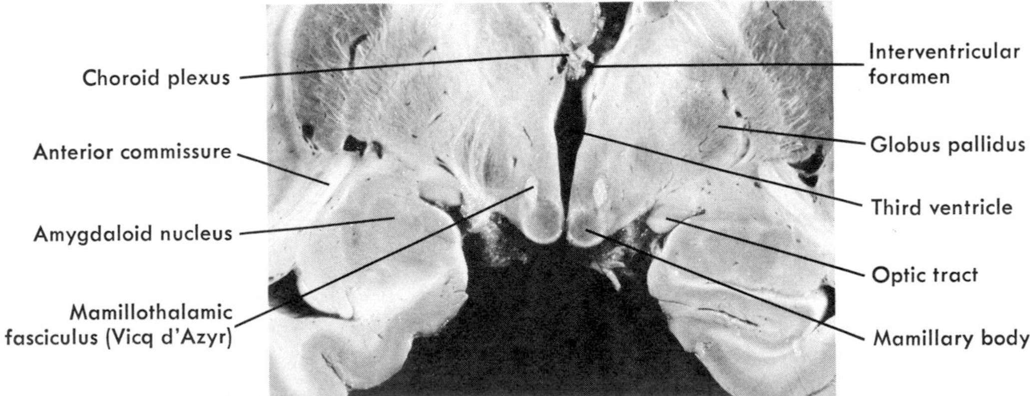

Fig. 4-9. Mamillary bodies and adjacent structures in coronal view.

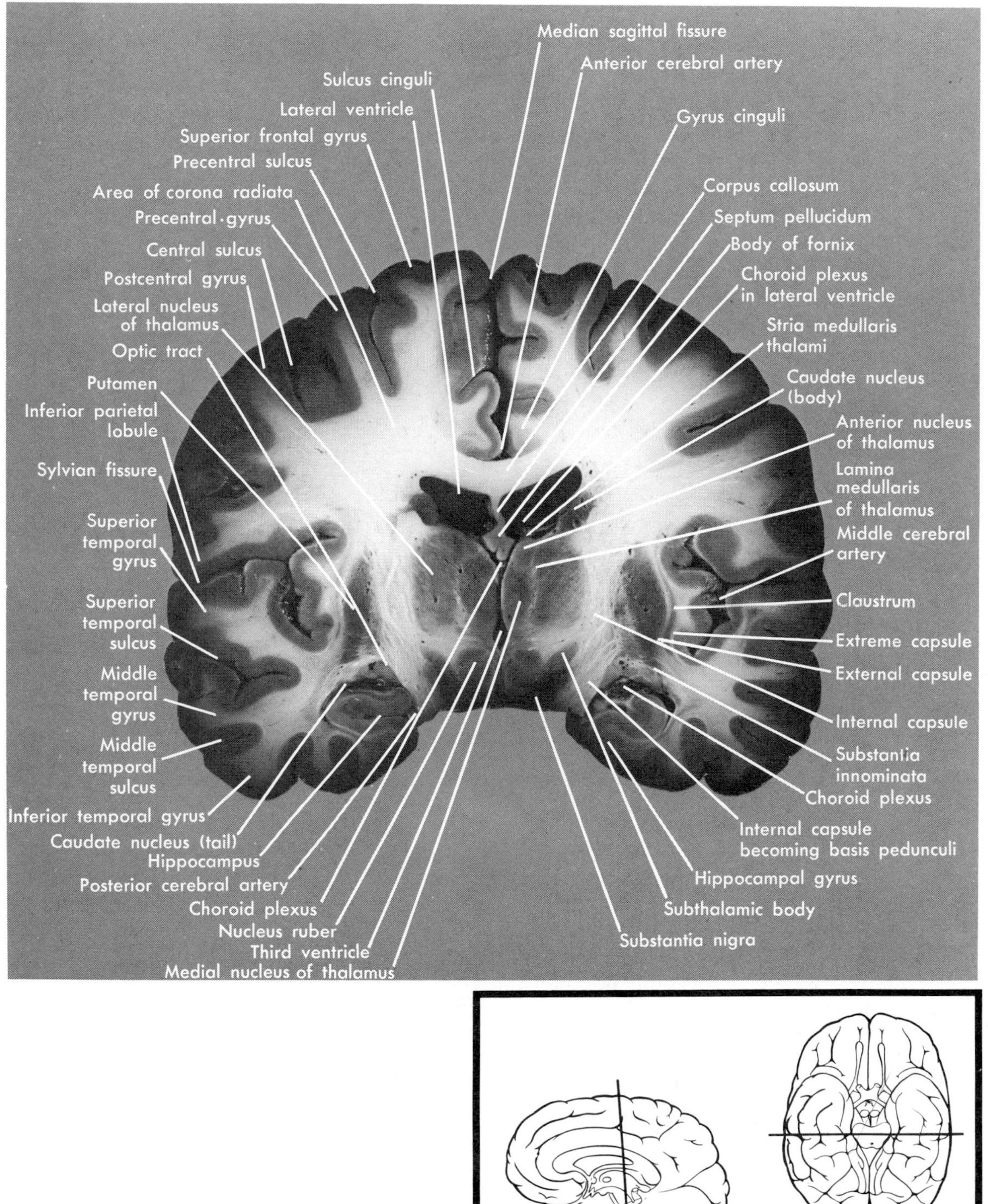
Median sagittal fissure
Anterior cerebral artery
Sulcus cinguli
Lateral ventricle
Gyrus cinguli
Superior frontal gyrus
Precentral sulcus
Area of corona radiata
Corpus callosum
Precentral gyrus
Septum pellucidum
Central sulcus
Body of fornix
Postcentral gyrus
Choroid plexus in lateral ventricle
Lateral nucleus of thalamus
Stria medullaris thalami
Optic tract
Putamen
Caudate nucleus (body)
Inferior parietal lobule
Anterior nucleus of thalamus
Sylvian fissure
Lamina medullaris of thalamus
Superior temporal gyrus
Middle cerebral artery
Superior temporal sulcus
Claustrum
Extreme capsule
Middle temporal gyrus
External capsule
Internal capsule
Middle temporal sulcus
Substantia innominata
Choroid plexus
Inferior temporal gyrus
Caudate nucleus (tail)
Internal capsule becoming basis pedunculi
Hippocampus
Hippocampal gyrus
Posterior cerebral artery
Subthalamic body
Choroid plexus
Nucleus ruber
Substantia nigra
Third ventricle
Medial nucleus of thalamus

Fig. 4-10. Plane through center of midbrain peduncle.

sultant *corona radiata* is displayed better in dissections, appearing as vertically projecting fibers of the capsule (Fig. 4-22).

Plane through the level of the mamillary bodies (Fig. 4-7)

The lateral ventricular outline in this level is typically triangular, with a slight bulge in the inferolateral side from the caudate nucleus. The caudate is smaller at this level, due to the reduction in size from head to body to tail as the sections continue posteriorly. The *third ventricle* is outlined in full depth, with the inferior slit appearing between the *mamillary bodies* as part of the hypothalamic floor. At a slightly more posterior level is the variable massa intermedia, which bridges the ventricle from side to side (Fig. 4-8). In the roof of the ventricle, to the bottom of this picture, the granular *choroid plexus* is apparent in the enlargement (Fig. 4-8). Note the opening to the right (Fig. 4-9) where the plane of section has caught the *interventricular foramen* of Monro, interconnecting lateral and third ventricles. Choroid can also be identified, extending along the floor of the lateral ventricle on the left side of the picture. The bodies of the fornices are fused and are connected to the corpus callosum by the septum pellucidum. Note that the *columns of the fornices* have disappeared into the mamillary bodies. This relationship of the columns to the mamillary bodies is shown better in Fig. 4-6. The *mamillothalamic tract* (Vicq d'Azyr) is visible as it moves away from the mamillary bodies. This extension to the *anterior nucleus of the thalamus* is just beyond the plane of section. The anterior limb of the internal capsule has extended to the genu of the capsule at this level (see transverse section, Fig. 4-26). The main bulk of the hypothalamic wall lies adjacent to the lower part of the third ventricle.

The basal nuclei, at the area of maximum width, lie lateral to hypothalamus. The *putamen* is the darker, lateral segment of the *lentiform nucleus,* which includes as its second major segment the *globus pallidus* (the pallid or paler medial segment). This comes to an apex leading into a fiber bundle, the *ansa lenticularis,* which curves around the internal capsule slightly posteriorly and downward to join the subthalamic and midbrain area. This continues into the next level (Fig. 4-10). As seen in Fig. 4-7, this bundle is closely related to the anterior commissure, lying immediately behind it. Note that the optic tract has moved laterally (see Fig. 4-6) and is wedged between the globus pallidus and amygdala. At this point, the lentiform nucleus and amygdala are closely apposed. It is seen from the relationship shown in Fig. 4-10 that the tail of the caudate nucleus has also blended with the amygdala as it continues forward in the temporal lobe (see the reconstructed basal nuclear diagram in Fig. 2-12, *B*). The outlying claustrum and its associated capsules stand out well at this level.

The cortical patterns now include the central sulcus and parts of the postcentral gyrus (general sensory area) of the parietal lobe. The *motor cortex* is the thickest of the layers and can be identified in this way, if not cut on the bias (Fig. 2-11). Both middle cerebral and anterior cerebral arteries and their usual relationship to Sylvian and median sagittal fissures, respectively, are well shown. The corpus callosum and centum display the same topography as in the forward levels. The *inferior, or temporal, horns of the lateral ventricles* are seen on either side. The peculiar configuration of the hippocampus is in view on the right. This is better seen in more posterior cuts. The lateral and posterior continuation of the anterior commissure stands out prominently.

Plane through the level of the middle of the cerebral peduncles (Fig. 4-10)

At this level the lateral ventricles are flattened superoinferiorly, and the third ventricle is a narrow slit with slight widening anterosuperior to the midbrain channel. The bilaterally fused body of the fornix has moved close to the corpus callosum and is attached to it by a stubby *septum pellucidum.* The choroid plexus and attachments are better demonstrated in a drawing (see Fig. 3-7). The *caudate nucleus* has narrowed to a small body superiorly and to the barely perceptible tail in the temporal region. The putamen is the principal part of the remaining lenticular nucleus and is moved far laterally by the lateralized posterior limb of the internal capsule (see transverse section, Fig. 4-26). An isolated gray field, *substantia innominata,* appears inferior to the putamen at this level (right side of picture).

The most conspicuous feature is the prominence of the thalamus that lies adjacent to the third ventricle, between the ventricle and the posterior limb of the internal capsule. The principal *nuclear groups of the thalamus* proper can be distinguished as anterior, medial, and lateral. The *massa intermedia* is displayed in Fig. 4-8. The *posterior nucleus,* extending into *pulvinar,* is shown in Fig. 4-18, and in transverse section in Fig. 4-26. The nu-

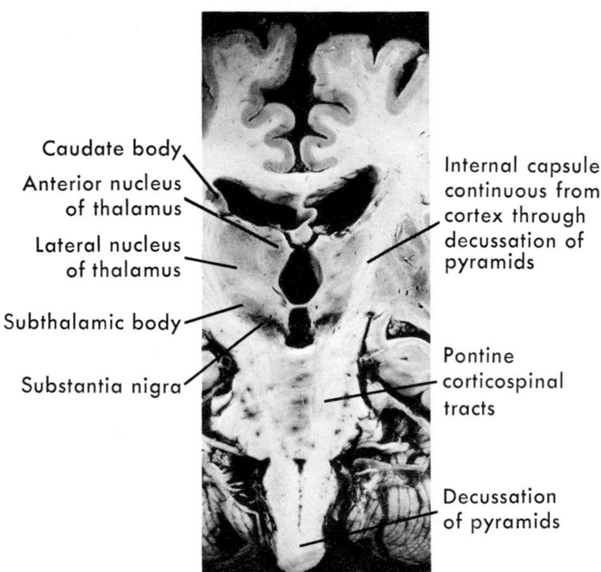

Fig. 4-11. Oblique plane between coronal and transverse to show continuity of internal capsule. Brain atrophic.

clear components of the thalamus proper are separated by the *medullary laminae* of the thalamus. This section (Fig. 4-10) displays to best advantage the continuity of tracts from cortex to internal capsule to basis pedunculi. (See Fig. 4-11, which includes, on a slightly different plane, continuation of the tracts through pons and into the pyramids of the medulla.) Inferior to the thalamus is the thalamic peduncle, which connects thalamus proper with subthalamus and midbrain. The *subthalamic body* (of Luys) stands out superior to the *substantia nigra* and lateral to the *nucleus ruber*. This nucleus and the *thalamic peduncle* are the main constituents of the subthalamus. The substantia nigra, nucleus ruber, and basis pedunculi are parts of the midbrain.

The temporal field lateral to the basis pedunculi takes on new configuration at this level. The optic tract has moved laterally to enter its thalamic receptive area, the *lateral geniculate body* (Fig. 4-12). The *tail of the caudate nucleus* has narrowed and become a slight gray mass on the superolateral aspect of the inferior (temporal) horn of the lateral ventricle. Branches of the posterior cerebral artery are conspicuous, projecting along the medial aspect of the temporal lobe as they extend posteriorly from the basal cistern area. The following associated distribution areas of the three principal superficial cerebral arteries are visible in the same plane: (1) the *anterior,* associated with the median sagittal fissure and corpus callosum; (2) the *middle,* associated with the Sylvian fissure; and (3) the *posterior,* associated with the medial aspect of the temporal and occipital lobes. The remarkable configuration of the *hippocampus* and the associated inferior horn are best revealed in a magnified photograph of the area (Fig. 4-13). The *tela choroidea* and *choroid plexus* of the inferior horn stand out clearly on each side, as do the optic tract and caudate tail marginal to the ventricle. The layer of white matter underlying the lenticular remnants is the *sublenticular part of the internal capsule,* which is most prominent on the left side of this picture.

The hippocampal area (Fig. 4-13) includes a *hippocampal gyrus, hippocampal fissure,* a buried *dentate gyrus, dentate fascia, fimbria, choroid fissure, choroid plexus,* and the *alveus,* which projects as a medial prominence into the wall of the inferior horn of the ventricle. A diagrammatic representation is shown in Fig. 4-14. Note that the fimbria is posteriorly continuous with the crus of the fornix (Fig. 4-18). The gyral configurations at this level include numerous parietal parts. An enlarged photograph (Fig. 4-15) shows the radiating fibers extending from thalamus to the cortex, via the posterior limb of the internal capsule. These are en route to the general sensory area of the postcentral gyrus. In this illustration fibers that interconnect lentiform and thalamic nuclei can be seen.

Plane through the level of the lateral midbrain sulcus (Fig. 4-12)

At this level, the bodies of the lateral ventricles are almost rectangular in outline, with the long dimension transverse. The *septum pellucidum* is short, and *fornices* are fused centrally. Choroid plexus attachments are evident in the floor of the bodies of the lateral ventricles, in the roof of the third ventricle, and in the inferior horns of the lateral ventricles. The third ventricle is limited below by the *posterior commissure,* which overlies the start of the *cerebral aqueduct.* The *habenular complex* shows somewhat, but is better seen in Fig. 4-16. Here the *stria medullaris thalami* leads to the habenular trigone on either side. The trigones are interconnected by the *habenular commissure.* The habenular complex, together with the pineal body (Fig. 4-16), constitute the epithalamus. The posterior commissure is also seen well in transverse section (Fig. 4-29). The relationship of the *superior colliculi* of the midbrain and the thalamic nuclei, as contributors to the posterior commissure, are demonstrated in Figs. 4-12 and 4-29.

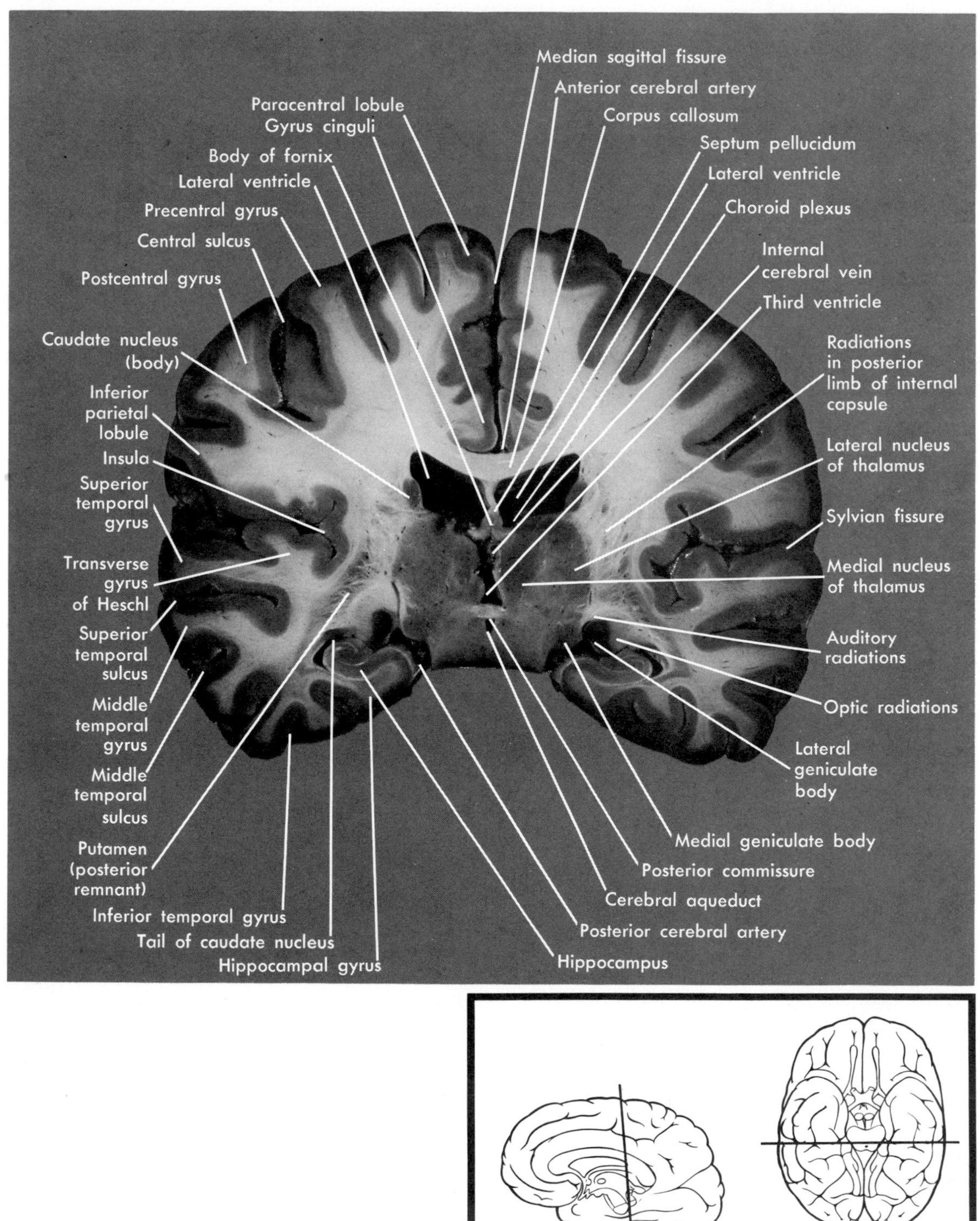
Median sagittal fissure
Anterior cerebral artery
Corpus callosum
Septum pellucidum
Lateral ventricle
Choroid plexus
Internal cerebral vein
Third ventricle
Radiations in posterior limb of internal capsule
Lateral nucleus of thalamus
Sylvian fissure
Medial nucleus of thalamus
Auditory radiations
Optic radiations
Lateral geniculate body
Medial geniculate body
Posterior commissure
Cerebral aqueduct
Posterior cerebral artery
Hippocampus
Paracentral lobule
Gyrus cinguli
Body of fornix
Lateral ventricle
Precentral gyrus
Central sulcus
Postcentral gyrus
Caudate nucleus (body)
Inferior parietal lobule
Insula
Superior temporal gyrus
Transverse gyrus of Heschl
Superior temporal sulcus
Middle temporal gyrus
Middle temporal sulcus
Putamen (posterior remnant)
Inferior temporal gyrus
Tail of caudate nucleus
Hippocampal gyrus

Fig. 4-12. Plane through the lateral midbrain sulcus.

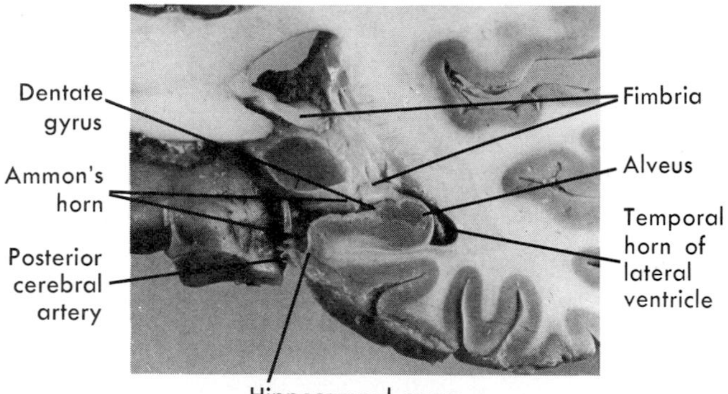

Fig. 4-13. Hippocampal area, right, viewed from behind.

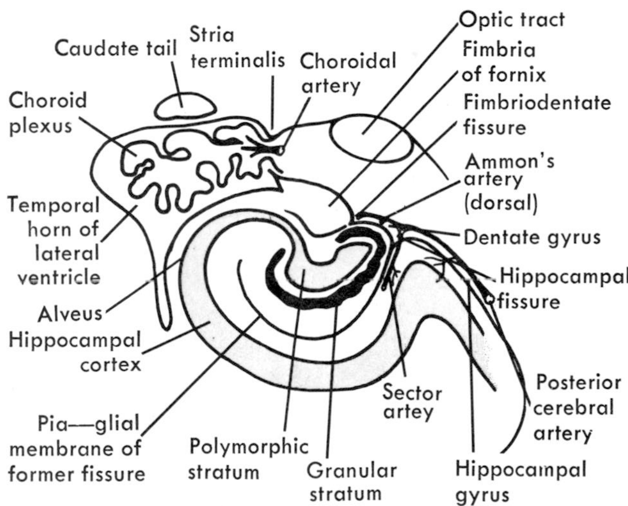

Fig. 4-14. Diagram of hippocampal complex, left, viewed from behind.

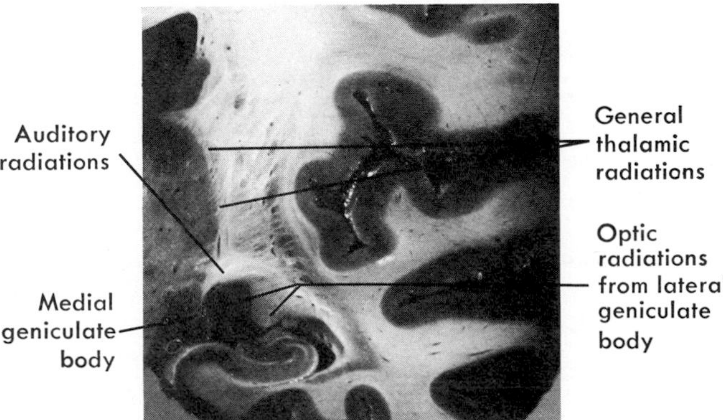

Fig. 4-15. Thalamic radiations.

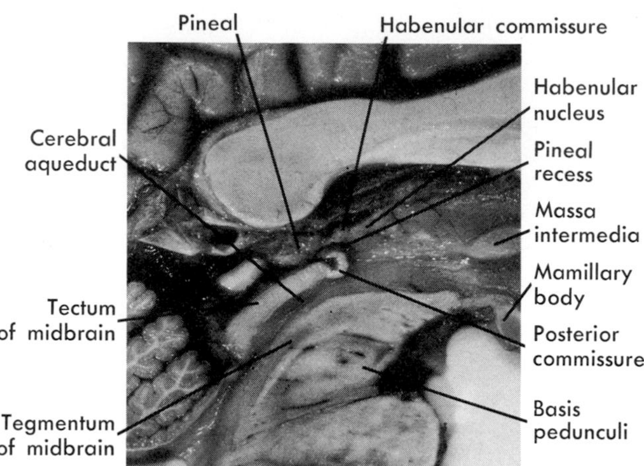

Fig. 4-16. Habenular complex, midsagittal view.

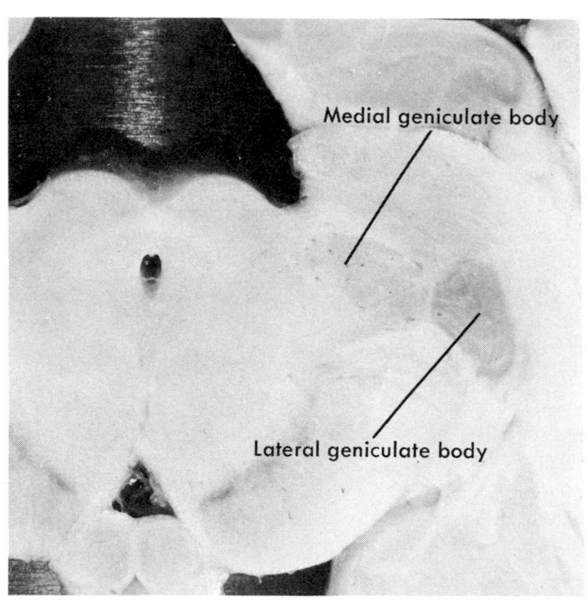

Fig. 4-17. Lamination of lateral geniculate body.

This level displays the *metathalamus* to best advantage. The nuclei of this part include the somewhat isolated *lateral geniculate body*. This appears in the line of the optic tract that has been traced back from the chiasm in Fig. 4-4. The outline of the lateral geniculate body has been likened to Napoleon's hat. In gross magnification (Fig. 4-17) it appears laminated. It radiates to the occipital cortex (Fig. 4-12), posterior to the lenticular nucleus, which shows very faintly lateral to the thalamus. The *optic radiation* is thus in the retrolenticular part of the internal capsule. The *thalamo-occipital radiations* and projections are shown well in transverse sections (Fig. 4-26). In this transverse section the cortex of the medial aspect of the occipital lobe along the *calcarine fissure* represents the visual cortex.

The second major component of the metathalamus is the *medial geniculate body*. This projects from the posterior and inferolateral part of the posterior (pulvinar) nucleus of the thalamus proper. In this level it is medial to the lateral geniculate body. In gross display (Figs. 2-1 and 2-14), it lies as a projecting nodule that is connected to the inferior colliculus of the midbrain by the *brachium of the inferior colliculus*. This complex is a principal relay series in the auditory pathway. In the same way (Fig. 4-28), the lateral geniculate body is related to the superior colliculus by the *brachium of the superior colliculus*. This complex is a relay series of major importance in the visual system (see Chapter 20). In Fig. 4-15, the auditory radiations extend from the medial geniculate body through the sublenticular part of the internal capsule to the gyri on the superior part of the temporal lobe (*Heschl's gyri*). This cortical area represents auditory cortex. These auditory gyri are oriented somewhat transversely across the temporal lobe and show well in the dissection displaying the insula (Fig. 2-8).

The hippocampus is well organized at this level, and the tail of the caudate continues in its posterolateral relationship to the inferior horn (Fig. 4-12). A prominent area of parietal cortex is represented,

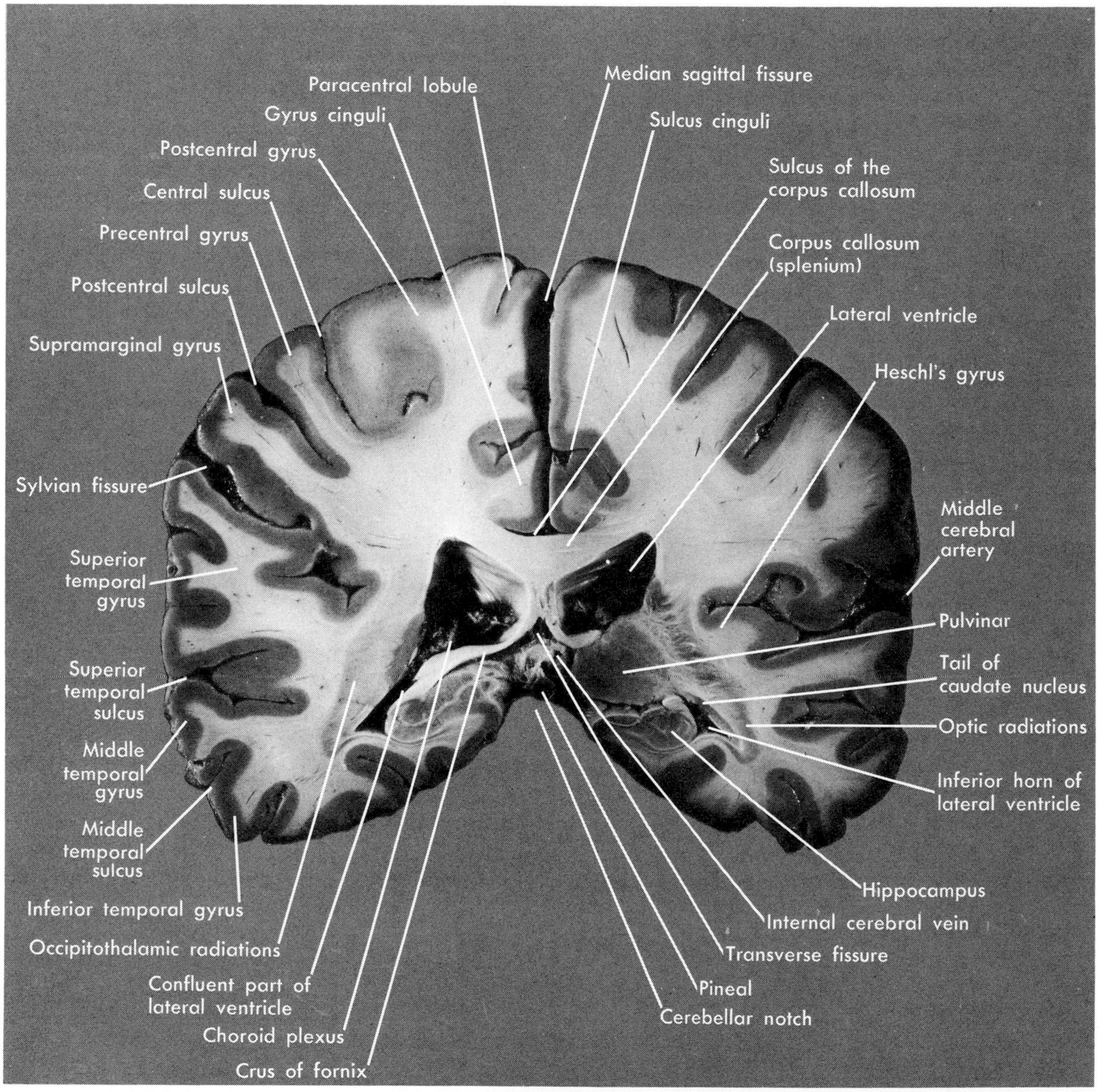

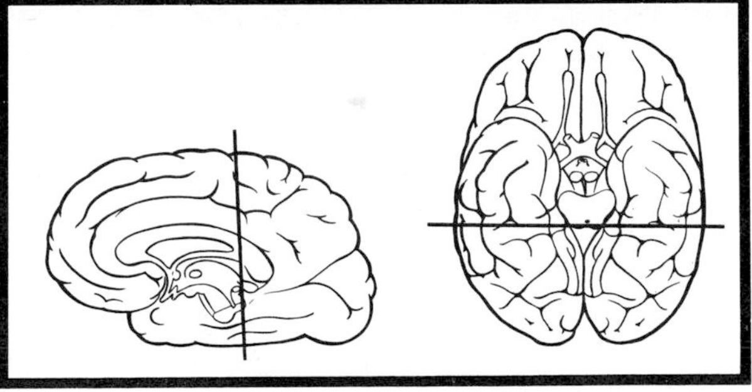

Fig. 4-18. Plane posterior to aqueduct carrying through the confluent ventricle region.

including postcentral *somesthetic area* and parts of the inferior parietal (supramarginal) lobule. The anterior part of the *paracentral lobule* is usually part of this section level. The relationships of anterior cerebral artery to median sagittal fissure persist. The middle cerebral arterial complex is seen in the Sylvian fissure. The posterior cerebral vessels are in the deep sulcus, between the temporal lobe and the brainstem. Note also the *internal cerebral veins,* which aggregate in bulk along the roof of the third ventricle. These are en route to join the great vein of Galen to eventually enter the straight sinus (Fig. 3-23).

Plane through the level of the superior colliculi behind the cerebral aqueduct (Fig. 4-18)

This plane displays the *confluent part of the lateral ventricle* on the left of Fig. 4-18. On the right, the extremity of the posterior extending pulvinar is in view. The thalamo-occipital bundle is apparent on both sides. In this bundle the pulvinar contributes a significant segment. The continuity of the fornix, through the crus to the fimbria, is apparent on the left of the picture. The bulge of the hippocampus that runs into the inferior horn of the ventricle is apparent in Fig. 4-18. This forms the *alveus* as the tracing is carried forward to the section of Fig. 4-7. This view permits the inspection of the terminus of the corpus callosum in the *splenium.* Note that the *crura of the fornix* come together under the splenium. The crossing fibers of the *hippocampal commissure* are located in this union of the crura. Note on the left the extending fibers of the corpus callosum as they pass over the upper and outer surface of the confluent part of the ventricle. These continue as the *tapetum* pos-

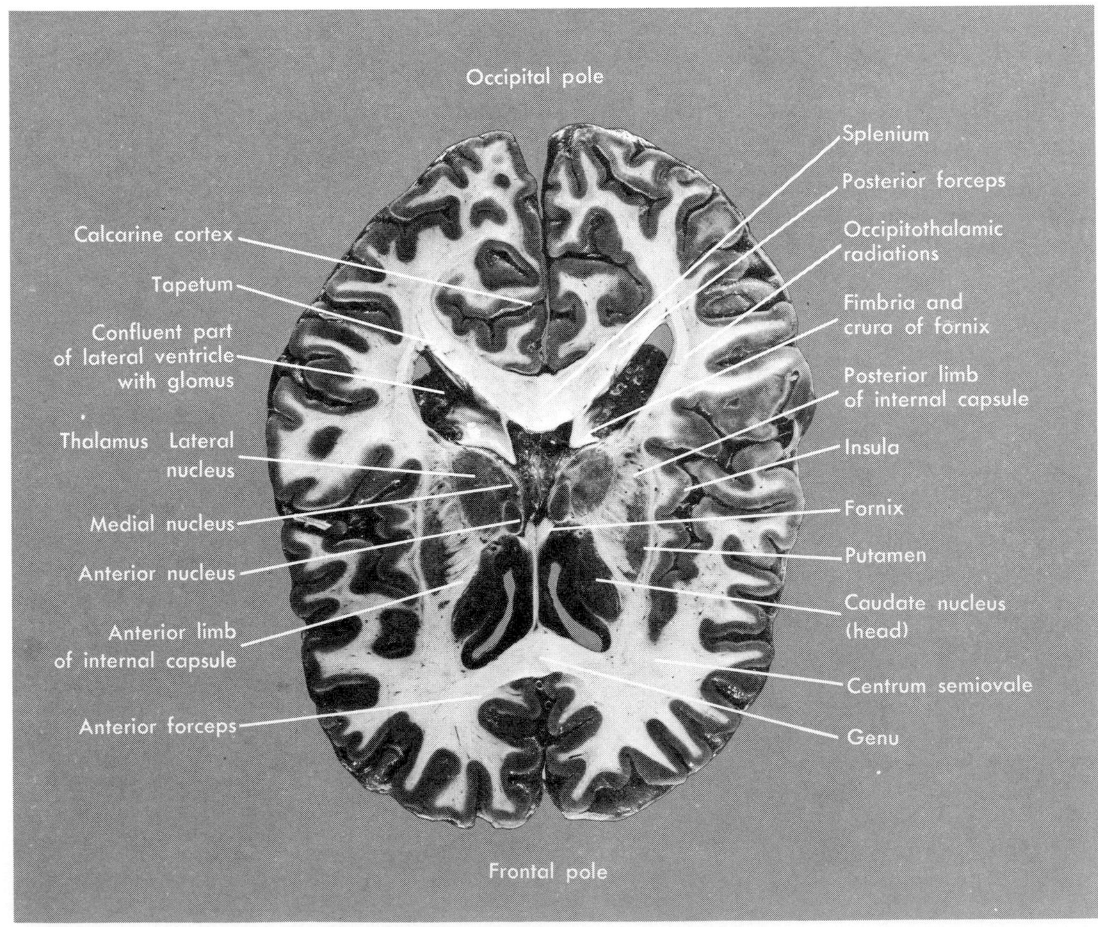

Fig. 4-19. Transverse plane through glomus.

teriorly along the lateral wall of the posterior horn of the lateral ventricle (Fig. 4-20). The tapetum underlies the *occipitothalamic radiations* and projections and is equally apparent in transverse sections (Fig. 4-25). The posterior continuation of the fibers of the corpus callosum form the *posterior forceps.* These fibers are not unlike the fibers of the same source at the genu that form the anterior forceps (Fig. 4-25).

The *cerebellar notch* is prominent at this level and peaks into the area of the *pineal body.* Here the internal cerebral and basal vessels converge to the *great vein of Galen* and thence to the straight sinus. The bulk of cerebral surface at this level is parietal, but some precentral tissue may be included in this section. The extremity of the Sylvian fissure is reached here, and parts of both supramarginal and angular gyri occur along the lateral surface. The continuity of choroid plexus from body to inferior horn is apparent in this section (left). Frequently the plexus exhibits cystic change at this level, and vessels are cavernous (*glomus of the choroid*) (Fig. 4-19). The arterial relationships continue in the manner described in previous levels.

Plane through the occipital lobes (Fig. 4-20)

The topographic relationship of the two lobes displays the cerebellar notch. The *posterior horn of the lateral ventricle* occupies this level and is devoid of choroid plexus. The bulge of the infolding calcarine fissure produces the *calcar avis* in the medial wall of the horn. The lateral border of the ventricle is covered by tapetum that is the extension of the corpus callosum. Lateral to this is the occipitothalamic bundle, including optic radiations. The visual cortex is oriented around the calcarine fissure and is distinguished grossly by inclusion of the pale thin *line of Gennari.*

TRANSVERSE SECTIONS OF FOREBRAIN

For the objectives of this book four transverse section levels of the forebrain are reviewed in the following sections. Other transverse views are mainly described in the legends of the illustrations.

Plane through the level above corpus callosum (Fig. 4-21)

This section shows the derivation of the term *centrum semiovale* in the central half-oval of white

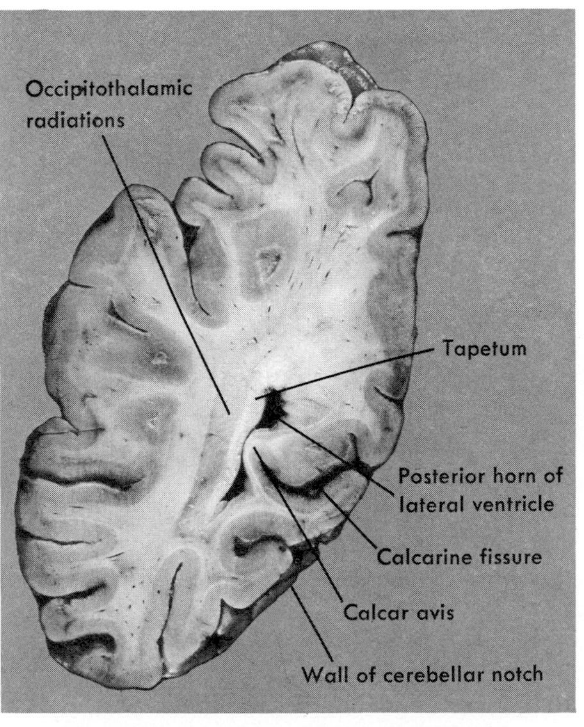

Fig. 4-20. Coronal plane through occipital lobe.

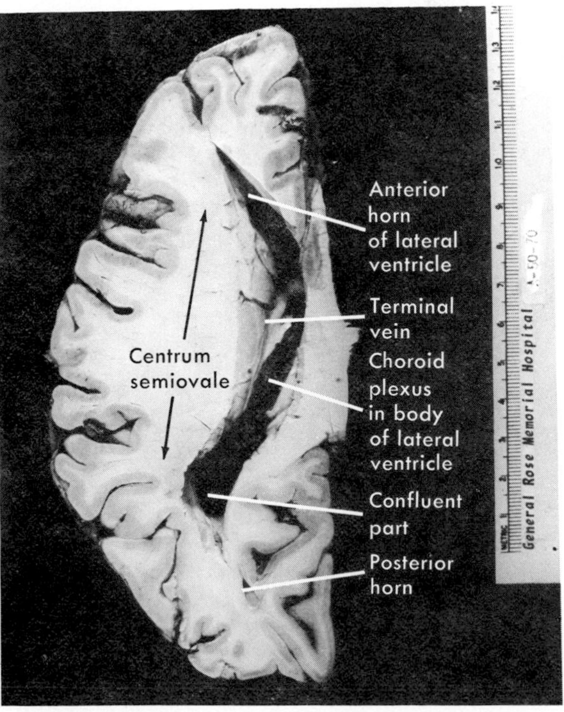

Fig. 4-21. Transverse level above corpus callosum showing contour of lateral ventricle.

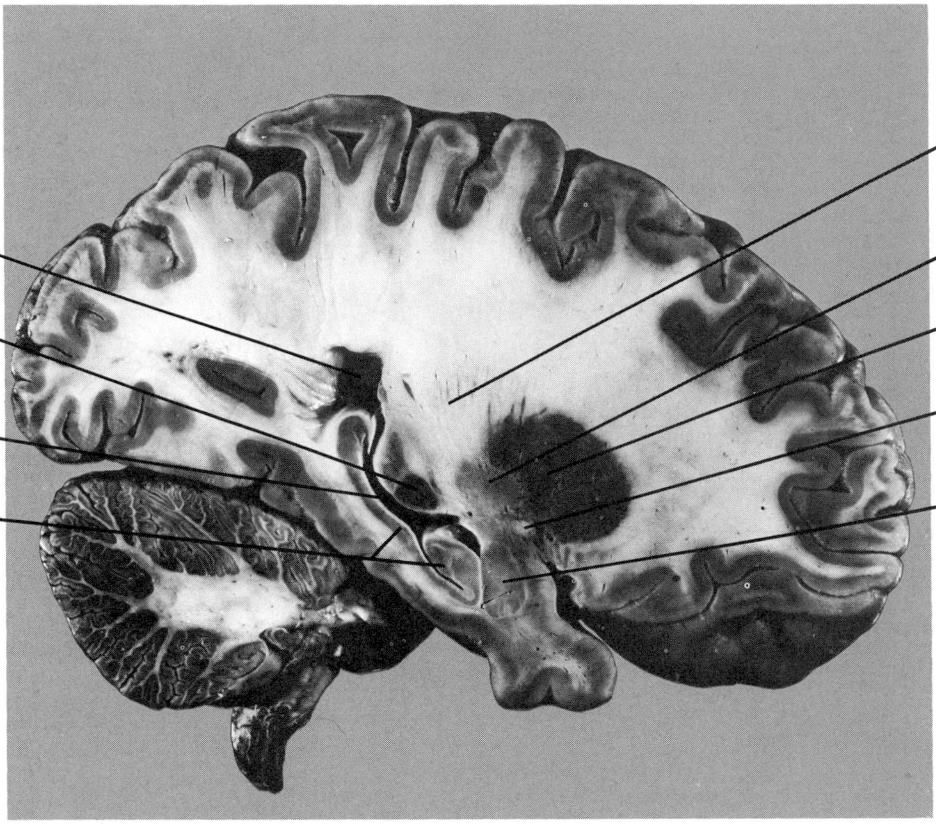

Internal capsule projecting upward as corona radiata

Globus pallidus

Basal nuclei (putamen)

Anterior commissure

Amygdaloid nucleus

Confluent part of lateral ventricle

Lateral geniculate body

Temporal horn of fourth ventricle

Hippocampus

Fig. 4-22. Lateral parasagittal plane showing corona radiata sweeping upward internal capsule.

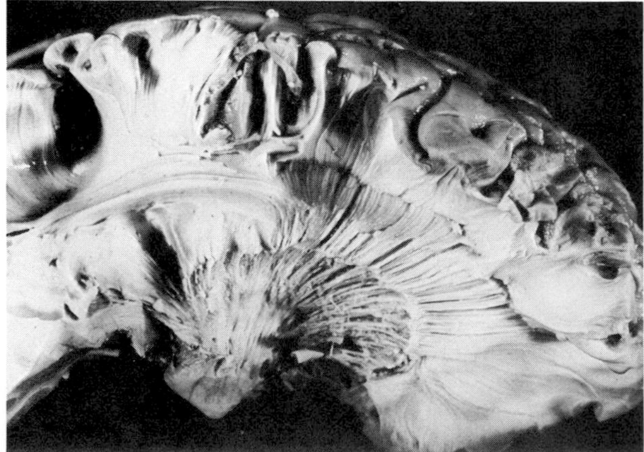

Fig. 4-23. Lateral dissection showing continuity of capsular fibers with peduncle and with cortex via corona.

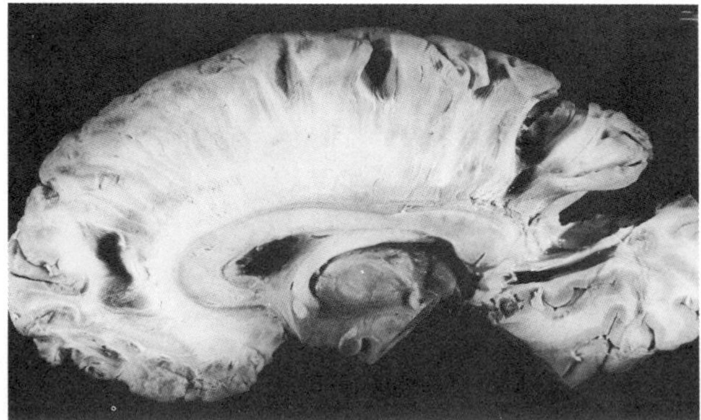

Fig. 4-24. Medial dissection showing sweep of callosal fibers upward to cortex. (Compare with Figs. 4-19, 4-25, and 4-26 for views of forceps.)

matter. The interdigitations of corpus callosum fibers with internal capsule are in this field but are not discernible without dissection (Fig. 4-22). The projecting *corona radiata* can best be seen in a lateral dissection (Fig. 4-23). The sweep of the corpus callosum is displayed in a dissection of the vertex and from a superior view (Fig. 4-24). The principal sulci and fissures are identified in **Fig. 4-19**. In Fig. 4-21 the left side the roof of the lateral ventricle has been lifted away to show the *stria terminalis* and *vena terminalis*. The course of attachment of the choroid plexus follows from the confluent part of the lateral ventricle to the interventricular foramen, as shown.

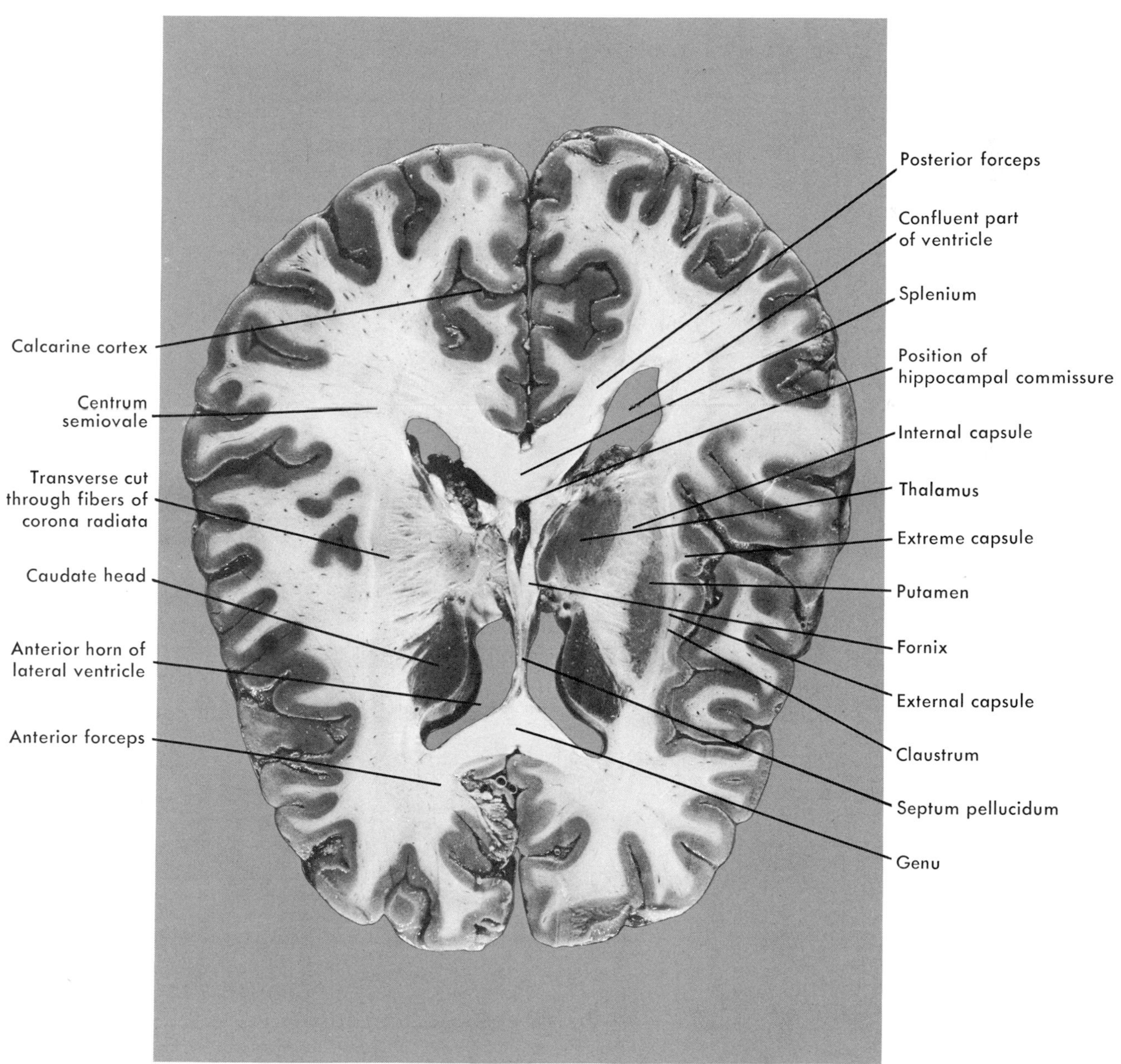

Fig. 4-25. Transverse level through genu and splenium.

Plane through the genu and splenium of the corpus callosum (Fig. 4-25)

The *anterior and posterior forceps* show clearly in the pincer outline of genu and splenium, respectively, as their fibers project to the related poles. The ventricular contour presents the divergent anterior horns marked by the lateral bulges of the caudate head. Posteriorly, the confluent part of the ventricle shows the line of the choroid. Anteriorly separating the ventricles is the *septum pellucidum.* The course of the two fornices that continue to the fimbria is apparent near the midline. As the fornices separate into the two pillars (*crura*), the fibers of the hippocampal commissure cross between them to form the *psalterium* (harp). The formation of the tapetum is well displayed by comparing the two sides. The posterior forceps on the left of the picture continues over the posterior horn of the ventricle. On the right, it forms the lamina of the tapetum as it follows the lateral contour of the horn medial to the occipitothalamic radiations. Both sides reveal the origination of the internal capsule in the fibers of the centrum semiovale. On the right, the capsule is starting to pass between thalamus, medially, and putamen, laterally, as the beginning of the posterior limb. Similarly, the anterior limb is beginning to divide the telencephalic *basal nuclei* into caudate head and putamen. The *external capsule* and *extreme capsule* are splitting over the *claustrum,* on the right. The cortical fields display the distinctive fissural pattern of the *calcarine area,* posteriorly, and the Sylvian fissure and insula, on the right side. The small gyri adjacent to the splenium mark the *isthmic portion of the limbic lobe.* They are continuous with the gyrus cinguli over the corpus callosum and with the hippocampal gyrus into the temporal lobe. Note the vessels of the anterior cerebral complex in the anterior part of the median sagittal fissure, the middle cerebral arteries in the Sylvian fis-

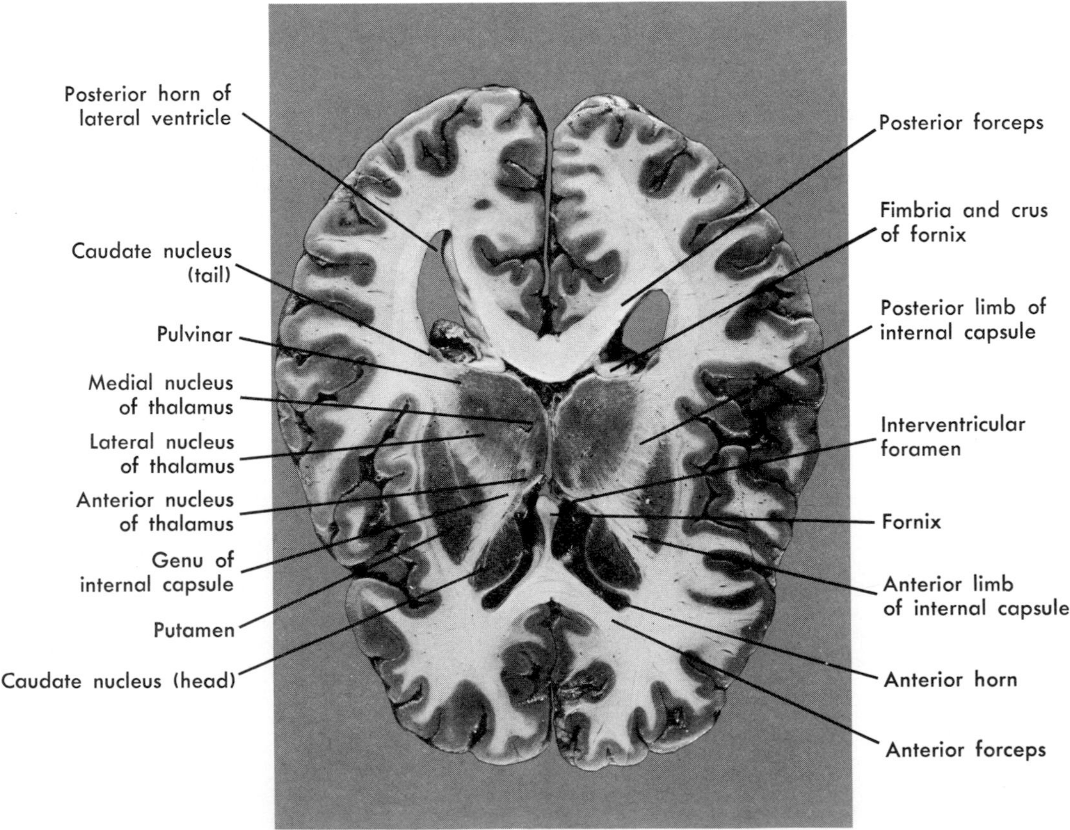

Fig. 4-26. Transverse level through interventricular foramen.

sure, and the posterior cerebral arteries in the posterior median sagittal fissure. (See Figs. 3-20 and 3-21 for relationship of distributions.)

Plane through the level of the interventricular foramen (Fig. 4-26)

This section displays the contour of the ventricular system from the posterior extremity of the third ventricle through the *interventricular foramen* to the end of the anterior horn. The fused fornices and the septum separate the ventricular bodies, and the extensions diverge into frontal lobes with the widening genu of the corpus callosum. The posterior horns are located between the calcarine gray mass and the occipitothalamic projections from the retrolenticular part of the capsule. The *caudate tail* is related to the anterolateral wall at the confluent part. At this level the *anterior* and *posterior limbs* of the internal capsule show clearly. The *genu of the capsule* is closely related to the anterior nucleus of the thalamus. This shows the subdivisions of thalamus proper to good advantage, and the *anterior, lateral, medial,* and *posterior (pulvinar)* parts are definable. Note the direct relationship of posterior thalamus to occipitothalamic fibers of the retrolenticular capsule and the direct association of posterior limb to occipitoparietal cortex. Similarly, the direct relationship of frontal cortex and anterior limb is apparent.

The familiar sectional contour of the telencephalic *basal nuclei* (claustrum, putamen, globus pallidus) are well displayed underlying the insula in Fig. 4-27. The extent of the cerebral cortex and the proportion buried are well displayed at this level.

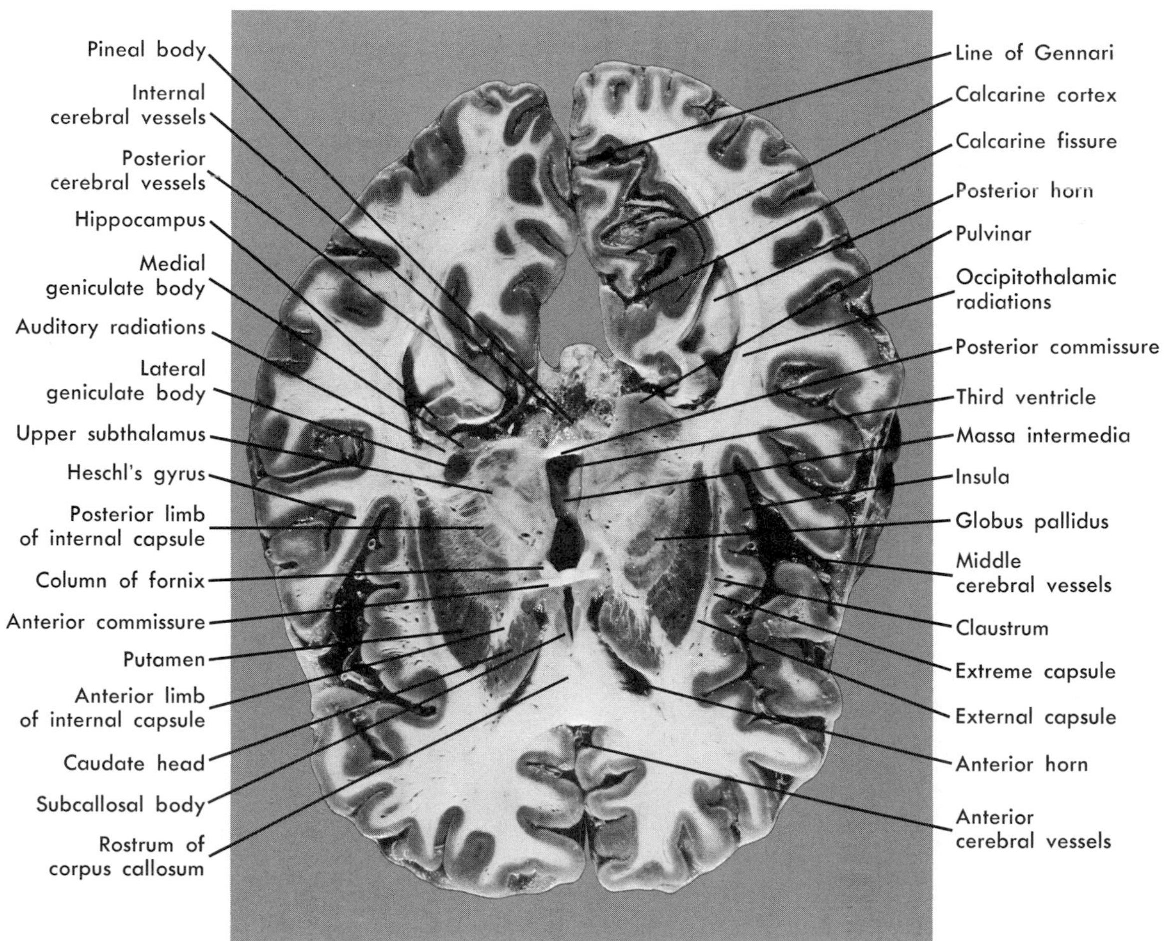

Fig. 4-27. Basal nuclei in transverse section.

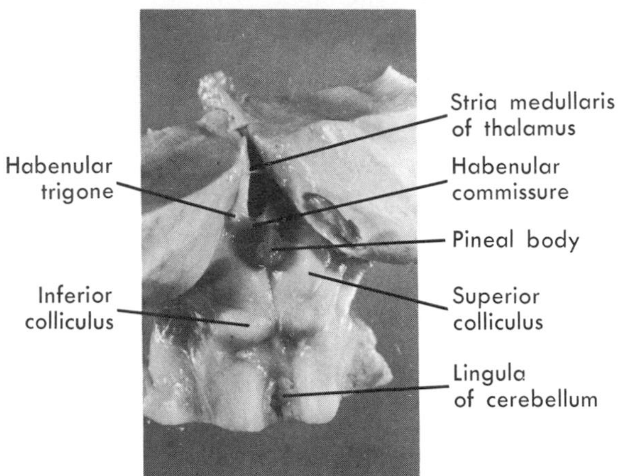

Fig. 4-28. Habenular complex, dorsal view.

The identity of the convolutions frequently requires tagging in side view because of the irregular courses of the sulci and fissures. The *calcarine complex* is identified by the *line of Gennari* as well as by location. The Sylvian fissure is unmistakable because of size and relationship to the island of Reil. Frequently the central sulcus of Rolando is less easily identified, and a lateral section must be made. The pineal body and the habenular complex frequently show well in this level but require magnification for clarity (Fig. 4-28).

Plane through the anterior and posterior commissures (Fig. 4-29)

The central depths of the third ventricle are bridged by the *massa intermedia.* Immediately underlying the *posterior commissure* is the continuation of the ventricle, leading into the *cerebral aqueduct* (see also Fig. 4-12). The relationship of the *columns of the fornices* and the *anterior commissure*

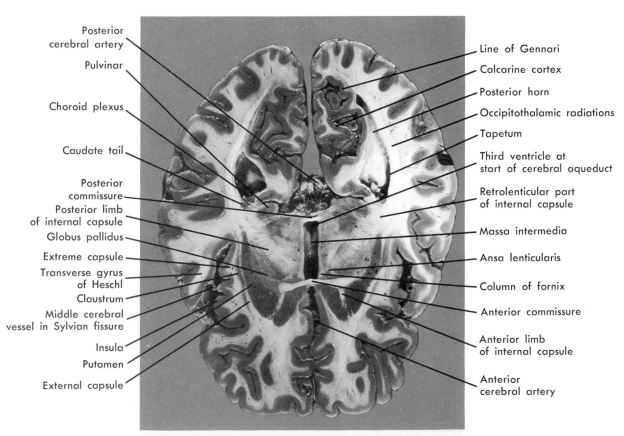

Fig. 4-29. Transverse plane through anterior and posterior commissures.

is shown better in Fig. 4-27. Note that the commissure passes just below the anterior limb of the capsule, near the genu. This establishes a close relationship between the commissure and the *ansa lenticularis,* which also passes downward, medially, and posteriorly around the capsule and enters the subthalamus and midbrain underlying this level. The thalamic peduncle is also funneled into the subthalamus and midbrain near this point, but it is seen better in other views (Fig. 4-10). The *pulvinar* shows well at this level. The *metathalamus* is displayed better at a slightly lower level (Fig. 4-30). Here the *optic radiations* from the lateral geniculate body join the occipitothalamic tracts, en route to the calcarine cortex. The *auditory radiations* from the medial geniculate body pass in the sublenticular part of the internal capsule to *Heschl's gyri* in the temporal lobe. Returning projections from the cortex to the thalamus and midbrain follow the same route. Vascular and cerebral markings continue the same relationships described for the preceding level.

The continuity of fiber traffic is shown in Fig. 4-11, which is cut through the transverse sections just shown. Note that this plane through the forebrain lies between coronal and transverse sections, in order to display the fiber continuity in the long axis of the brainstem.

PARASAGITTAL SECTIONS

Parasagittal planes are difficult to cut uniformly in gross material because of their size and the tendency for parts to fall away. They are perhaps best studied in large Weigert preparations. Considerable information is available however from unstained gross parasagittal planes, as illustrated in the two following levels. Note that the descriptive material applies to substantial plane depth and is suited

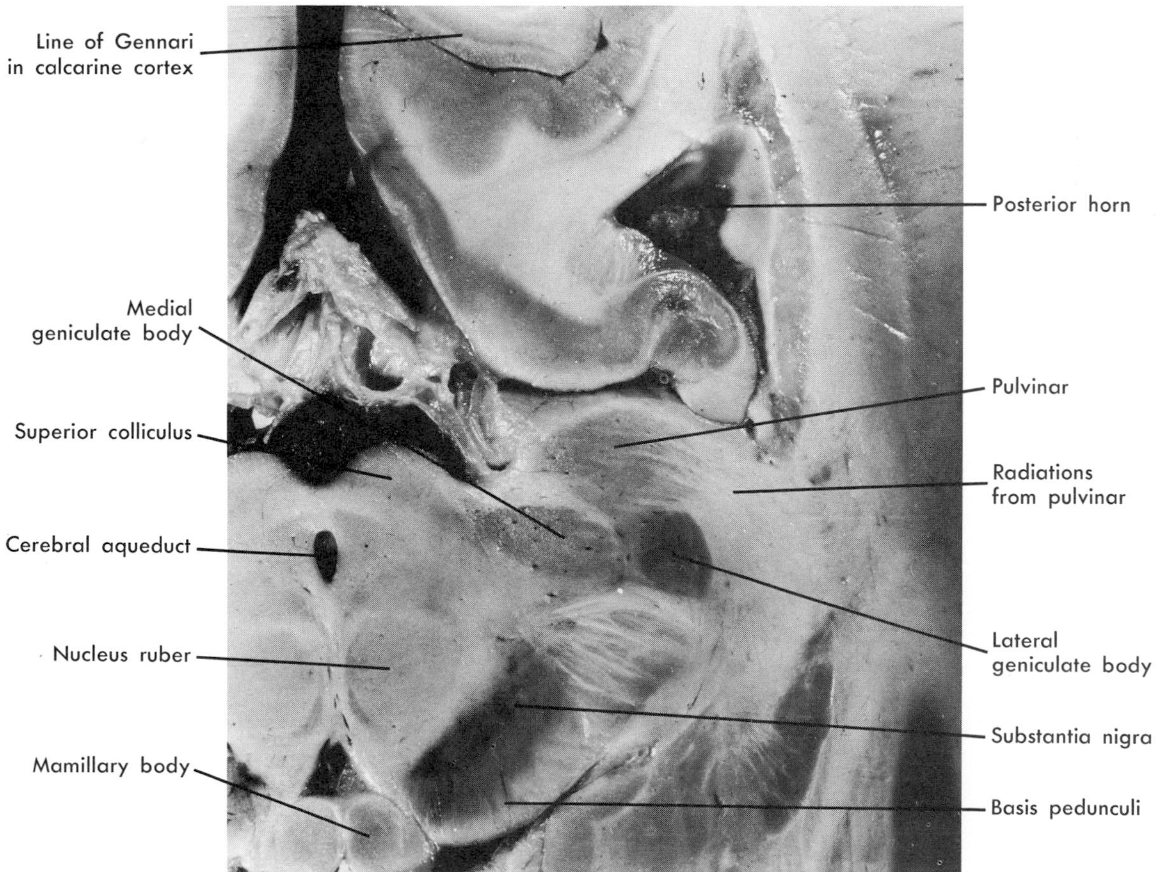

Fig. 4-30. Metathalamus and upper midbrain.

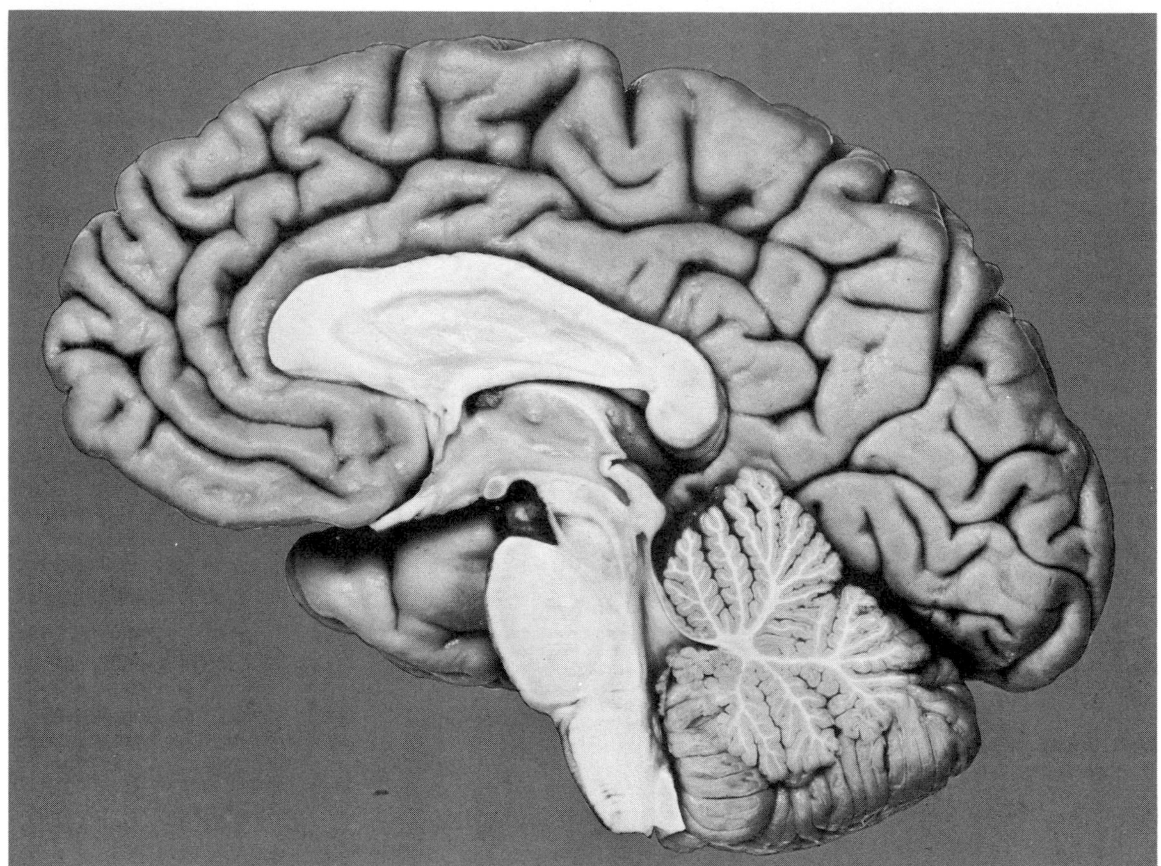

Fig. 4-31. Slightly parasagittal plane to left of midline.

to ranges of 4 to 6 mm. from midline in the first plane and from 7 to 10 mm. from midline in the second. The variation depends upon the size and conformation of the brain and upon variations inherent in sectioning. Fig. 4-31, cut just slightly to the left of midline (through the mamillary body), is included for comparison. The septum pellucidum is intact.

Plane 4 to 6 mm. from midsagittal plane
(Fig. 4-32)

The gyral pattern does not usually contribute significantly in this plane. The *corpus callosum* and its relationship to the body of the fornix is well displayed. The position of the *hippocampal commissure* in transverse section between the posterior columns of the fornix shows well beneath the splenium. The *anterior commissure* and the *anterior column of the fornix* are prominent, and this plane will frequently display the fornix reaching to the mamillary body. The course of the *mamillothalamic fasciculus* and the nuclear subdivisions of the *thalamus* are clarified further in this plane. Of particular note here is the *pretectal region,* which lies dorsal to the nucleus ruber and superior to the quadrigeminal bodies of the tectum. The tracts in the stem are difficult to delineate in unstained specimen. The *superior cerebellar peduncle* and its relationship to cerebellar nuclei are displayed in Fig. 4-33. The complex fiber traffic through the pons stands out clearly, and some of the tracts of the pontine tegmentum are differentiated in this view. The *inferior olive* is clearly in view, and the prominence of the *nucleus cuneatus* identifies this cell cluster (Fig. 4-32).

Plane 7 to 10 mm. from midline
(Figs. 4-33 and 4-34)

As in the first parasagittal plane, little is revealed in this level that contributes to the structural de-

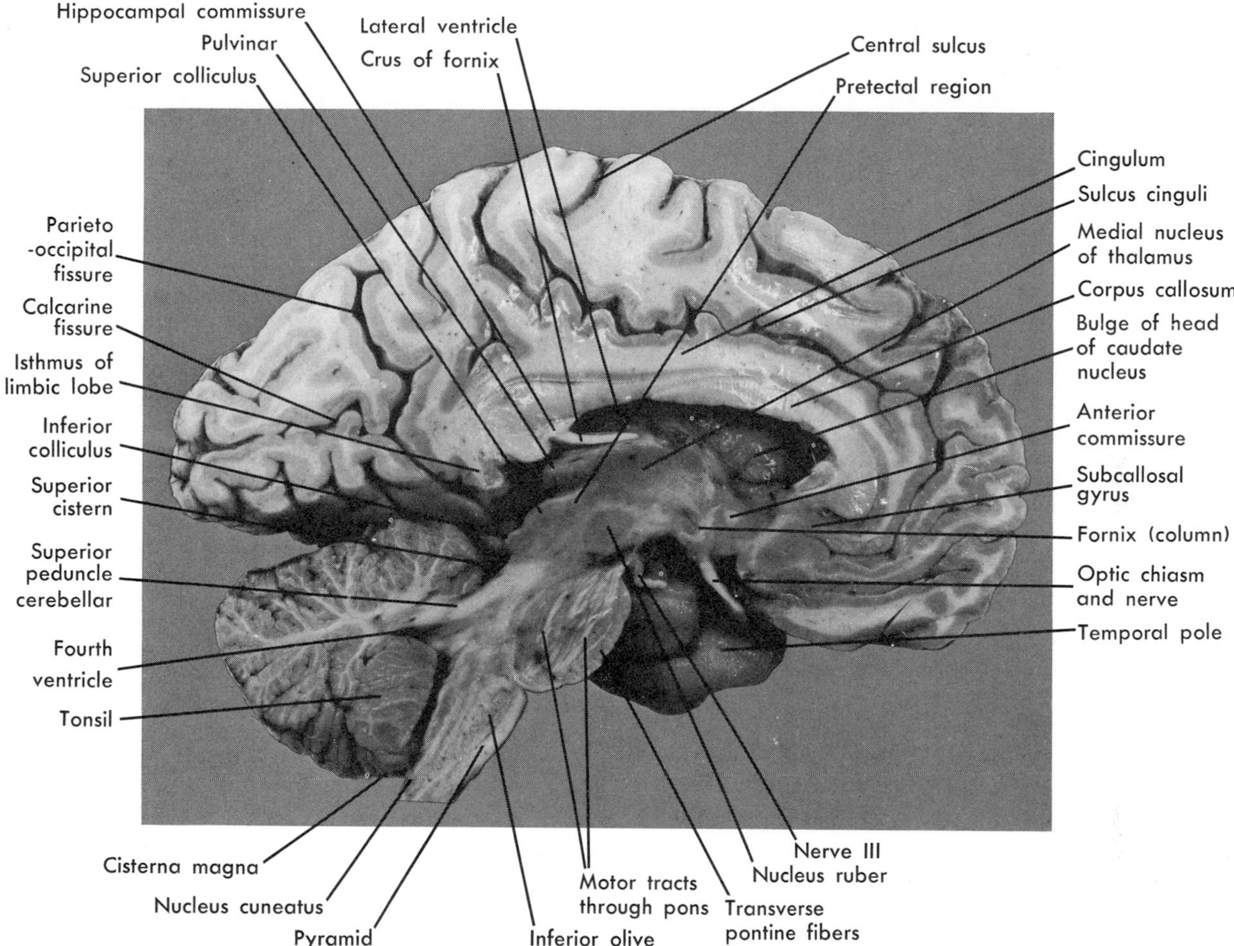

Fig. 4-32. Parasagittal plane 4 to 6 mm. off midline.

tails of the cortex and gyral patterns. The corpus callosum remains well delineated in all its parts, and the *crus of the fornix* attaches to the undersurface of its splenium. Familiar landmarks permit identification of the *caudate head,* which rises into the anterior part of the lateral ventricular floor. The anterior commissure stands out clearly, and normally the fibers of the *thalamic peduncle* are distinct behind it. The *ansa lenticularis* passes in a posterior direction immediately above the diverging fibers of the basis pedunculi. This tract enters the pretectal region and the area of the *nucleus ruber, subthalamic body,* and *substantia nigra.* The posterior extension of the thalamus into the pulvinar is well shown. Both the *superior colliculus* and its brachium are usually displayed well. The lateral part of inferior colliculus or its brachium may be evident. The *lateral lemniscus* comes prominently to view as it comes into relationship with the dorsal part of the basis of the pons. The lateral lemniscus usually reappears in this plane below the *superior cerebellar peduncle* (brachium conjunctivum), which crosses it medially at the level of the middle of the pons. Remnants of the *dentate nucleus* are evident in the cerebellum at this level. The belly of the pons is prominently subdivided by the fascicles of the *corticospinal tracts* that extend from the basis pedunculi. While tracts in the lower medulla are hard to discern in the fresh brain, the topography of the *inferior cerebellar peduncle* (corpus restiforme) is well displayed. The plane in Fig. 4-35 passes laterally to the inferior olive. This shows the continuity of the internal capsule, basis pedunculi, and pontine fibers. A more lateral plane is shown in Fig. 3-5 for the contour of the inferior horn.

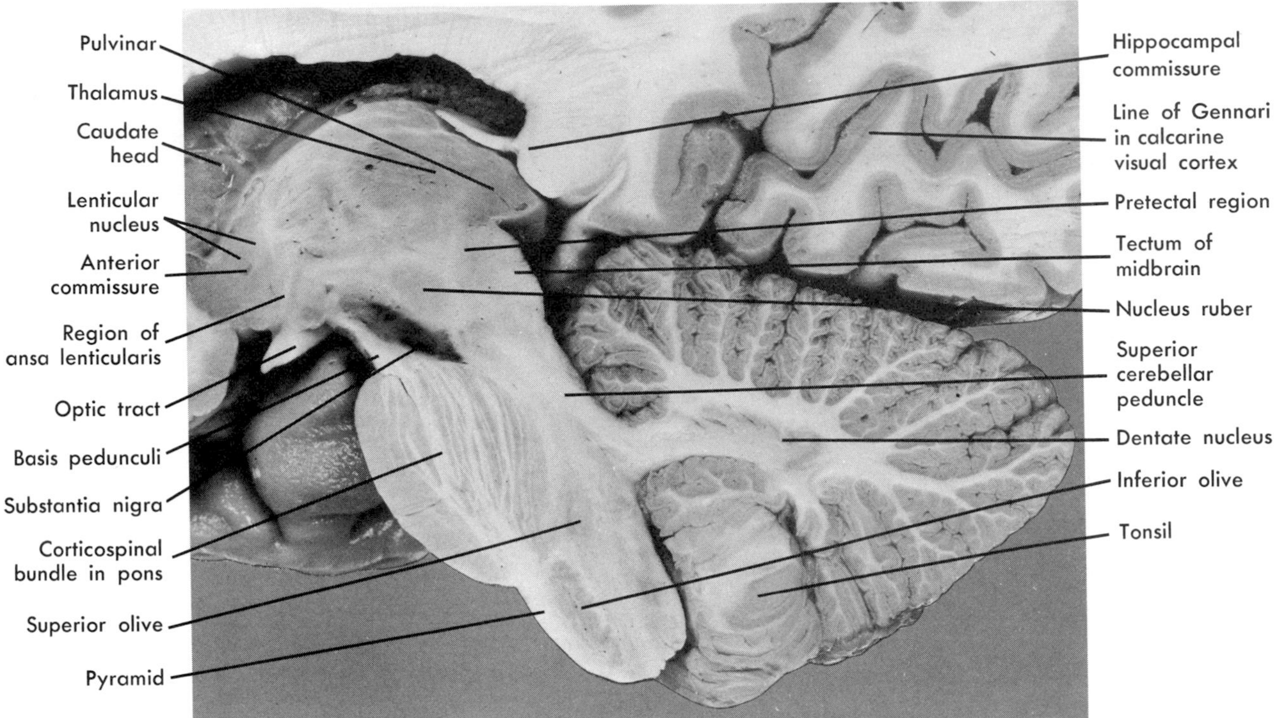

Fig. 4-33. Parasagittal plane, enlarged, 7 to 10 mm. off midline.

TRANSVERSE SECTIONS OF BRAINSTEM

Seven levels of the brainstem are utilized to display the major anatomy.

Plane through the level of the superior colliculus (Fig. 4-36)

Transverse section at this level of the brainstem displays the two uppermost posterior projections of the corpora quadrigemina, the *superior colliculi,* which are major midbrain relay stations functioning primarily in the visual pathway. Immediately lateral to the superior colliculus on either side is the *medial geniculate body* and varying representations of the *brachium* of the inferior colliculus. This brachium interconnects the inferior colliculus and the medial geniculate body (Fig. 4-16). This complex is the main midbrain and diencephalic way station for impulses traveling the auditory pathways. A coronal plane through the *cerebral aqueduct* of Sylvius and periaqueductal gray matter defines the *tectum* dorsally and the *tegmentum* ventrally. The *oculomotor nuclear* density appears faintly anterior to the aqueduct. Filaments of the *oculomotor nerve* (cranial III) traverse this section from the nucleus to the *interpeduncular fossa.* The *nucleus ruber* stands out clearly on either side in unstained sections, as does the dark *substantia nigra.* The *basis pedunculi* (cerebral peduncle) is clearly defined apart from the tegmentum as the continuing white fibers of the internal capsule. In the unstained specimen, it is impossible to clearly define the many functionally separate fascicles running longitudinally in the white matter. At the highest levels, the mamillary bodies are closely apposed to the interpeduncular walls.

Plane through the level of the inferior colliculus and upper pons (Fig. 4-37)

At this level the tectum contains, in addition to the aqueductal and periaqueductal tissue, the *inferior colliculi,* their dorsally coursing *commissure,* and the faintly visible *lateral lemnisci.* The last, as the main ascending auditory pathways, come into relationship with the inferior colliculi at this level. The *brachium of the inferior colliculus* (Fig. 4-16) usually produces a visible ridge in the lateral midbrain sulcus at this level. The nuclear masses that are the origin of the *trochlear* nerves (cranial IV) are faintly visible in the anterior periaqueductal gray matter. These nerves turn dorsally to

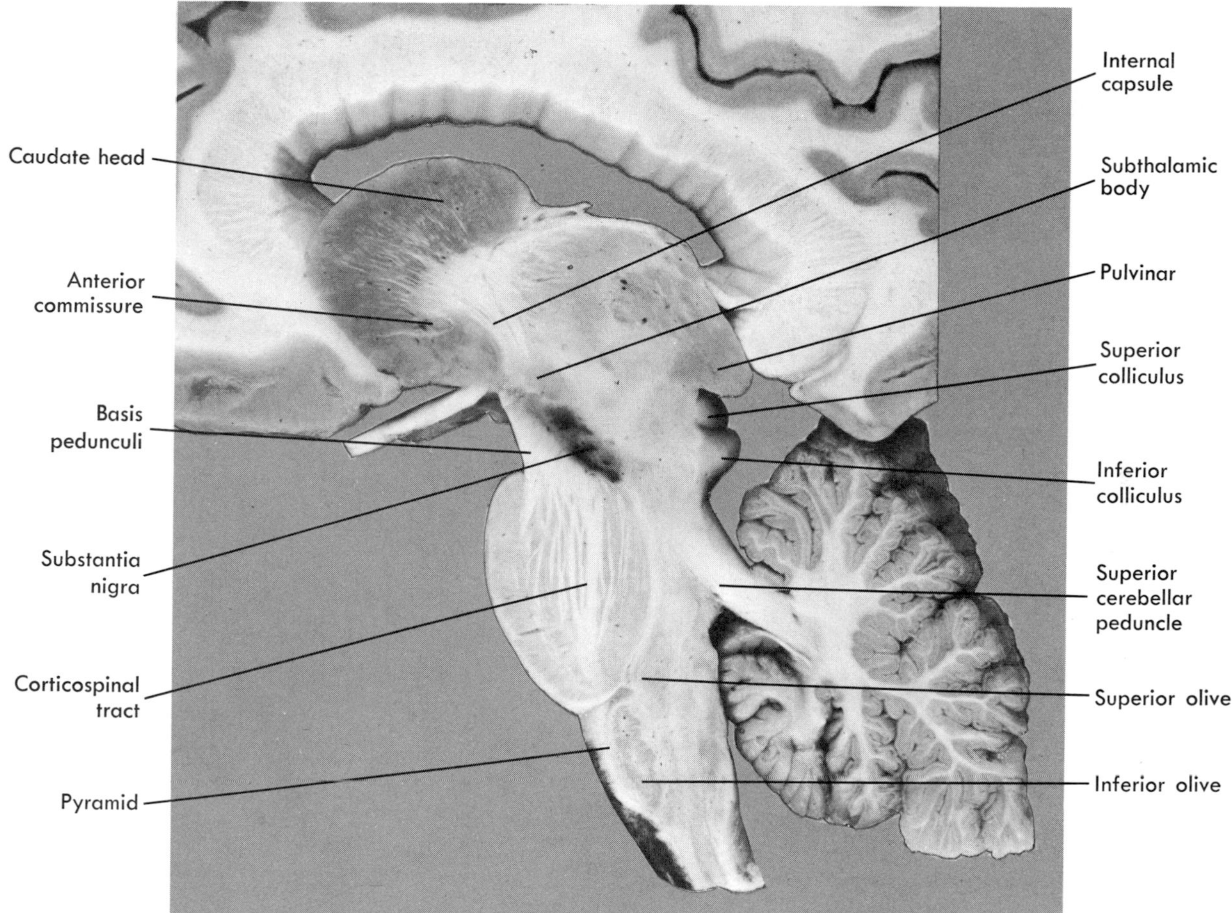

Fig. 4-34. Parasagittal plane of brainstem, 7 to 10 mm. off midline.

exit on either side of the dorsum of the midbrain, just below the inferior colliculi. Frequently, the *posterior recess* of the interpeduncular fossa is included in this section. The *decussation of the brachium conjunctivum* (superior cerebellar peduncle) stands out as a mass of fibers in the central tegmentum. The tegmentum carries fibers from the cerebellar dentate nucleus to the nucleus ruber and beyond. The *basis pontis* is disrupted by crossing *pontine fibers* that become more dense as the pons is more deeply transected.

Plane through the level of the trigeminal nerve (Fig. 4-38)

At this level the aqueduct is widened into the upper part of the *fourth ventricle*. The cavity formed is roofed by the anterior (superior) medullary velum and is bordered laterally on either side by the *brachium conjunctivum*. The tegmentum at this level contains many longitudinal bundles that are difficult to delineate in unstained sections. The *basis pontis* has unusual bulk at this level. The *brachium pontis* stands out prominently as the middle cerebellar peduncle, which conveys fibers from the pons to cerebellar cortex of the opposite side. The crossing of these fibers in the midline produces a fibrous mass (*median raphe*). *Cranial nerve V* penetrates the brachium pontis and is grossly visible as it runs transversely to terminate near gray masses (nerve V nuclei). At this level the longitudinal *corticospinal* and *corticobulbar* bundles (continuous with the basis pedunculi above) stand out clearly in the unstained pons. The smaller *lemnisci* (medial, lateral) and *longitudinal fasciculi* are less clear in the unstained specimen.

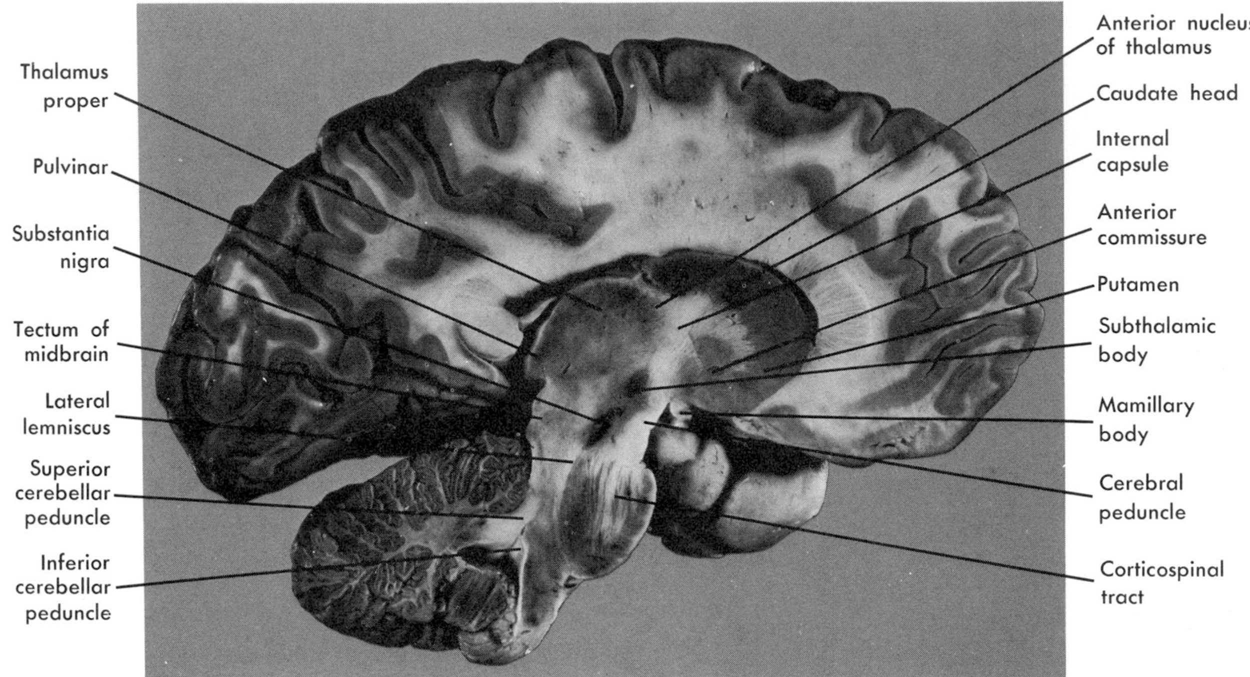

Fig. 4-35. Parasagittal plane, 7 to 10 mm. off midline.

Plane through the level of the lower pons through the superior olive (Fig. 4-39)

At this level the fourth ventricle is wider than above. The marginal *brachium conjunctivum* is more dorsally placed. Note that both *brachium pontis* and *corpus restiforme* are evident; thus all *three peduncles of the cerebellum* appear in the same plane. At the junction of tegmentum and basis pontis, a robust transverse bundle pattern is grossly evident. This pattern comprises the *trapezoid body,* an important part of the auditory pathway. Near the lateral extremities of, and slightly dorsal to, the trapezoid body are bilateral gray, wrinkled areas representing the *superior olivary complex,* a nuclear group important in the auditory system. In the unstained specimen it is usually possible to discern the *genu* (knee) of the *facial nerve* (cranial VII), lying in a medial position to the nucleus of the *abducens* nerve (cranial VI). Filaments of nerve VII can be seen passing from the nucleus of nerve VII toward the genu. Filaments of the nerve VI dorsoventrally cross the tegmentum on their way to exit immediately below the bulge of the pons. The corticospinal tracts are better described at this level as a definitive longitudinal bundle, mixed into the transversely oriented pontocerebellar fibers.

Plane through the level of cochlear nuclei and acoustic nerve (Fig. 4-40)

This plane includes the junction of metencephalon (pons) and myelencephalon (medulla). It is particularly important in the study of the auditory pathway, as it includes the *dorsal and ventral cochlear nuclei.* The dorsal nucleus elevates the floor of the fourth ventricle, producing the *acoustic tubercle.* The acoustic nerve (cranial VIII) attaches at the sides and grossly divides over the *corpus restiforme.* The *vestibular* division runs deep to the inferior peduncle (corpus restiforme) and the *cochlear* division, which are external to it both laterally and dorsally. Nuclei of nerves V, VIII (vestibular), and IX occupy the line of gray matter medial to the corpus restiforme that extends almost to midline in the floor of the fourth ventricle. Note that the ventricle opens into the *lateral apertures of Luschka* at this level. The upper part of the *inferior olive* frequently shows at this level. The pyramids form from the corticospinal tracts.

Plane through the midolive (Fig. 4-41)

The dominant features in unstained specimens at this level are the *inferior olives* and their accessory nuclei. The *pyramids* are distinctly outlined

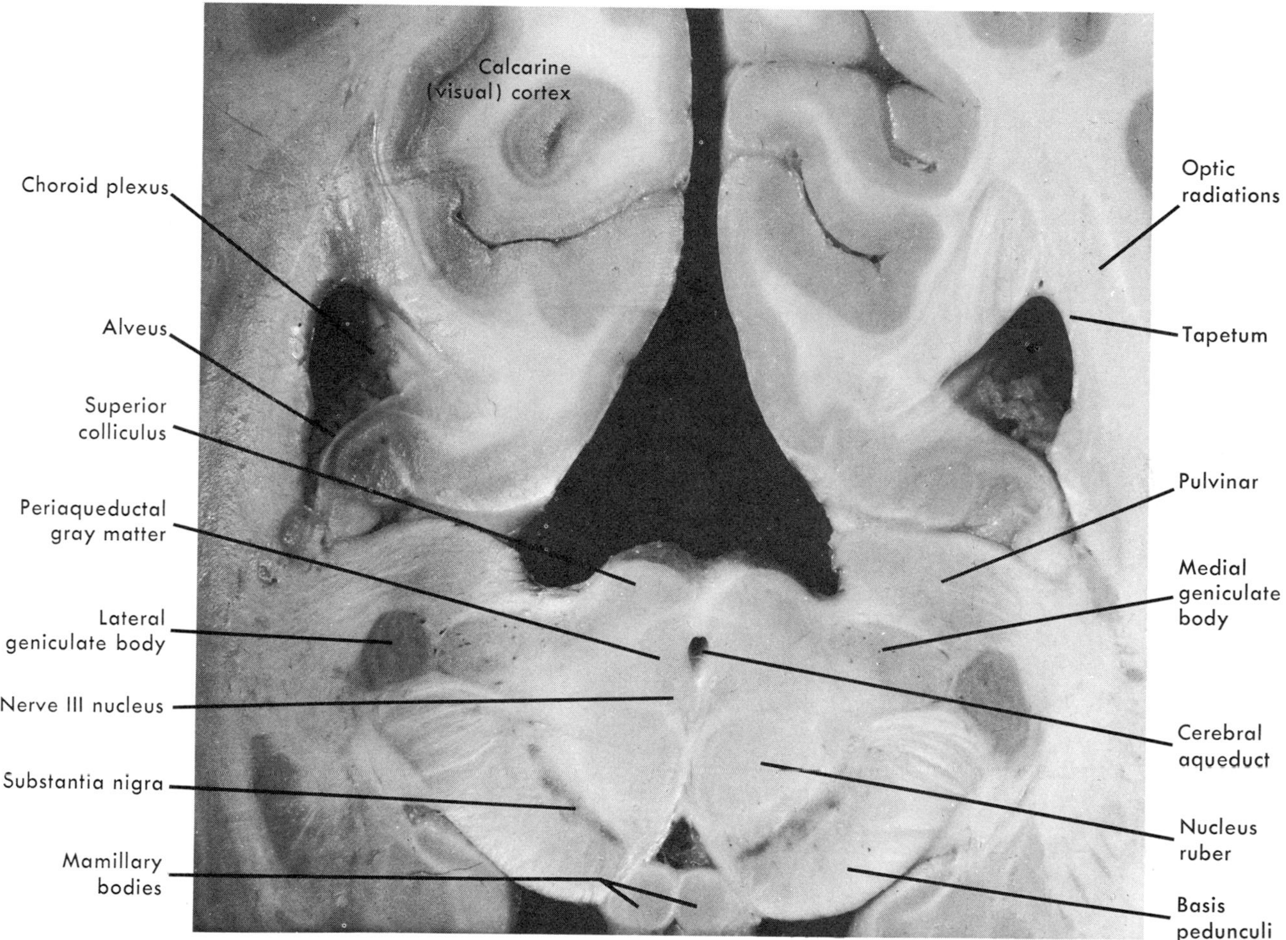

Fig. 4-36. Transverse section through upper midbrain (superior colliculus).

on either side of the *anterior median fissure.* The *solitary fasciculus* stands out clearly, and the *dorsal vagal nucleus* produces a bulge in the floor of the fourth ventricle dorsolateral to the hypoglossal nuclear mass. Depending on the level, the upper extension of the *nuclei* of the *posterior funiculi* (cuneatus and gracilis) of the spinal cord may be visible medial to the corpus restiforme.

Plane through the level of decussation of pyramids (Fig. 4-42)

Below the inferior olives the pyramids begin decussating most of their bulk. This moves the *corticospinal tracts* in most part to a dorsolateral position. The fourth ventricle is replaced by a central canal, and the cross-sectional contour is more like that of the spinal cord. Nuclear groups that are grossly evident are the *anterior gray matter,* upward extension of *substantia gelatinosa* (spinal cranial nerve V nucleus), nucleus *cuneatus,* and nucleus *gracilis.* The anterior *median fissure* and the *dorsal median septum* are grossly visible. Because these features show poorly in unstained photos, an enlarged drawing is provided (Fig. 2-27, *B*).

SECTIONAL ANATOMY—CEREBELLUM

Transverse section at the level of the fastigium (Fig. 4-43)

A transverse section of the cerebellum advantageously displays the roof nuclei, including the *fastigial, globosal,* and *emboliform* group and the *dentate nucleus.* The efferent fibers passing from the cerebellum arise in these nuclei (see also Figs. 2-23 and 4-37 to 4-41 and Chapter 22).

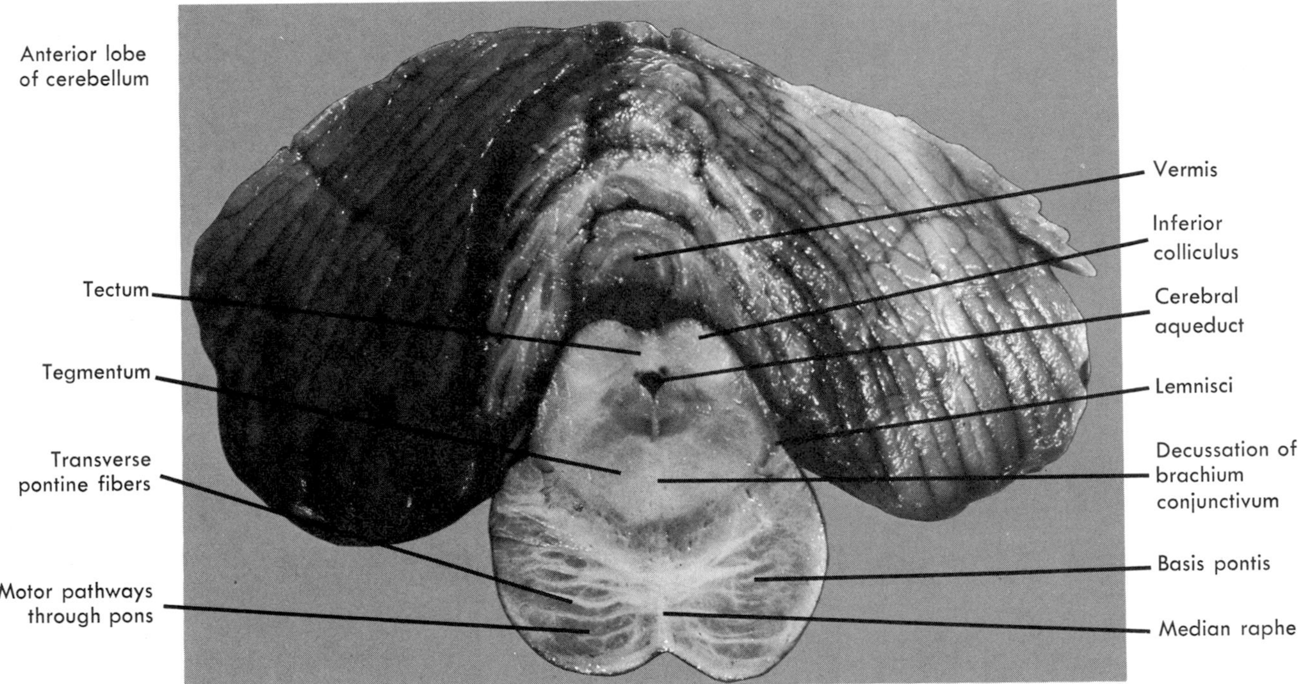

Fig. 4-37. Transverse section through inferior colliculus.

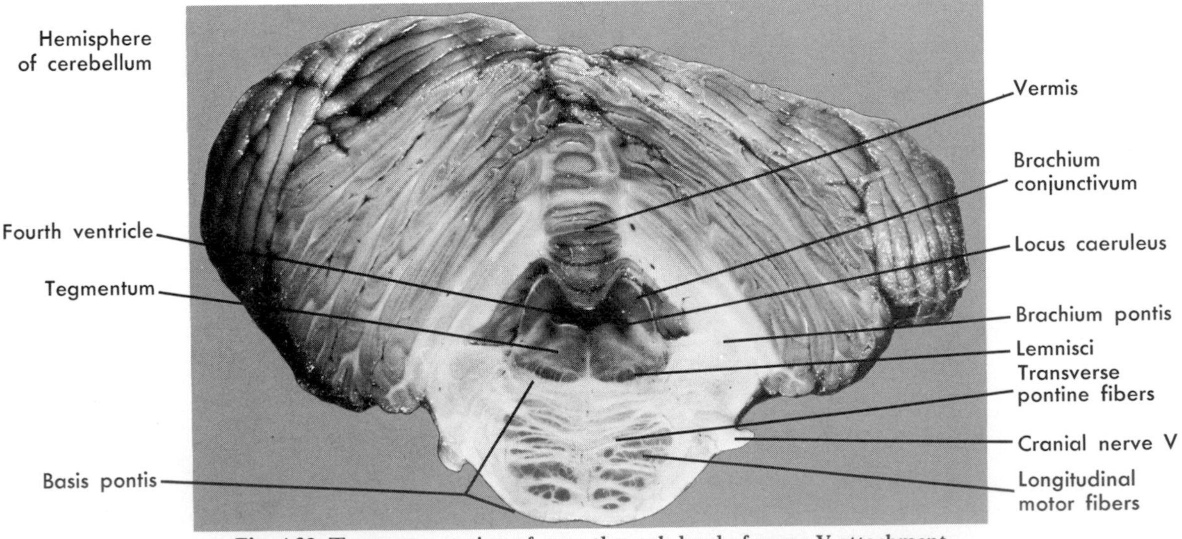

Fig. 4-38. Transverse section of pons through level of nerve V attachment.

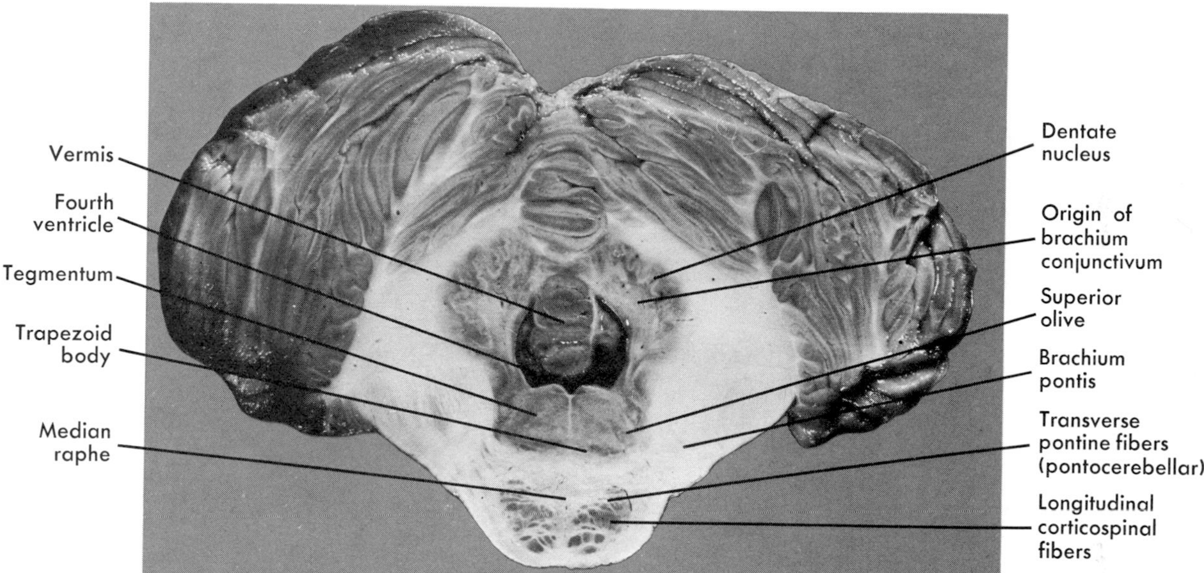

Fig. 4-39. Transverse section of lower pons through level of superior olive.

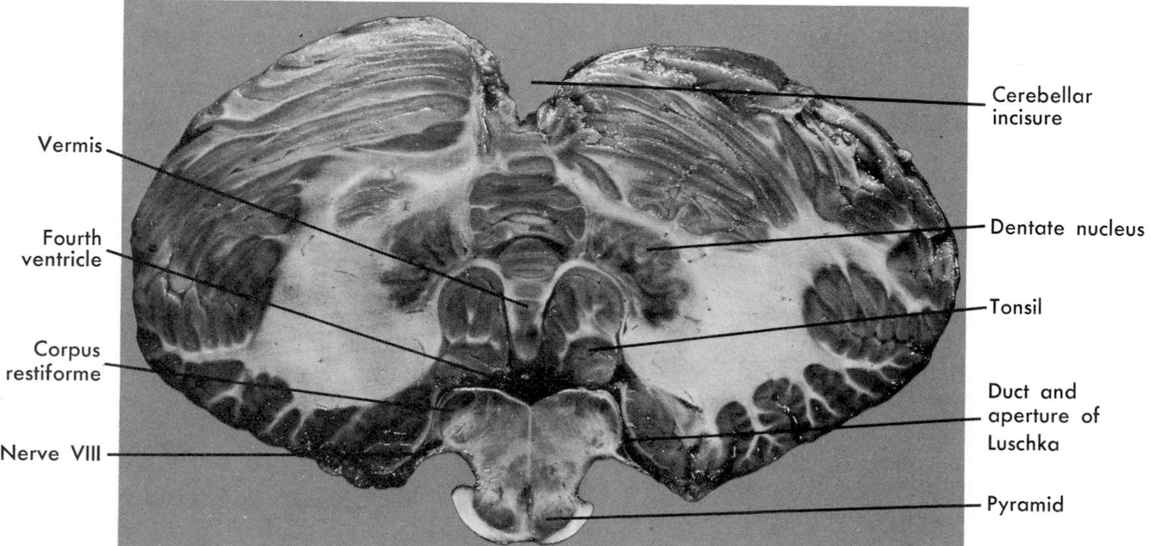

Fig. 4-40. Transverse section through medulla at the level of the cochlear nuclei.

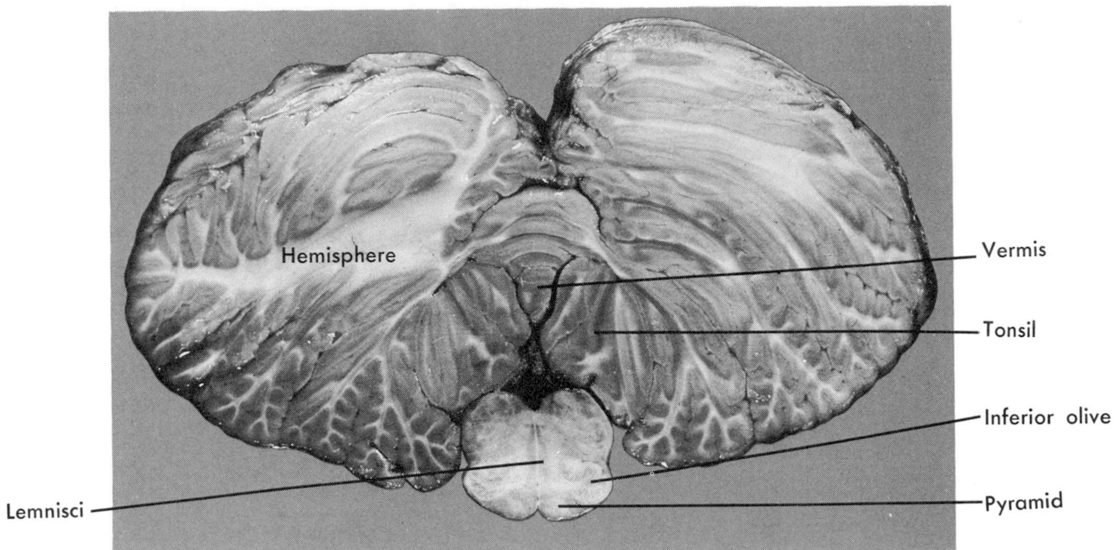

Fig. 4-41. Transverse section of medulla through midolive.

Sagittal section (Figs. 4-31 to 4-35)

The sagittal plane through the vermis of the cerebellum displays the principal lobular subdivisions, including the following: *lingula, central lobule, postcentral fissure, culmen, preclival fissure, declive, postclival fissure, folium vermis, great horizontal fissure, tuber, precentral fissure, postpyramidal fissure, pyramid, prepyramidal fissure, uvula, postnodular fissure,* and *nodule.* Note the *anterior (superior) medullary velum* and *posterior (inferior) medullary velum.* The last structure is associated with *choroid plexus.* The *great horizontal* fissure continues laterally from the area of the folium vermis. The midplane of the pons, the contour and continuations of the fourth ventricle, and the choroid plexus are evident (see also Fig. 2-22 and Chapters 3 and 22).

SECTIONAL ANATOMY—SPINAL CORD

Transverse sections of three levels are utilized in depicting the major sectional anatomy of the spinal cord (Fig. 4-44). (For details see Chapter 6.) Because the unstained parts show poorly in photographs, these illustrations are presented in drawings.

Section at the level of the cervical enlargement (Fig. 4-45, *A*)

The gross inspection of fissure patterns and gray matter is facilitated by use of a magnifying lens. In the unstained specimen, the *central canal* and gray matter and the *anterior* and *posterior gray horns* are detectable. Their pattern characterizes the cervical enlargement. Note the relatively large lateral component of the anterior horn (for housing nerve cells supplying the upper extremity). The division of the *posterior white funiculus* (dorsal white columns) into a medial *fasciculus gracilis* and a lateral *fasciculus cuneatus* is clearly shown. The *dorsal median septum* separates the two dorsal funiculi. Note the fissures and sulci, as described on p. 36.

Section at the level of the thoracic enlargement (Fig. 4-45, *B*)

This level displays the *intermediolateral nuclear column,* which houses the *visceral efferent* cells of the sympathetic system. In the unstained specimen, it is impossible to distinguish the subdivisions in the longitudinal bundles that make up the nervous pathways. The narrow *anterior horn* is characteristic in the thoracic planes (cells supply axial musculature only).

Section at the level of the lumbosacral enlargement (Fig. 4-45, *C*)

The lumbosacral enlargement exhibits relatively bulky gray horns, both posterior and anterior. The white columns are correspondingly reduced in bulk and exhibit no clearcut divisions in the unstained specimen. Note that the dorsal white column of this level and the thoracic levels becomes the fasciculus gracilis of the cervical levels.

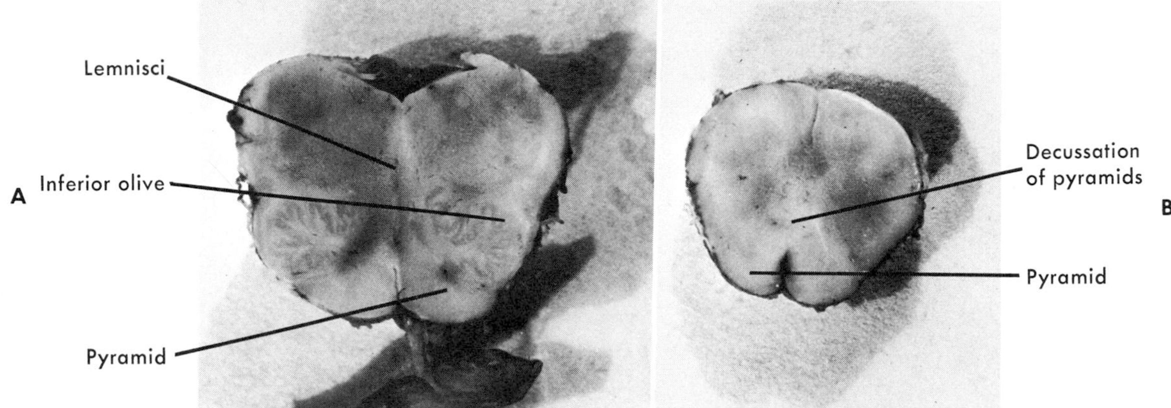

Fig. 4-42. A, Transverse section of medulla to show pyramids; **B,** transverse section showing decussation of pyramids.

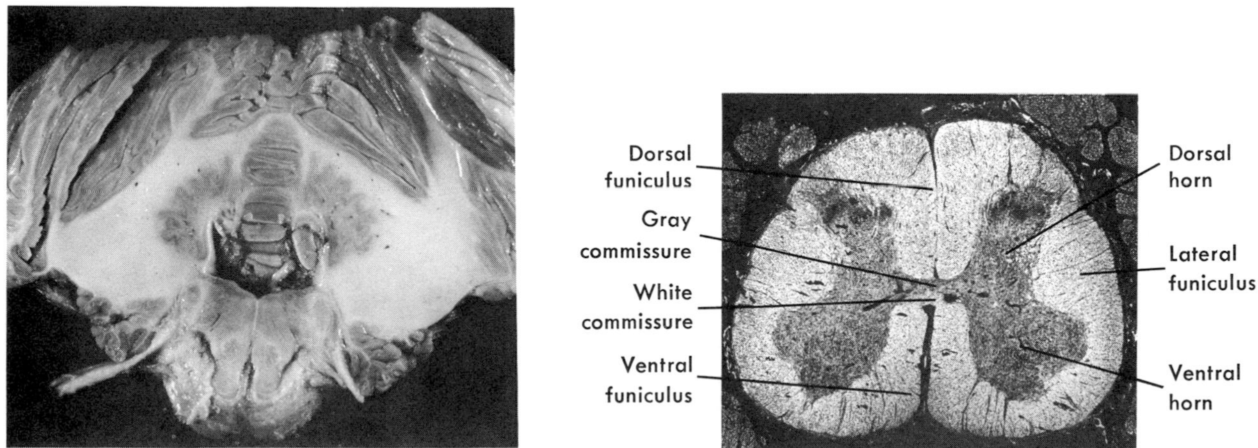

Fig. 4-43. Transverse section showing cerebellar nuclei, viewed from below (see Figs. 4-37 to 4-41).

Fig. 4-44. Prototype photo of transverse section of spinal cord.

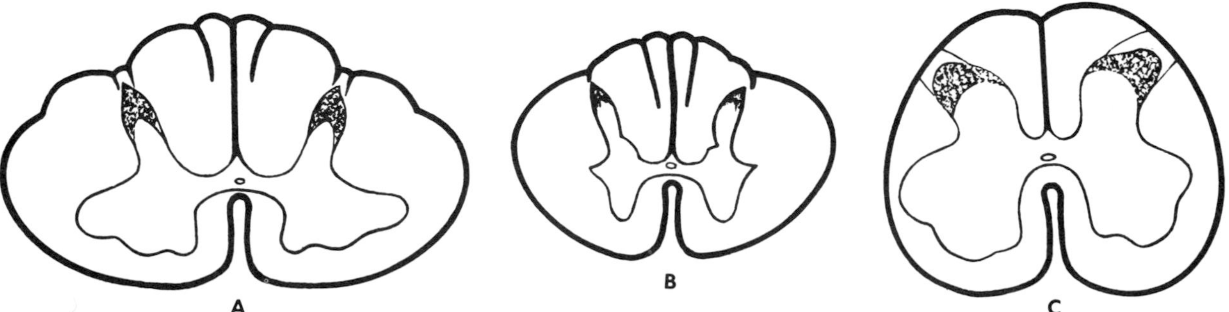

Fig. 4-45. Diagram of transverse sections of cervical, **A,** thoracic, **B,** and lumbosacral, **C,** planes of spinal cord. The outline of gray matter is characteristic of the region, as is the fasciculation of the white matter.

REFERENCES

1. Matzke, H. A., and Roofe, P. G.: Gross anatomy of the central nervous system. In Minckler, J., editor: Pathology of the nervous system, vol. I, New York, 1968, McGraw-Hill Book Co.
2. Miller, R. A., and Burack, E.: Atlas of the central nervous system in man, Baltimore, 1968, The Williams & Wilkins Co.
3. Riley, H. A.: An atlas of the basal ganglia, brain stem, and spinal cord, New York, 1960, Hafner Publishing Co., Inc.
4. Singer, M., and Yakovlev, P.: The human brain in sagittal sections, Springfield, Illinois, 1954, Charles C Thomas, Publisher.
5. Villiger, E.: In Piersol, editor: Brain and spinal cord, Philadelphia, 1912, J. B. Lippincott Co.

CHAPTER 5

INTRODUCTORY NEURORADIOLOGY

JOHN C. RILEY

TECHNIQUE

Arteriography

Depending on the available technical facilities, various procedures may be used to demonstrate the cerebral arteries and veins. An iodinated contrast medium can be injected by needle through the skin into the artery of interest in the neck. Serial frontal and lateral films of the head and neck are obtained on mechanical film changers. Two to four films per second are needed for complete evaluation. The time taken to complete the examination varies, but usually nine to ten seconds is adequate. When carotid puncture is difficult, or when demonstration of the vertebral and basilar artery anatomy is desired, these vessels may be filled by retrograde high-pressure injection of the right brachial artery. Injection of the left brachial artery usually fills only the left vertebral artery. The method of selective catheterization of the brachiocephalic vessels from the axillary or femoral artery route is now widely used and adds certain refinements not possible by direct needle puncture.

Pneumoencephalography

Injection of gas, usually air, into the lumbar region is easily accomplished in the sitting position. Air, being lighter than CSF, floats to the most superior surface available. By fractionated injection of the gas and by varying the patient's head position, selective ventricular or cisternal fill is obtained. Close scrutiny is necessary throughout this examination, so that cerebellar tonsillar herniation does not occur. Neurosurgical intervention is seldom needed.

Ventriculography

Frequently, air must be injected from above because of increased intracranial pressure. A small hole (burr hole) is made under sterile conditions in the parietal bone. A special needle is then passed through the hole, the meninges, and cerebral cortex, and into the lateral ventricular cavity. An appropriate amount of air is slowly injected. After adjusting the head to obtain desired location of the air, films are made in different projections, as seen in Figs. 5-14 through 5-22.

Myelography

Contrast evaluation of the spinal canal and its contents is obtained by intrathecal (subarachnoid) instillation of approximately 9 to 15 cc. of iophendylate (Pantopaque),* a substance that is radiopaque because of a high iodine content. Occasionally a radiolucent medium such as gas is used. Interpretation of these studies is usually more difficult and less definitive. Using a special table that can be placed at various degrees of angulation and with head either up or down, the fluoroscopist can adjust the radiopaque substance to the desired location. Radiographs are then obtained, as shown in Figs. 5-23 through 5-26.

Brain scanning

Nuclear medicine is one of the most rapidly developing fields of study. The use of radioactive nuclides (isotopes) is a very simple and almost totally harmless procedure for evaluating the CNS. The isotope may be injected intravenously or intrathecally. Scanners and/or cameras sensitive to the emitted gamma rays are then placed close to the head, and an image is produced via a complex of photoconductors and electronic gadgetry. Both

*E. M. Parker Co., Inc., Brookline, Mass.

the scanner and camera are similar in that the gamma rays are absorbed in a sodium iodide crystal, and the absorbed energy is transformed into light rays. These rays are then transposed through the complex photoconductor system and recorded on film. The scanner moves systematically across the surface of the head. The final result is a complex of dots characteristic of the isotope localized in the vascular spaces of the head. With the stationary camera the brain scan can be obtained much more rapidly.

The most frequently employed radiopharmaceuticals include technetium 99 and the mercurial compounds, 197 or 203 Neohydrin. Two examples are shown in Figs. 5-27 and 5-28. Under these normal circumstances, the technetium remains in the vascular spaces for varying periods of time, and the scan shows the various blood pools. Under abnormal conditions, such as in brain tumors, subdural hematomas, and brain abscesses, the blood-brain barrier is broken down, and more of the isotope collects in these abnormal locations. Collection in abnormal arteriovenous malformations is also frequently shown on brain scans.

Notice that on the lateral scan (Fig. 5-27) the predominant portion of the isotope is localized in the sinuses and temperofacial area, where the greater amount of blood normally circulates. The choroid plexus is occasionally seen and should not be confused with an abnormal mass lesion. On the posterior scan (Fig. 5-28), notice that the blood flows predominantly to the right side through the transverse sinus. This is most common. The superior sagittal sinus is clearly seen on both frontal and lateral scans. The thinner rind, as seen on the posterior scan (Fig. 5-28), represents the normal vasculature of the surface of the brain, diploic space, and scalp.

ARTERIAL SUPPLY OF THE CENTRAL NERVOUS SYSTEM

Carotid Arteries and Branches

Usually the right common carotid artery originates from the innominate artery, and the left originates independently from the aortic arch. Bifurcation into the external and internal carotids is usually at or around the level of the fourth cervical vertebra. Anastomotic channels exist with the internal carotid and vertebral arteries. Knowledge of external carotid anatomy therefore becomes important, especially in the presence of obstructive disease. Most meningeal supply is derived from the external carotid artery. Fig. 5-1 illustrates

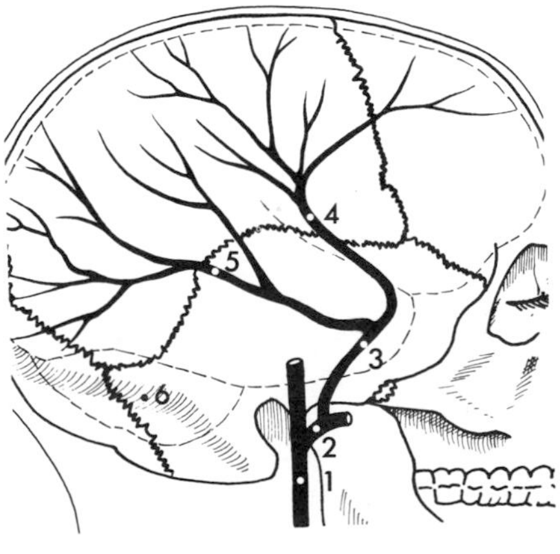

Fig. 5-1. Middle meningeal artery (diagram). *1,* External carotid artery; *2,* internal maxillary artery; *3,* middle meningeal artery; *4,* Anterior branch of middle meningeal artery; *5,* posterior branch of middle meningeal artery; *6,* transverse sinus.

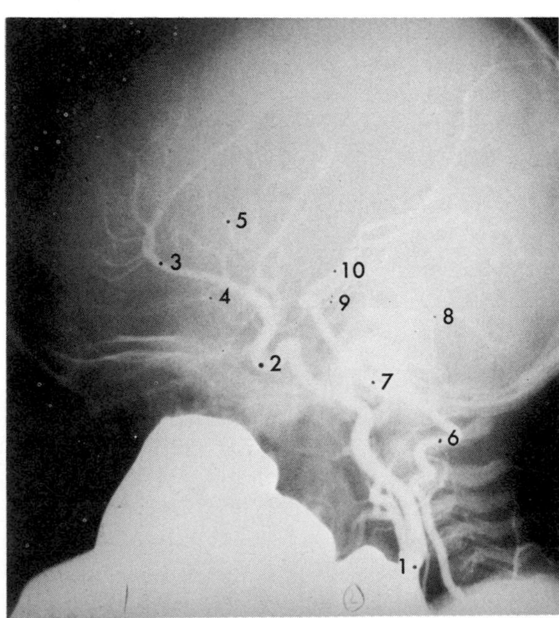

Fig. 5-2. Right retrograde brachial injection. *1,* **Bifurcation** of common carotid artery; *2,* cavernous portion of internal carotid; *3,* anterior cerebral artery; *4,* frontopolar artery; *5,* middle cerebral artery; *6,* vertebral artery; *7,* junction of two vertebral arteries; *8,* posterior inferior cerebellar artery (pica); *9,* superior cerebellar artery; *10,* posterior cerebral artery.

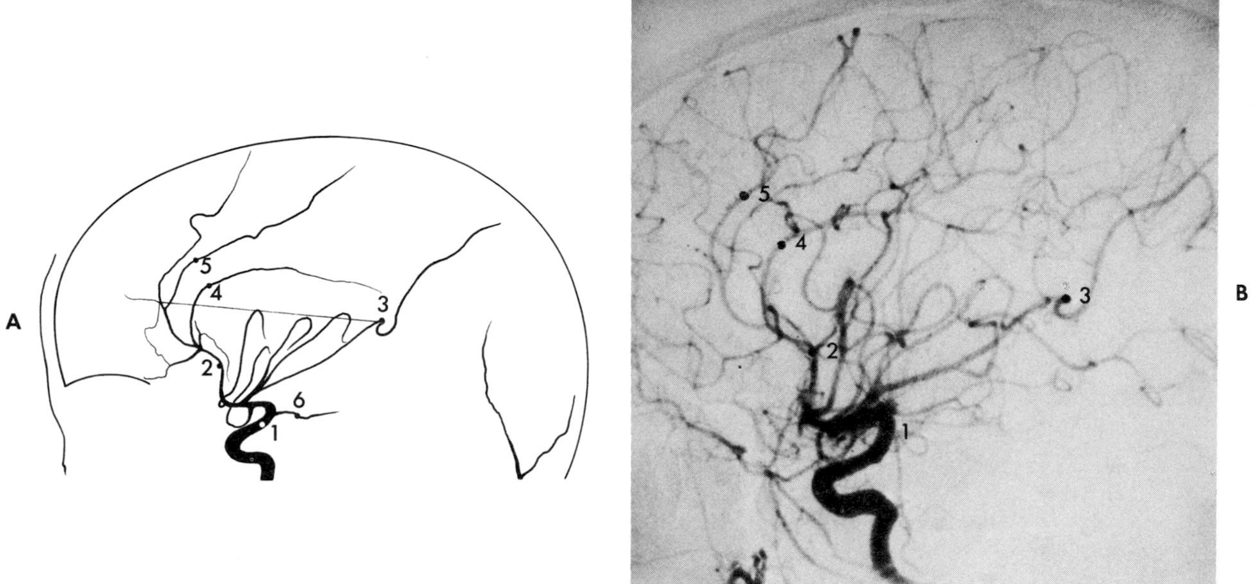

Fig. 5-3. A, Cerebral arteries, lateral view (diagram); **B,** subtraction study from carotid artery injection, lateral view. *1,* Internal carotid artery; *2,* anterior cerebral artery; *3,* posterior point of Sylvian triangle; *4,* pericallosal artery; *5,* callosomarginal artery; *6,* anterior choroidal artery.

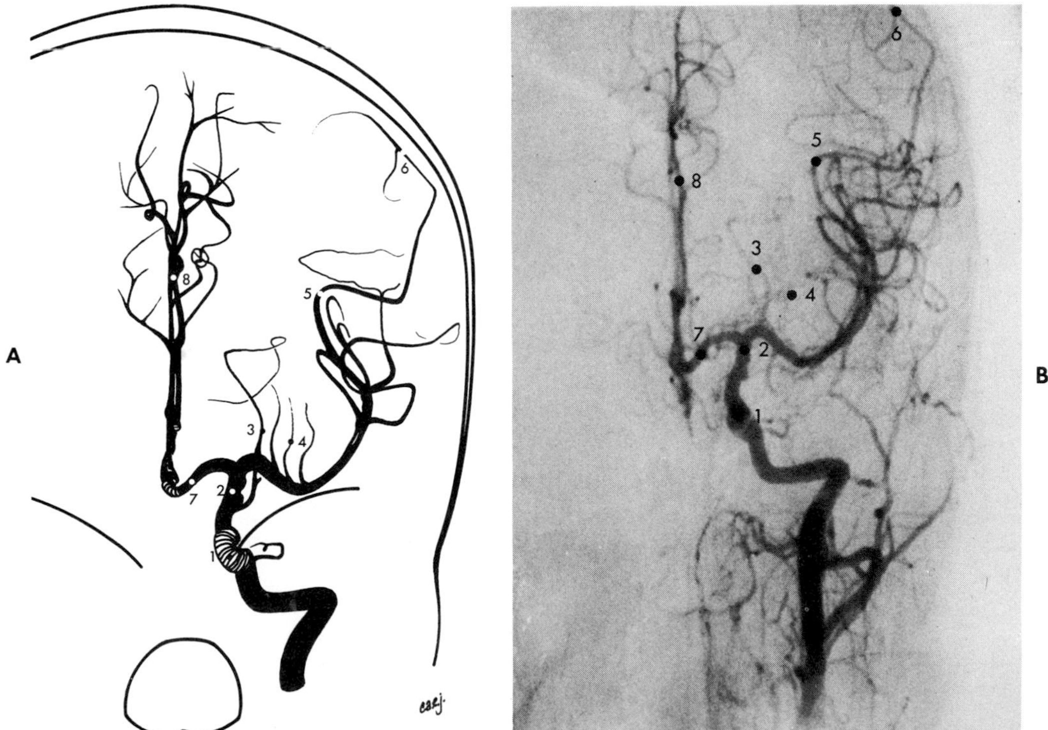

Fig. 5-4. A, Cerebral arteries, frontal projection (diagram); **B,** subtraction study from carotid injection, frontal projection. *1,* Internal carotid artery (cavernous); *2,* cerebral portion of internal carotid artery; *3,* anterior choroidal artery; *4,* lenticulostriate artery; *5,* Sylvian point; *6,* peripheral branches of middle cerebral artery; *7,* first portion of anterior cerebral artery; *8,* pericallosal and callosomarginal branches of anterior cerebral artery.

a middle meningeal artery that originates from the internal maxillary artery, passes through the foramen spinosum, and supplies blood to the predominant portion of the meninges. The infrequently mentioned anterior meningeal artery usually originates from the cavernous portion of the internal carotid artery, supplies the dura mater of the anterior cranial fossa, and anastomoses with other meningeal branches from the posterior ethmoidal artery.[1] The posterior meningeal artery is a branch of the occipital artery. It enters the skull through the jugular foramen and serves the dura mater of the posterior fossa.

The internal carotid artery is divided into four portions: cervical, petrous, cavernous, and cerebral. Fig. 5-2 shows the artery in a child. The cervical portion of the artery runs with the vagus nerve and internal jugular vein in the carotid sheath. There are no branches in this portion. The artery takes a medial and cephalad course, through the carotid canal in the petrous portion of the temporal bone. In the cavernous sinus the artery is covered by the dura. The artery curves upward, passes medial to the anterior clinoid, and pierces the dura mater (Figs. 5-2 and 5-5). This cerebral portion passes between the optic and oculomotor nerves and divides into the cerebral branches. There are several branches of the petrous and cavernous portions. The most important branch of the cavernous portion is the opthalmic artery. The posterior communicating artery is the first important branch of the cerebral portion. Immediately following is the anterior choroidal artery (Figs. 5-3 and 5-4). The internal carotid bifurcates into the anterior and middle cerebral arteries near the roof of the chiasmatic cistern (Figs. 5-3, *A*; 5-4, *B*; and 5-20), lateral to the optic chiasm. The anterior cerebral, usually the smallest of these terminal branches, passes medially and is usually joined with its contralateral artery at the long fissure, via the anterior communicating artery. (The portion of the brain supplied blood by the cerebral arteries is described on p. 55.) Important branches include the frontopolar (Fig. 5-1), callosomarginal, and pericallosal arteries (Fig. 5-3). The latter usually courses fairly close to the corpus callosum.

The middle cerebral, or Sylvian, group can be divided by location into four sections. The first is from the point of bifurcation of the internal carotid artery to the Sylvian fissure. The main branches usually arise in this first portion. Important minor branches of the first section include the lenticulostriate arteries (Fig. 5-4). The second section in-

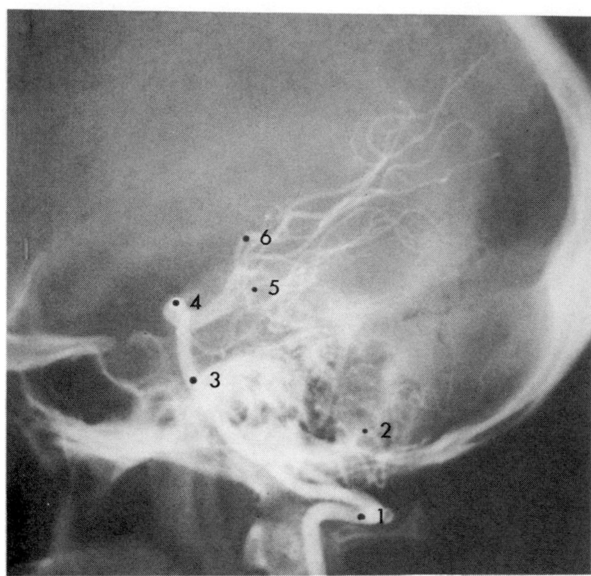

Fig. 5-5. Vertebral injection, lateral view. *1,* Vertebral artery; *2,* posterior inferior cerebellar artery; *3,* basilar artery in prepontine cistern; *4,* uppermost portion of basilar artery; *5,* superior cerebellar artery; *6,* posterior cerebral artery.

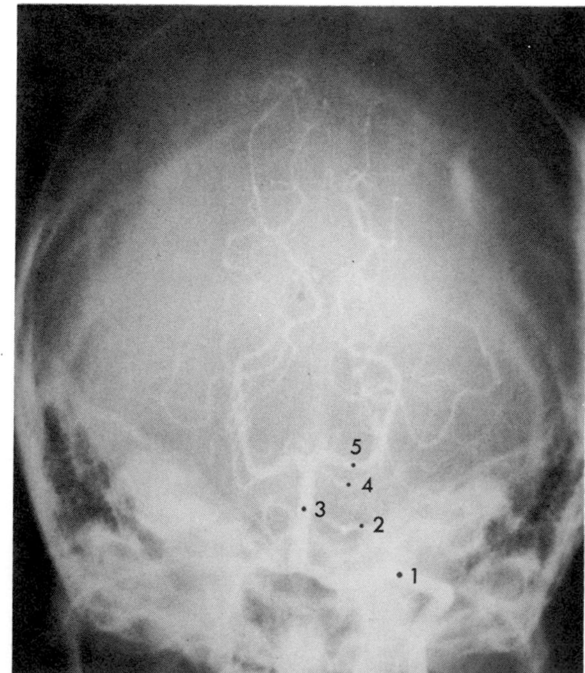

Fig. 5-6. Vertebral injection, frontal projection. *1,* Vertebral artery, left; *2,* posterior inferior cerebellar artery; *3,* basilar artery; *4,* superior cerebellar artery; *5,* posterior cerebral artery.

cludes all of the middle cerebral group as they cross the surface of the insula (Fig. 5-4, *A*). The third includes the lateral portion that runs over the operculum to the lateral cerebral surface. The fourth section includes the ramification of these vessels over the cerebral surface. As diagrammed in Fig. 5-3, *A*, a line is formed by joining the point of the five to eight middle cerebral arteries as each reaches the deepest portion of insula at the junction with the frontoparietal operculum. The anterior and posterior margins of this line, projected to the anterior portion of the trunk of the middle cerebral artery, form a triangle,[4] an important landmark in evaluation of cerebral angiograms. Correlation of the lateral with the frontal angiograms is in all cases of tantamount importance (Figs. 5-3 and 5-4).

Vertebral and basilar arteries

Figs. 5-5 to 5-7 illustrate much of the course of the vertebral arteries that arise from the first portion of both subclavian arteries. The vertebral arteries run cranially through the foramina of the transverse processes of vertebrae C_6 to C_1. They then bend abruptly in a medial direction across a groove on the superior surface of the posterior arch of the first cervical vertebra (Fig. 5-5). The vessel then enters the skull through the foramen magnum and joins the other vertebral artery to form the basilar artery (Figs. 5-1 and 5-6). Important branches of the vertebral arteries are divided into cervical (spinal and muscular) and cranial branches (meningeal, posterior spinal, anterior spinal, posterior inferior cerebellar artery, and medullary) (see Figs. 5-5 to 5-7).

Important branches of the basilar artery include the pontine, labyrinthine, anterior inferior cerebellar, superior cerebellar (Fig. 5-5), and posterior cerebral arteries (Figs. 5-5 through 5-7). Notice the position of the terminal portion of the basilar artery in the interpeduncular cistern (Figs. 5-5 and 5-20). The two posterior cerebral arteries run lat-

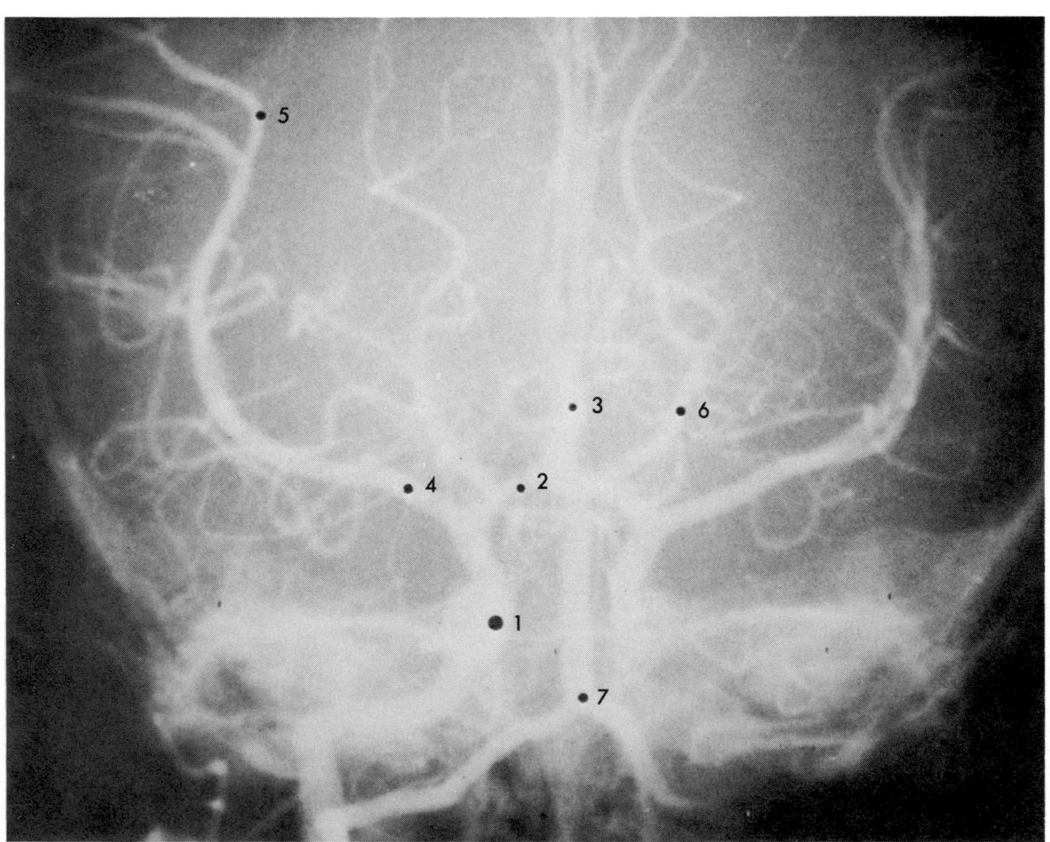

Fig. 5-7. Retrograde brachial injection, frontal projection. *1,* Cavernous portion of internal carotid artery; *2,* first portion of anterior cerebral artery; *3,* anterior cerebral artery; *4,* middle cerebral artery; *5,* Sylvian point, *6,* posterior cerebral artery; *7,* junction of vertebral arteries.

erally, and then turn posteriorly around the cerebral peduncles in the crural cisterns and around the midbrain in the ambient cisterns (Fig. 5-22). The point where the posterior cerebral arteries pass over the tentorium is important in evaluation of possible herniation of the uncus through this tentorial notch in certain supratentorial lesions. The superior cerebellar artery takes a similar course, as seen on both frontal and lateral projections (Figs. 5-5 and 5-6), and is not to be confused with the other vessels.

VENOUS DRAINAGE

Deep group

The internal cerebral veins are paired vessels that traverse the roof of the third ventricle (Figs. 5-8 and 5-9). The thalamostriate and septal veins join at the venous angle, which localizes the interventricular foramen of Monro (Figs. 5-8 to 5-11). Tributaries of the thalamostriate veins run along the wall of the anterior horn and body of the lateral ventricle and are frequently well demonstrated

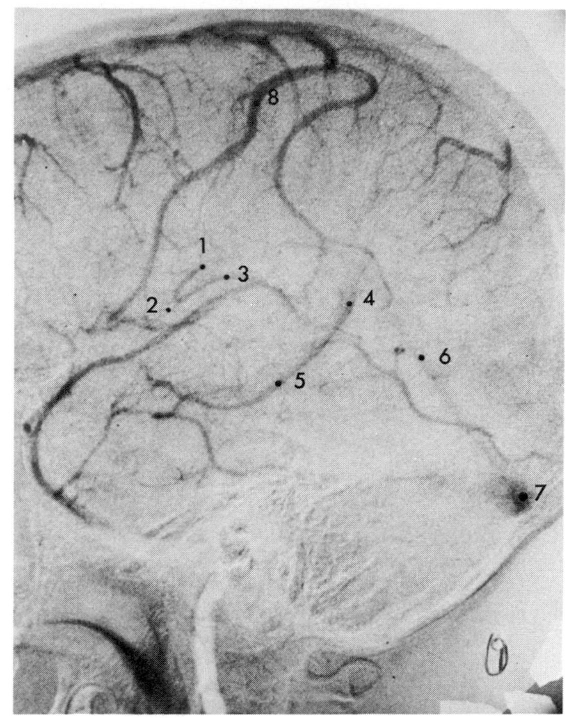

Fig. 5-8. Venous phase of circulation, lateral view. *1,* Thalamostriate vein; *2,* septal vein; *3,* internal cerebral vein; *4,* great cerebral vein (of Galen); *5,* basilar vein (of Rosenthal); *6,* straight sinus; *7,* torcular Herophili; *8,* superior cerebral vein (of Trolard).

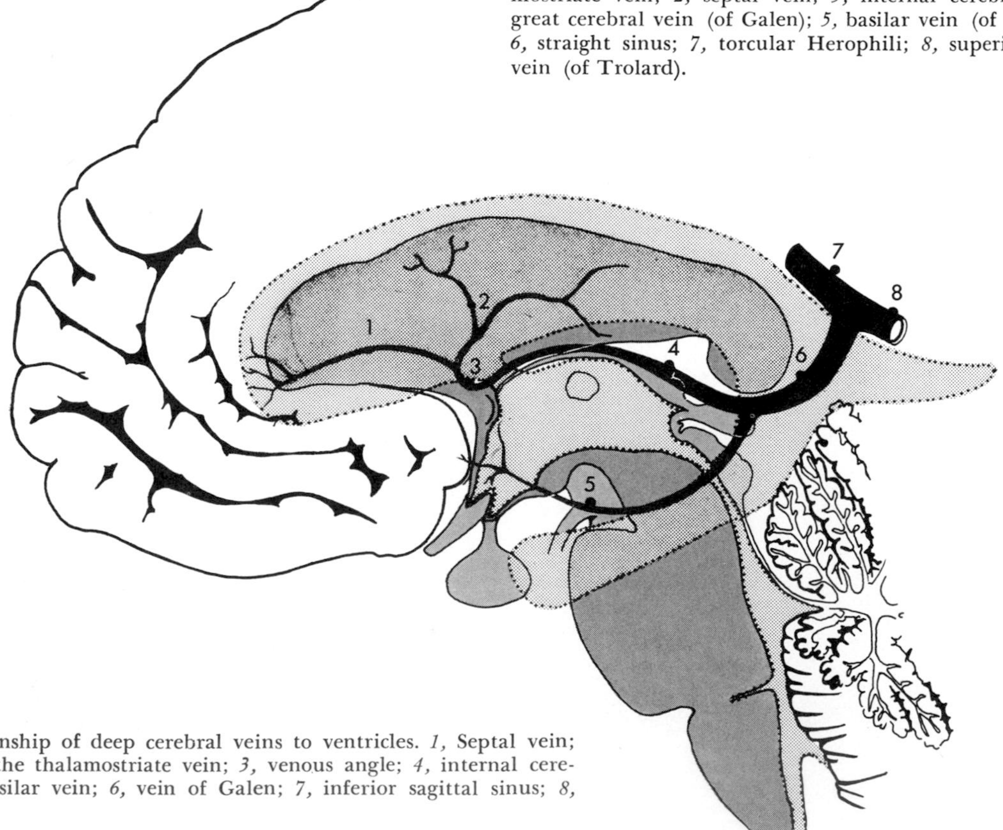

Fig. 5-9. Relationship of deep cerebral veins to ventricles. *1,* Septal vein; *2,* tributary of the thalamostriate vein; *3,* venous angle; *4,* internal cerebral vein; *5,* basilar vein; *6,* vein of Galen; *7,* inferior sagittal sinus; *8,* straight sinus.

in the later venous phase of a cerebral angiogram (Figs. 5-9 to 5-11). The two internal cerebral veins join and form the single midline vein of Galen in the quadrigeminal cistern (Figs. 5-9 and 5-20). The basal vein (of Rosenthal) arises from tributaries in the anterior perforated substance, insular region, and corpus striatum. It passes posteriorly around the cerebral peduncle and follows a course similar to the posterior cerebral artery (Fig. 5-9). This basilar vein then joins either the internal cerebral vein or the vein of Galen (Figs. 5-8 and 5-9). Notice the convex course of the vein of Galen around the splenium of the corpus callosum (Fig. 5-9). The vein of Galen enters the straight sinus at the junction of the tentorium and falx cerebri (Figs. 5-8 and 5-9). The inferior sagittal sinus in the inferior margin of the falx also joins the straight sinus at this point. Blood then flows to the torcular herophili, through the transverse and sigmoid sinuses, and through the jugular foramen to form the internal jugular vein (Figs. 5-10 to 5-12).

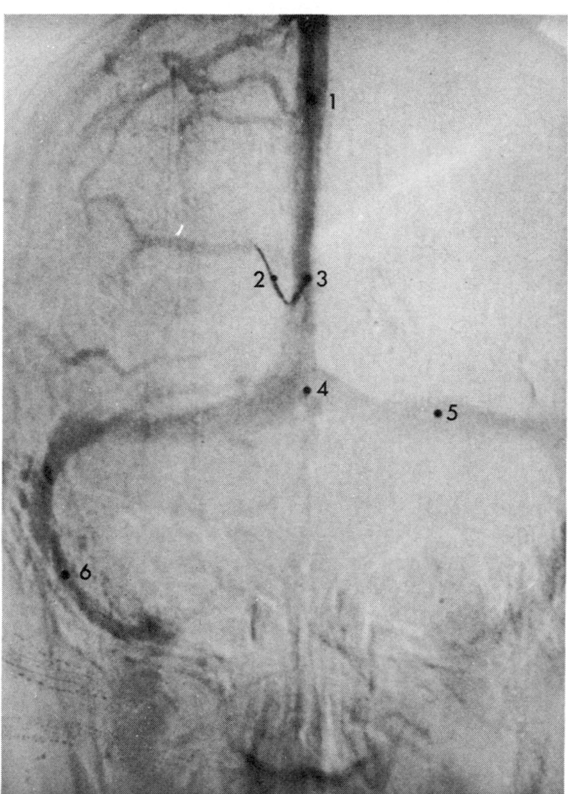

Fig. 5-11. Venous circulation, frontal projection. *1,* Superior sagittal sinus; *2,* thalamostriate vein; *3,* internal cerebral vein; *4,* torcular Herophili; *5,* transverse sinus; *6,* sigmoid sinus.

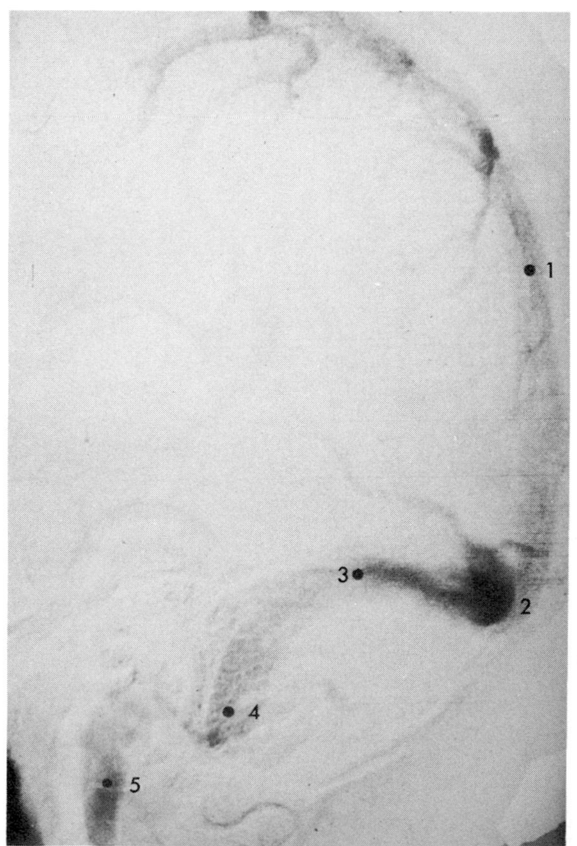

Fig. 5-10. Venous phase showing sinuses, lateral projection. *1,* Superior sagittal sinus; *2,* torcular Herophili; *3,* transverse sinus; *4,* sigmoid sinus; *5,* internal jugular vein.

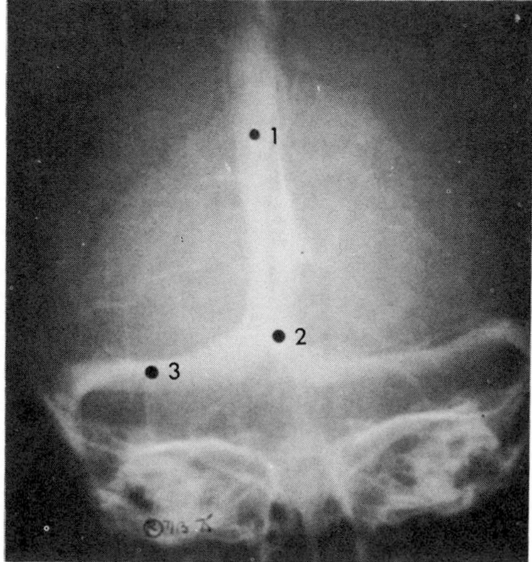

Fig. 5-12. Venous sinuses in child, frontal projection. *1,* Superior sagittal sinus; *2,* torcular Herophili; *3,* transverse sinus.

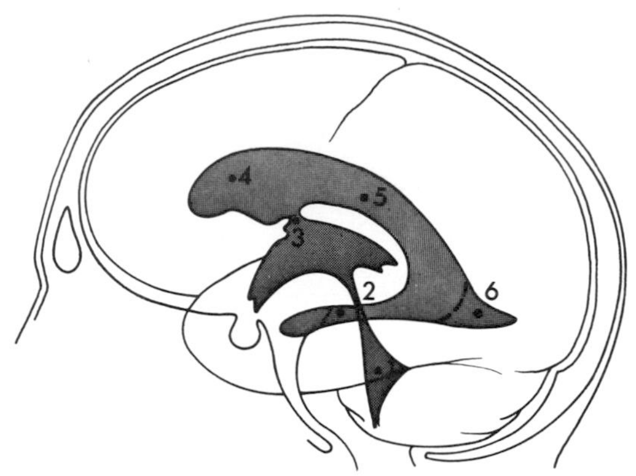

Fig. 5-13. Abstract of ventricular system. *1,* Fourth ventricle; *2,* aqueduct; *3,* foramen of Monroe; *4,* anterior horn of lateral ventricle; *5,* body of lateral ventricle; *6,* occipital horn; *7,* temporal horn.

Superficial group

As depicted in Fig. 5-8, these vessels receive tributaries from the cerebral surface, cross the meninges, and drain into the dural sinuses. Nomenclature for these vessels is not important because anatomic landmarks are seldom critical, and variation is the rule. It should be remembered however that there is free communication between the deep and superficial veins, and reversal of flow may occur under certain circumstances. The major superficial cerebral veins are generally divided into: (1) superior anastomotic vein of Trolard; (2) middle vein of the Sylvian fissure; and (3) the inferior cerebral vein of Labbé. The minor veins either drain into one or these major vessels or penetrate independently into the dural sinuses. The cerebellar veins, superior and inferior, usually drain to the nearest sinus (Figs. 5-8 to 5-12).

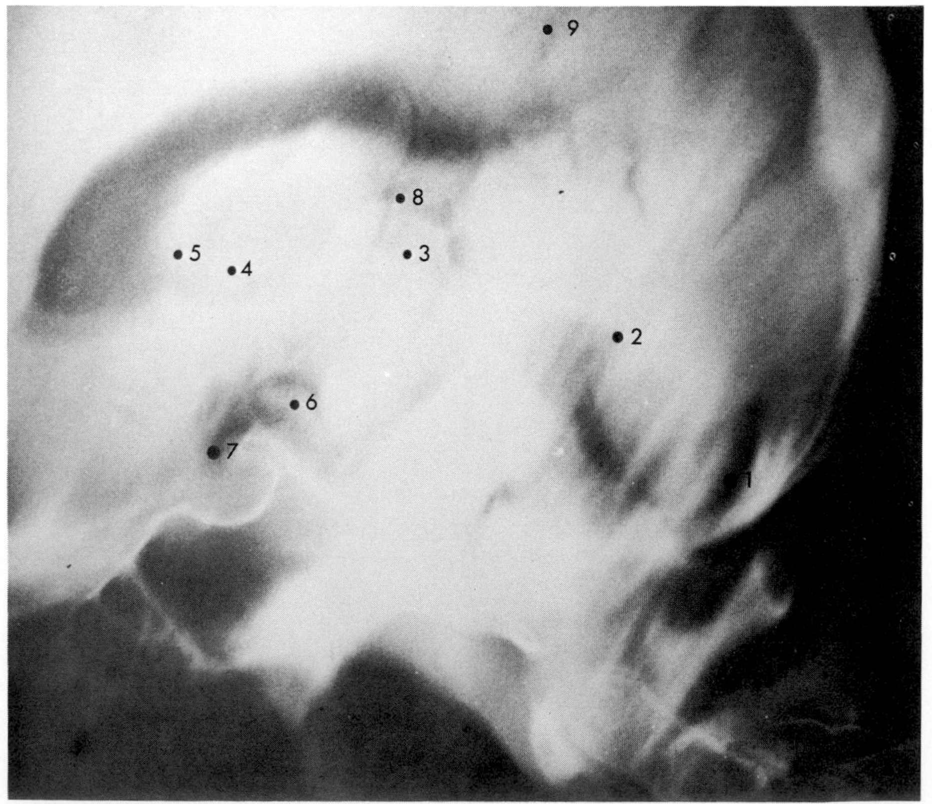

Fig. 5-14. Tomogram taken during pneumoencephalography. *1,* Cisterna magna; *2,* fastigium of fourth ventricle; *3,* aqueduct; *4,* massa intermedia; *5,* foramen of Monroe; *6,* basilar artery in prepontine cistern; *7,* suprasellar cistern; *8,* quadrigeminal cistern; *9,* subarachnoid gas over cerebrum.

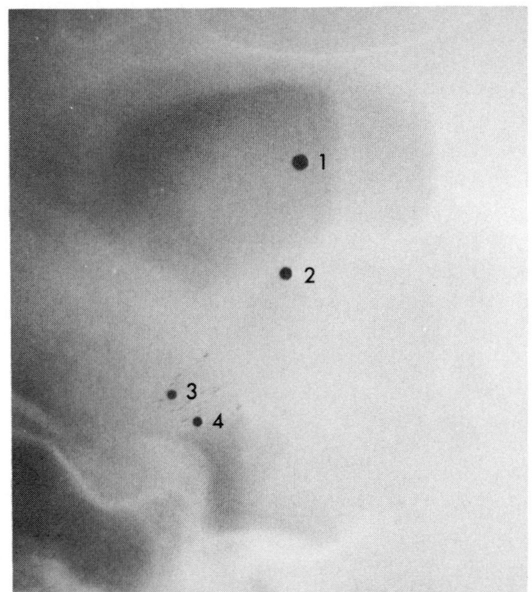

Fig. 5-15. Brow-up projection, lateral view. *1,* Anterior portions of lateral ventricles; *2,* foramen of Monroe; *3,* optic recess of third ventricle; *4,* infundibular recess of third ventricle.

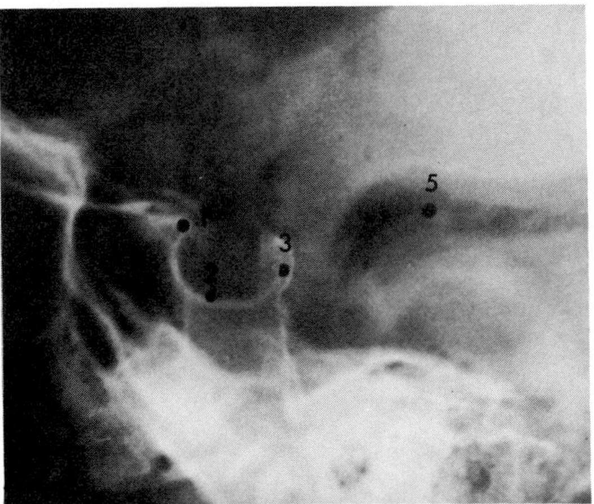

Fig. 5-16. Lateral film from pneumoencephalogram. *1,* Tuberculum sellae and anterior clinoids; *2,* floor of sella; *3,* dorsal clinoids; *4,* sphenoid sinus; *5,* air in temporal horn of lateral ventricle.

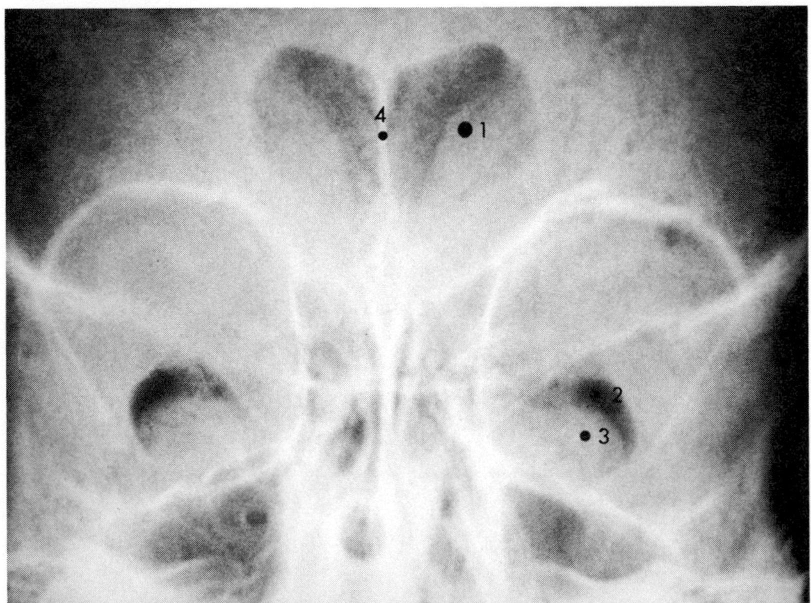

Fig. 5-17. Brow-up with air in temporal horns, frontal projection. *1,* Caudate nucleus; *2,* temporal horn of lateral ventricle (horizontal and vertical clefts); *3,* hippocampal gyrus; *4,* septum pellucidum.

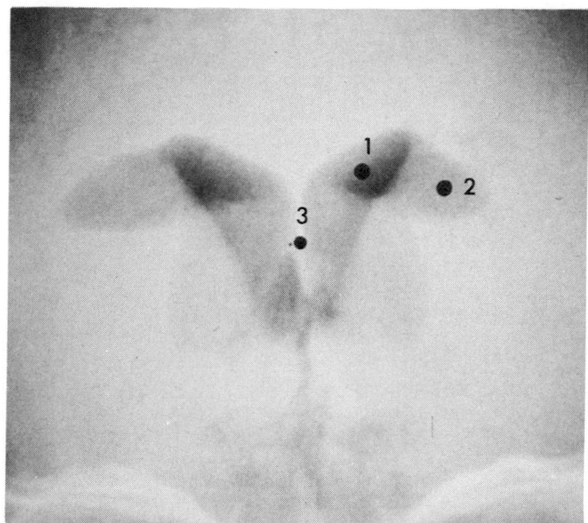

Fig. 5-18. Ventricles as seen on frontal projection. *1,* Body of lateral ventricle; *2,* anterior horn of lateral ventricle; *3,* septum pellucidum.

PNEUMOENCEPHALOGRAPHY

Ventricular system

The lateral film of the lower skull and cervical spine in Fig. 5-21 was taken immediately following instillation of air. Notice the normal position of the cerebellar tonsils. Following displacement of CNS fluid from the cisterna magna and securement of the head in a flexed position, gas begins to pass through the vallecula and into the fourth ventricle by way of the midline foramen of Magendie. The lateral recesses of the fourth ventricle contain the foramina of Luschka. These three appertures are the only normal communications between the ventricular system and the cisternal or subarachnoid space.

The floor of the fourth ventricle consists of the medulla oblongata and the lower pons (Figs. 5-14, 5-20, and 5-21). The anterior medullary velum makes up the anterior portion of this tent-shaped ventricle. The caudal portion consists of the posterior medullary velum and the choroid plexus. The appearance of the fourth ventricle in frontal projection (Fig. 5-19) and lateral projection in a roentgenogram (Figs. 5-14 and 5-21) is extremely

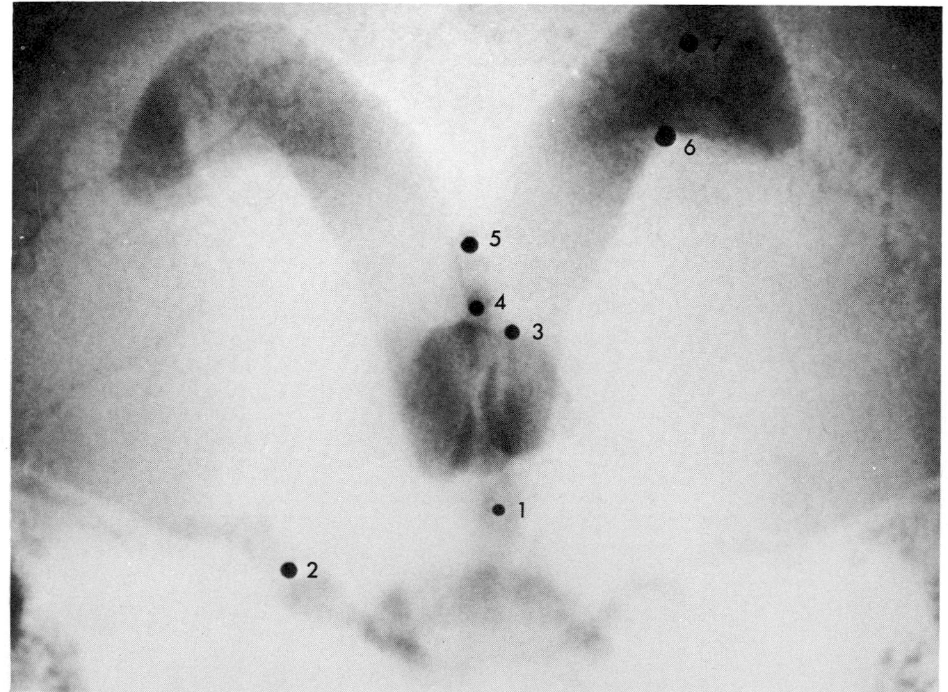

Fig. 5-19. Brow-down, frontal half, axial projection. *1,* Vallecula; *2,* cerebellopontine angle cistern; *3,* roof of fourth ventricle; *4,* aqueduct; *5,* third ventricle; *6,* floor of lateral ventricle; *7,* occipital horn of lateral ventricle.

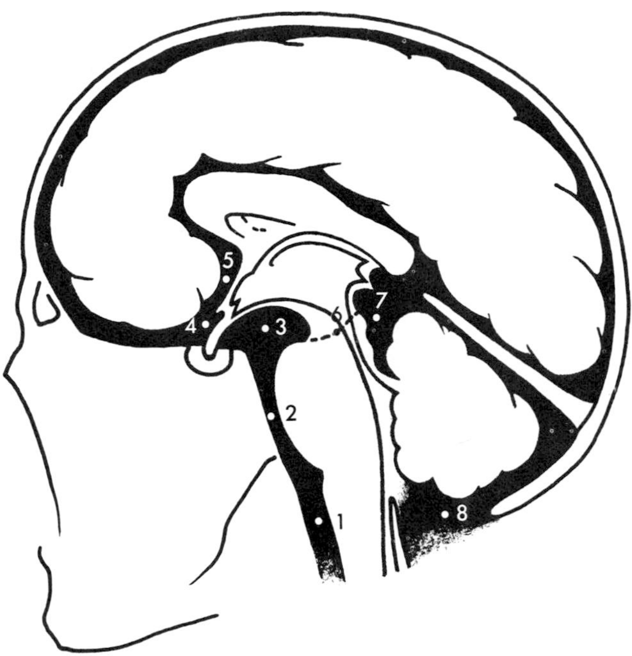

Fig. 5-20. Cisternal anatomy (diagram). *1,* Premedullary cistern; *2,* prepontine cistern; *3,* interpeduncular cistern; *4,* chiasmatic cistern; *5,* cistern of the lamina terminalis; *6,* retrothalamic cistern; *7,* quadrigeminal cistern; *8,* cisterna magna.

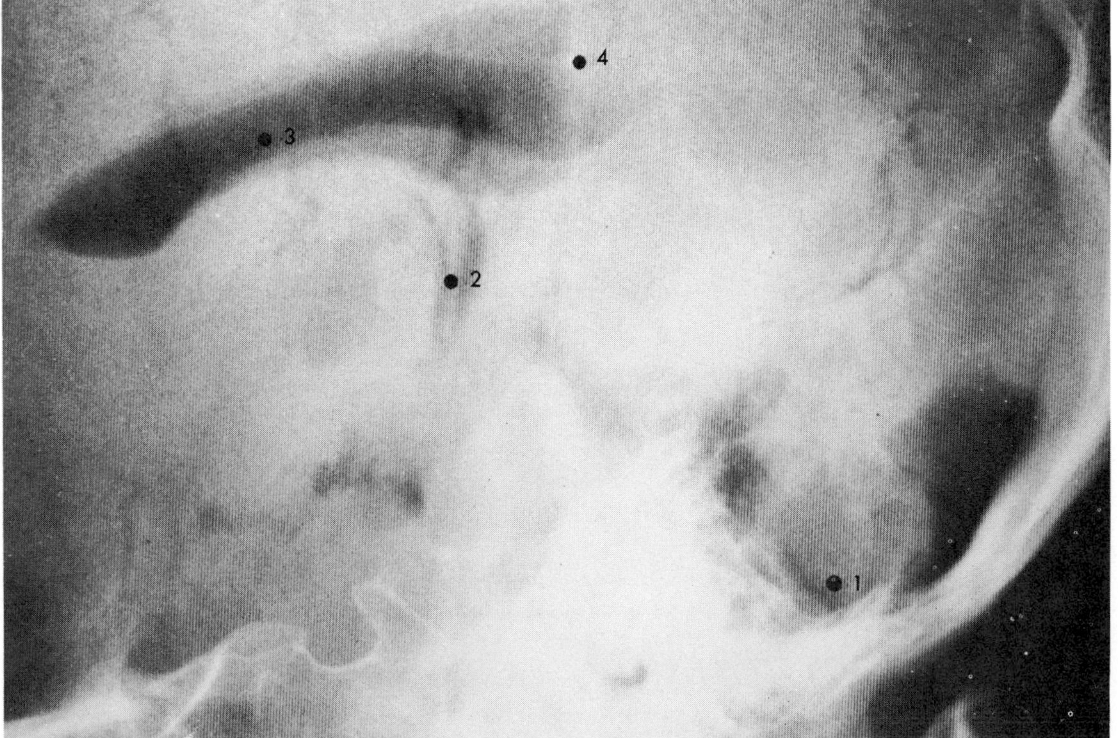

Fig. 5-21. Lateral projection. *1,* Normal position of cerebellar tonsils; *2,* retrothalamic cistern (wings of ambient cistern); *3,* body of lateral ventricle; *4,* glomus of the choroid plexus.

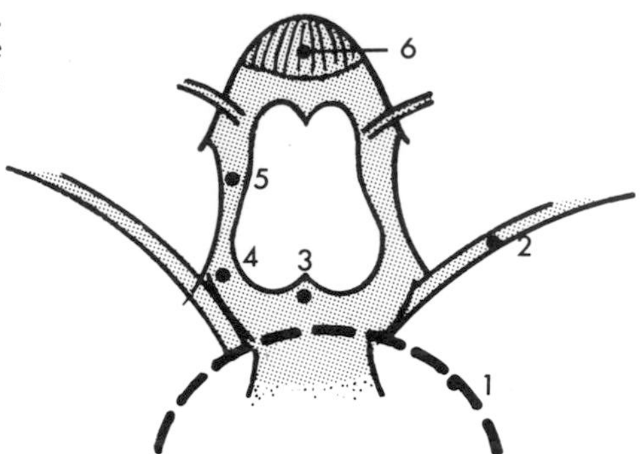

Fig. 5-22. Abstract for cisternal anatomy, frontal projection. *1,* Posterior rim of foramen magnum; *2,* cerebellopontine angle cistern; *3,* interpeduncular cistern; *4,* crural cistern; *5,* ambient cistern; *6,* quadrigeminal cistern.

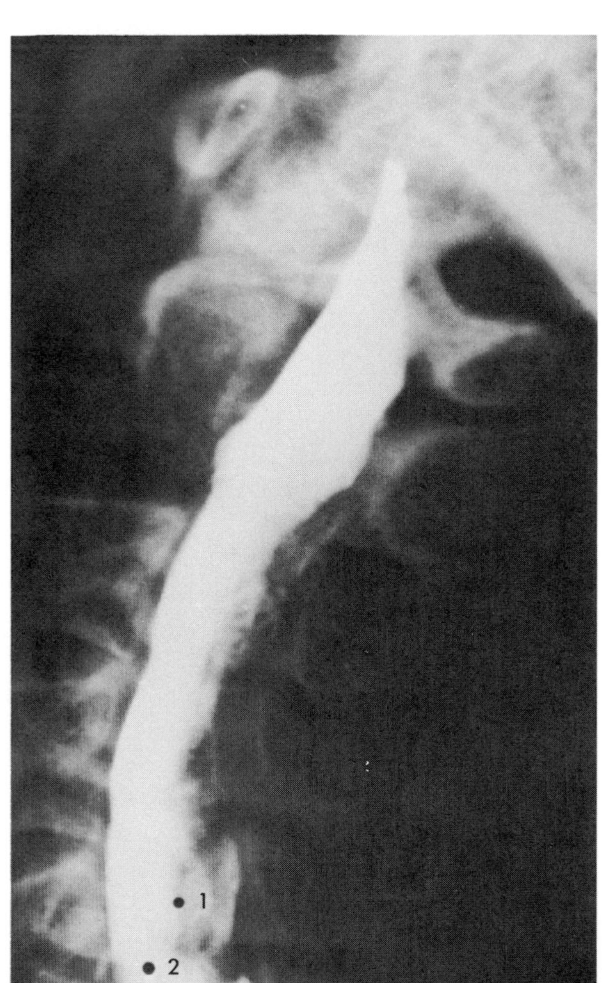

Fig. 5-23. Lateral projection, cervical myelogram. *1,* Attachment of dentate ligaments; *2,* ventral border of spinal cord; *3,* defect from slight hypertrophy of the ligamentum flavum; *4,* spinous process of C7.

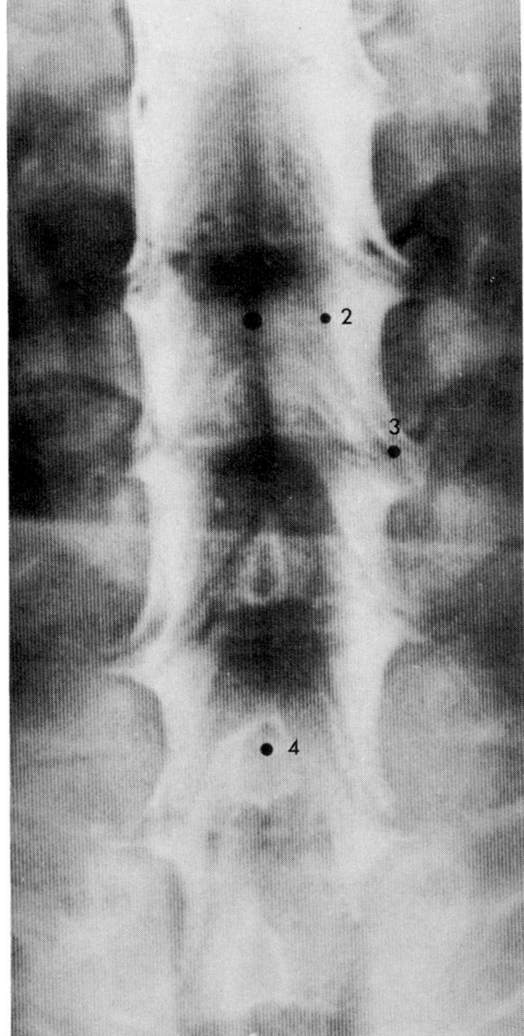

Fig. 5-24. Frontal projection, cervical myelogram. *1,* Anterior spinal artery outlined by Pantopaque column; *2,* lateral border of spinal cord; *3,* nerve rootlets of C6 emerging through intervertebral foramen; *4* spinous process of C7.

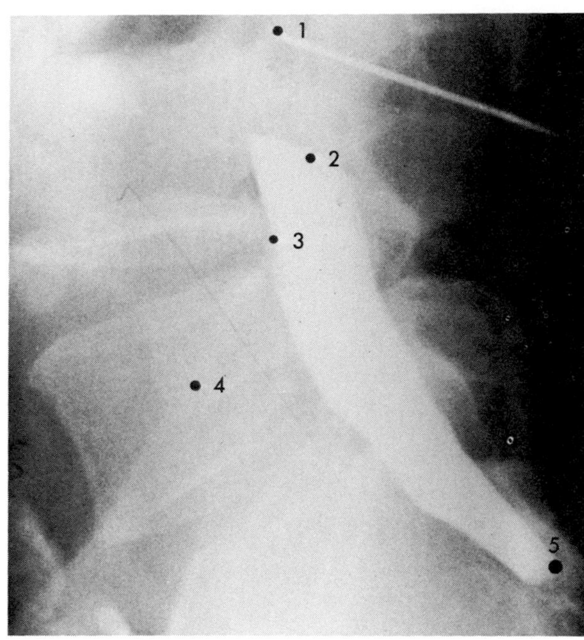

Fig. 5-25. Standing lateral projection, lumbar myelogram. *1,* Needle tip in subarachnoid space (L3 to 4); *2,* fluid level of Pantopaque column; *3,* normal appearance of subarachnoid space at disk space; *4,* body of L4; *5,* caudal extension of subarachnoid space.

important, especially in evaluation of posterior fossa anatomy.*

The cerebral aqueduct (of Sylvius) is a structure of communication between the upper part of the fourth and posteroinferior part of the third ventricles. The floor consists of the midbrain and upper pons. The roof consists of the superior and inferior colliculi (quadrigeminal bodies). The single third ventricle is at midline and is complex in contour. On lateral projection (Figs. 5-9, and 5-13 to 5-15) the numerous recesses and the relationship of surrounding structures, such as the pineal gland, optic chiasm, massa intermedia, and vascular structures, are evident. As stated on p. 44; the walls of the third ventricle consist of the thalamus above and hypothalamus below. A band of tissue connects both halves of the thalamus and is evident on most pneumograms (Fig. 5-14). The anterior wall consists of the anterior commissure and lamina terminalis. The optic chiasm joins the floor of the third ventricle immediately beneath the optic recess. The floor consists of the middle and posterior hypothalamus and the subthalamus.[6] The roof consists of the velum interpositum, which is invaginated by the choroid plexus. The relative position to the body and splenium of the corpus callosum is also important (Figs. 5-9 and 5-20).

Fluid passes from the third to the lateral ventricles and from the lateral to the third ventricles via the foramen of Monro, located in the anterior

*For normal measurements and relationship of the fourth ventricle to the bony structure see references 2 and 4.

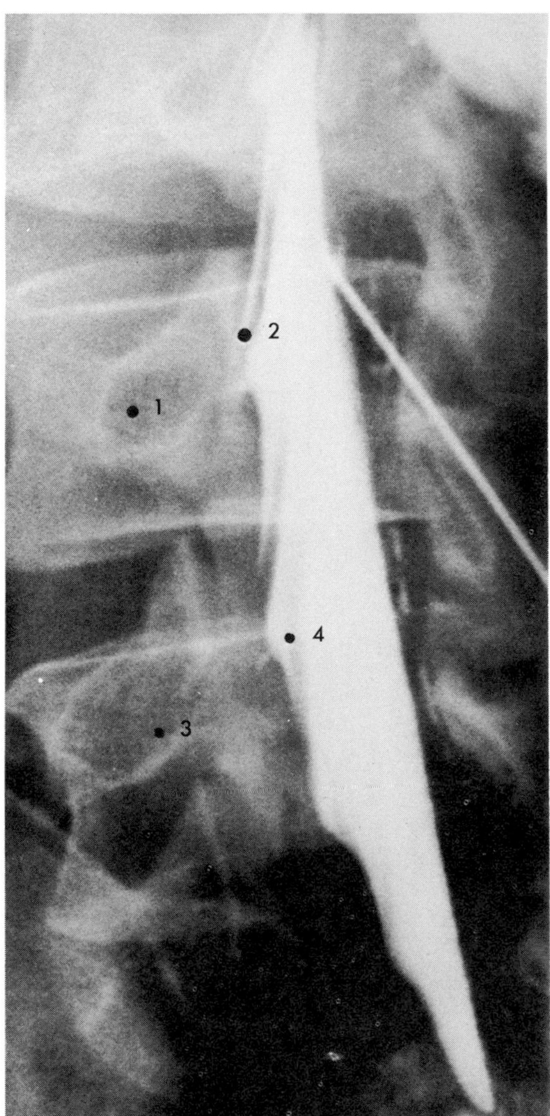

Fig. 5-26. Oblique projection, lumbar myelogram. *1,* Body of L4; *2,* fourth lumbar nerve; *3,* body of L5; *4,* fifth lumbar nerve.

and lateral portion of the third ventricle (Fig. 5-14). As stated previously, this is the usual position of the venous angle. Lateral ventricular anatomy is also complex. For simplicity, each ventricle can be divided into: (1) anterior horn; (2) body; (3) posterior horn; and (4) temporal horn. Depending on the position of the head when the roentgenogram is obtained, either of the compartments can be selectively filled for evaluation of size, position, filling defects, or asymmetery. Correlation with gross anatomy is especially important in pneumographic study of the lateral ventricles. Figs. 5-13 to 5-21 correlate ventricular anatomy in frontal and in lateral projections. Correlation with cross-sectional anatomy also should be attempted for more thorough understanding.

Note that the septum pellucidum separates the frontal horns, and the corpus callosum forms the roof. Note the position of the caudate nucleus and thalamus on anterior projection. The temporal horns are well illustrated in Figs. 5-16 and 5-17. Occasionally the choroid plexus is noted as a filling defect near the junction of the body and temporal horns. The occipital horns probably vary more in size and appearance than the other portions of the lateral ventricles.

Subarachnoid spaces (Cisternal system)

Normally the subarachnoid space and ventricular system communicate by way of the apertures of the fourth ventricle. The spinal and cranial subarachnoid space is continuous. Study of the cranial subarachnoid space is complex, and only a brief introduction and classification is presented here. One important feature to understand however is that these spaces are more accurately demonstrated

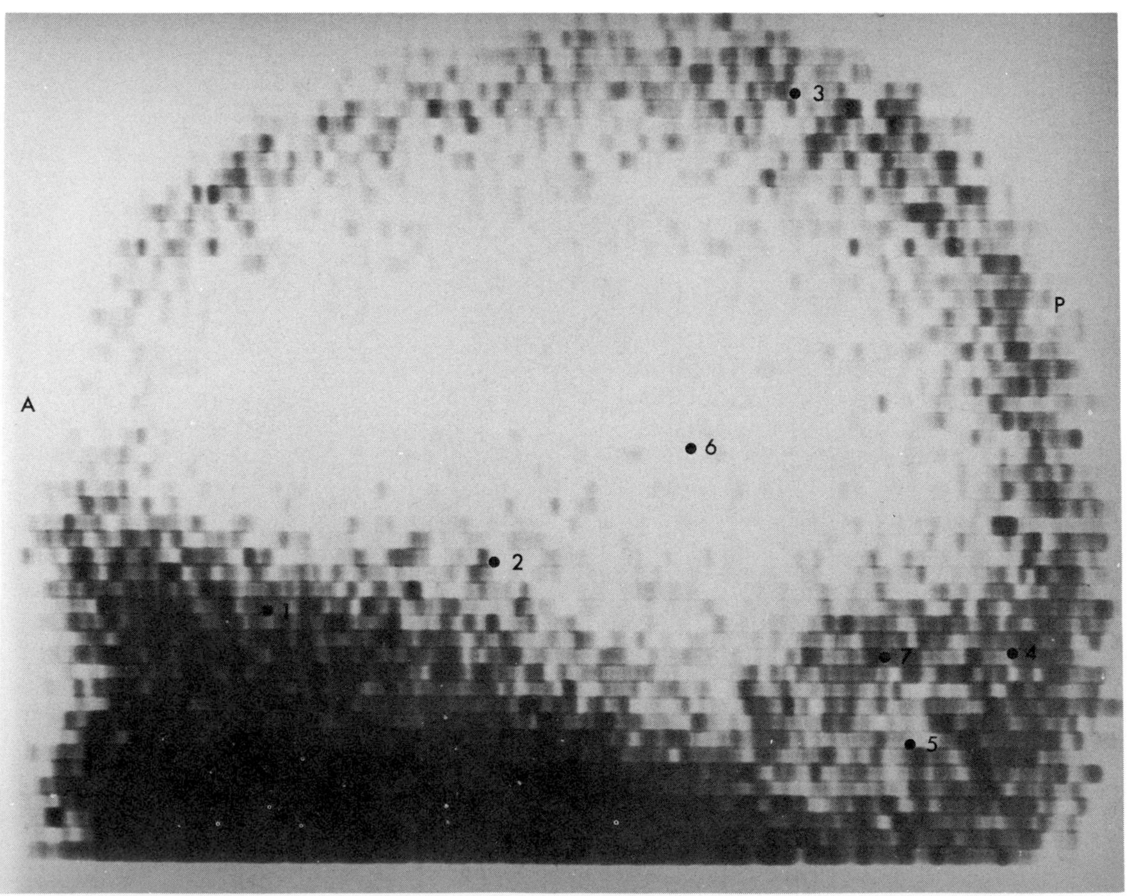

Fig. 5-27. Brain scan, lateral view, (technetium). *1,* Facial area; *2,* temporal muscle mass; *3,* superior sagittal sinus; *4* confluence of sinuses; *5,* posterior fossa; *6,* area of choroid plexus; *7,* transverse sinus.

on film than at autopsy. At autopsy, many of these cisterns appear only as potential spaces, rather than as they exist in life.

The subarachnoid cisterns may be divided into: (1) posterior fossa cisterns; (2) suprasellar cisterns; and (3) cisterns around the tentorial notch.* Nomenclature for the most part is based upon the surrounding anatomic structures. For example, the interpeduncular cistern is the space between the cerebral peduncles. Lateral to the interpeduncular cistern are the crural cisterns (Fig. 5-22), which are the spaces between the peduncle and uncus of the temporal lobe. The structure communicating with the more dorsally situated cisterns are called the cisterna ambiens. The quadrigeminal cistern (cistern of the great vein of Galen) communicates anteriorly with the space above the third ventricle (cavum velum interpositum) and posteriorly with the superior cerebellar cistern (Fig. 5-14).

*For a more complete understanding of cisternal anatomy see reference 1.

Knowledge of cisternal anatomy is extremely important. Without this knowledge, a true understanding of CNS fluid dynamics and structural relationships of the brain is unlikely.

Spinal canal and its contents

Fig. 5-23 is a lateral film of the cervical spine, taken during cervical myelography. The attachment of the dentate ligament and ventral border of the cervical spinal cord are evident. On the anteroposterior (AP) film (Fig. 5-24) the overall width of the spinal cord at this level is about two-thirds that of the spinal canal. The nerve roots, emerging through the intervertebral foramina, are well illustrated on this view. The anterior spinal artery is also outlined by the Pantopaque column.

Myelographic evaluation of the thoracic subarachnoid space is more difficult. A fairly complete examination can be accomplished however, especially if enough contrast media is used, and films in the decubitus position are obtained.

Since the spinal cord terminates in the upper

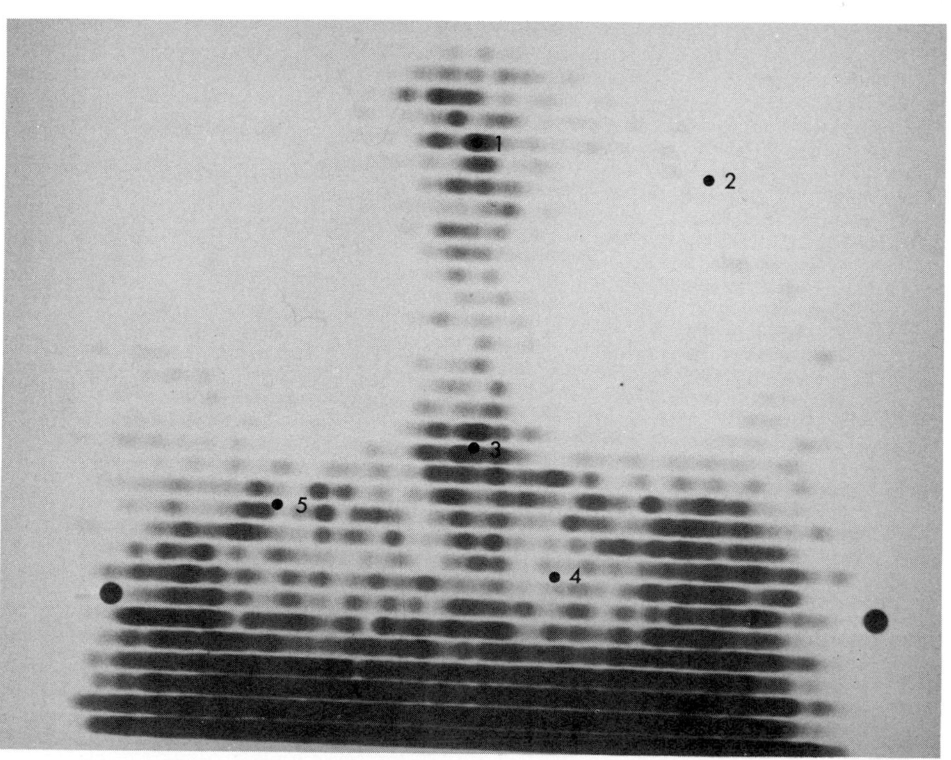

Fig. 5-28. Brain scan, posterior view. *1,* Superior sagittal sinus; *2,* vascularity over cerebrum; *3,* confluence of sinuses; *4,* posterior fossa: *5,* transverse sinus.

lumbar region, the rest of the lumbar subarachnoid space contains only nerve roots (Fig. 5-25). Note that the subarachnoid space extends to the second sacral segment in this patient. The subarachnoid space, outlined by this Pantopaque column, is continuous with the posterior surfaces of the vertebral bodies and disk spaces in the normal patient (Fig. 5-25). Any deviation from this normal relationship suggests possibility of a herniated nucleus pulposus or of some other space-occupying lesion. As in the cervical area, Fig. 5-26 shows the nerve roots emerging from the subarachnoid space.

REFERENCES

1. Hodges, F. J. III: Seminar, Roentgenology 5:101, 1970.
2. Meschan, I.: Atlas of normal radiographic anatomy, Philadelphia, 1959, W. B. Saunders Co.
3. Shapiro, R.: Myelography, ed. 2, Chicago, 1968, Year Book Medical Publishers, Inc.
4. Taveras, J., and Wood, E. H.: Diagnostic neuroradiology, Baltimore, 1964, The Williams & Wilkens Co.
5. Wagner, H.: Principles of nuclear medicine, Philadelphia, 1968, W. B. Saunders Co.
6. Wilson, M.: The anatomical foundation of neuroradiology of the brain, Boston, 1963, Little, Brown and Co.

CHAPTER 6

PERIPHERAL NERVOUS SYSTEM

JEFF MINCKLER

For descriptive purposes it is convenient to group the gross components of the peripheral nervous system into *cranial nerves* and *spinal nerves.* The quantitative characteristics of these structures are presented in Chapter 7. The cranial and spinal nerves will be divided into *motor* and *sensory* categories when applicable. This will require that the *motor nucleus* be identified in the CNS with the motor distribution pattern to the peripheral end-organ supplied. The course and topography of motor nerves en route to the end-organ can be found in text books of gross anatomy. The objective here is to establish the relationship between the central nucleus and the peripheral terminal target. In relating *motor nuclei* to end-organ, it is helpful to keep in mind the basic functional separations: *somatic efferent, special visceral efferent,* and *general visceral efferent* (see p. 10). A separate, summarizing section will deal with general visceral efferent nuclei. Their overlapping motor patterns are separated into *parasympathetic* (craniosacral division) and *sympathetic* (thoracolumbar division) components. The gross *sensory* neuroanatomic features of prime importance include: assignment of *peripheral distribution* of sensory areas to both segments and nerves; location of *sensory ganglia;* and location of *primary sensory nuclei,* or central receiving cell masses, to which the afferent impulses are first carried. Again, subdivisions into functional afferent units will be observed; that is: *general somatic afferent, special somatic afferent, general visceral afferent,* and *special visceral afferent.* Many of the nerves are *mixed,* conveying both afferent and efferent impulses.

CRANIAL NERVES

A basal view of the brain displays the twelve cranial nerves in their take-off positions (Fig. 6-1). From times long gone, students have adapted "On Old Olympus's Towering Top A Fat Auld German Viewed A Hop" to their own tastes as a device to facilitate memorizing the cranial nerves. The numerical, "classical" representation of the cranial nerves as given in Fig. 6-1 and in the following paragraphs is probably not the most accurate, but it is almost universally used. Exceptions to the numerical classification that might be proper include: (1) *nervus terminalis,* which is first in line but often overlooked; (2) *vomeronasal nerve,* a primitive nerve that supplies the vestigial vomeronasal organ (of Jacobson); (3) *masticator nerve,* which is a separate motor unit but is usually regarded as the motor division of the trigeminal nerve (V); (4) *nervus intermedius* (glossopalatine, or nerve of Wrisberg), which is an independent nerve typically tied to the facial nerve (VII); (5) separation of *vestibular* and *auditory* parts of the acoustic nerve (VIII); and (6) *Benedikt's "thirteenth"* cranial nerve, which represents special fibers traveling with central cranial nerve (X) fibers to supply the choroid plexus. With these modifications there would be eighteen cranial nerves in man. In light of the above poem so well known to thousands, this would be wholly untenable.

Terminal nerve (cranial nerve O)

This nerve appears as a definitive bundle in the olfactory trigone and passes peripherally to the nasal mucous membrane along side the olfactory tract. The fibers continue from the region of the crista galli through the cribriform plate, along with the olfactory filaments and the vomeronasal nerve. The function of the terminal nerve is not well understood. It seems to have an efferent, or possibly visceral efferent, component leading to glands or vessels in the nasal mucous membrane. These

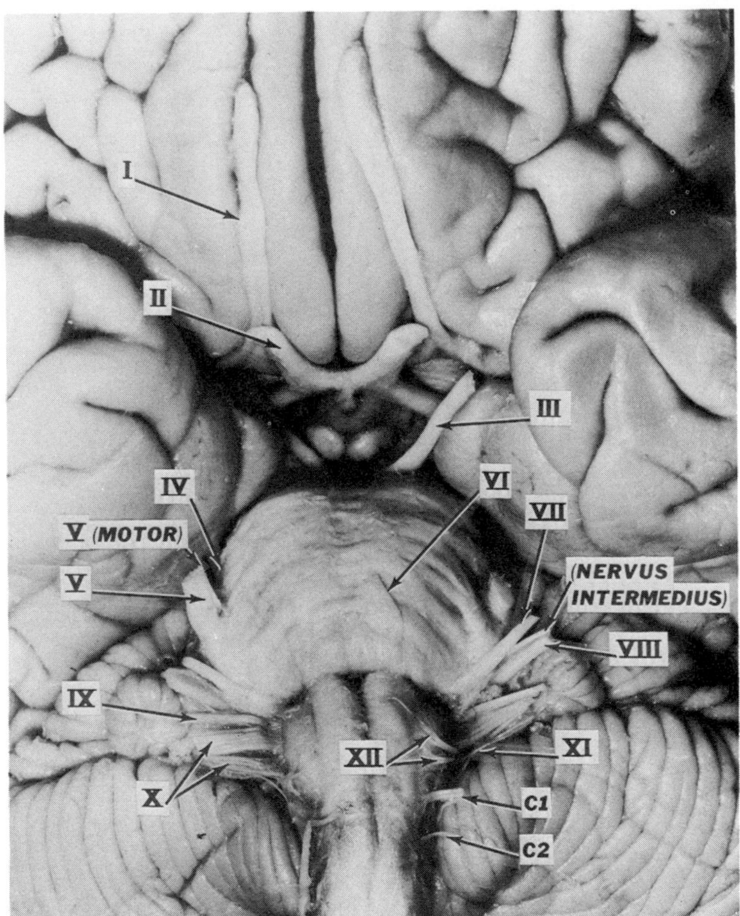

Fig. 6-1. Ventral view of brain and nerves.

visceral fibers arise in the supraoptic region and synapse en route with ganglion cells.[4] The remaining fibers appear to be sensory, with ganglion cells located along the peripheral parts of the nerves and near the olfactory bulbs (*terminal ganglia*). Centrally they pass to primary receptive areas in the septum pellucidum, the olfactory cortical areas, and the posterior commissural region.

Vomeronasal nerve (vestigial)

This nerve arises in the vomeronasal *organ of Jacobson,* which is an embryonic neuroepithelial organ in the anterior nasal septum. It persists in the adult only as a rudiment, if at all. It probably represents a special odor-sampling organ in lower forms, such as reptiles. In man it occasionally provides the originating tissue of neurogenic tumors in the nose. In the embryo the nerves pass with olfactory filaments to *accessory olfactory bulbs.* These nerves disappear in later embryonic life.

Olfactory nerve (I) (Fig. 6-1)

The olfactory nerves are aggregated into eighteen or twenty filaments on either side that pass through the foramina of the cribriform plate and terminate in the olfactory bulbs. They arise as extensions of special *olfactory cells,* which possess hair-like processes that project into the nasal cavity. These cells are bipolar chemoreceptors with cell bodies located in the olfactory epithelium. The peripheral distribution is to the upper third of the nasal mucous membrane covering both septum and side walls (Fig. 6-2). The primary receptive nucleus is in the olfactory bulb, which, together with its tract, is an extension of the CNS. A point of considerable interest is the continuity of the *peri-*

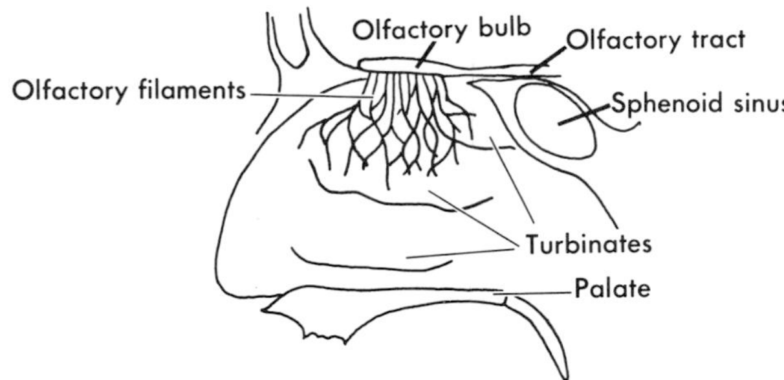

Fig. 6-2. Distribution of olfactory fibers.

neuronal spaces around olfactory filaments with the subarachnoid space of the brain (see Chapter 3). This provides a presumed route of spread for noxious agents and accounts for leakage of CSF into the nose in fractures of the cribriform plate. (See Chapter 17 for pathways and histology of the system.)

Optic nerve (II) (Fig. 6-1)

The optic nerve as represented is actually a tract of the CNS. It conveys approximately one million fibers from the retina to the diencephalon and midbrain in the bulky "nerve." This is attached to the eyeball approximately 3 mm. inferomedial to the posterior pole and enters the cranial cavity through the optic foramen. The nerve is covered with meninges in the same pattern as the brain, and the spaces are continuous with those of the brain. The cell bodies giving rise to optic nerve fibers are the *ganglion cells of the retina* (see Chapter 20). The nerve continues into the *chiasm,* in which the fibers from the nasal half of each globe cross to the opposite side. These fibers join the fibers from the temporal half of the opposite eye in the optic tracts. The *optic tracts* encircle the peduncles (Fig. 6-3) and terminate in three areas: (1) the *lateral geniculate body;* (2) the *superior colliculus,* via the brachium of the superior colliculus; and (3) the *pretectal area* of the midbrain. These terminations are not primary receptive areas for the visual system. The equivalent of primary receiving nuclei such as in the olfactory bulb are within the retinal layers themselves (see Chapter 20). In some animal forms, other fibers are added to the optic tracts and chiasm. These include the *medial geniculate commissure of Gudden,* by which the medial geniculate bodies of the auditory system are presumedly interconnected. There is uncertainty concerning the identity of this tract in the human optic system. It is possible also that visceral efferent fibers travel from the midbrain to the retina via the optic nerves. These have not been demonstrated in man, and more appropriate pathways for such supply are known to exist (for example, autonomic nerves along vessels).

The blood supply to the optic nerve travels through the *central artery of the retina.* The central artery, a branch of the ophthalmic artery, enters the nerve a few millimeters posterior to the attachment of the nerve to the bulb. A *central vein*

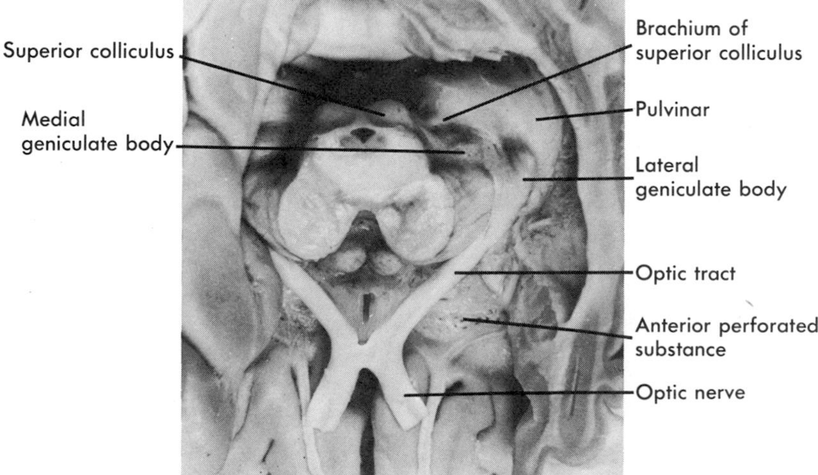

Fig. 6-3. Dissection of optic tract.

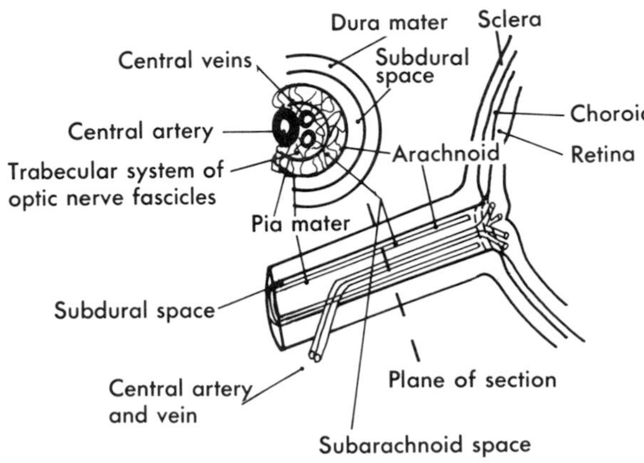

Fig. 6-4. Diagram of optic nerve and vessels.

accompanies the artery. These two vessels are subject to the effects of intracranial pressure, since they traverse the meningeal spaces that are continuous with those covering the brain (Fig. 6-4). The difference in compressibility between artery and vein plays a part in the congestive features of the retina in the event of elevated intracranial tension. (See Chapter 20 for details of the visual pathway.)

Oculomotor nerve (III) (Fig. 6-1)

Cranial nerve III arises superficially in the oculomotor sulcus within the interpeduncular fossa on the medial side of each peduncle. The efferent part of the nerve carries *somatic efferent* fibers and *parasympathetic general visceral efferent* fibers. The *somatic efferent* fibers arise in the somatic nucleus. The somatic nucleus is in the gray matter ventral to the cerebral aqueduct, and extends from the parasympathetic nucleus above downward to the nucleus of cranial nerve IV. The extent of the nucleus (about 5 mm. of length) roughly corre-

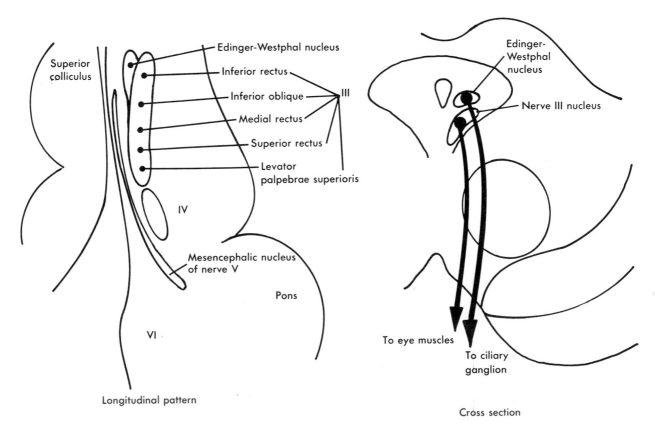

Fig. 6-5. Presumed somatotopic pattern of oculomotor nuclear complex. Left, side view; right, cross section.

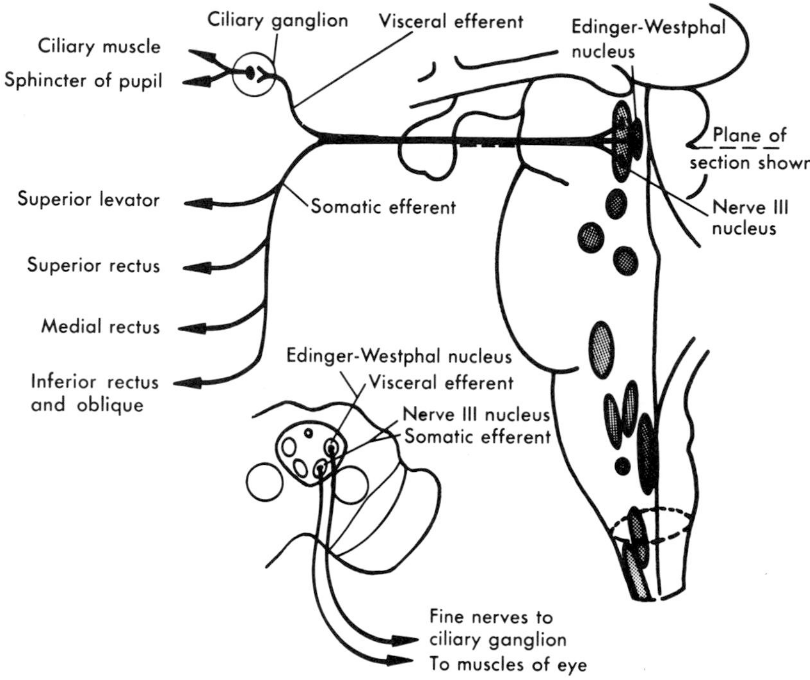

Fig. 6-6. Distribution of cranial nerve III (oculomotor).

sponds to that of the superior colliculus. From above downward the nucleus in cats exhibits a *somatotopic order* in relation to the extrinsic eye muscle supplied. This order is as follows: inferior rectus, inferior oblique, medial rectus, superior rectus, and levator palpebrae superioris. The same order appears to apply to monkeys. Projected to the human nucleus, it would provide the somatotopic pattern represented in Fig. 6-5. In cross section the somatic nucleus is dorsoventrally elongate and has a triangular shape. The nerve III fibers arising in it pass through and around the adjacent midbrain structures (nucleus ruber and longitudinal fasciculus) to reach the oculomotor sulcus (Fig. 6-6). In an extramedullary position it passes between the superior cerebellar artery and posterior cerebral artery (Fig. 3-19) and penetrates the dura mater at the point of attachment of the tentorium. It runs in the lateral wall of the cavernous sinus and enters the orbit through the superior orbital fissure. Here it supplies the levator palpebrae superioris and all the extrinsic ocular muscles except the superior oblique and lateral rectus (inferior rectus, inferior oblique, medial rectus, superior rectus). The nerve supply to the levator has a bilateral origin. The superior rectus muscle is supplied by fibers from the opposite nucleus, while the other muscles are supplied by fibers from nuclei on the same side.

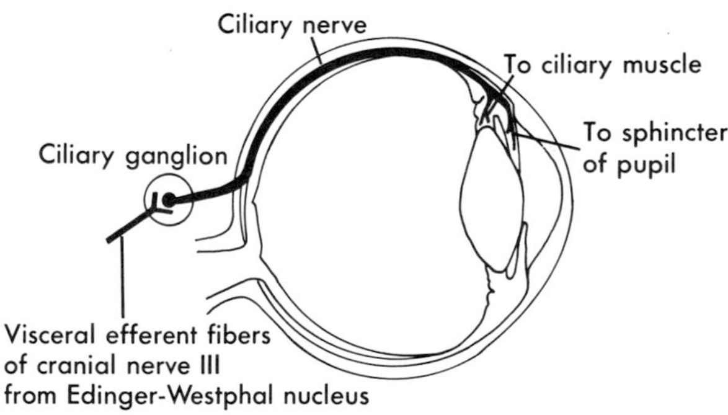

Fig. 6-7. Innervation of ciliary muscle and pupillary sphincter from ciliary ganglia.

The *visceral efferent fibers* (parasympathetic) are presumed to arise in the *Edinger-Westphal nucleus,* although direct evidence for this relationship in man is lacking. This nucleus lies dorsal and superior to the bilateral parts of the somatic nucleus.

It has a small midline part superiorly and isolated bilateral parts in a more posterior position (Fig. 6-5). The fibers are believed to leave the midbrain with nerve III proper, but this also has not been clearly demonstrated. The fibers of this origin presumably represent parasympathetic components of the autonomic system and are preganglionic, with termination in the *ciliary ganglion* (Fig. 6-7). The postganglionic fibers pass from the ciliary ganglion to the *ciliary muscle,* for the most part, with a few innervating the *sphincter of the pupil.*[8]

Deep sensibility (somatic afferent) in ocular muscles is known to exist, although its pathways are uncertain. Some of the cells of the somatic nucleus proper resemble those of the mesencephalic nucleus of the trigeminal nerve[5] and may therefore represent unipolar sensory cells that mediate ocular muscle sense. A second possibility is that deep sensibility (*proprioception*) for these muscles is mediated by nerve V itself with cell bodies in the mesencephalic nucleus, which lies dorsolateral to the nerve III nucleus (Fig. 6-5). Afferent fibers might reach the nucleus either over nerve III or nerve V.

Trochlear nerve (IV) (Fig. 6-1)

Cranial nerve IV has its superficial origin in the superior part of the anterior medullary velum, posterior to the inferior colliculus and on either side of the dorsum of the midbrain. It is the smallest of the cranial nerves and passes around the cerebral peduncles into the orbit via the lateral wall of the cavernous sinus and the superior orbital fissure. The trochlear nerve supplies the superior oblique extrinsic ocular muscle (trochlear muscle). The *somatic motor nucleus* of the trochlear nerve is continuous with that of the oculomotor. It lies in the ventral gray matter of the cerebral aqueduct, at the level of the inferior colliculus (Fig. 6-8). Its fibers pass inferiorly and turn dorsally to cross in the anterior (superior) medullary velum. After crossing, the fibers issue just below the inferior colliculus at the sides of the frenulum of the velum. Deep-sensibility fibers for the trochlear muscle are believed to travel either in nerve IV itself or in nerve V. They are related to intramedullary unipolar cells, occupying either the nerve IV nucleus or the mesencephalic root of nerve V.

Trigeminal nerve (V) (Fig. 6-1)

Nerve V is the largest of the cranial nerves. It is mixed and complex, possessing the following: (1) a *special visceral efferent* component to the muscles of mastication; (2) a very large *somatic afferent* component distributed both to skin and mucous membranes; and (3) the unusual *deep sense*

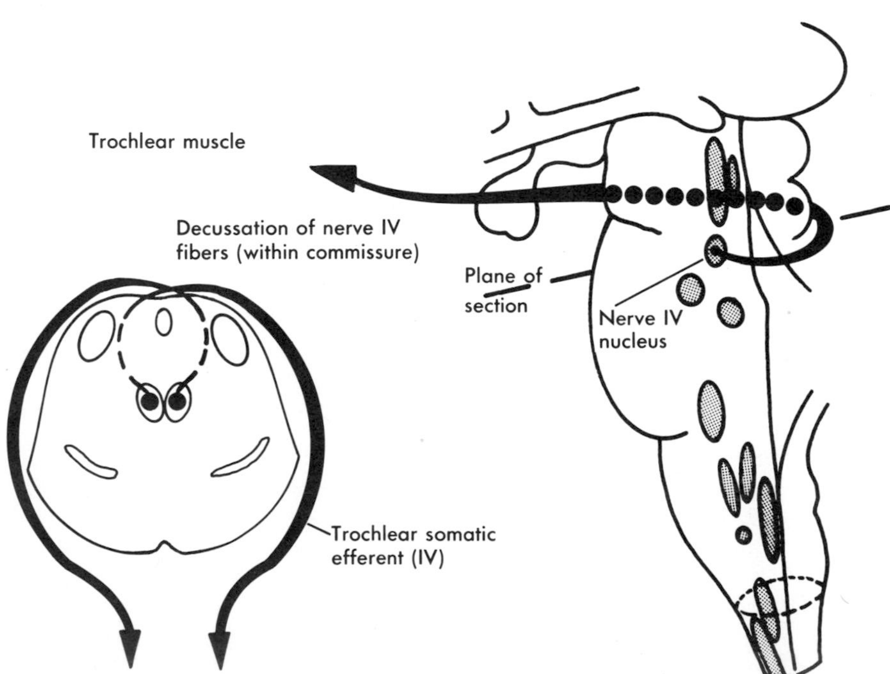

Fig. 6-8. Distribution of cranial nerve IV (trochlear).

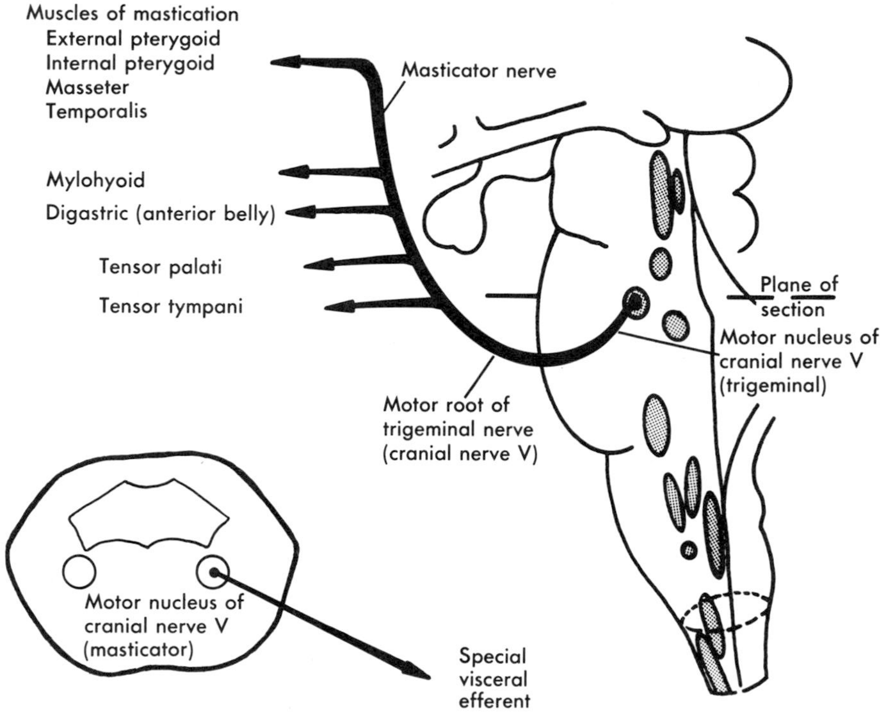

Fig. 6-9. Distribution of motor root of cranial nerve V (trigeminal).

afferent components (from the branchial muscles) that have ganglion cells placed within the brainstem. The superficial origin is on either side of the pons, with bulky fibers issuing through the middle cerebellar peduncle near its base. The special visceral motor root (*masticator nerve*) arises slightly superior and ventral to the sensory root and is separated from it by a few transverse pontine fibers. It passes into Meckel's cave and runs as a separate strand, medial to the semilunar ganglion. It joins the mandibular sensory division immediately after passing through the foramen ovale. The masticator nerve is distributed to the muscles of mastication (external pterygoid, internal pterygoid, masseter, and temporalis muscles). Other motor branches supply the mylohyoid and anterior belly of the diagastric muscle, as well as the tensor palati and tensor tympani. The muscles supplied originate in branchial arches. This feature establishes the nerve supply as special visceral efferent. The nucleus of origin of the masticator nerve is the *motor nucleus* of the trigeminal. This nucleus is located in the lateral tegmentum of the pons (Fig. 6-9) near the floor of the ventricle at the level of the pontine attachment of nerve V roots (Fig. 6-1). As

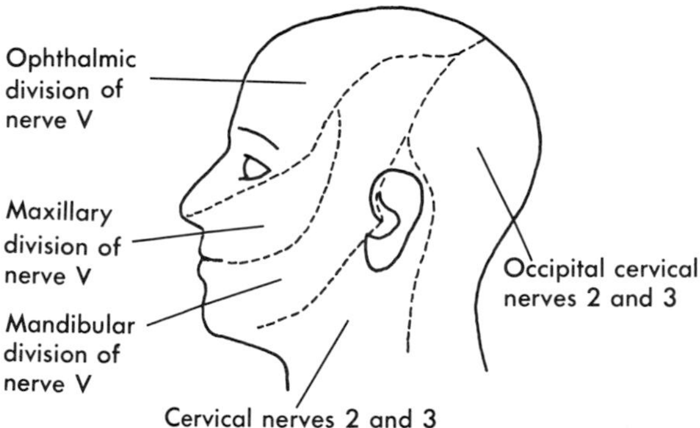

Fig. 6-10. Cutaneous nerve supply to head region.

special visceral efferent fibers these are final-common-path in character and have no intervening postganglionic cell between the motor nucleus and the end-organ.

The *somatic sensory root* of the trigeminal nerve enters the pons slightly inferior and dorsal to the motor root. The root's cell bodies (unipolar) are located in the *semilunar ganglion,* which occupies Meckel's cave. The distal afferent fibers of the nerve are distributed in three large divisions, *oph-*

thalmic, maxillary, and *mandibular.* The ophthalmic division gives off a recurrent branch to the tentorial dura and enters the orbit through the superior orbital fissure. Through elaborate branches it provides sensory nerves to the orbit and the related mucous membranes and glands and to the nasal mucous membranes and sinuses (frontal and ethmoidal). The distribution to the skin of the face is displayed in Fig. 6-10. The maxillary division gives off a middle meningeal branch, which follows the course of the middle meningeal artery, and leaves the cranial cavity via the foramen rotundum. The main branch is distributed to the skin of the face, from lower eyelid to upper lip. The maxillary division also supplies sensory fibers to the mucous membranes of the upper gums, roof of the mouth, soft palate, tonsilar area, maxillary sinus, lower nasal area, and nasopharynx. In addition, it supplies the upper teeth. The mandibular division passes through the foramen ovale and gives off a meningeal branch that turns back into the foramen spinosum for sensory distribution to the dura. The sensory mandibular division supplies the lower teeth, the mucous membrane of the mouth associated with the lower jaw and tongue, the external auditory meatus and tympanic membrane, and the skin in preauricular, mandibular, and posterior temporal areas.

The primary receptive nuclei for the somatic afferent components of nerve V include two major clusters, the *chief sensory nucleus* and the *nucleus of the descending root.* The *chief nucleus* is lateral and superior to the motor nucleus (Fig. 6-11) and receives touch and discriminative sense impulses from the short ascending divisions of the incoming sensory fibers. The longer divisions turn downward into the descending (spinal) tract. The descending fibers terminate in relationship to the cells of the associated nucleus of the *descending (spinal) trigeminal tract.* The *descending (spinal) nucleus* is continuous above with the chief sensory nucleus; at this point the nucleus ceases. The nucleus of the descending tract is continuous downward with the *substantia gelatinosa* of the spinal cord (Fig. 6-11). The descending tract is concerned with pain and conduction of temperature from skin, mucous membranes, and meninges. It is probable that fibers mediating these sensations from nerves VII, IX, and X also join the descending root of nerve V and terminate in its nucleus. Fibers of the descending root of mandibular origin continue as far down as the medulla. Fibers of maxillary origin continue somewhat farther, and those of ophthalmic origin probably run as far as to upper cervical segments.

The special *deep sensibility* afferent fibers mediating muscles sense of the visceral striated muscle supplied by nerve V have special interest. These fibers pass the trigeminal (semilunar) ganglion, probably with the fibers of the motor root, and are associated with cell bodies located along the *mesencephalic root* of the nerve. This root turns superiorly near the motor nucleus and extends upward to the level of the superior colliculus (Fig. 6-11). In cross section through the upper

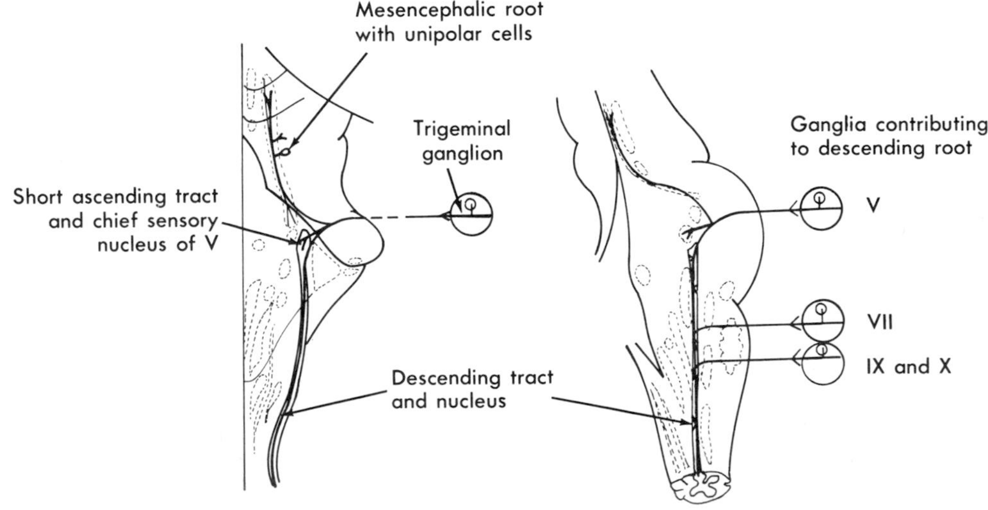

Fig. 6-11. Intramedullary sensory patterns of cranial nerve V (trigeminal). Note contributions to descending root from nerves VII, IX, and X.

pons, the mesencephalic nucleus lies between the ventricle and the superior cerebellar peduncle. It remains lateral to the cerebral aqueduct in the midbrain. The cells of the mesencephalic nucleus are unipolar and are believed to represent sensory cell bodies that have not migrated into the customary outlying sensory ganglionic position. It is possible that this nucleus also mediates deep muscle sense (proprioception) for muscles supplied by nerves III, IV, VI, and VII.[5,6]

Abducens nerve (VI) (Fig. 6-1)

The superficial origin of nerve VI is in the sulcus between the upper end of the pyramid and the inferior border of the pons. The nerve passes upward and anteriorly, paralleling the basal artery. It then enters the dura to course in the medial wall of the cavernous sinus. It enters the orbit through the superior orbital fissure and supplies the lateral rectus muscle. The *somatic motor nucleus* lies beneath the facial colliculus in the floor of the fourth ventricle (Fig. 6-12). Its fibers pass transversely and inferiorly through the reticular formation, trapezoid body, pontine fibers, and pyramidal tracts of the pons. The fibers reach the pontomedullary sulcus and exit on the same side as the nucleus (Fig. 6-1). It should be noted that the abducens nerve nucleus lies in the same line as the nuclei of nerves III and IV, and functions with them in controlling eye movements. Deep sense supply to the lateral rectus muscle is obscure, but the afferents probably either run among the fibers of the nerve VI efferents or join the ophthalmic division of nerve V to find their way to the mesencephalic root.

Facial nerve (VII) (Fig. 6-1)

The superficial origin of the nerve VII is in the lateral part of the sulcus between pons and medulla. It arises as a larger *motor root,* which is medial to the smaller, hair-like *nervus intermedius.* On gross inspection the latter is closely related to nerve VIII. The motor root is *special visceral efferent* in supplying muscles of branchial origin. The motor division of nerve VII passes into the internal auditory meatus with the nervus intermedius and nerve VIII. At the extremity of the meatus, it enters the facial canal to emerge at the stylomastoid foramen, where it enters the substance of the pa-

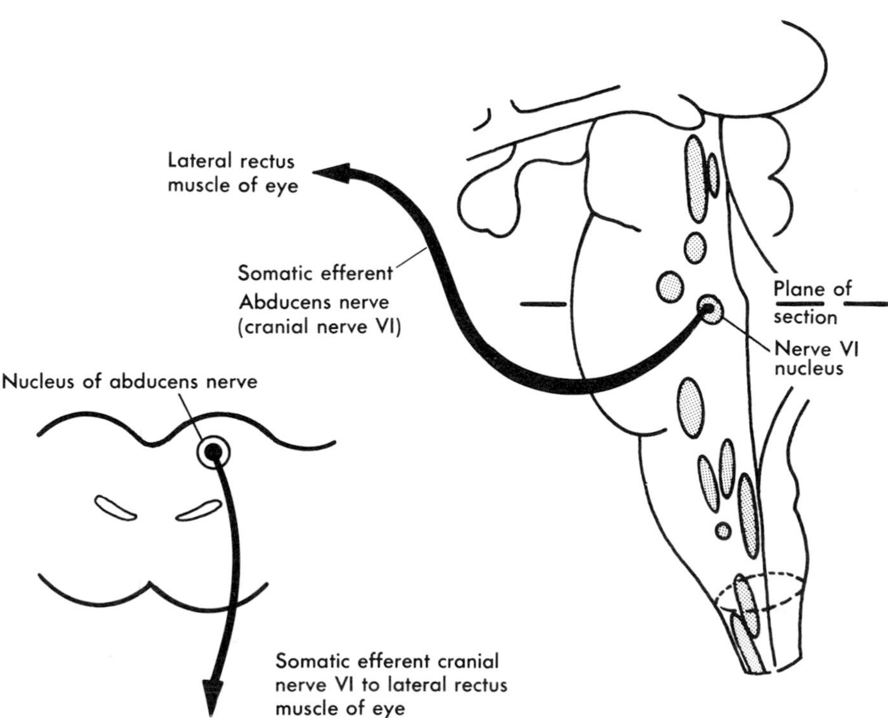

Fig. 6-12. Distribution of cranial nerve VI (abducens).

rotid gland. En route it gives off the nerve to the stapedius muscle, and branches to the posterior belly of the digastric muscle and to the stylohyoid muscle. The motor nerve is then distributed to the muscles of facial expression. These include the following muscles: auricular, occipitofrontal, procerus, corrugator, nasal, zygomatic, levator of the angle of the mouth, depressor of nasal septum, orbicularis oris, risorius, buccinator, depressor of angle of mouth, depressor of lower lip, mentalis, and platysma. The motor nucleus lies in the lateral part of the medullary tegmentum, just lateral to and above the superior pole of the inferior olive. At a higher level (in lower pons) it lies immediately dorsal to the nuclear clusters of the superior olivary complex (Fig. 6-13). The fibers of the nerve pass dorsally to the floor of the fourth ventricle, where they turn upward and then anteriorly, arching over the nucleus of the abducens nerve to form the *internal genu,* or knee, which produces the bulge of the facial colliculus in the floor of the ventricle (Fig. 2-1, *A*). The fibers continue inferolaterally and anteriorly, passing close to the nucleus; they emerge on the same side in the lateral pontomedullary sulcus.

Deep sensibility afferent fibers from the distribution of the motor root of nerve VII probably run centrally in either the motor division of VII or with nerve V fibers to become part of the mesencephalic root.

Somatic afferent fibers in nerve VII arise in the skin of the external ear and in the tympanic membrane. They convey impulses along nerve VII within the facial canal and have their cell bodies in the *geniculate ganglion.* They join the descending tract of the nerve V centrally and terminate in its nucleus.

Nervus intermedius (glossopalatine nerve or nerve of Wrisberg) is described as part of nerve VII, although its character would justify classification as a distinct cranial nerve. It is a mixed motor and sensory nerve, with *general visceral efferent* (parasympathetic) and *general* and *special visceral afferent* components. The general visceral efferent fibers arise in the *superior salivatory nucleus,* which is lateral to the nerve VI nucleus and dorsal to the motor nucleus of nerve VII (Fig. 6-14). The fibers pass directly out of the *medulla* close to the motor fibers of nerve VII. They continue into the internal auditory meatus and divide near the genu of nerve VII into the *greater superficial petrosal* and the

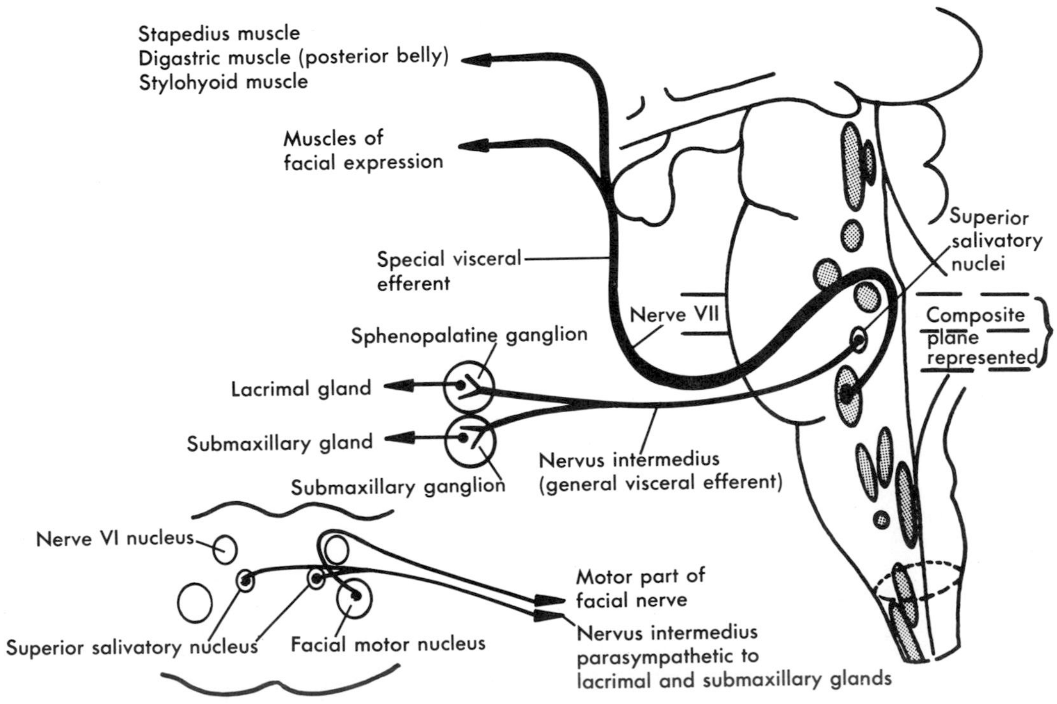

Fig. 6-13. Distribution of motor parts of cranial nerve VII (facial).

efferent part of the *chorda tympani.* The greater superficial petrosal conveys parasympathetic preganglionic fibers to the *sphenopalatine ganglion.* Postganglionic fibers from this ganglion innervate the *lacrimal gland* in the orbit and mucous glands in the nose and mouth. The efferent components in the chorda tympani are the preganglionic secretory parasympathetic fibers to the *submandibular ganglion.* The postganglionics from this ganglion supply secretory fibers to both the *submandibular* (submaxillary) and *sublingual* salivary glands and to mucous glands of the mouth. Vasodilator fibers pass to the same areas as secretory postganglionics.

General visceral afferent fibers from blood vessels of the face and meninges are conveyed through the nervus intermedius and have their cell bodies in the *geniculate ganglion.* These fibers terminate centrally in the nucleus of the *solitary fasciculus* (Fig. 6-14). The *special visceral afferent* fibers of the nervus intermedius arise in taste buds in the anterior two-thirds of the tongue and pass centrally via the chorda tympani. Their cell bodies are located in the *geniculate ganglion,* and their central processes terminate in the nucleus of the solitary fasciculus. The solitary tract lies dorsolateral to the central canal in the lower medulla. This tract moves laterally in position as it is traced upward to the level of the inferior part of the facial motor nucleus (Fig. 6-13). The nucleus related to the solitary tract receives visceral afferent impulses from nerves IX and X as well as from nerve VII (see following paragraphs).

Acoustic nerve (VIII) (Fig. 6-1)

The acoustic nerve is the combination of *vestibular* (equilibration) and *cochlear* (hearing) divisions. The two gross divisions combine at the superficial origin of nerve VIII, at the lateral extremity of the pontomedullary sulcus. The combined nerve passes into the external auditory meatus and redivides. The cochlear division goes to the cochlea and the vestibular division to the semicircular

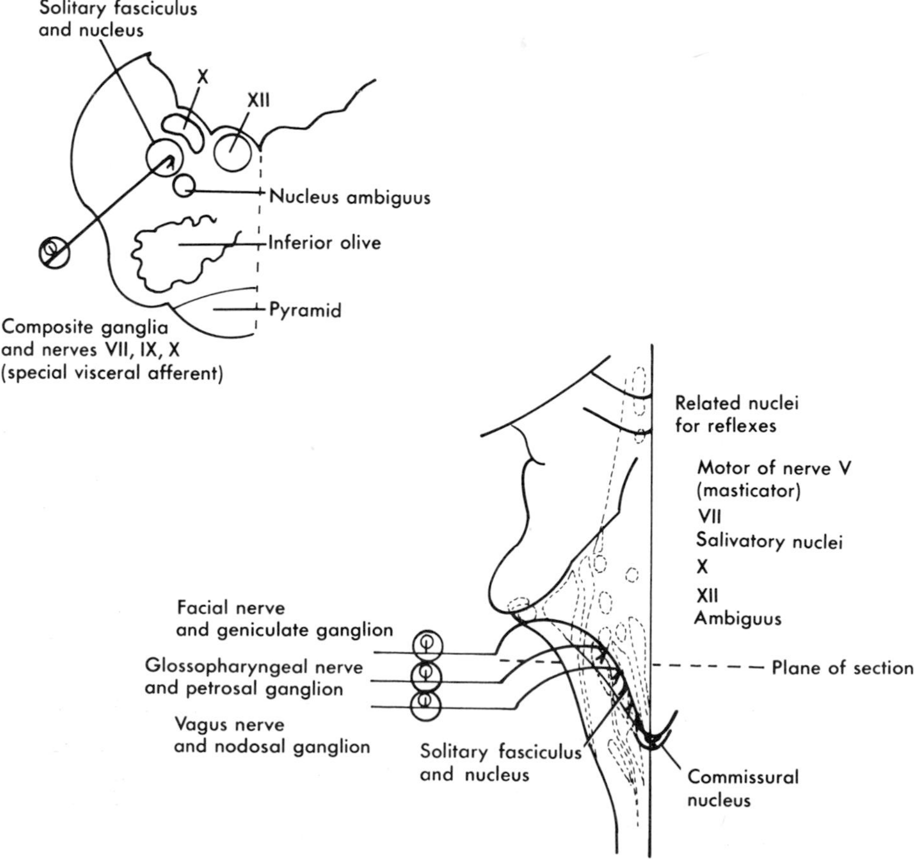

Fig. 6-14. Solitary fasciculus and related nuclei.

canals, utricle and saccule (Fig. 6-15). The vestibular division arises from fibers in the maculae and cristae of the equilibratory apparatus. The fibers have their cell bodies (bipolar) in the vestibular ganglion (of Scarpa), in the depths of the internal auditory canal (Fig. 6-15). The nerve passes to the medulla and penetrates deep to the corpus restiforme, terminating in the *vestibular nuclei.* (See Chapter 19 for details.) The cochlear division arises from fibers within the cochlea. Its ganglion (of Corti) lies in a spiral pattern at the base of the modiolus and is made up of bipolar cells. It joins the vestibular nerve in the internal auditory canal and passes to the brainstem, where it turns over (external to) the corpus restiforme (Fig. 6-15). The cochlear nerve terminates in the *dorsal* and *ventral cochlear nuclei,* with a few fibers going to the *superior olivary complex* (Fig. 6-15). Nerves of uncertain type pass in an efferent direction in the vestibulocochlear complex. The best

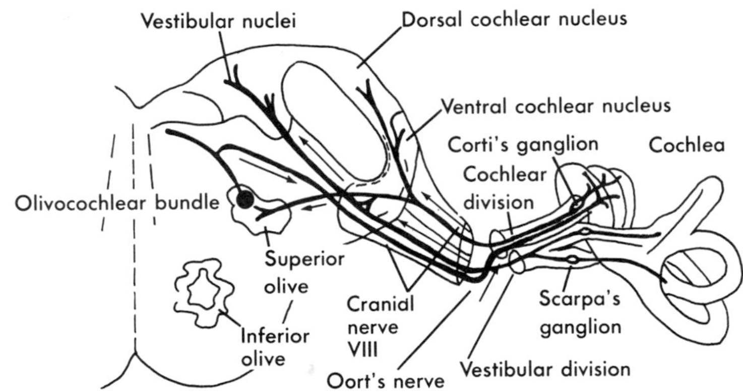

Fig. 6-15. Sensory patterns of cranial nerve VIII (auditory).

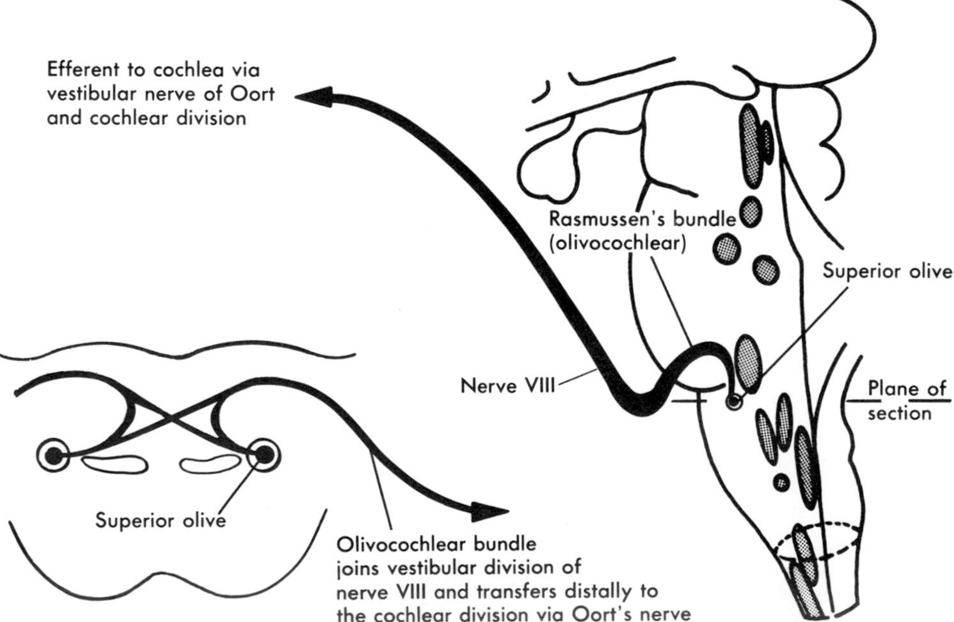

Fig. 6-16. Probable olivocochlear pattern of cranial nerve VIII.

known efferent component is the *olivocochlear bundle* (of Rasmussen) (Fig. 6-16). A small bundle of nerves (of Oort) interconnects the vestibular and cochlear divisions distally. (See Chapter 19 for details.)

Glossopharyngeal nerve (IX) (Fig. 6-1)

The superficial origin places this complex mixed nerve as the uppermost in the "vagal group" (nerves IX, X, and XI). It includes *special visceral efferent, general visceral efferent, special visceral afferent,* and *general somatic afferent* fibers. The peripheral course is through the jugular foramen. The nerve possesses two sensory ganglia, the *superior* (related to somatic afferent) and the *petrosal* (related to the general and special viceral afferent systems). *Special visceral efferent* fibers are represented by the nerve supply to the stylopharyngeus muscle, a branchial derivative. The nucleus of the special visceral efferent fibers lies in the lateral part of the medulla as the upper part of the *nucleus ambiguus* (Figs. 6-17 and 6-18). This is also the nucleus of origin for the special visceral efferent fibers of nerve X. *General visceral efferent* fibers arise in the *inferior salivatory nucleus,* which is a discrete cell cluster medial to the solitary fasciculus (Fig. 6-14). These efferent fibers are parasympathetic preganglionic and terminate in the otic ganglion. From the otic ganglion they are relayed by postganglionic fibers as secretory fibers to the *parotid* salivary gland (Fig. 6-17). Like the other parasympathetics these secretory fibers are also vasodilators. *General visceral afferent* impulses are carried in nerve IX from the tongue, tonsil, eustachian tube, middle ear, and portions of nasopharynx and oropharynx. The cell bodies are located in the inferior, or petrosal, ganglion and terminate in the solitary nucleus. The visceral afferent fibers that supply the carotid sinus and body are of particular note, as they are important in regulation of blood pressure. *Special visceral afferent* fibers with cell bodies located in the inferior ganglion convey taste from the posterior third of the tongue through nerve IX. These fibers enter the solitary tract and terminate in the adjacent solitary nucleus (gustatory). *Somatic afferent* fibers arise in the external auditory meatus and have their cell bodies in the superior, or jugular, ganglion. They terminate by joining the descending tract of nerve V, ending in relationship to cells of its nucleus. Deep sense arising in the stylopharyngeus muscle is presumed to reach the

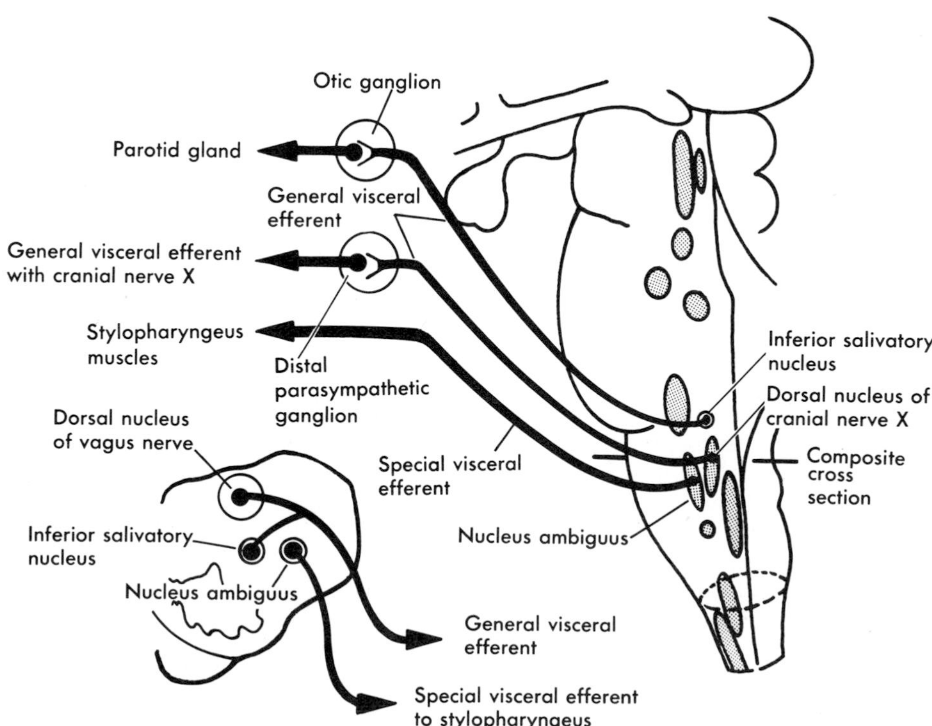

Fig. 6-17. Distribution of cranial nerve IX (glossopharyngeal). Note mixture with nerve X.

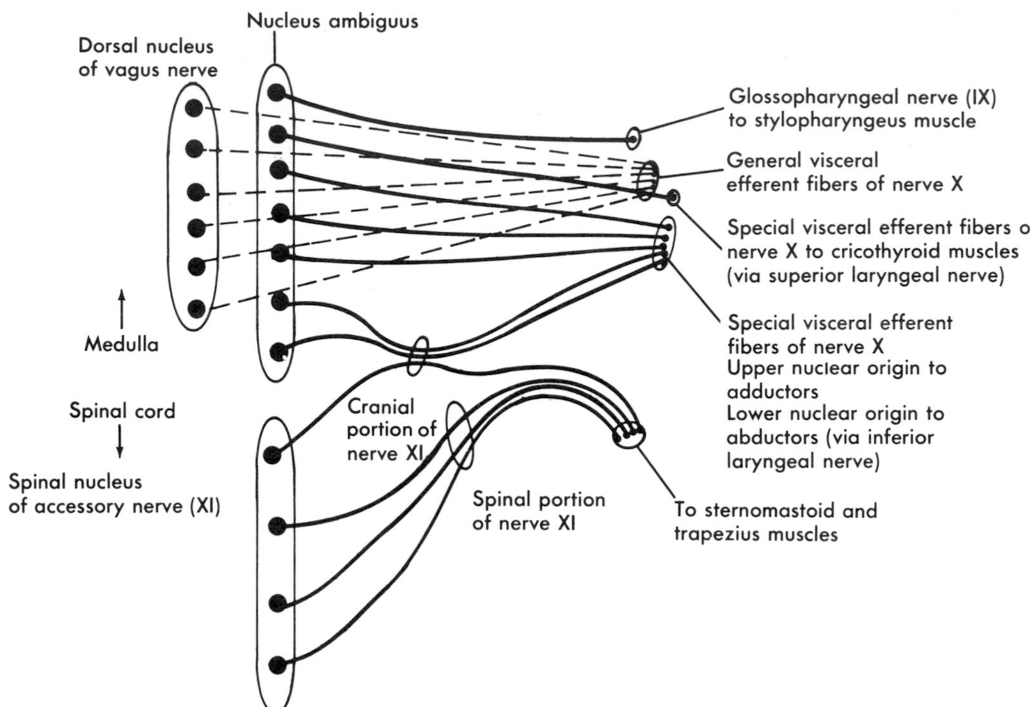

Fig. 6-18. The vagal complex in the brainstem, with presumed somatotopic pattern in nucleus ambiguus.

mesencephalic root of nerve V. There is some uncertainty regarding an admixture of nerve IX and X nuclear origins in the supply to muscles of the pharynx. The two nerves are closely related.

Vagus nerve (X) (Fig. 6-1)

The vagus is a complex mixed nerve with extensive gross distribution. Its superficial origin is immediately inferior to nerve IX through eight to ten filaments in the postolivary sulcus. The nerve leaves the cranial cavity as a bound bundle through the jugular foramen and possesses two sensory ganglia, an upper *jugular* and a lower *nodose,* which are respectively within and outside the opening in the skull. The vagus nerve is the most important nerve in point of extent of distribution among the cerebral nerves of the *general visceral efferent* system (nerves III, VII, IX, and X). It also contains *special visceral efferent* fibers to the branchiogenic muscles of the pharynx and larynx.

Autonomic fibers of uncertain character pass from nucleus ambiguus to the choroid plexus (Benedikt's "thirteenth" cranial nerve). Other fibers pass directly from the medulla to the choroid of the fourth ventricle; these are probably not vagal.[7]

Afferent limbs include both *visceral* and *somatic* components. In the peripheral course the right and left vagi take significantly different routes. The *right vagus* runs in the neck to the level of the subclavian artery, which it passes in an anterior position. Here it gives off the right recurrent (laryngeal) nerve. It descends in the mediastinum to the posterior aspect of the right main bronchus and travels through the diaphragm on the posterior surface of the esophagus. The right nerve spreads over the posterior surface of the stomach and continues to the viscera (intestines, pancreas, spleen, kidneys) through the celiac plexus without interruption. The *left vagus* passes through the neck and crosses the arch of the aorta anteriorly. At this level it gives off the left recurrent (laryngeal) nerve and proceeds to the posterior aspect of the left main bronchus. The left nerve then forms a plexus on the anterior surface of the esophagus that interconnects with the posterior esophageal plexus. It is conveyed through the diaphragm aggregated as a trunk and spreads over the anterior surface of the stomach. The left nerve extends grossly to the liver and somewhat to the intestines,

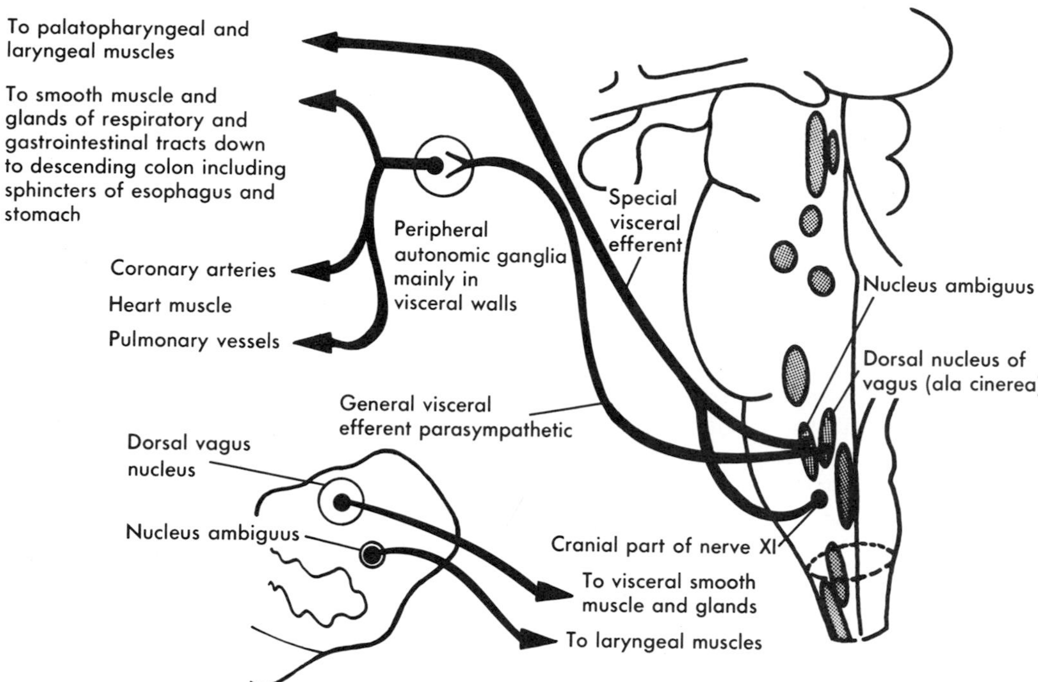

Fig. 6-19. Distribution of cranial nerve X (vagus).

but its principal route to the small bowel is in commingling with the right vagus in the esophageal plexus. The vagus nerves on either side en route provide branches to the meninges, auricle, pharynx, larynx (superior and inferior), bronchi, lungs, heart, pericardium, esophagus, stomach, liver, biliary tree, pancreas, spleen, kidney (smooth muscle in pelvis), small intestine, and large bowel to the level of the left colic flexure (Fig. 6-26).

The *general visceral efferent* fibers of the vagus nerve are preganglionic and terminate in relationship to parasympathetic ganglion cells within the organs supplied. Short postganglionics supply the end-organs (glands and smooth muscles). The central nucleus for these fibers is the dorsal motor nucleus of nerve X. This produces the ala cinerea in the floor of the fourth ventricle (Fig. 6-19). The dorsal motor nucleus lies close to the central canal in the lower medulla and migrates somewhat laterally in higher levels, as seen in cross section. It is possible that cells of the ala cinerea supply the cardiorespiratory areas and the lower nuclei supply the abdominal region.

The *special visceral efferent* components of nerve X arise in nucleus ambiguus (Fig. 6-18) and pass to the branchiogenic musculature of the pharynx and larynx. The palatopharyngeal muscles supplied include the *constrictors* of the pharynx (*palatoglossus palatopharyngeus, salpingopharyngeus, uvular,* and *levator veli palatini*). These muscles are principally concerned with deglutition and articulation. The upper segment of nucleus ambiguus supplies fibers through nerve IX to the *stylopharyngeus* muscle. A somatotopic pattern is apparent in the nuclear origin of nerves supplying the intrinsic muscles of the larynx that regulate speech. The part of the nucleus below the origin of nerve IX supplies nerve X fibers through the superior laryngeal nerve to the *cricothyroid* muscle. The remaining vagal fibers that supply the intrinsic muscles of the larynx (inferior laryngeal from recurrent nerves) are related to the caudal extremity of the nucleus ambiguus. Those fibers that innervate abductors are placed higher than those supplying adductors. The abductor action is carried out principally by the *posterior cricoarytenoids* and adduction principally by the *lateral cricoarytenoids* and the *arytenoids,* both oblique and transverse. The lateral portion of the *thyroarytenoids* also assists in narrowing the rima glottidis, and, during deglutition unrelated to voice, the glottis is partially closed by the combined action of the *thyroarytenoids, arytenoids,* and *aryepiglottics.* The *cricothyroids* tense and elongate the vocal fold, and these muscles oppose the action of the *thyroarytenoids,* which shorten and relax the folds. The *vocalis* component of the thyroarytenoid muscle inserts obliquely into the vocal ligament and helps regulate its tension and length. The *thyroepiglottic* muscle, a subdivision of the thyroarytenoid, and the *ventricular* muscle are sometimes considered individual muscles. All the above intrinsic muscles are supplied by the vagus nerve, originating in the nucleus ambiguus (Fig. 6-19).

The *general visceral afferent* fibers of the vagus mediate unconscious reflex sensory impulses from the viscera mentioned in the preceding paragraphs. The cell bodies of these sensory neurons are located in the nodose (inferior) ganglion. The fibers turn downward in the solitary tract and terminate in the solitary nucleus (Fig. 6-14). It is uncertain whether visceral afferent nerves arising below the stomach actually join the vagus complex. These may be routed through spinal nerves. *Special visceral afferent* fibers mediate taste from the region of the epiglottis and probably terminate in the solitary nucleus as a primary receiving nucleus (see Chapter 17). *Somatic afferent* components arise in the meninges around the transverse sinus, the external auditory meatus, and the lower posterior aspect of the auricle. These have their cell bodies in the jugular (surperior) ganglion and terminate in the nucleus of the descending root of the trigeminal nerve by turning into the spinal tract of that nerve (Fig. 6-14). *Deep muscle sense* (proprioception) from the branchiogenic muscles supplied by the vagus remains obscure in course and termination. It is presumed to be mediated by nerves with cell bodies in the jugular (superior) ganglion and to terminate in or near the nucleus ambiguus.

Accessory nerve (spinal accessory, XI) (Fig. 6-1)

In the classical sense nerve XI has two superficial origins, a *cranial* and a series of *spinal* roots. The cranial root arises from the medulla in the postolivary sulcus just below the fibers of the vagus nerve. It is joined immediately by the ascending spinal root and enters the jugular foramen. The fibers of cranial origin separate from the trunk of nerve XI just beyond the jugular foramen and join the vagus (Fig. 6-20). For this and other reasons most students regard this root as part of the vagus nerve. This view is strengthened by the fact that the *special visceral efferent* fibers in the cranial

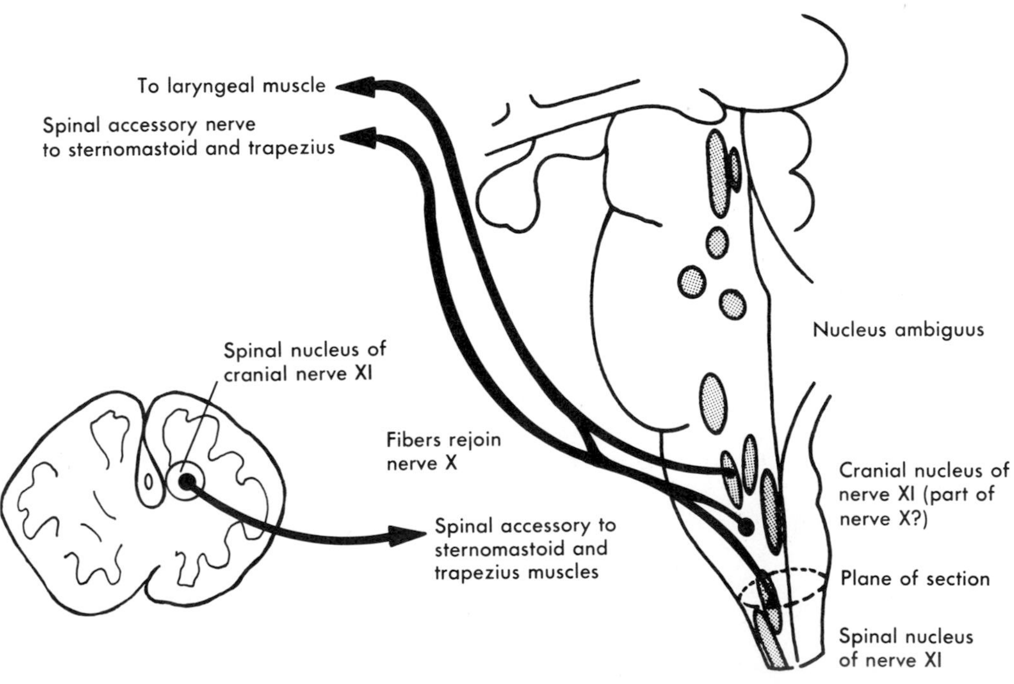

Fig. 6-20. Distribution of cranial nerve XI (spinal accessory).

root arise in the lower part of nucleus ambiguus and distribute to the laryngeal muscles as part of a vago-accessory complex (Fig. 6-18). Similarly, *general visceral efferent* fibers arising in the dorsal motor nucleus of nerve X travel through the cranial root of nerve XI. The *visceral afferent* fibers routed over the cranial segment of nerve XI travel to the nucleus solitarius and have their cell bodies in the nodose ganglion, a feature of identity with cranial nerve X. *Deep sense afferent* parts of the cranial segment are unknown.

The distinctive characteristic of nerve XI is its *spinal* component, which appears to be purely motor. It arises in a dorsolateral column of nerve cells in the ventral horn of the upper six cervical segments of the spinal cord (Fig. 6-20). This column of nerve cells is variously regarded as the *nucleus of the spinal accessory* and as part of the *supraspinal nucleus,* which also gives rise to motor elements of the first cervical nerve. The rootlets are assembled by a series of contributing filaments to form an ascending nerve that passes through the foramen magnum, joins the cranial root, and enters the jugular foramen. Just outside the foramen the cranial root leaves the spinal accessory to join the vagus (see above), and the main accessory trunk continues into the neck to supply the *sternocleidomastoid* and part of the *trapezius* muscles. The spinal accessory nerve is usually regarded as *special visceral efferent,* although the branchial origin of the two muscles it supplies is subject to question. *Deep muscle sense* (proprioception) in the distribution of the spinal part of the nerve XI has two possible routes: (1) travelling with nerve XI, with ganglion cells scattered along the rootlets or (2) via spinal nerve dorsal roots.[3,6] By either route, they seem to reach the fasciculus solitarius and its nucleus.

Hypoglossal nerve (XII) (Fig. 6-1)

Nerve XII emerges from the brainstem by ten to fifteen filaments in the preolivary sulcus. The fused filaments pass through the hypoglossal canal to supply the extrinsic and intrinsic muscles of the tongue (transverse, vertical, inferior and superior longitudinal, styloglossus, hyoglossus, and genioglossus) (Fig. 6-21). The hypoglossal nerve is joined peripherally by a branch of the first cervical nerve to form the descending hypoglossal limb of a loop that continues into a descending cervical limb (from C2 and C3). The pattern produces the ansa hypoglossi or ansa cervicallis, through which

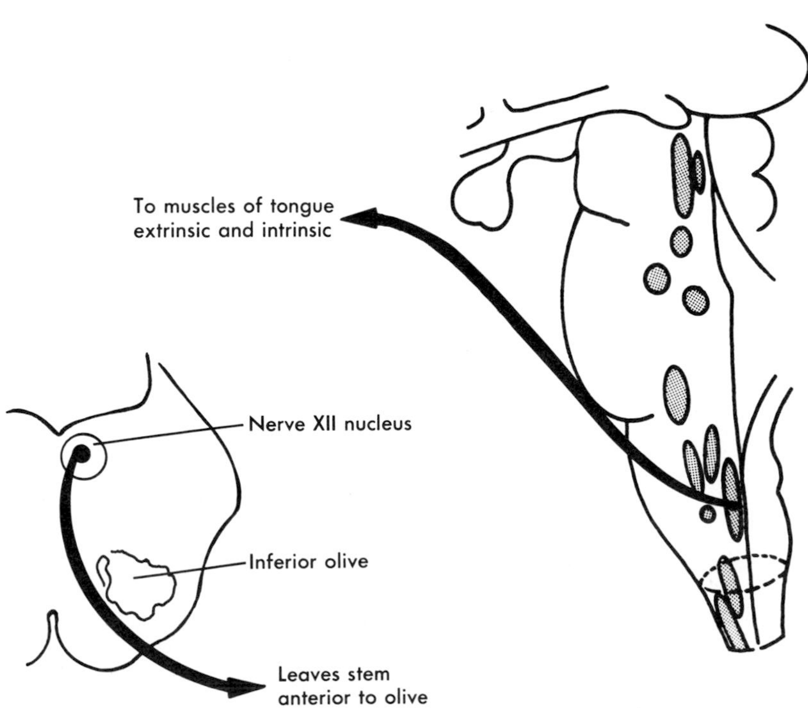

Fig. 6-21. Distribution of cranial nerve XII (hypoglossal).

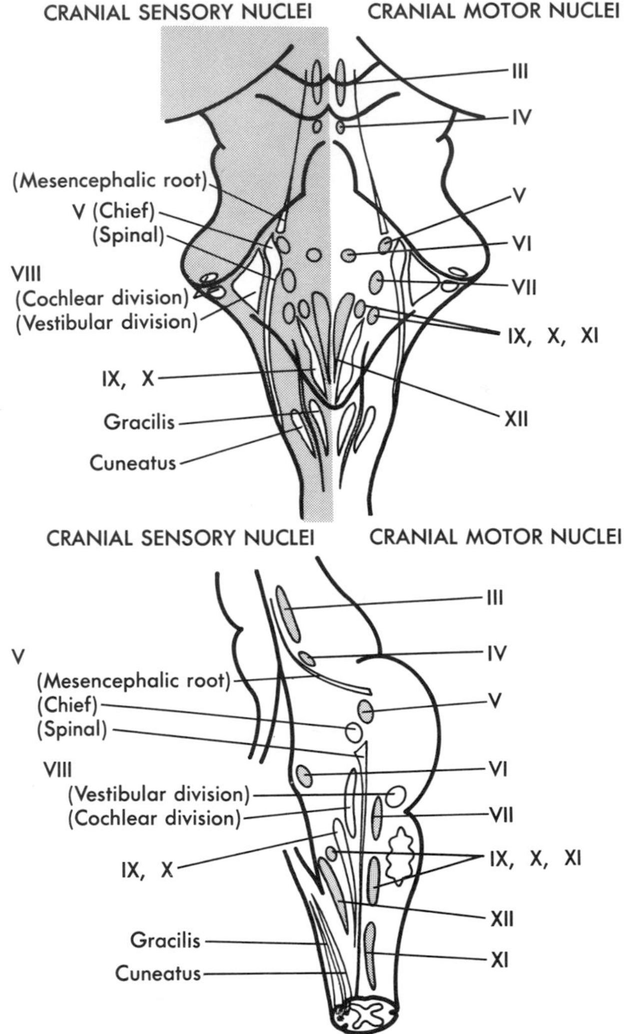

Fig. 6-22. Composite summary of motor and sensory nuclei of the brainstem.

cervical nerves join the hypoglossal for distribution. The hypoglossal is *somatic efferent* and arises in the hypoglossal nucleus, which underlies the hypoglossal trigone. *Proprioception* may be conveyed in hypoglossal fibers with cell bodies located in an intramedullary position.[6] Muscle sense may also pass in the ansa hypoglossi via the upper cervical nerves with cell bodies in the dorsal root ganglia.

See Fig. 6-22 for summary of cranial nerve nuclei.

SPINAL NERVES

The spinal nerves arise segmentally from the spinal cord as thirty-one pairs that are grouped as cervical (C) (eight pairs), thoracic (T) (twelve pairs), lumbar (L) (five pairs), sacral (S) (five pairs), and coccygeal (Co) (one pair). The segmentation and gross relationships of spinal cord to nerves to vertebral bodies and intervertebral foramina are reviewed in Chapter 2 (Figs. 2-28 and 2-29). Note that the sulci (dorsolateral and ventrolateral) exhibit almost uninterrupted emerging *rootlets* that coalesce into *roots.* Each root is related to a spinal *segment.* The segment vary considerably in length. The dorsal rootlets are larger than the ventral and contain more nerve fibers by several fold. (See Chapter 7 for the quantitative features of the peripheral nerves.) The general arrangement of the spinal nerves in relation to both the spinal cord and end-organs is basically the same in all segments. Each nerve, on both sides, is separated into a sensory, or afferent, dorsal root and a motor, or efferent, ventral root. The *sensory root* and *motor root* combine laterally just distal to the dorsal root ganglion into a *trunk,* which is mixed motor and sensory. The coalescence of the two roots occurs in most levels within the intervertebral foramen, external to the ganglion. (Exceptions are the sacral nerves whose ganglia are within the vertebral canal, and the coccygeal nerve, the ganglion for which is within the dural sheath.) The trunk gives off a *recurrent* branch to the spinal meninges and divides into a *posterior primary division,* an *anterior primary division,* and a *communicating* branch. The posterior primary divisions pass dorsally to supply skin, muscles, and glands of the posterior aspect of the body. The anterior primary divisions run laterally and anteriorly to supply the sides and ventral aspects of the body including the extremities. The communicating branches represent the visceral supply and reach the viscera by two grossly differentiable filaments, a white communicating and a gray communicating branch. The white branch is myelinated and the gray unmyelinated (Fig. 6-23).

Like the cranial nerves, the spinal nerves possess components that are functionally separable (Fig. 6-23). The spinal nerves, however, convey no special sense and therefore have fewer subdivisions: (1) *somatic afferent* (no special somatice afferent equivalent to visual, auditory, and equilibratory senses exist in spinal nerves); (2) *visceral afferent* (no special visceral afferent equivalent to gustatory and olfactory senses exist in spinal nerves); (3) *visceral efferent* (no branchial musculature is supplied as in the special visceral efferents of the cranial nerves); and (4) *somatic efferent.* The *somatic afferent* components convey cutaneous senses (pain,

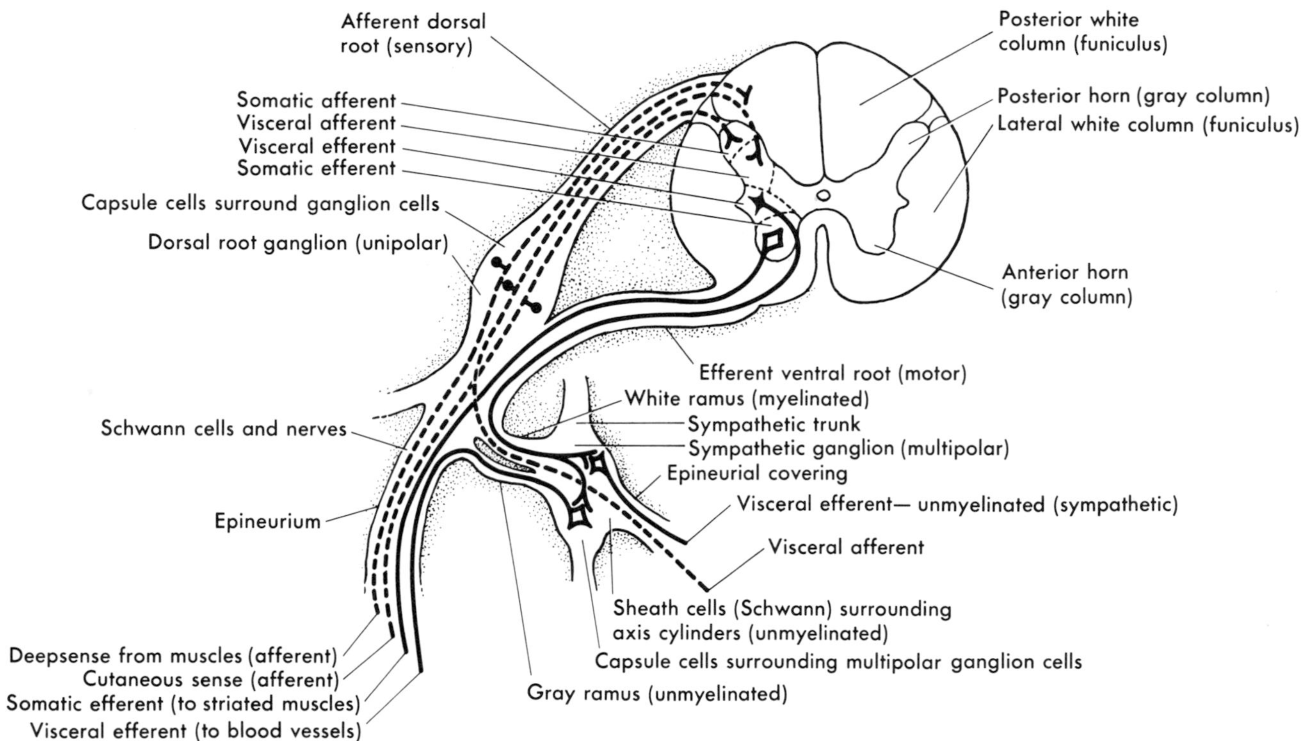

Fig. 6-23. Functional subdivisions of the spinal nerve.

temperature, and light touch) and deep sensibility (muscle, tendon, bone, joint, vibratory), as well as discriminative sense (two-point, texture, size, shape, stereognosis). The peripheral distribution of the cutaneous nerves is displayed in segments (dermatomes) in Fig. 6-24. Deep sensibility distribution is peripherally the same as the somatic efferent. The ganglia of these sensory fibers are in the dorsal roots (Fig. 6-23). The primary receptive nucleus for spinal nerves mediating cutaneous sense is either the substantia gelatinosa or the nuclei gracilis and cuneatus. The substantia gelatinosa runs the length of the spinal cord at the dorsolateral extremity of the dorsal horns (Fig. 6-25). This nucleus is continuous above with the nucleus of the descending root of cranial nerve V (Fig. 6-11). Nucleus gracilis and nucleus cuneatus are reached by fibers ascending in the dorsal white funiculus. It is believed that deep sensibility and discriminative sense terminate around cells of the nucleus dorsalis (Clarke's column) or in the nuclei cuneatus and gracilis. Cell bodies of the fibers mediating these impulses are located in the dorsal root ganglia (see Chapter 16).

Visceral afferent components of the spinal nerves arise in nerve endings in the thoracic and abdominal viscera. They reach the spinal cord through cervical nerve 4 (via the phrenic nerve from the diaphragm), through thoracic nerves 1 through 12 and lumbar nerves 1 through 3 (via white communicating branches), and through sacral nerves 2 through 4 (via the pelvic nerves). The cell bodies of the visceral afferent fibers are located in dorsal root ganglia of the segments mentioned. The primary receptive nuclei for visceral afferent fibers reaching the spinal cord remain somewhat obscure. For cervical nerve 4 and for sacral nerves 2, 3, and 4, the visceral receptive areas are called Stilling's cervical and sacral nuclei, respectively. In cross section these nuclei are located in the medial part of the base of the dorsal horn (Fig. 6-25). Stilling's nuclei are commonly regarded as extensions of the nucleus dorsalis (Clarke's column), although there is considerable uncertainty regarding this assertion (see Chapter 16). In longitudinal dimension the nuclei are limited to the segments indicated in Fig. 6-25. The visceral afferent fibers that arise in endings within thoracic

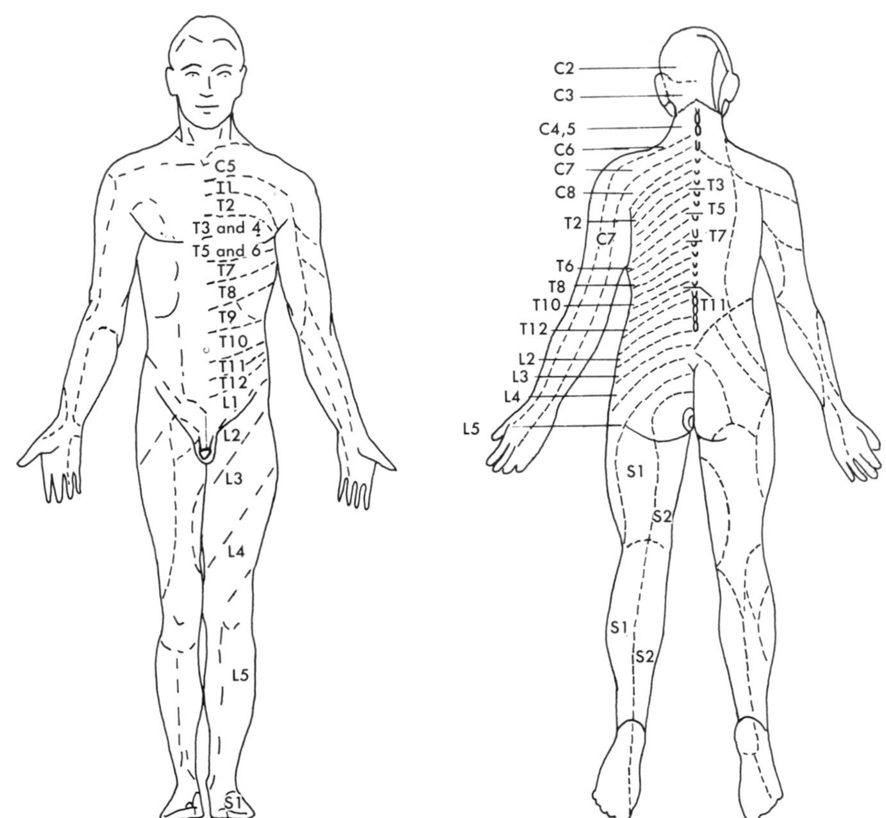

Fig. 6-24. Segmental distribution. Perineum supplied by C4, 5, and Co 1.

and abdominal structures and terminate in segments T1 through L2 end in relationship to cells in the medial aspect of the base of the dorsal horn. The coincidental location of nucleus dorsalis in this area (Fig. 6-25) has stimulated the notion that this nucleus is the primary receptive field for visceral afferent impulses. In general however the nucleus dorsalis is regarded as the primary receptive area for deep sensibility although the relationship remains uncertain. Visceral afferent fibers from blood vessels probably course inward with all segmental nerves and have their cell bodies in dorsal root ganglia. They participate in important vasal reflexes, but their actual route and primary termination are unknown (Fig. 6-23).

Visceral efferent fibers in the spinal nerves arise in the intermediolateral column of cells in the ventral horn of segments from the first thoracic through the second lumbar (Fig. 6-23). They emerge with the ventral roots and leave the trunks of the nerves of these segments as *sympathetic fibers* of the general visceral efferent or autonomic system. These are myelinated preganglionic fibers that pass via the white communicating branch to sympathetic ganglia or directly to adrenal. Postganglionics extend from the sympathetic trunk to the viscera via sympathetic nerves and plexuses or rejoin the main spinal nerves through gray communicating branches (Fig. 6-23). They innervate smooth muscles and glands in the viscera and skin, and the walls of blood vessels. Other spinal visceral efferent fibers are part of the *parasympathetic* division of the autonomic system. These arise in the visceral efferent column (Fig. 6-25) of the second, third, and fourth sacral segments and pass via the pelvic nerves to the descending colon and pelvic viscera. They function with the cranial division of the parasympathetic system, particularly with cranial nerve X (Fig. 6-19).

Somatic efferent fibers innervate the general striated musculature of the body. These fibers arise in the cell columns of the ventral horn (Fig. 6-25). On cross section these cells are disposed in a *medial group* that supplies axial musculature and a *lateral*

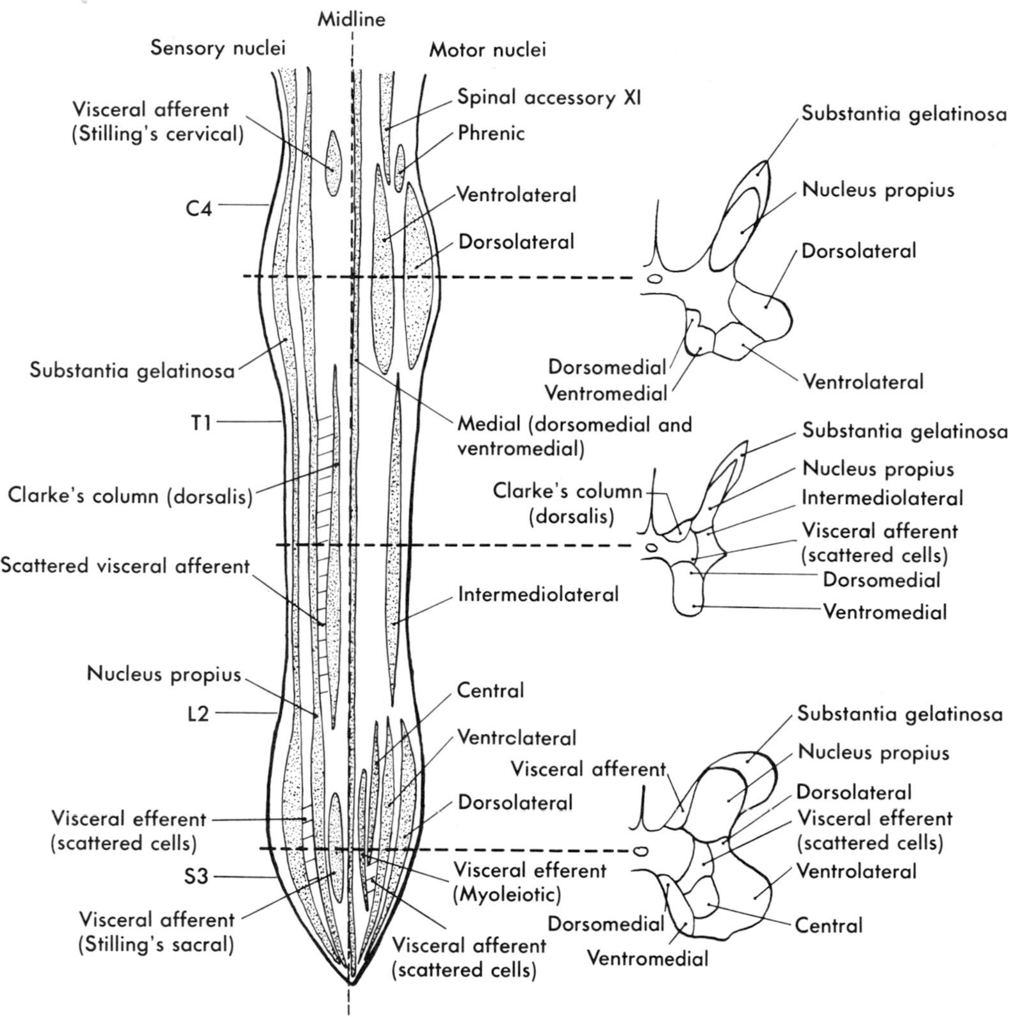

Fig. 6-25. Composite summary of motor and sensory nuclei of spinal cord.

group that supplies appendicular musculature. The medial group thus extends throughout the length of the cord. In the enlargements it is crowded toward midline and elsewhere spreads out over the full width of the ventral horn. The medial group presents dorsomedial and ventromedial cell clusters, but a definite somatotopic relationship to specific muscles has not been established for these groups. The *lateral group* of cells in the ventral columns occurs only in the enlargements of the spinal cord. In the cervical enlargement (the fourth cervical to the first thoracic segments) the lateral group is separable into *dorsolateral* and *ventrolateral* columns. The dorsalmost cells supply the distal musculature of the upper extremity (forearm and hand), and the ventrolateral group supplies the more proximal muscles (shoulder and arm). The more peripherally placed cells may go to the extensors and the more centrally placed cells to the flexors. A retrodorsolateral cluster of cells stands out clearly in the eight cervical to the first thoracic segments. These cells supply the small muscles of the hand. In the lumbosacral enlargement (second lumbar to third sacral segments) the same general columns appear in the lateral group of the ventral horn. The leg and foot are supplied by *dorsolateral* cells, and the hip and thigh by *ventrolateral* cells. The small muscles of the foot and toes are related to a *retrodorsolateral* cluster (from the first to the third sacral segment). A *central nucleus* (lumbosacral) appears from the second lumbar to the second sacral segment, but its somatotopic pattern is not certain. The origin of phrenic motor fibers is in the *phrenic* nucleus, located in the fourth and fifth cervical segments. The cells are mixed with the medial group of cells for axial muscular supply.[3] (See Fig. 6-25 for summary of motor and primary receptor nuclei of the spinal cord.)

Plexuses of anterior divisions of nerves issuing from the spinal cord account for the cabling patterns in the segmental distribution through definitive peripheral nerves. The plexuses of major importance include *cervical* (first through fourth cervical segments), *brachial* (fourth through eighth cervical and first thoracic segments), *lumbar* (first through fourth lumbar segments), *sacral* (fourth and fifth lumbar and first through third sacral segments), *pudendal* (second through fourth sacral segments), and *coccygeal* plexuses (fourth and fifth sacral and first coccygeal segments).*

A few exceptions to the general pattern of distribution are noteworthy. The first cervical nerve does not always possess a dorsal root. Thus the first cervical segment does not appear on the map of cutaneous distribution (Figs. 6-10 and 6-24). The first cervical nerve is the suboccipital nerve, which passes above the first vertebra. The remaining cervical nerves pass over vertebral pedicles of the same number. Cervical nerve 8 passes over the first thoracic vertebral pedicle. The remaining spinal nerves pass under the pedicle of the same-numbered vertebra. In the diagrams displaying peripheral distribution to skin (dermatomes) and muscles (myotomes), the overlap in each segment should be noted. In skin segments each nerve extends in part over approximately half the adjacent skin segment above and below. Only the short-trunk muscles possess a nerve supply from a single segment; most are supplied by two to four segmental nerves.

AUTONOMIC SYSTEM

In the preceding review of the peripheral nerves, *general visceral efferent* components were designated as the motor nerves supplying smooth muscles, glands, heart, and blood vessels. These efferent nerves make up the *autonomic system*. They are distinctive in possessing two neural units in the delivery system, one passing from the CNS to an outlying ganglion or paraganglion (*preganglionic fiber*) and a second neuron passing from the ganglion where the cell body lies to the end-organ (postganglionic fiber). The autonomic system is anatomically separable into a *craniosacral division* and a *thoracolumbar division*. As the name implies, the craniosacral division arises in cranial and sacral nuclei and travels via cranial and sacral nerves to the effectors. Similarly, the thoracolumbar division arises in thoracic and lumbar spinal nuclei and emerges in the related spinal nerves. The craniosacral division possesses long preganglionic fibers with its ganglia located close to the organ supplied. By contrast the thoracolumbar division possesses relatively short preganglionic fibers; its ganglia are located closer to the CNS. For the same reason, the craniosacral division has short postganglionics and the thoracolumbar division longer postganglionics.

The peripheral distribution of the two divisions of the autonomic system is practically the same, and almost all viscera are innervated by both systems. In general the two oppose each other functionally. For example, stimulation of one division will cause secretion of a gland, and stimulation of the other division will depress secretion. This functional divergence has generated opposing terms for the divisions, *sympathetic* for the thoracolumbar division and *parasympathetic* for the craniosacral division. The functional separation has a neurohumoral basis inasmuch as sympathetic postganglionics liberate an adrenalin-like substance on stimulation (*adrenergic*), while parasympathetic postganglionics liberate acetylcholine on stimulation (*cholinergic*). Stimulation of preganglionics in both divisions produces acetylcholine as the transmitter substance at the synapse in the ganglion (see Chapter 12). Because the autonomic system has to do primarily with unconscious reflex responses, it is also referred to as the *involuntary nervous system*. The autonomic system also plays a prominent role in basic functions of growth and nutrition (metabolism, neuroendocrine influences, etc.) and is therefore also called the *vegetative nervous system*.

The *craniosacral division* is diagrammed in Fig. 6-26 to display the continuity from CNS through the parasympathetic ganglia to the effectors. The peripheral pathways include four cranial visceral efferent nerves and their related ganglia and the three segments of sacral nerves whose fibers complete the coverage of the pelvic and abdominal viscera. The role of cranial nerves III, VII, IX, and X in the craniosacral division has been noted previously in this chapter. The pelvic nerves (nervi erigentes) leave the sacral segments of the spinal cord with ventral roots from their origin in the visceral efferent nucleus. They pass as preganglionics through the hypogastric plexus to reach

*See textbooks of anatomy for makeup and course of plexuses.

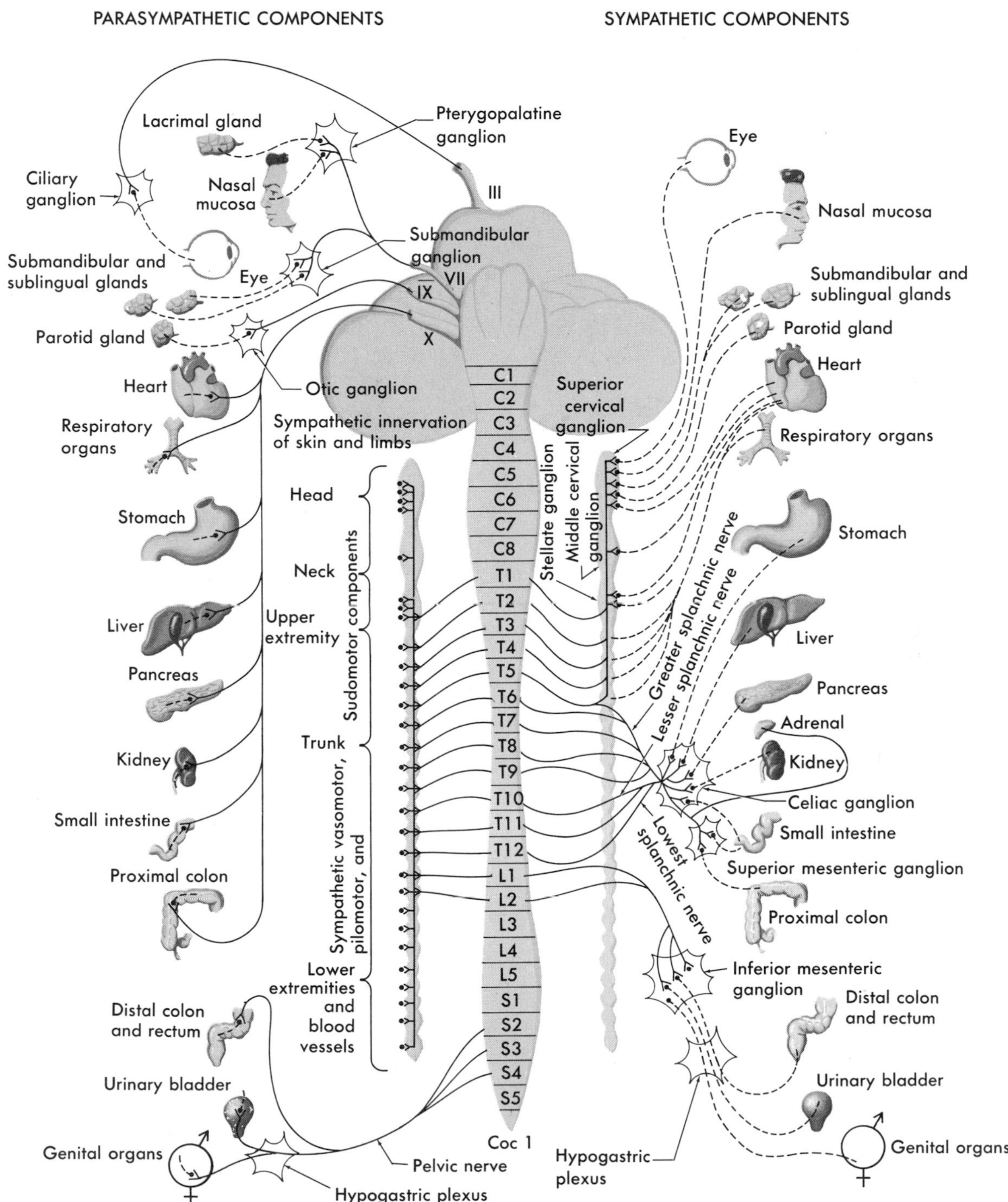

Fig. 6-26. Diagram of the autonomic nervous system. (From Richins, C., and Saccomanno, G. In Minckler, J., editor: Pathology of the nervous system, New York, 1968, McGraw-Hill Book Co.)

the walls of pelvic viscera and the descending colon to synapse with ganglia within the viscera. Short postganglionics innervate the effectors (see Chapter 22) (Fig. 6-26).

The *thoracolumbar division* arises from the first thoracic to the second lumbar segments in the intermediolateral cell column. The fibers emerge with the ventral roots and leave the main nerve trunk as preganglionic sympathetic fibers. They pass via the *white communicating branches* and terminate in sympathetic ganglia. These ganglia form a paravertebral sympathetic chain on either side of the vertebral column. They also form a series of large cell masses that are more distally located (Fig. 6-26). In the makeup of the sympathetic chain it will be noted that a ganglion forms from T1 down, which roughly corresponds to each spinal segment. Since the visceral efferent connections to the chain terminate at the second lumbar segment, the ganglia below this level are reached by elongate preganglionic fibers arising above that level of the cord. In the cervical region there are usually only three ganglia, an *inferior,* a *middle,* and a *superior.* The inferior cervical ganglion is commonly combined with the first thoracic to form the stellate ganglion. Since no direct preganglionics reach these ganglia above the first thoracic segment, these cells are reached by fibers from segments below this level. Some of the preganglionic fibers from between the first thoracic and the second lumbar segments pass through the sympathetic chain without synapsing and extend to the more distal sympathetic ganglia in the thoracic and abdominal cavities (Fig. 6-26). Preganglionic fibers pass directly to the paraganglia without interruption.

Postganglionic sympathetic fibers arising in the sympathetic chain take one of three courses. Some continue to the viscera via sympathetic nerves. Others rejoin the spinal nerves through *gray communicating branches* and are distributed peripherally to smooth muscles, glands, and vessels with the nerves. These pass to all the spinal nerves; unlike the preganglionic fibers, these fibers are not restricted to the segmental representatives of T1 to L2. The third route taken by sympathetic postganglionic fibers is joining vessel walls as plexuses and being carried peripherally in this manner. This last route represents the principal mode of travel for postganglionic sympathetic fibers to the head region. These travel to the head via the carotid arteries (Fig. 6-26).

(See Chapter 22 for details of the autonomic system as a motor unit and the character of the visceral efferent final-common-paths.)

REFERENCES

1. Bender, M. B., and Weinstein, E. A.: Functional representation in the oculomotor and trochlear nuclei, Arch. Neurol. Psychiat. **49**:98, 1943.
2. Furstenberg, A. C., and Magielski, J. E.: A motor pattern in the nucleus ambiguus, Ann. Otol. **64**:788, 1955.
3. Keswani, N. H., and Hollinshead, W. H.: Localization of the phrenic nucleus in the spinal cord of man, Anat. Rec. **125**:683, 1956.
4. Larsell, O.: Studies on the nervus terminalis; mammals, J. Comp. Neurol. **30**:1, 1918.
5. Olszewski, J., and Baxter, D.: Cytoarchitecture of the human brain stem, Basel, 1954, S. Karger. Ag.
6. Pearson, A. A.: Further observations on the mesencephalic root of the trigeminal nerve, J. Comp. Neurol. **91**:147, 1949.
7. Tennyson, V. M., and Pappas, G. D.: Choroid plexus. In Minckler, J., editor: Pathology of the nervous system, vol. I, New York, 1968, McGraw-Hill Book Co.
8. Warwick, R.: Oculomotor organization, Ann. Roy. Coll. Surg. Eng. **19**:6, 1956.

CHAPTER 7

GROWTH, BIOMETRICS, AGING

TATE M. MINCKLER

Neural tissue exhibits a unique and precocious growth pattern in comparison with other body tissues (Fig. 7-1). This precocity results in a relative preponderance of nervous tissue in early life (Tables 7-1 and 7-2). The nervous system is already one-quarter its adult weight at birth, but the whole body is only five percent its eventual mass.

THE CENTRAL NERVOUS SYSTEM

The development of the *brain* as reflected by weight change is presented in Fig. 7-2. The percentage of weight contributed by each component is graphed in Fig. 7-3. At birth the *cerebrum* weighs 325 grams (ninety-three percent of brain weight), and the *cerebellum* weighs 20 grams (five and one-half percent). It should be noted that by one year of postnatal age the relative percentage of each part is within one percent of its final adult value.

Until the total brain reaches a weight of approximately 1,000 grams, there is no discernible sex difference. Among adults however there is a significant variation in brain weight related to sex (Fig. 7-4). The male brain is 125 to 150 grams heavier than the female brain at any given body stature.

Convolutional development begins in the cerebrum at about five lunar months and is complete at about two years of age (Fig. 7-5). The mature cerebrum contains approximately 1,650 sq. cm. of total cortical surface area. Of this total about 560 sq. cm. are free or visible cortex, and the remainder is buried in convolutions (Fig. 7-6). Fissural development of the cerebellum begins somewhat earlier and provides around 1,100 sq. cm. of cortical surface in the adult brain.

The quantitative development of *gray matter* in the cerebrum follows the general pattern of nervous tissue, reaching the adult quantity of 550 grams by the second postnatal year. Of this amount, ten percent is basal nuclei, and the rest is cortex. *White matter* has a slower rate of increase, probably due to the late addition of myelin. Adult cerebral white matter weighs slightly over 500 grams. Values for gray and white matter in the cerebellum and brainstem are not available.

Weights of the *hypophysis* during development and at maturity are given in Fig. 7-7. Pregnancy may produce a temporary increase of 1,000 mg. or more in the anterior lobe in the female.

The *pineal body* undergoes a slight, steady weight increase throughout life, due to mineral deposit. It weighs 8 mg. at birth, 100 mg. by five years of age, and averages from about 150 to 160 mg. in adults.

The relative rate of *bone growth* in relation to brain development is usually measured by the sequence and timing of fontanelle closure (Fig. 7-8).

Growth in the length of the spinal cord and relationship of the cord to the vertebral column are illustrated in Fig. 7-9. Available data suggest that increases in length are proportionate straight line functions both before and after birth. The spinal cord of the newborn baby averages 15.4 cm. and weighs about 2.5 grams. The adult cord measures about 41 cm. and weighs 28 grams; this includes about 5 grams of gray matter and 23 grams of white substance. The thoracic segments measure about fifty percent of the total cord length at any age, cervical segments twenty-five percent, lumbar segments fifteen percent, and sacral segments about ten percent. The diameter of the thoracic unit is 1 cm. transversely and 0.8 cm. anteroposteriorly. The cervical and lumbar bulges increase these measurements by twenty to forty percent.

The *ventriculomeningeal system* includes an in-

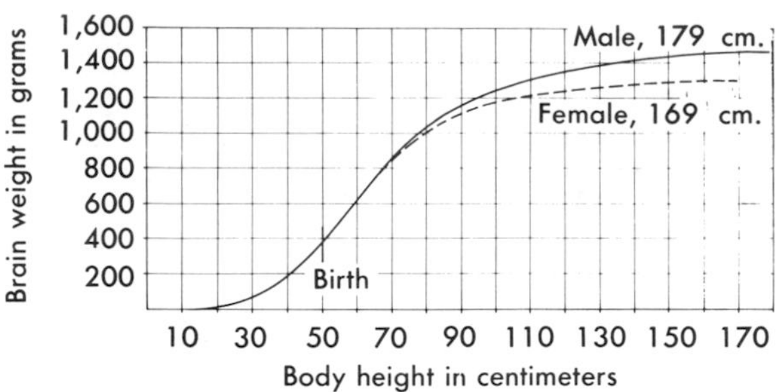

Fig. 7-2. Brain weight related to body height.

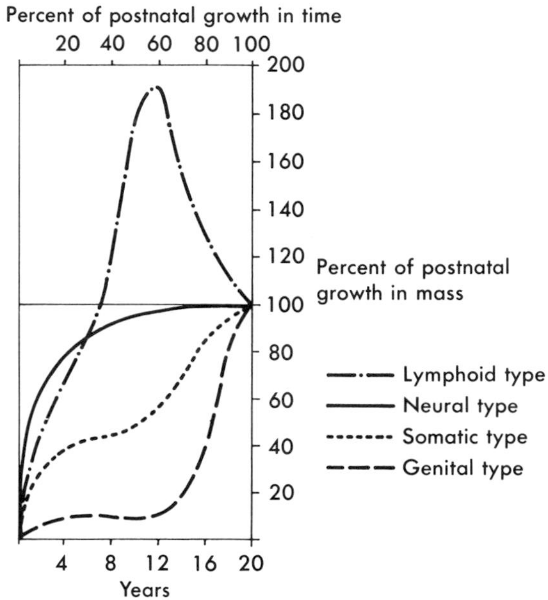

Fig. 7-1. Comparative growth curves of four tissue systems.

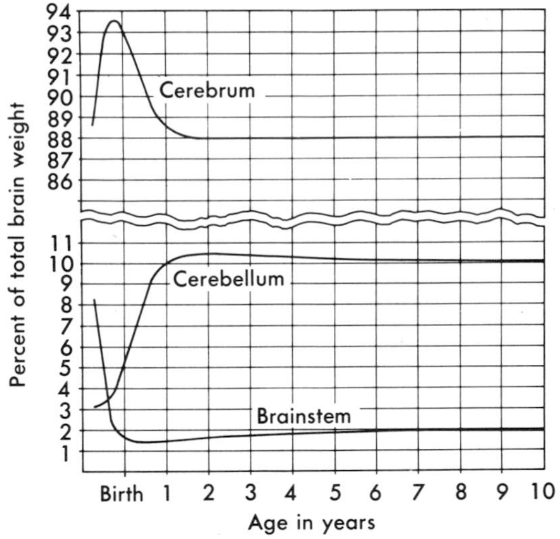

Fig. 7-3. Percent of total weight of brain contributed by its major parts at different ages.

Table 7-1. Weights of parts of the central nervous system

Structure in CNS	Average weight in grams	
	Newborn infant	Adult
Brain	350	1,350
Cerebrum	325	1,185
Cerebellum	20	140
Brainstem	5	25
Spinal cord	2.5	28
Meninges	22	65

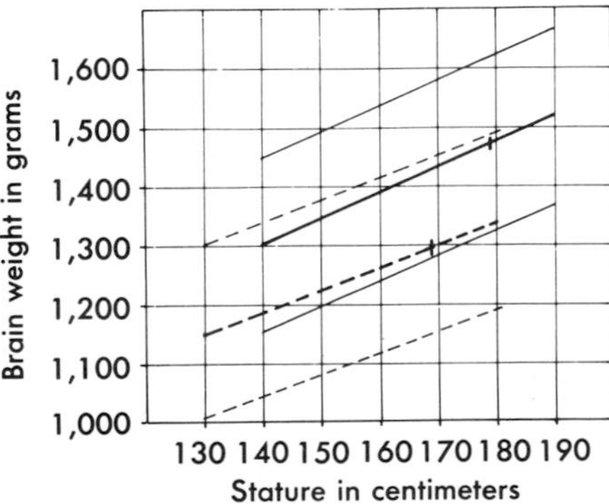

Fig. 7-4. Brain weight related to height for males (solid lines) and females (dotted lines). Heavy lines represent average, light lines the two standard deviation limits for each sex.

Table 7-2. Percentage of body composition of various tissues during development.*

Tissue	Six fetal months	Birth	Adult
Nervous tissue	21	15	3
Viscera	16	16	11
Skeleton	22	18	18
Skin and fat	16	26	25
Muscle	25	25	43

*After Wilmer.

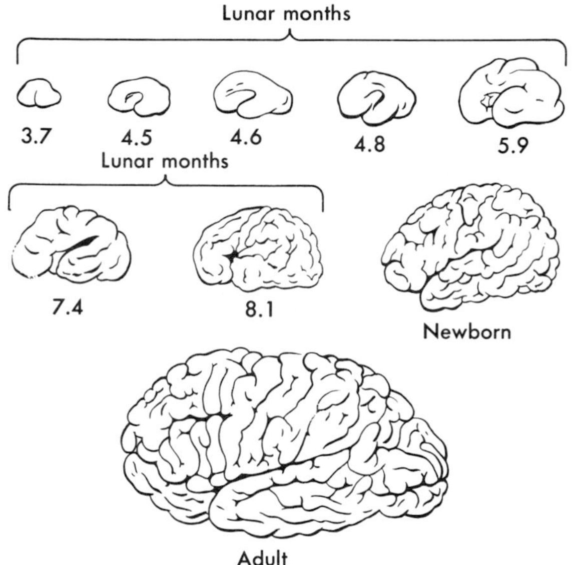

Fig. 7-5. General convolutional patterns as viewed laterally. (After Hesdorffer and Scammon.)

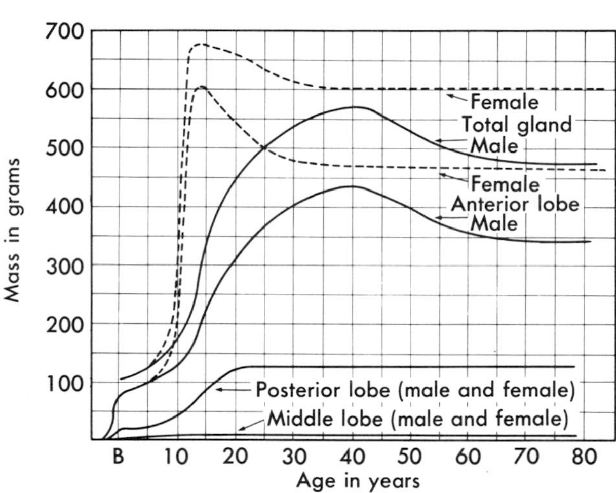

Fig. 7-7. Growth of the pituitary. (After Rasmussen.)

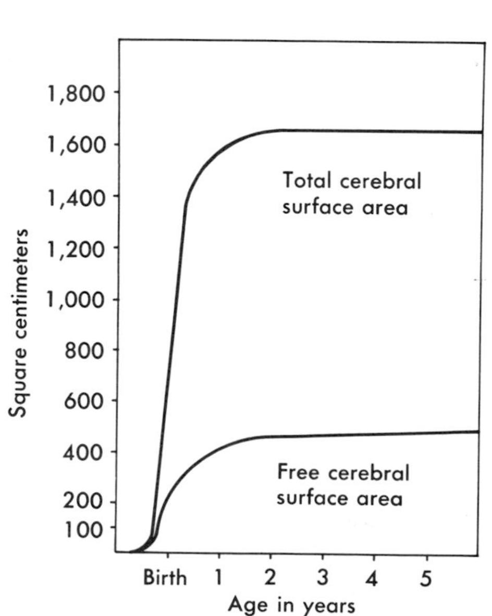

Fig. 7-6. Visible and total cerebral surfaces during growth. (After Hesdorffer and Scammon.)

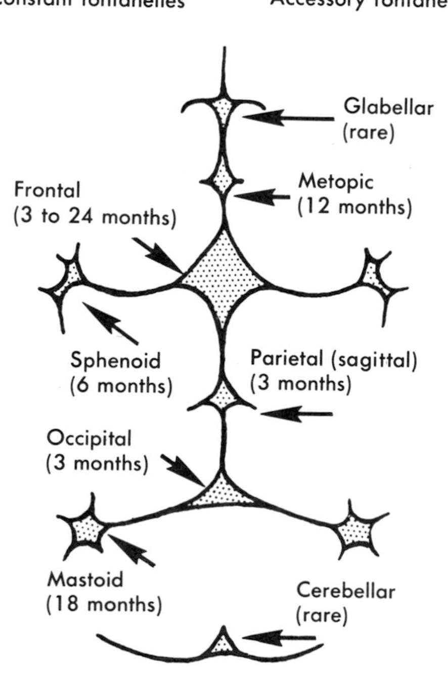

Fig. 7-8. Fontanelle closures.

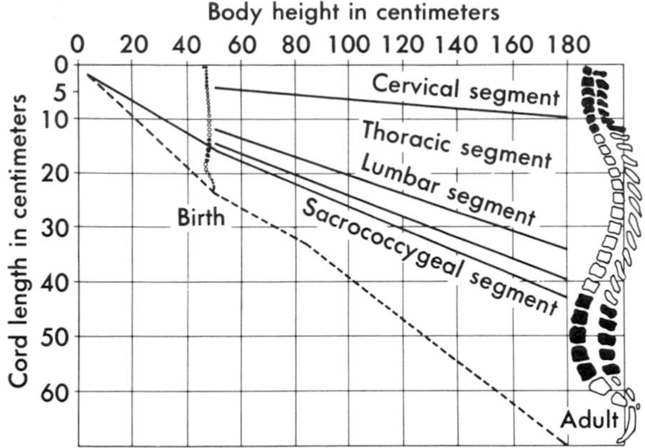

Fig. 7-9. Relationships of spine and cord by age. (From Minckler, T., and Boyd, E. In Minckler, J., editor: Pathology of the nervous system, vol. I, New York, 1968, McGraw-Hill Book Co.)

Table 7-3. Measurements of the eye during growth

Structure in eye	Birth	Adult
Globe		
(diameter)	17 mm.	24 mm.
(volume)	3.4 cc.	7.7 cc.
Anterior chamber	64 cu. mm.	116 cu. mm.
Posterior chamber	30 cu. mm.	64 cu. mm.
Vitreous body	1466 cu. mm.	4585 cu. mm.

traventricular volume of approximately 35 cc. (15 cc. in each lateral ventricle and 5 cc. in the third and fourth ventricle and the aqueduct). The volume of the meningeal tissues and spaces of the cranium is estimated at 110 cc., of which 85 cc. are filled by meningeal tissues and 25 cc. by subarachnoid fluid space. The volume of spinal subarachnoid fluid is estimated at 75 cc., and that of spinal leptomeninges at 4 cc. Thus the total circulating volume of CSF is 135 cc., and the volume of meninges is 89 cc. Fluid is formed at a rate of between 15 and 500 cc. per 24 hours; the actual rate is dependent upon physiologic state and the vagaries in manner of determination.

The special sense organs, *eye* and *ear,* exhibit noteworthy growth characteristics. The *eye* of the newborn has already attained nearly half its adult size (compared to one-fourth for the rest of the nervous system). The globe measurements are given in Table 7-3. A striking change in convergence of the optic tracts and globes occurs; from 180 degrees at the second lunar month (eyes point laterally), the tracts and globes converge to approximately 68 degrees in the adult. At birth the convergence is slightly less (73 degrees) than in the adult. This places the optic nerve heads of the newborn in a relatively more medial position. The lens is unusual in its growth pattern, as it exhibits continuous increase in weight throughout life. It also becomes increasingly flat, probably due to loss of elastic fibers. The optic nerve is 2.7 mm. thick in the newborn, compared to a thickness of 3.2 to 3.5 mm. in the adult.

The *internal ear* seems to attain its full stature by the fifth fetal month. There is however some adjustment of the planes of the semicircular canals; posterior canals of the newborn diverge laterally 55 degrees from midline. This angle of divergence is 45 degrees in the adult. The semicircular canals measure from 7 to 8.5 mm. in maximum dimension, and the cochlea has a vertical length of 7.5 mm.

THE PERIPHERAL NERVOUS SYSTEM

The peripheral nervous system has a growth pattern that remains unknown because of its diffuse distribution and the difficulty inherent in obtaining accurate measurements. The total mass is estimated to be half that of the CNS at birth and three-quarters of the adult CNS mass (approximately 1,000 grams of mature peripheral nerve tissue). The individual nerves are plotted according to their average diameters in Fig. 7-10. Note that the sensory components are larger than the motor components, due to the larger number of fibers. The entire system is estimated to carry approximately two and a half million fibers to and from the CNS, with unequal distribution side to side. This distribution is probably predominantly to the right. Of this total number of fibers, approximately two million are recognized as sensory, and the remainder as motor (slightly more than half a million). The accuracy of these estimates is highly questionable, particularly in regard to the counting of the small unmyelinated fibers. The usual counting technique has been to compare osmic preparations (for myelinated fibers) with silver impregnations (for axis-cylinders); this technique separates myelinated and unmyelinated fibers. Several dependable reports that quantitate these nerves are available.[2]

The fiber counts in nerves and in cell bodies in ganglia are discussed in the following paragraphs. The vagaries arising from tissue techniques and counting samples for estimation should be kept in mind.

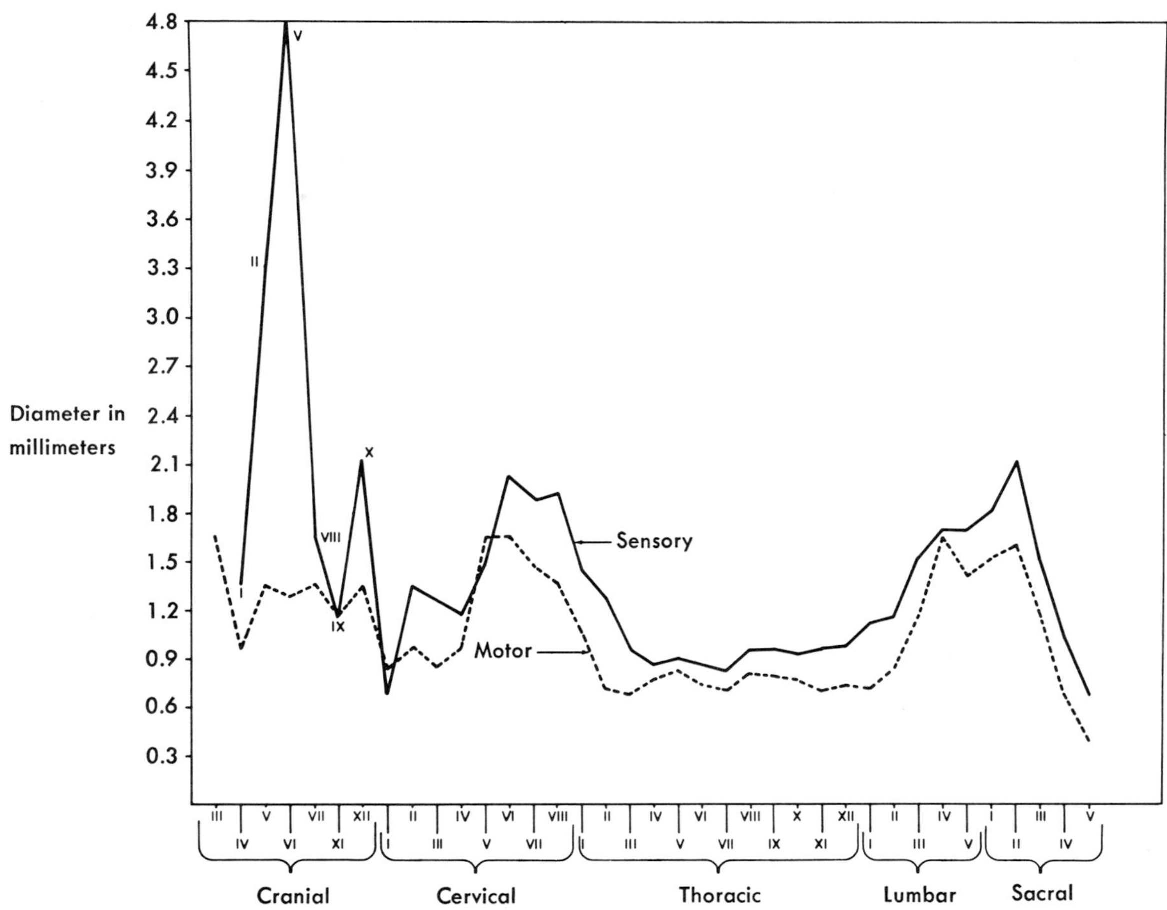

Fig. 7-10. Mean diameters of cranial spinal nerves. (From Minckler, T., and Boyd, E. In Minckler, J., editor: Pathology of the nervous system, vol. I, New York, 1968, McGraw-Hill Book Co.)

Cranial nerves

The *nervus terminalis* contains an unknown quantity of both afferent and efferent fibers, and the *vomeronasal nerve* (of Jacobson) possesses an unknown number of fibers during its transient existence.

There are approximately 200 million *olfactory receptors.* The central processes are aggregated in eighteen to twenty gross afferent filaments on each side. These fibers distribute to the mitral receptive cells of the olfactory bulbs; each cell receives impulses from approximately 18,000 receptors. This complex arrangement is effected by coalescence of the fibers leading from the chemoreceptors into the olfactory filaments and by elaborate branching within the olfactory bulb. There appears to be a continuing decrease in number of olfactory fibers with age.

Each *eye* contains from about 3.8 to about 6.8 million cones and from about 75 to about 175 million rods. These sensory cells lead via the neuronal links within the retina into approximately 800,000 to 1 million fibers in each *optic nerve.* As stated previously, the optic nerve is actually a central tract.

Nerve III contains 25,000 to 35,000 fibers that arise from the same number of cells in the oculomotor nuclei. Of the nuclear cells, 10 to 15 thousand on each side are Edinger-Westphal cells.

Nerve IV contains from 3,000 to 3,500 fibers that arise in the same number of cells in the trochlear nucleus on each side.

Nerve V is made up on each side of approximately 140,000 sensory fibers and 8,100 motor fibers. The motor nucleus probably possesses the same number of cells as the motor root contains fibers.

Estimates are somewhat lower, however, ranging from 4,500 to 5,500 fibers. The chief sensory nucleus contains about 35,000 cells, and the mesencephalic nucleus about 5,700 cells. No estimates are available on the number of cells in the receptive nuclei of the descending root.

Nerve VI contains between 2,400 and 3,600 fibers. The nuclei contain on each side roughly twice as many cells as the number of fibers emerging with the nerve.

The motor nucleus of nerve VII contains 8,000 cells that give rise to the same number of fibers. These fibers emerge on each side as nerve VII. The geniculate ganglion is reported to contain from 1,100 to 3,100 cells, and the nervous intermedius has the same number of fibers. The number of primary receptive cells for nerve VII fibers has not been established.

Nerve VIII is separated into two major divisions, cochlear and vestibular. The cochlear division is related on each side to an estimated 25,000 hair cells. The spiral ganglion cells number about 30,000, and the cochlear nerve contains the same number of fibers. The primary receptive nuclei for the cochlear division (dorsal and ventral combined) contain approximately 200,000 cells on each side. There are about 19,000 vestibular fibers that terminate in vestibular nuclei. These nuclei contain approximately 250,000 cells. It is assumed that the vestibular ganglion of each side contains the same number of cells as the fibers issuing from it.

Nerve IX contains between 3,500 and 4,000 fibers. The ganglia are presumed to contain the same number of cells as there are sensory fibers, but estimates are not available.

Nerve X contains between 32,000 and 36,000 fibers. Of these, about 2,000 are thought to arise in the nucleus ambiguus, and about 17,000 in the dorsal motor nucleus. The remaining 15,000 fibers are presumed to be sensory or to arise from other motor sources. No estimates of ganglion cells and sensory components are available.

Nerve XI is estimated to contain 3,500 fibers.

Nerve XII contains between 5,500 and 7,500 fibers, and the nucleus of each side is presumed to house the same number of cells.

The cranial nerves of each side are aggregations of an estimated 1,300,000 afferent fibers and 72,000 efferent fibers. Excluding the olfactory and optic nerves, there are approximately 300,000 sensory fibers extending into the brain, compared to 72,000 motor fibers emerging from the brain; thus the ratio of sensory to motor fibers is approximately 4:1. Large variations occur in all the reported studies. Frequently large differences occur in comparing left and right sides. The veracity and significance of this observation are not known, but counts are usually greater on the right. Fibers counts appear to be lower in females than in males. Numbers of ganglion cells and fibers in cranial nerves probably change with age. Certainly the number of demonstrable myelinated fibers increases through childhood, probably as a feature of growth. These diminish after middle age, but it remains uncertain whether axis-cylinders (axons) disappear as well as stainable myelin.

Spinal nerves

The spinal nerves are estimated to contain on each side 1 million fibers in their posterior roots and 210,000 fibers in their anterior roots. There is up to fifty percent variation between sides. In any single segment the ratio of sensory to motor fibers varies from 2:1 up to 10:1. The dorsal root ganglia of the cervical segments average 50,000 cells; those of the thoracic segments average 25,000 cells; and those of the lumbosacral segments average about 35,000 cells. The fifth sacral dorsal root ganglion of one side contains 3,500 cells. Of the 1 million entering fibers, 290,000 fibers enter the cervical segments, 210,000 enter the thoracic segments, 425,000 enter the lumbosacral segments, and 75,000 enter the sacrococcygeal segments. No accurate figures exist on the primary receptive nuclei for these fibers. The total number of sensory and internuncial cells available to these incoming impulses is approximately 5.6 million. Of the 210,000 efferent fibers, it is estimated that from 40,000 to 57,000 arise in cervical segments, 73,000 to 96,000 in thoracic segments, and between 52,000 and 70,000 in lumbosacral segments. There are presumably as many cells of origin (final-common-path cells) as there are issuing fibers (an approximate total of 500,000 fibers). However, estimates vary up to four times that many concerning the number of cells in the ventral horns. It is assumed that most of these are connecting cells. The estimates are crude and will probably be subject to major revision as improved quantitative methods are developed. The spinal nerves respond to growth and aging in the same manner as cranial nerves. Demonstrable myelinated fibers may diminish from twenty-two to twenty-seven percent after age fifty. Again, it is uncertain whether the axons disappear also. Certainly it is unnecessary to assume so to explain failing neural function beyond that age.

Myelination

Myelination of fibers occurs in some measure as a sign of maturation. The entire concept of the myelin sheath has been revised with the advent of the electron microscope (see Chapter 10). The histologic demonstration of myelin is dependent upon the depth of the wrapping of axons by cell membranes; it seems to occur as a function of size of the axis-cylinder. Small fibers, which are predominant in total number, possess a similar sheath but not in an amount sufficient to be displayed by myelin stains. Consequently, the specific relationship of neural function to the appearance of myelin has been greatly overplayed, since most of the nervous system possesses no myelin. Myelin growth studies have made possible the identity of related tracts and have figured prominently in anatomic studies of the embryonic brain. The studies continue, but they are strikingly altered in their contribution to basic information about myelin, its function, and its sustenance in disease. The first appearance of myelin in the human nervous system is in ventral roots during the end of the fourth month of gestation. It makes a new appearance in some spinal nerves as late as the second year after birth. The myelin sheaths continue to expand in some nerves into adulthood. In other nerves, both central and peripheral, myelin never appears in stainable form (unmyelinated fibers), although similar cell membrane sheathing appears in all nerves (see Chapter 10). The sequence of myelination in major tracts is presented in Table 7-4.

Table 7-4. The appearance of myelin in various areas and tracts*

Neural structure	Weeks of gestation						
	16	20	24	28	32	36	40
Ventral spinal roots	X	X	X	X	X	X	X
Dorsal spinal roots		X	X	X	X	X	X
Oculomotor (III), trochlear (IV) and abducens nerves (VI)		X	X	X	X	X	X
Vestibular nerve		X	X	X	X	X	X
Trigeminal nerve (V)		X	X	X	X	X	X
Facial nerve (VII)		X	X	X	X	X	X
Medial longitudinal fasciculus		X	X	X	X	X	X
Ventral commissure or cord			X	X	X	X	X
Hypoglossal nerve (XII)			X	X	X	X	X
Auditory nerve (VIII)			X	X	X	X	X
Vestibulospinal tract			X	X	X	X	X
Gracilis and cuneatus tracts			X	X	X	X	X
Tectospinal tract				X	X	X	X
Spinocerebellar tract				X	X	X	X
Olivocerebellar tract				X	X	X	X
Spinothalamic tract				X	X	X	X
Vermis of cerebellum				X	X	X	X
Hemispheres of cerebellum					X	X	X
Pontocerebellar tract					X	X	X
Dentatorubral tract					X	X	X
Frontopontine tract					X	X	X
Afferent tract to thalamus					X	X	X
Afferent tracts to cerebral cortex					X	X	X
Optic nerve (II)						X	X
Olfactory (I) tracts						X	X
Rubrospinal tract						X	X
Corticospinal tract						X	X
Correlation area of thalamus						X	X
Correlation areas of cerebral cortex						X	X

*After Scammon, 1933.

AGING

In the present context, aging is represented as a continuing biologic process, and in the usual view is the terminal segment of the spectrum of living in point of time. The period of the aged is that of senescence or normal involution, and it is rather distinctly separable from—although continuous with —the periods of the embryo, fetus, postnatal growth, and maturity. While anatomic and physiologic decline is implied in aging, the present representation avoids the area of pathology, or tissue disturbances to the point of disease or threatened life, which are, admittedly, often concomitant with aging. It should be recognized that aging is species-peculiar (in a rather broad range); that is, man has a life expectancy of from fifty to one hundred years, in comparison to a dog's expectancy of from eight to fifteen years, a mayfly's life expectancy of one day, a rat's expectancy of two or three years, and a sea turtle's life expectancy of several hundred years. The rate of senescence varies greatly from person to person, and the various tissues within any individual will vary remarkably in their degree of involution at any age.

The aging process is dependent upon many factors, no one of which can be held accountable in the usual sense of etiology. Certainly heredity plays a role in governing the onset and rapidity of involution. The impact of environment on aging is somewhat less certain and remains controversial. Of the many associated phenomena, the following merit extended consideration as modifiers of species-specific *abiotrophy,* or the natural tendency to decline or involution in cellular structure. This natural involution ideally should be clearly distinguished from pathologic processes, which notoriously take their toll in the aged. Such a distinction is often not possible, and degenerative processes due to disease are not easily distinguished from those of abiotrophy. Following are some factors that can operate in aging in the absence of recognizable disease. These factors apply not only to the nervous system but, as well, to other complex organ systems. It should be clearly understood that the nervous system is not an isolate as tissues go, but almost more than others is dependent for its vitality on the proper functioning and integrity of all other tissues.

1. *Heredity* seems to bear directly on aging, not only in terms of longevity but also on the organ system that manifests the aging process most prominently. The genetic constitution governs metabolic potential as protein makeup. This affects the growth and maintenance of cells and, in like manner, the management of intracellular metabolic waste accumulation and riddance. These by-products of living accumulate within the nerve cells as lipochromes and as possible deterrants to proper metabolism. Their collection within cells might well signal the gradual onset and continuing sequence of senescence (the "constipation" concept of aging).

2. *Mutagenic agents* are those environment factors that are known to be capable of inducing somatic mutations in protein makeup. Responding cells, which undergo division, would tend to cancel this influence through exfoliation of the newly produced cells. On the other hand, the same mutagenic effect on postmitotic cells (such as nervous tissue) might well represent one factor in aging. The best recognized mutagenic agents that contribute continuing influence on many organisms are *radiations, viruses,* and *chemicals* (such as drugs).

The fundamental alterations in tissue activity that arise either through genetic or mutagenic influences are brought about by *endocrine dysfunction,* altered *homeostatic mechanisms,* disturbed cellular *membrane permeability,* changing *vascular factors,* and nonlethal intracellular *metabolic changes.* The functions in aging cells are frequently altered in measurable ways in accordance with the above listing. Occasionally these altered functions are demonstrable in structural changes.

3. *Environment factors other than mutagenic agents* are frequently considered as factors in the etiology of aging. Malnutrition is commonly associated with both food deprivation and excess. Stress and strain as part of living are also suspected of contributing to aging phenomena in cells. Conversely, rest is thought to abate the aging process, perhaps only because physiologic stability is best represented under resting conditions. There are many behavioral peculiarities in the aged that are obscure in basic cause. Many of these behavioral problems center in the sensory processes (vision, hearing) and in neural responses, particularly those of complex nature. It would appear that the behavioral features represent a consequence or organic changes incident to aging, although these are frequently obscure.

Age changes

Physicochemical aging is a concept directed to all body systems but with several special connotations in regard to nervous tissues. The tendency for colloids and water to separate in tissues is greater in the aged (syneresis). This may generate the so-called congophilic changes of aging, which include amyloid deposits. Alterations in the selective permeability in the barrier systems of the brain (dyshoric changes) are prone to occur in the aged. The ability of nervous tissue to withstand chemical insult appears to be compromised, and control systems effecting homeostasis seem less adept. Hyden has shown that the content of ribonucleic acid in neurons falls after about fifty years of age, while lipochromes continue to increase in amount after that age.[10] It is probable that these chemical changes have a definite relationship to metabolic capabilities in the cells. What parts of these alterations represent aging and what parts disease are sometimes difficult to assess.

In general, the brain *loses weight,* and *pigments tend to accumulate* in nerve cells with age. Little else appears to be specifically related. Alterations in peripheral nerves are less conspicuous, but functional loss of neuromuscular type is a definite aging phenomenon. The effects of aging on the nervous system are probably best regarded as a composite result of both the associated tissue defects and inherent changes in nervous tissues themselves. These alterations related to loss of weight of the brain are summarized in their pathogenesis as: (1) reduction in size of cells (atrophy); (2) reduction in number of cells; (3) increase in relative amount of stroma (supporting tissue) over parenchyme (tissue typical of the area); (4) shrinkage and condensation of intercellular material; and (5) increase of intracellular metabolic product deposits. Once again, it is difficult to be certain to what degree these represent uncomplicated expressions of senescence (Fig. 7-11). The list of changes reads very much like the consequences of disease processes. Often, aging in the nervous system is represented as the culminating product of previous disease. This is a little hard to accept entirely, since most disease experience, particularly of the infectious

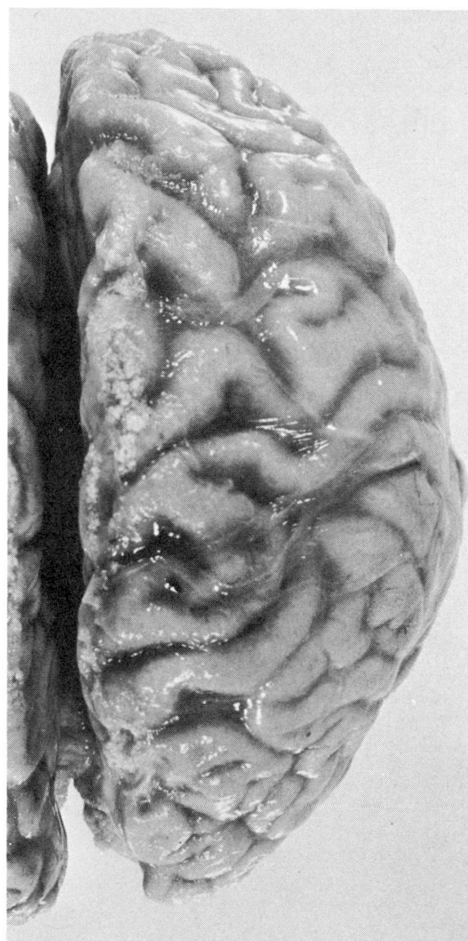

Fig. 7-11. Macroscopic view of aging brain (ninth decade). Accentuation of sulcal volume, reduction of gyral volume, and slight opacity of frontal arachnoid are characteristic.

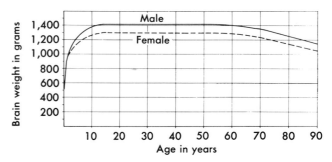

Fig. 7-12. Relationship between brain weight and age.

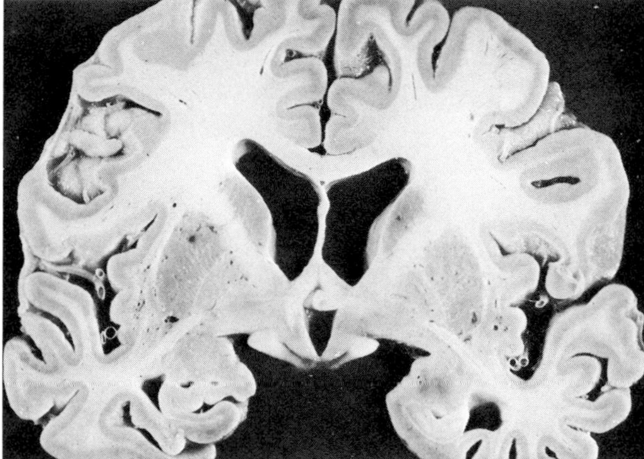

Fig. 7-13. Coronal section of aged brain (ninth decade). Triangular shape of lateral ventricles, slight enlargement of ventricles, pitting of ventricle surface, increased sulcus volume, and narrow gyri are characteristic.

type, seems to impart a measure of resistance to further inroads. Further, the notion implies that a nervous system unsullied by disease might live forever. The subject is reviewed nicely by McMenemey.[14] From whatever causes, however, the brain of the aged presents the following characterizing gross features of interest to anatomists.

The brain diminishes in *weight* beginning in the fourth decade of life (Fig. 7-12). This reduction, however, appears to be no different from the reduction in height that also occurs with age (Fig 7-4). The change is such that the brain of a 90-year-old man might be expected to weigh approximately the same as that of a 3-year-old child. This diminution in size is generally regarded as a combination of reduction of size in nerve cells, loss of nerve cells, condensation of intercellular substance, and loss of myelin in white matter. Sections of the brain of the aged therefore present less centrum semiovale, and the white part of the convolutions may be relatively reduced (Fig. 7-13). This *atrophy* accentuates the sulcus volume at the expense of the gyri. It is commonly most prominent over the frontal lobes. The leptomeninges of the area often are thickened, tough, and opaque. There is a tendency to cicatricial contraction of cerebral substance with production of *corrugations* along the ventricular surfaces (Fig. 7-13). The *ventricular volume* is somewhat enlarged, as is the subarachnoid space. The contour of the ventricular cavities in sections is therefore slightly altered (Fig. 7-13). There is some probability that either the membrane permeability or valving effect at the arachnoid granulations might be impaired with age. Embarrassment of CSF absorption in such a case would contribute to the occurrence of communicating hydrocephalus as mentioned. In this condition both the subarachnoid and ventricular spaces distend at the expense of cerebral substance.

No unanimity in opinions exists regarding the loss of nerve cells and their individual reduction in size. These alterations with age appear to vary greatly from area to area in the same brain and even more from brain to brain. The further microscopic findings in intercellular spaces, deposits of intercellular fibers, and loss of myelin are touched upon in Chapter 10 and have been reviewed extensively elsewhere as pathologic changes. As previously mentioned, deposits of *lipochromes* (lipofuscin) within nerve cells are an accompaniment to aging (see Chapter 10). It is not surprising that considerable speculation has been given over to the probability that loss of nerve cells is the main feature of aging in the brain. This seems a logical means of explaining the functional failure of the brain, which is so conspicuous as people grow older. With little supporting evidence, various estimates of daily nerve cell dropouts have been attempted (up to 150,000). As an attrition feature of aging past the middle years this would leave the usual human being (with probably 20 billion nerve cells normally) completely brainless at the approximate age of 400 years. Such a statistic is of real moment only to the dyed-in-the-wool longevity fan. The notion behind it, however, has nurtured the concept of the neuron as an isolated container of intelligence, communicative ability, and general neural well-being. To explain these things in terms of human behavior, it is already abundantly clear that neuronal interrelationships, quantitative and qualitative features of their synapses, and the physicochemical activities attending their reactions are equally as important as the neurons themselves. Neuroscientists thus far have barely touched these items in their investigations, but the eventual understanding of the aging process must encompass such information.

REFERENCES

1. Andrew, W.: Cellular changes with age, Springfield, Illinois, 1952, Charles C Thomas, Publisher.
2. Blinkov, S. M., and Glezer, I. I.: The human brain in figures and tables, New York, 1968, Plenum Publishing Corporation.
3. Broman, T., and Steinwall, O.: Blood-brain barrier. In Minckler, J., editor: Pathology of the nervous system, vol. I, New York, 1968, McGraw-Hill Book Co.
4. Campain, R., Jaeger, M., and Minckler, J.: The auditory cortex and area 22, a quantitative study. (In preparation.)
5. Corbin, K. B., and Gardner, E. D.: Decrease in number of myelinated fibers in human spinal roots with age, Anat. Rec. **68:**63, 1937.
6. Cowdry, E. V., editor: Problems of aging, ed. 2, Baltimore, 1942, The Williams & Wilkins Co.
7. Crace, R., Jaeger, M., and Minckler, J.: The human cochlear nuclei. (In preparation.)
8. Gardner, E.: Decrease in human neurons with age, Anat. Rec. **77:**529, 1940.
9. Grenell, R. G., and Scammon, R. E.: An iconometrographic representation of the growth of the central nervous system, J. Comp. Neurol. **79:**329, 1943.
10. Hyden, H.: The neuron, New York, 1967, American Elsevier Publishing Co., Inc.
11. Igarashi, M.: Inner ear end organs. In Minckler, J., editor: Pathology of the nervous system, vol. II, New York, 1970, McGraw-Hill Book Co.
12. Jaeger, M., Crace, R., and Minckler, J.: A quantitative study of the medial geniculate body. (In preparation.)
13. Luse, S.: The Schwann cell. In Minckler, J., editor: Pathology of the nervous system, vol. I, New York, 1968, McGraw-Hill Book Co.
14. McMenemey, W. H.: Neuropathology of the aging brain. In Minckler, J., editor: Pathology of the nervous system, vol. II, New York, 1970, McGraw-Hill Book Co.
15. Minckler, J., editor: Pathology of the nervous system, vols. I and II, New York, 1968-1970, McGraw-Hill Book Co.
16. Minckler, T. M., and Boyd, E.: Physical growth. In Minckler, J., editor: Pathology of the nervous system, vol. I, New York, 1968, McGraw-Hill Book Co.
17. Polyak, S.: The retina, Chicago, 1942, University of Chicago Press.
18. Powers, M., and Minckler, J.: The VIIIth nerve of man; a quantitative study. (In preparation.)
19. Quarton, C. G., Melnechuk, T., and Schmitt, F. O.: The neurosciences, New York, 1967, The Rockefeller University Press.
20. Rasmussen, A. T.: The growth of the hypophysis cerebri and its major subdivisions during childhood, Amer. J. Anat. **80:**95, 1947.
21. Scammon, R. E.: A summary of the anatomy of the infant and child. In Abt's pediatrics, Philadelphia, 1923, W. B. Saunders Co.
22. Sinclair, I. G.: A developmental study of the fourth cranial nerve, Texas Rep. Biol. Med. **16:**257, 1958.
23. Tomasche, J., and Etemandi, A. A.: Human hypoglossal nucleus, J. Comp. Neurol. **119:**105, 1962.
24. Tourtellotte, W. W.: Cerebrospinal fluid and its reactions in disease. In Minckler, J., editor: Pathology of the nervous system, vol. I, New York, 1968, McGraw-Hill Book Co.
25. van Buskirk, E. C.: The seventh nerve complex, J. Comp. Neurol. **82:**303, 1945.
26. Weinberg, E.: The mesencephalic root of the fifth nerve, J. Comp. Neurol. **46:**249, 1928.
27. Wolman, M.: Myelin structure, ultrastructure, and degeneration. In Minckler, J., editor: Pathologic of the nervous system, vol. I, New York, 1968, McGraw-Hill Book Co.

PART II Microanatomy

CHAPTER 8

ELECTRON MICROSCOPY

RONALD COWDEN

There are physical limitations to the resolving power of the light microscope. In the most favorable material and using the best lens systems available, the light microscope can resolve structures with a diameter of 0.25 μ. Since the development of the electron microscope and suitable techniques for preparing biologic material, it has become possible to examine an entire class of structures that previously lay beyond the grasp of cytologists.[12] The fundamental unit of measure in studying ultrastructure is the Ångstrom (Å), which is .00001 μ. The instruments currently used are able to resolve structures of about 5Å. Therefore, the electron microscope can resolve structures that are 2×10^3 times smaller than objects resolved by the light microscope. This increased resolving power carries certain increased preparative demands. Rather than cutting specimens embedded in paraffin or celloidin or cutting fresh frozen material, it is necessary to embed material being prepared for electron microscopy in relatively hard plastics, such as Epon 812, and to section these on a special microtome that is designed to cut sections of from 200 to 300 Å thickness. Thicker sections would absorb or scatter electrons used under the voltage conditions of most electron microscopes (50 to 100 kV); therefore there is a limitation on the thickness of a structure to be examined. This means that only very small areas can be examined at a particular time, that many fields must be examined to gain insight into the cellular population of a tissue, and that sections at different levels are required to obtain some idea of the three-dimensional structure of a cell. The fact that the very thin specimen is bombarded by a beam of electrons causes further difficulties; under this bombardment the specimen is unstable and often curls up.

The tedious and painstaking preparation completed before introducing the specimen into the electron microscope is the most important step of this process. Most scientists prefer either buffered gluteraldehyde or paraformaldehyde for fixation. Very small tissue blocks of about 1 mm. square are used. After an hour of treatment at ice water temperature (4° C.), the tissues are washed in buffered, osmotically balanced solutions (usually sucrose) and treated with cold buffered osmium tetroxide (OsO_4). Formerly osmic acid was used as a primary fixative, but the two aldehydes currently used have proven to ensure the best preservation of fine structure. However, osmium is a heavy metal; therefore electrons hitting osmium atoms do not penetrate through the tissue and are scattered away. This material is added to the tissue block to increase contrast, providing an electronopaque stain.

Following the osmium treatment, the small tissue blocks are washed in cold water (or in buffered, balanced salt), and water is slowly removed by short sequential treatments with increasing strengths of alcohol. It is often necessary, particularly in climates with high humidity, to remove water absorbed from the atmosphere from the absolute alcohol with silica gel or *molecular sieve*. Then the tissues are given a final dehydration treatment with propylene oxide and placed in gelatin capsules in a monomer mixture of the plastic in which they are to be hardened.

The following are examples of plastics currently in use: Araldite, Vestopol, Maraglas, Epon 812, and various methacrylates. Certain accelerators must be added to the monomer mixture to ensure polymerization, which causes hardening of the plastic. The extent of polymerization can to a certain degree be controlled by the amount of accelerator added. It is necessary to treat the monomer-accelerator mixture with either heat or ultraviolet light to ensure proper polymerization.

The tissue embedded in the polymerized plastic is then cut on an ultramicrotome using a specially broken fresh glass knife. In many laboratories a knife made of industrial diamond is substituted for the glass knife. The cutting face of the ultramicrotome is designed to cut tissues of about 1 mm. square. The tissues are placed in such a way that the sections float onto dilute alcohol held in a depression behind the cutting surface. They are floated onto fine wire mesh plates (grids) and dried. The grids are often coated with a film of carbon to give the fragile thin section further support. This is particularly true when a wider mesh grid is used. After drying, sections on the grid are sequentially stained in lead citrate and uranyl acetate. Both of these treatments are designed to introduce additional heavy, electron-scattering atoms into the tissue and thus to act as electronopaque stains.

It should be clear by now that the electron microscope acts on a similar principle to that of the light microscope. In the light microscope rays of light are bent and focused by glass lenses. In the electron microscope a beam of electrons is bent by electromagnetic lenses. The light microscope possesses a condenser, an objective lens, and an ocular lens; counterparts in the electron microscope are the condenser (usually two in better instruments), the objective lens, and the projective lens. In direct light microscopy, contrast in the specimen is caused by dyes introduced by staining procedures. The dyes selectively absorb certain wavelengths of light. In electron microscopy contrast is caused by the inability of electrons to penetrate certain structures; thus the light is scattered away and never reaches the film upon which the image is recorded. Electron scattering is to a considerable extent dependent on the atomic weight of the atoms the electrons hit. Most biologic material is composed of atoms of low atomic weight, such as carbon (12), oxygen (16), nitrogen (14), and hydrogen (1). Heavy metals are introduced as stains to increase electron scattering and thus improve contrast in the picture. Unlike the light microscope, the electron microscope does not provide for direct visual observation as the major method of examining a specimen. The image is projected on a removable phosphor screen; then it can be examined with a conventional stereo microscope for focusing and selecting a field for photography. The fluorescent screen is then removed and a picture taken. Initial magnifications may be low (in the hundreds) or up to about 300,000, but photographic enlargement is necessary for further magnification. For example, a picture taken of an image that is magnified 200,000 times may be enlarged five times to give a picture with a total 1 million times enlargement.

The conventional electron microscope is just one of the many types of electron microscopes now in use. Quite recently several ultrahigh voltage (600,000 to 1 million kV) electron microscopes have been developed. These instruments have the advantage of allowing photography of thicker sections (up to 1 μ), because the higher accelerating voltage allows deeper penetration. These instruments are very new, and less than a dozen are currently in use in the United States. Another type now in use is the scanning electron microsope. This instrument, like a television tube, passes a stream of electrons rapidly over a specimen. When the electrons hit the specimen, certain types of energy are emitted that are picked up by photometric devices and used to construct a picture on a television display tube. The display tube picture is then photographed. While maximum resolution with this instrument is only from 100 to 200 Å, it is considerably better than the resolution that can be obtained with a light microscope. The scanning electron microscope offers particular advantages in the examination of three-dimensional structure and of the detailed surface structure of biologic materials.

GENERAL ULTRASTRUCTURE (Fig. 8-1)

Unit membrane

The cell is bounded by a plasma membrane. Like most biologic membranes, this consists of an outer and an inner layer of protein and lipids, separated by a highly lipid layer (Figs. 10-14 and 10-15). In each of these layers, the outward-directed portion consists of protein, with the hydrophilic pole of a lipid associated with the protein, while the hydrophobic end is directed toward the intervening lipid layer (Fig. 10-18).[6,16] When viewed with the electron microscope using moderately high resolution, protein-dense layers appear as two thin lines representing the outer and inner protein borders. These trilaminar layers are called unit membranes. The surface of a cell is seldom smooth. Often microvilli are seen as evaginations of the surface (Fig. 8-2). These are particularly abundant on the surface of kidney cells and intestinal cells. It is through these microvilli that the cell ingests larger molecules that cannot readily pass through

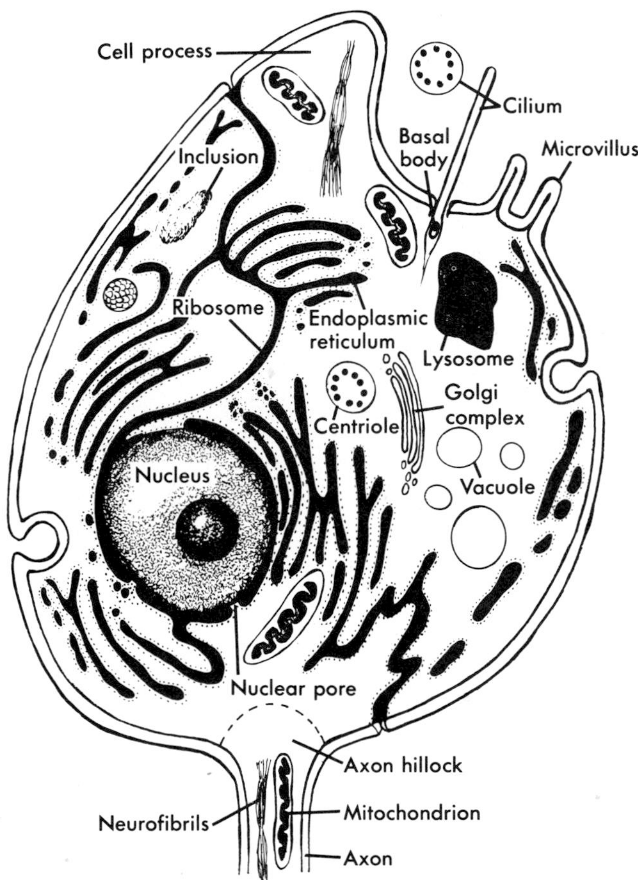

Fig. 8-1. Composite diagram of a neural cell with components, as seen in electron microscopy.

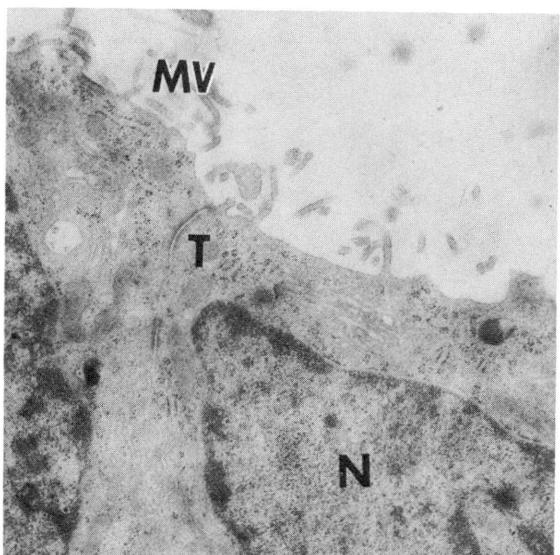

Fig. 8-2. Microvilli (*MV*) on ependymal surface. *T,* tight junction; *N,* nucleus.

the plasma membrane. These molecules are folded in by the microvilli, pass into the body of the cell, and are finally pinched off into vesicles, in which they are subsequently broken down by enzymatic action.

Junctions

Cell surfaces also have other specializations. In mature tissues, close connection and approximation between cells is maintained by two types of surface structures, *tight junctions* and *desmosomes* (Fig. 8-3).[8] Tight junctions are internal modifications that rigidify the membrane over several hundred angstroms in the membranes of two adjacent cells. In the electron microscope these structures appear as thickenings. The desmosomes also represent thickened areas in adjacent cells. They are shorter and thicker than tight junctions, and tonofibrils extend perpendicularly from these thickenings into the cell bodies. No material has been observed extending from one cell to the other, or lying between the tight junction or desmosome complexes of adjacent cells. Nevertheless these structural modifications have considerable adhesive capacity and inhibit the passage of other material in the space between adjacent cells.

Cilia

The cellular organelles of motility, the cilia and flagellae, are also considered modifications of the cell surface.[8] The cilia consist of a basal body, a filamentous portion, and tonofibrils that exhibit a periodic striated pattern extending into the cell body. In cross section a cilium consists of nine outer pairs of microtubules and a central pair of microtubules oriented perpendicular to the direction in which the cilium beats (Fig. 8-3). The basal body swells and is a bit larger than the filamentous portion, but it contains no central pair of microtubules. A flagellum differs in that in addition to the microtubule system of the cilium, an additional pair of microtubules is wrapped around the system. This allows for circular movement in addition to the single axis of movement of the cilium (Fig. 10-33).

Mitochondria

In light microscope preparations the mitochondria, which house the enzymes required for oxidative phosphorylation, lie near the limits of resolu-

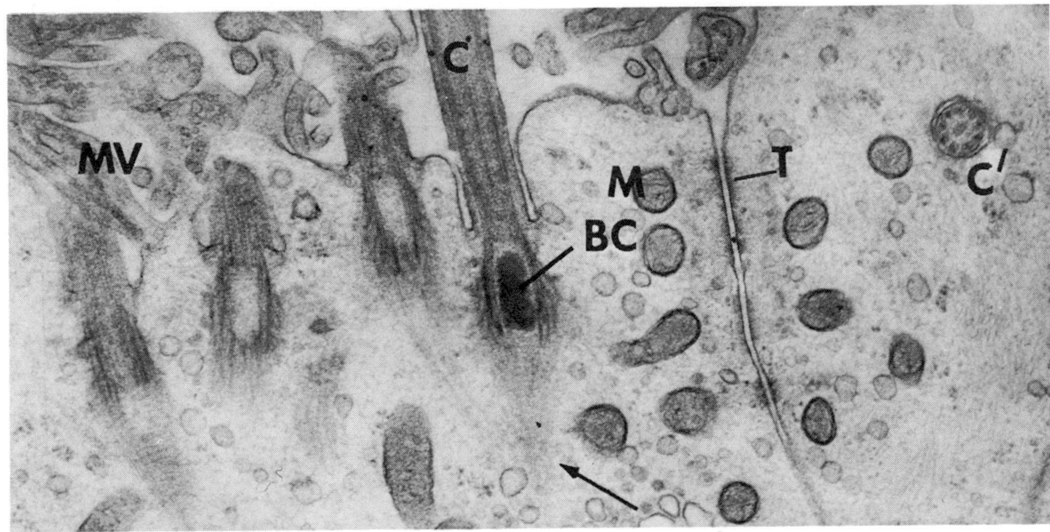

Fig. 8-3. Cilia (*C*) with basal corpuscle or body (*BC*) on ependymal cell. *C'*, cilia in cross section *MV*, microvillus; *T*, tight junction. Arrow joints to less dense filaments at base of shaft. (From Tennyson, V. M., and Pappas, G. D. In Minckler, J., editor: Pathology of the nervous system, vol. I, New York, 1968, McGraw-Hill Book Co.)

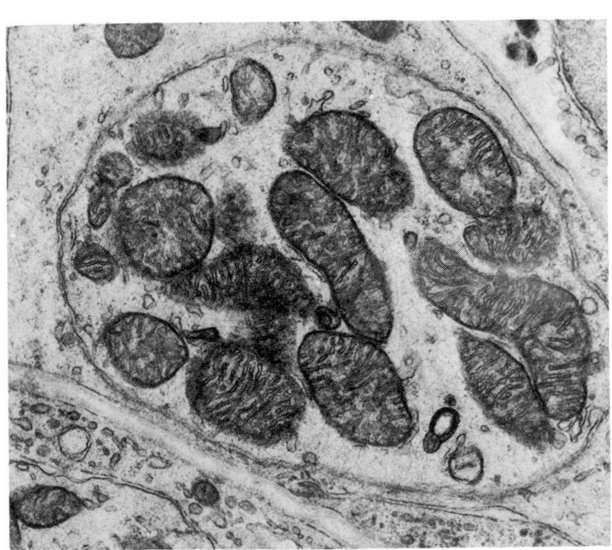

Fig. 8-4. Mitochondria in axoplasm. (From Luse, S. In Minckler, J., editor: Pathology of the nervous system, vol. I, New York, 1968, McGraw-Hill Book Co. Courtesy Anthony D'Agostino.)

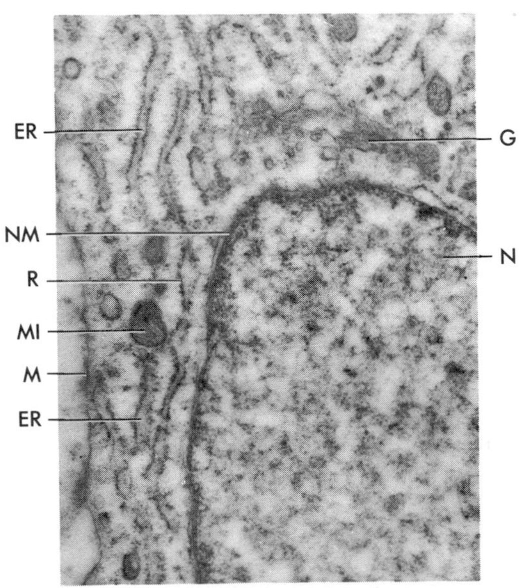

Fig. 8-5. Electron micrograph showing nucleus (*N*), nuclear membrane (*NM*), Golgi apparatus (*G*), endoplasmic reticulum (*ER*) with attached ribosomes (*R*), mitochondrion (*MI*), and surface membrane (*M*). (×30,000.) (From Hager, H. In Minckler, J., editor: Pathology of the nervous system, vol. I, New York, 1968, McGraw-Hill Book Co.)

tion. As such they are very difficult to see. In the electron microscope they appear as oval structures bound by a unit membrane with internal projections that are also constructed of unit membranes (cristae). The shape of mitochondria and the form of the cristae vary in different kinds of cells (Fig. 8-4). Mitochondria are the first organelles in the cell to be affected by anoxia or cell damage.[17] The conditions are usually manifested by mitochondrial swelling, which is a frequent finding in pathologic cells. Small amounts of DNA have also been localized within these structures. In the electron microscope it appears as internal helically coiled filaments.

Nucleus

The nucleus is bound by a unit membrane that is modified by the presence of pores (Figs. 8-1 and 8-5).[8] Although the detailed structure of the pores is not yet completely understood, it seems certain that they are not simply pores. They may take the form of octagonal cylinders projecting beyond the membrane both above and below. Some form of diaphragm may also be located within the pore; this possibility has been debated. In any event, the nuclear membrane does not function as a simple osmometer. Modifications in the nuclear membrane are directed toward selective transport of materials in and out of the nucleus.

Endoplasmic reticulum

Unit membrane material proliferates from the surface of the nuclear membrane and may in certain types of cells fill a considerable portion of the cytoplasm (Fig. 8-5).[12] This membrane, the endoplasmic reticulum, is particularly abundant in cells that synthesize lipoproteins or secretory proteins. In cells synthesizing the former the endoplasmic reticulum is smooth, but in cells producing the latter it becomes studded with spherical structures of about 180 Å diameter. These structures are called the ribosomes. Ribosome-studded endoplasmic reticulum is called *rough endoplasmic reticulum.* In certain types of neurons rough endoplasmic reticulum is so densely packed that the aggregations can be seen with the light microscope as *Nissl bodies.* Some workers contend that the endoplasmic reticulum may begin at the nuclear surface, ramify through the cytoplasm, and eventually connect with the plasma membrane. This model would offer a direct connection between the nucleus and cell surface, but such a pattern has not been observed. In many cells, particularly embryonic cells, there is very little endoplasmic reticulum. In these cells ribosomes are usually abundant and are free of connection with membranes.

Ribosomes

The ribosomes are spherical particles of about 180 Å diameter; on their surface protein synthesis occurs (Fig. 8-5).[3] They contain two subunits that appear to be held together by positively charged magnesium ions. Removal of magnesium ions causes these subunits to dissociate. The whole ribosome structure and its subunits contain about fifty percent RNA and fifty percent protein. In electron micrographs they may be seen as free ribosomes or attached to unit membranes (endoplasmic reticulum). In some instances a number of ribosomes will appear as a round cluster held together by a filament. These structures are called polyribosomes (polysomes) and are thought to represent a number of ribosomes sharing a single long strand of messenger RNA. Polyribosomes are normally abundant in cells that do not contain an abundance of endoplasmic reticulum.

Golgi complex

Secretory proteins are synthesized on the ribosomes embedded in the walls of the endoplasmic reticulum. They accumulate in the space within the unit membranes, the *cisternal space,* and may eventually move into a smooth portion of the endoplasmic reticulum that is modified into a series of flat, stacked (lamellae) plates. This series is called the Golgi complex.[8] In the Golgi complex, the final packaging of this protein material into secretory granules occurs (Fig. 8-5). This package is subsequently pinched off and the granules come to lie free in the cytoplasm.

Lysosomes

The cytoplasm also contains another type of inclusion that appears to be bound by a single rather than a unit membrane and that contains the major collection of hydrolytic enzymes.[8] The single membrane theory is now disputed. These structures, the lysosomes, often appear as homogeneously electron-dense structures (Fig. 8-6). They may engulf damaged or worn-out organelles. Thus it is not unusual to find a portion of a mitochondrion or some other structure included within a lysosome. Lysosomes containing other structures are called *phagosomes.* By concentrating the hydrolytic enzymes in a specialized structure, the cell preserves the capacity to digest foreign or worn-out structures, and the material is not liberated within the cell to impair its normal function.

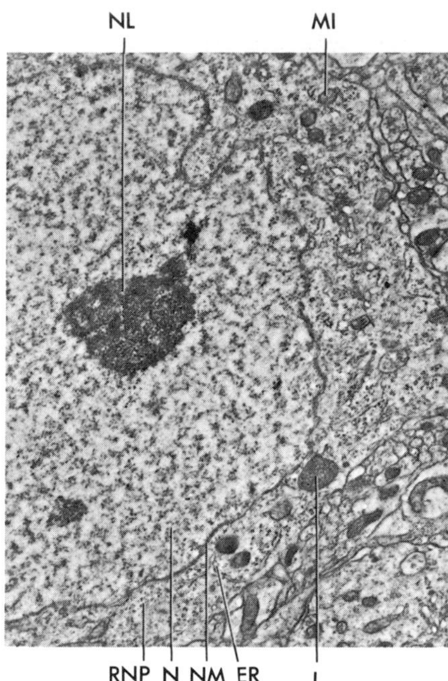

Fig. 8-6. Electron micrograph of nucleus (*N*), nucleolus (*NL*), lysosome (*L*), ribonucleoprotein (*RNP*), nuclear membrane (*NM*), endoplasmic reticulum (*ER*), and mitochondrion (*M*) in neuron. (From Hager, H. In Minckler, J.: editor: Pathology of the nervous system, vol. I, New York, 1968, McGraw-Hill Book Co.)

Mitosis

When cell division occurs the nuclear membrane breaks down, and the mitotic spindle is formed. The polar attachments of the spindle is to a pair of *centrioles* (Fig. 8-1) lying at opposite ends of the cell and representing the poles in which the cell will divide. The ultrastructure of the centriole is identical to that of the basal body of cilia and flagella. The centriole possesses nine pairs of external microtubular filaments but no internal filaments. Replication occurs at right angles to the centriole. This occurs during prophase, and at the time of division only two centrioles are normally present. Additional centrioles would cause multipolar division and considerable abnormality in the distribution of chromosomes into the daughter cells.[8]

Chromatin

The nuclear membrane has already been discussed. In most cells types the nucleoplasm appears as more or less homogeneous, fine granular material. It appears either darker or lighter than the cytoplasm, depending upon the concentrations of nucleoplasmic protein. In some instances other nucleoplasmic materials, such as accumulated glycogen granules, may be observed. In virus-infected nuclei, virus particles or the accumulated products of viral activity may also be seen. In some ways the electron microscope has not been a particularly useful instrument for studying the structure of chromosomes. The latter are too dense and too large. It is known that chromosomes are composed of fibrils of about 100 Å diameter; the fibrils appear to represent the DNA double helix and histone associated with it. The ultrastructural studies however have not been able to clarify whether the chromosomes' linear integrity is due to a single very long and coiled filament of DNA, or if DNA and protein alternate throughout its length. A distinction can be made by the electron microscope between fine or extended chromatin and coarser, condensed chromatin. Some of the chromatin tends to lie against the nuclear membrane.[8]

Nucleoli

Nucleoli arise from certain regions on the chromosomes, the nucleolar organizers, which contain genes encoding precursors to ribosomal RNA. In a sense these organelles represent the manifestations of the activation of these genes. Nucleoli are not present in all cell nuclei; they are found only in cells actively synthesizing ribosomal RNA. They are usually quite prominent in neurons. With the electron microscope the nucleolus is seen to contain a filamentous component and a granular one, the *pars amorpha* (Fig. 8-6). They may, in parts of their functional cycles that are not yet completely understood, develop a central vacuole. When viewed with the electron microscope this vacuole is manifested as a region of finer granules less dense than the predominant granules within the nucleolus. Because replacement of damaged neuronal processes leads to a series of nucleolar changes, nucleolar alterations that occur during chromatolysis and restructuring has been of interest not only to neurologists but also to cell biologists.[3]

Microtubules

The mitotic spindle, which forms completely after the nuclear membrane breaks down in late prophase, is composed of bundles of microtubular elements attached to both the chromosomes (at the centromeres) and the polar centrioles. The microtubular nature of these fibers should be emphasized, since they will be encountered repeatedly in cellular structures associated with contraction and movement; these structures are cilia, flagellae, muscles, centrioles, and the neurofibrillar networks of neurons (Figs. 8-1 and 10-47).[8]

Inclusions

There are vast numbers of specialized cytoplasmic inclusions characteristic of one cell type or another. These would generally be dealt with best if and when these structures are encountered. Within nerve cells however there are two particular structures that should be discussed before describing the nerve cells proper. Some neurons produce hormonal substances, the *neurosecretory granules.* These granules are of relatively uniform size and spherical shape when mature, but unfinished stages in their assembly may be found, particularly in the Gogi complex. These granules are of intermediate density, usually not quite as electron-dense as lysosomes. They are found only in certain neurons, and these neurons may be filled with, partially filled with, or completely free of neurosecretory material, depending upon their position in the general hormonal secretory cycle. Neurons may possess multiple laminated bodies, including a whorl with filamentous structure, sometimes laminated filamentous structure, and both fine and coarse granular components. The role of these structures is presently a complete mystery, but they are generally present in neuron cytoplasm and are sometimes located in the cytoplasm of associated glial cells.[8]

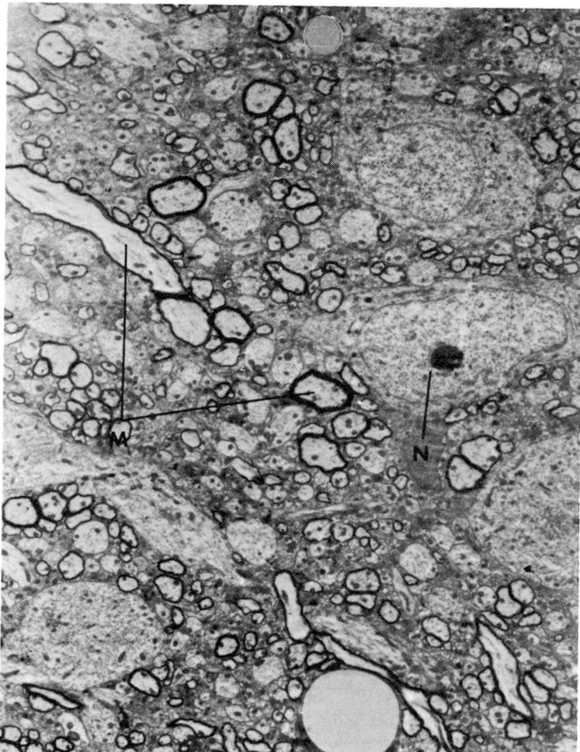

Fig. 8-7. General low-power electron microscopic view of CNS tissue. *N,* Neuron; *M,* thin myelinated axis-cylinder with elongated mitochondria. Much of intervening substance is made up of glial processes.

CELLULAR ULTRASTRUCTURE

It would be foolish to attempt anything other than a highlighted summary of the ultrastructure of the nervous system (Fig. 8-7); comprehensive treatment would require several volumes. Instead, an attempt will be made to describe the neuron, the major recognized types of glial cells, some of the major nonneuronal elements of the peripheral nervous system, and selected sensory cells. (For details of ultrastructure see Chapter 10.)

Neuron

The neuron should be examined in its major parts—the cell body with the nucleus, and the axonal and dendritic processes. The rather large neuronal nucleus is surrounded by cell body cytoplasm, the perikaryon (Fig. 8-6).[13] Before going further, it should be noted that there are different kinds of neurons. The very large neurons include the Purkinje cells and pyramidal cells of the cortex, and some of the neurons of ganglia. The CNS abounds with smaller neurons, which in size and appearance are virtually indistinguishable when viewed with the light microscope from glial elements (see Chapter 10). The neuronal nucleus is usually spherical or ovoid, with condensed bits of chromatin dispersed throughout. This is particularly true of the nuclei of larger neurons. In smaller neurons chromatin tends to be somewhat more compact. There is usually a single relatively large nucleolus, which may display alterations in detail as the cell undergoes specific metabolic phases (as in regeneration), requiring rapid synthesis of new ribosomes. The structures of nuclear membrane and pores are for all practical purposes identical to these structures in other types of cells.

Within the perikaryon, certain organelles can be identified by light microscopy. These structures include the neurofibrillar network, mitochondria, Nissl bodies, and Golgi elements, as well as some special types of inclusions that vary with cell type. In light microscopy it has been demonstrated that the neurofibrillar network not only abundantly fills the perikaryon, but also extends into the axonal and dendritic processes.[18] With the electron microscope these neurofibrils are seen to consist of cylinders of about 100 Å diameter, with lumens of 40 Å. Evidence indicates that these structures are microtubules identical to the contractile units of the mitotic spindle and cilia.

The rough endoplasmic reticulum of the neuron reaches considerable density in some types of neurons and not in others. The accumulations of endoplasmic reticulum (containing RNA) are manifested under the light microscope as Nissl substance where the Nissl bodies stain due to the presence of RNA.[8] The presence of such densities of endoplasmic reticulum gives further evidence that the neuron is active in the production of secretory material. The same consideration applies to the presence of Golgi elements in the neuron cell body.

Perikarya also contain mitochrondria. However, as in the case of the neurofibrillar network, mitochrondria extends into the nerve processes and may become abundant in the axonal cytoplasm (axoplasm) (Figs. 8-4 and 8-7). Mitrochondria in both locations are conventional in appearance.

Neurons ingest extracellular material that is sometimes passed on to them by associated glial cells.[20] As such the neuronal cytoplasm may display both pinocytotic vesicles and lysosomes. Other, more complex inclusions may also be observed. Many such inclusions have fine complicated fibrous whorls or lattice structures as well as fine and coarse granular components. In certain neurons (such as those of the ventral horn spinal ganglia) accumulations of lipofuscin granules may be found. As such these granules are unit membrane–bounded, somewhat irregular structures containing a filamentous internal component as well as a granular component. With increasing age these pigments tend to accumulate and may impair normal neuronal function. Glycogen granules may also be evident in the neuronal cytoplasm.

There are both myelinated and unmyelinated neuronal processes in the nervous system.[1,9] In the CNS these myelin investments are provided by oligodendroglial cells; in the peripheral nervous system the myelin is produced by Schwann cells.[1] There is an important distinction in the two myelin sources. As hypermature derivatives of neural ectoderm, oligodendroglia are not capable of mitotic proliferation and therefore cannot replace degenerated myelin; Schwann cells also appear to be of neuroectodermal origin but may be replaced by cell division. In both instances the manner in which myelin sheaths form is almost identical. The main difference lies in the fact that Schwann cells place an elaborate wrap on only one axon or house many nonmyelinated fibers, while oligodendroglia relate to several axonal filaments (see Chapter 10).[1] The plasma membrane of the enveloping cell extends and rolls inself repeatedly around the axon in the manner of a jelly roll (Figs. 10-13 through 10-18).[10,15,19] This plasma membrane surface becomes thicker so that sections through myelin investments give the impression that apposed, thickened unit membrane surfaces are present (Fig. 10-15). As one might expect, the cells involved in the elaboration of myelin characteristically display high densities of rough endoplasmic reticulum and abundant mitochondria.

The *nodes of Ranvier,* which can be seen with the light microscope, represent the borders of individual Schwann cells and the areas of least electrical insulation. If there are lateral outgrowths of the axon, these will occur at the nodes. While the jelly-roll profile of the Schwann cells is well known, the longitudinal profile indicates that these protoplasmic extensions terminate as loops, with the outermost layer extending farthest toward the neighboring Schwann cell (Fig. 10-17).[7,14]

The axons usually undergo considerable terminal arborization, ending in swellings, the terminal buttons *(boutons terminaux).* Terminal buttons are characterized by considerable accumluations of mitochondria and vesicles, the synaptic vesicles (Figs. 10-47, 10-49, and 10-50).[5] These vesicles are found only in the axonal terminals and not in the dendrites, and are thought to represent areas of reduced electrical resistance in the cell membranes. If the axon is damaged proximal to the terminal buttons, the buttons and the mitochondria will swell, and the vesicles will become obliterated.

Neuroglia

In addition to the neurons proper, there are three types of supporting cells that appear in the CNS; these are the oligodendroglia and the astrocytes, both called neuroglia or macroglia, and the microglia. Both oligodendroglia and astrocytes are derivatives of the neuroepithelium, while the microglia are of mesodermal origin.[11,20]

As noted earlier, oligodendroglia take over the myelin-producing role of the Schwann cells in the CNS. As such they possess relatively high levels of rough endoplasmic reticulum, a Golgi complex, and a number of mitochondria (Fig. 10-30). These cells are often found associated with neuron cell bodies, and processes from these cells frequently invaginate or notch the surface of neurons, sending processes deep into the perikaryon.[2] Oligodendroglia are believed to have some role in the maintenance of neurons by passing material taken from capillary circulation into the neuron, although astrocytes are probably more important in such transport.

Both oligodendroglia and the Schwann cells of the peripheral nervous system produce myelin sheaths through proliferation of their cell membranes. These sheaths progressively enfold the axon (CNS) or bundles of axons (peripheral nervous system) in jelly-roll fashion (see Chapter 10).* Careful examination of high magnification electron micrographs indicates that this type of configuration could be expected from formations of jelly-roll type produced by external cellular unit membranes (Fig. 8-8). Further experimental evidence was developed from experiments in which the jelly roll was induced to unroll.[19]

There are two types of astrocytes. There are fibrous astrocytes, which contain an abundance of fibrous strands running through the cytoplasm, forming an intracellular web not unlike the neurofibrillar network of neurons, and protoplasmic astrocytes, which display a characteristically large number of fine processes with extensive arborization (Fig. 10-27). These distinctions are largely drawn from observations with the light microscope of the results of silver staining and appear to be based on microenvironmental conditions that influence the shape of these cells. These two types of astrocytes are indistinguishable with the electron microscope. Characteristically they contain few mitochondria, very little endoplasmic reticulum, and few other organelles associated with high levels of protein synthesis. The intracellular fibrillar complex appears to be composed of material very similar or identical to protocollagen fibrils in fibrocytes. There is a possibility that these structures may be in some way related to microtubules, but this has not yet been established.[10,20]

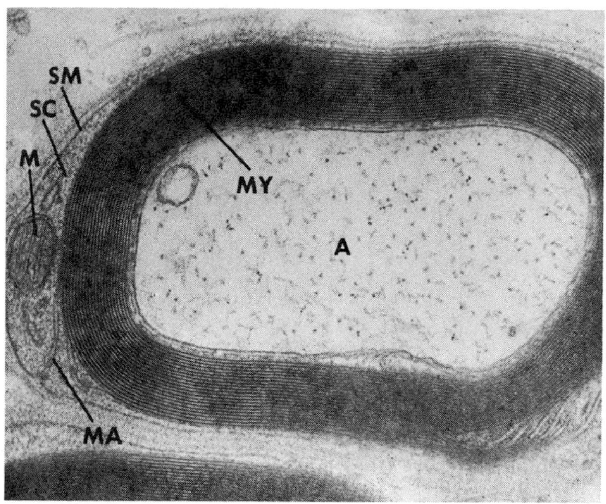

Fig. 8-8. Myelinated axon (*A*) showing mesaxon (*MA*), myelin laminae (*MY*), mitochondria (*M*) in Schwann cell cytoplasm (*SC*), and Schwann cell membrane (*SM*). (From Luse, S. In Minckler, J., editor: Pathology of the nervous system, vol. I, New York, 1968, McGraw-Hill Book Co.)

Microglia

Microglia are virtually indistinguishable in function and ultrastructure from macrophages (Fig. 10-25). Indeed, there are some who suggest that they are simply macrophages of the CNS. As such they contain variable but usually small amounts of rough endoplasmic reticulum. They seldom contain Golgi complexes, but normally possess lysosomes.[20]

Ependyma

The CNS develops from ectodermal epithelium that becomes enclosed as a simple tube of epithelium, the neural tube, early in embronic life. For a considerable portion of the subsequent development of the CNS to a many-cell, layered system, an inner epithelial layer, the ependymal layer, persists. During the development stages cells move from the periphery of the neural tube to the ependyma to undergo mitosis, then they go back into the cell mass. The choroid plexus, though convoluted, retains this simple epithelial nature in the adult.

In the embryo the ependyma is ciliated. The cilia have the characteristic ultrastructural configuration that has already been described. In adult life some ciliated ventricular ependymal surfaces may persist.

The ependyma persists in adult life as special glial elements. These cells form a palisade of elongated epithelial cells associated at their lateral margins by a series of desmosomes. They line the surfaces of the cerebral ventricles. As in the astrocytes of adults, ependymal cells exhibit only a small amount of ergastoplasm and fewer mitochondria than oligodendroglia. The ependymal cells are relatively broad at the ventricular surface, but they taper, sending thin processes into the underlying neural tissue. The nuclear pattern is typical of a metabolically inactive cell and generally lacks a nucleolus. In some cells a complex filamentous system passes through the length of the cell. These cells will form the internal limiting membrane of

*See references 1, 4, 6, 8, 10, 15, 16, and 19.

the ventricle, which is constructed of extracellular amorphous fine granular material with some fine fibrous elements. In those instances where ependymal cells extend from the internal surface of the neural tube to the external surface, they may also form an external limiting membrane of the same material.[20]

These cells are very active in pinocytosis and as such may exhibit a convoluted surface with many microvilli. These microvilli extend inward into the cell, pinch off as pinocytotic vesicles, and may be digested by lysosomes.

Intercellular space

Some organs or organ systems are characterized by considerable amounts of extracellular space. This is true of the loose connective tissues, for example. A good deal of this space is often filled by an extracellular (exoplasmic) material, loosely termed *amorphous ground substance*. This material is really a very heterogeneous mixture of proteins (largely serum proteins) and mucoproteins. Probably the highest content, or at least the components by which this material can best be characterized, are the acid mucoproteins *chondroitin sulfate* and *hyaluronic acid*. In light microscopy these are relatively simple to identify by selective staining and enzyme predigestion methods.

There is not much amorphous ground substance in the nervous system. Actually some authors feel that there is not more than two to three percent extracellular space. This figure is based on electron microscopic surveys of nervous tissue in which the space between cells has been calculated from serial or semiserial sections. This interpretation has been contested on indirect evidence that was obtained from measurements of electrical resistance and conductivity from electrodes placed some distance apart in the brains of rats. Similar measurements were made under the same conditions but during perfusion of the brains with various perfusion fixation mixtures. The combined measurements led to the conclusion that the amount of extracellular space in the CNS must be considerably higher than the usual low percentage estimated from measurements of gaps between cells (Fig. 8-9). The ergastoplasm, which *may be* continuous from nuclear membrane to plasma membrane, thus represents the best possible source of this additional functional space. In this concept the ergastoplasmic cisterna functions as extracellular space. The matter is still disputed and far from settled.

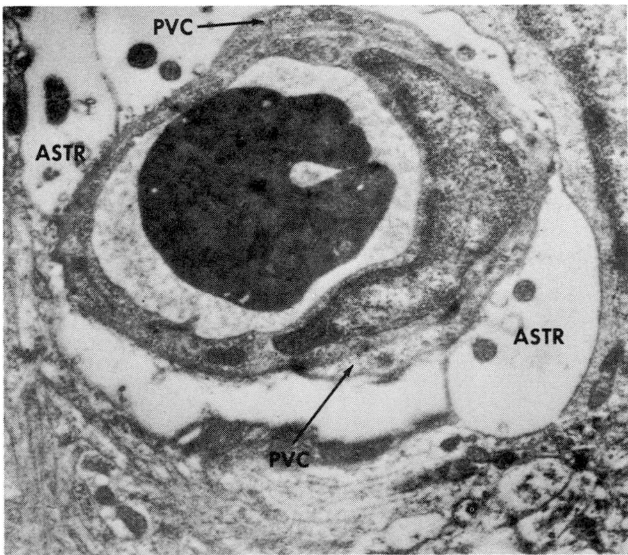

Fig. 8-9. Electron micrograph of capillary showing surrounding astroctyes (*ASTR*) and perivascular cells (*PVC*). Note minimal evidence of intercellular space. (From Woollam, D. H. M., and Millen, J. W. In Minckler, J., editor: Pathology of the nervous system, vol. I, New York, 1968, McGraw-Hill Book Co.)

REFERENCES

1. Bischoff, A., and Moor, H.: Ultrastructural differences between myelin sheaths of peripheral nerve fibers and CNS white matter, Z. Zellforsch. **81**:303, 1967.
2. Blunt, M. J., Wendell-Smith, C. P., and Baldwin, F.: Glia-nerve fiber relationships in mammalian optic nerve, J. Anat. **99**:1, 1965.
3. Busch, H., and Smetana, K.: The nucleolus, New York, 1970, Academic Press, Inc.
4. Causey, G.: The cell of schwann, Edinburgh, 1960, E. and S. Livingstone, Ltd.
5. De Robertis, E.: Synaptic complexes and synaptic vesicles as structural and biochemical units of the central nervous system. In Rodahl, K., and Issekutz, B., editors: Nerve as a tissue, New York, 1966, Harper & Row, Publishers.
6. Finean, J. B.: The molecular structure of nerve myelin and its significance in relation to the nerve membrane. In Richter, D., editor: Metabolism of the nervous system, London, 1957, Pergamon Press Ltd.
7. Geren-Uzman, B., and Nogueira-Graf, G.: Electron microscope studies of the nodes of Ranvier in mouse sciatic nerves, J. Biophys. Biochem. Cytol. **3**:589, 1957.
8. Hama, K.: Nervous system. In Yamada, E., and others, editors: Fine structure of cells and tissues electron microscope atlas, vol. IV, Tokyo, 1968, Igaku Shoin.
9. Hess, A.: The fine structure and morphological organization of nonmyelinated nerve fibers, Proc. Roy. Soc. **144B**:496, 1956.
10. Luse, S. A.: Formation of myelin in the central nervous system of mice and rats as studied with the electron microscope, J. Biophys. Biochem. Cytol. **2**:777, 1956.

11. Mugnaini, E., and Walberg, F.: Ultrastructure of neuroglia, Ergebn. Anat. Entwicklungsgesch. **37**:193, 1964.
12. Palade, G. E.: The endoplasmic reticulum, J. Biophys. Biochem. Cytol. **2**:85, 1956.
13. Palay, S. L., and Palade, G. E.: The fine structure of neurons, J. Biophys. Biochem. Cytol. **1**:69, 1955.
14. Pease, D. C.: Nodes of Ranvier in the central nervous system, J. Comp. Neurol. **103**:11, 1955.
15. Robertson, J. D.: Molecular structure and contact relationships of cell membranes, Progr. Biophys. **10**:343, 1960.
16. Robertson, J. D.: The unit membrane of cells and mechanisms of myelin formation, Res. Publ. Ass. Res. Nerv. Ment. Dis. **4**:94, 1962.
17. Rouiller, C.: Physiological and pathological changes in mitochondrial morphology, Int. Rev. Cytol. **9**:227, 1960.
18. Schmitt, F. O., and Samson, F.: Neuronal fibrous proteins, Neurosci. Res. Prog. Bull. **6**:113, 1968.
19. Smart, I.: Reconstruction of myelinated Schwann cells by "unrolling," J. Anat. **99**:212, 1965.
20. Windle, W. F.: Biology of neuroglia, Springfield, Illinois. 1958, Charles C Thomas, Publisher.

CHAPTER 9

DEVELOPMENTAL BIOLOGY

ROBERT LASHER

Like all phases of embryonic development, vertebrate neurogenesis is a dynamic process. Starting at the time of gastrulation with primary embryonic induction, morphogenesis proceeds through reorganization of neuroepithelial structure, cell proliferation and migration, cell differentiation, and formation of specific synaptic connections. These last two events are accompanied by differentiation of nervous function, which is closely paralleled by development of behavior and regulation of vital functions.

NEURAL INDUCTION AND EARLY PATTERN FORMATION IN THE CNS

The basic pattern of the CNS is laid down at the time of primary embryonic induction. Induction is achieved through apposition of the prechordal plate and chordamesoderm with the overlying ectoderm during gastrulation. Although the mechanics of gastrulation differ markedly in the various vertebrate phyla, the process of induction appears to remain the same. For example, in amphibians and fish the ectoderm becomes neuralized in a *caudocranial* direction through craniad extension of the chordamesoderm and simultaneous caudal expansion of the ectoderm (Fig. 9-1). However, in birds (and probably in mammals) neuralization of the ectoderm proceeds in a *craniocaudal* direction through caudad extension of the chordamesoderm, promoted by regression of Hensen's node and the primitive streak (Fig. 9-2). Thus, while the mechanics of gastrulation in these two groups of vertebrates lead to initiation of induction from opposite directions in the anterior-posterior axis, it is still achieved through progressive interaction of ectoderm and mesoderm.

A variety of studies have indicated that the following two main factors are required for neural induction: (1) that one or more stimuli be passed from the prechordal plate and chordamesoderm to the overlying ectoderm, and (2) that the ectoderm be in the proper state of responsiveness (competence) at the time the stimulus is given. The exact nature of the inducing factors and their mode of action is still unknown. The primary factors are thought to be proteins or ribonucleoproteins that act either directly on the genetic or epigenetic apparatus of the responding cells or by modifying their permeability to other effecting agents, such as ions.* The exact basis of neural competence is also unknown, but certain characteristics have been established. Ectodermal responsiveness varies quantitatively with time, being high at the beginning of gastrulation and dropping off sharply by its completion.[50] It also varies qualitatively with time. Thus, a uniform stimulus presented to competent ectoderm at different times during gastrulation will elicit qualitatively different types of neural differentiation.[4,5] The neural induction process involving any one area of ectoderm is therefore expressed as the temporal summation of all stimulus-competence interactions in that area.

The temporal nature of the induction process has been examined experimentally by separating ectoderm and mesoderm at different times during gastrulation and after neural plate formation. In all cases it has been found that interaction of prechordal plate and competent ectoderm leads to formation of prosencephalic (forebrain) structures. However, further interaction with notochordal mesoderm leads to differentiation of more caudal brain structures. The type of brain structure eventually formed appears to depend on both the length of interaction and the region of notochordal mesoderm

*See references 5, 34, 50, and 58.

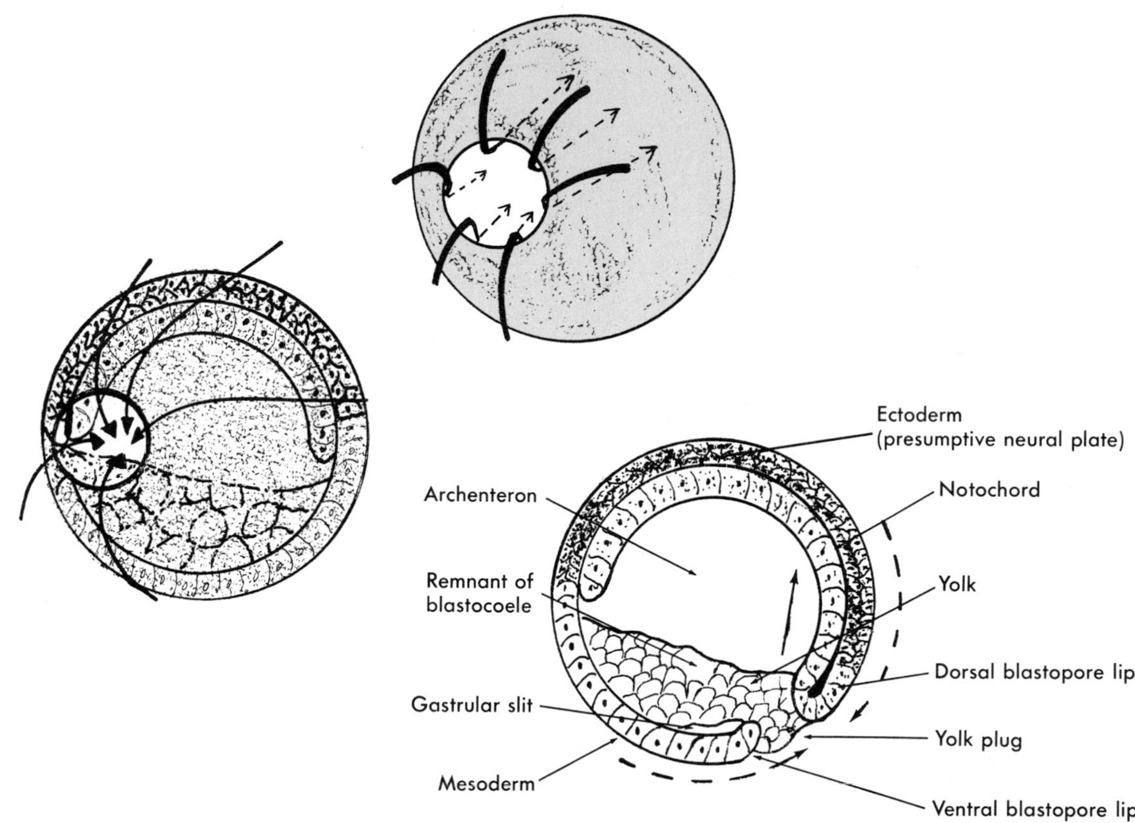

Fig. 9-1. Morphogenetic movements leading to induction in the late frog gastrula. Presumptive mesoderm cells migrate inward over the lip of the blastopore and under the ectoderm in a craniad direction.

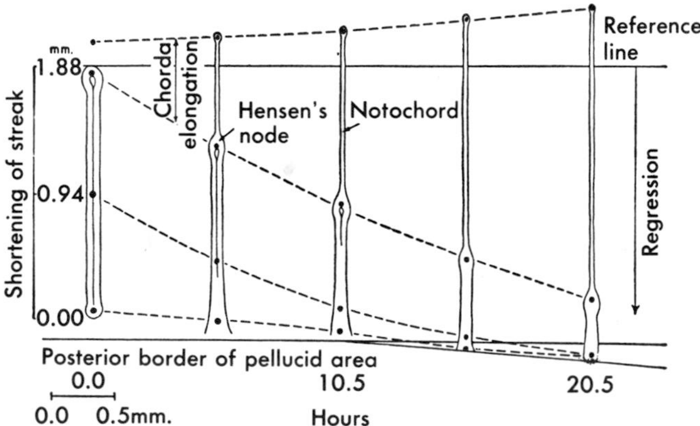

Fig. 9-2. Formation of the chorda-mesoderm during gastrulation in the chick embryo. As the primitive streak regresses, presumptive mesoderm cells invaginate at its anterior end, coming to underlie the ectoderm in a craniocaudal direction. (After Romanoff, A. L.: The avian embryo, New York, 1960, The Macmillan Co.)

involved, with successively more caudal regions of mesoderm first inducing mesencephalon (midbrain), then rhombencephalon (hindbrain), and then spinal cord and possibly muscle tissue. Thus, by the time of neural plate formation, the primary embryonic axis is formed, with forebrain, midbrain, hindbrain, and spinal cord differentiation tendencies established in the neural plate in a craniocaudal sequence.[45,48,50] Further specification and stabilization of future histotypic and organotypic patterns is brought about both by continued interaction of neuroepithelium with somite and chordamesoderm and by interaction of cells within different regions of the neuroepithelium.[37,45]

FORMATION OF THE NEURAL TUBE AND NEURAL CREST

Soon after gastrulation is completed, an elongated, flattened area, the neural plate, forms over the region of the prechordal plate and notochordal

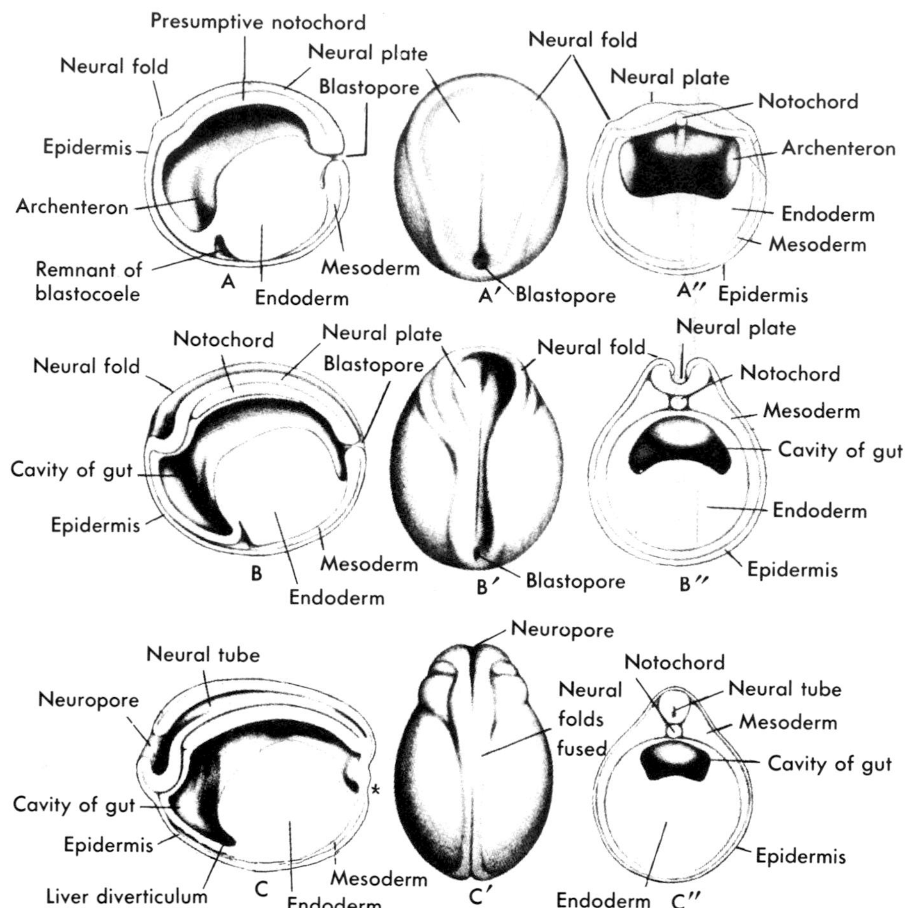

Fig. 9-3. Neurulation in the frog embryo. *A, A'*, and *A″* represent the early neural plate stage in median sagittal and top and median transverse views. *B, B'*, and *B″* and *C, C'*, and *C″* represent similar views of middle and late neurula stages. (From Balinsky, B. I.: An introduction to embryology, ed. 2, Philadelphia, 1965, W. B. Saunders Co.)

mesoderm. Its shape varies from an elongate pear in amphibians to a slipper in birds and mammals (Fig. 9-3). The cells of the neural plate proliferate, forming a pseudostratified epithelium. Formation of the neural tube from the neural plate involves a large number of morphogenetic processes: thickening, thinning, infolding, elongation, fusion, and detachment. These tissue changes in turn result from specific cellular events, such as elongation, shortening, enlargement, constriction, dissociation, cell migration, and adhesion. Ultrastructural analysis of cellular changes during neurulation in amphibians suggests correlations between cellular dynamics and subcellular function such as microtubule support (elongation), filament-dependent contraction (apical contraction), ameboid movement (cell migration), attachment devices (cell migration and fusion), and cell recognition (specific fusion, migration).[3,9,51]

Neurulation begins with the formation of a neural groove running the length of the neural plate. The groove results from the deformation of neuroepithelial cells from a columnar to a bottle shape in the median region of the plate. This change probably involves both elongation of microtubules and contraction of apical filaments, events initiated during the preceding induction period. After the neural groove is formed, neural folds arise from the lateral part of the neural plate. This appears to result from a microtubule-mediated elongation of cells in both the medial and lateral parts of the neural plate and in the mesodermal cells of the myotomes. The resulting dorsomedial components of force help to elevate the neural folds. Along with

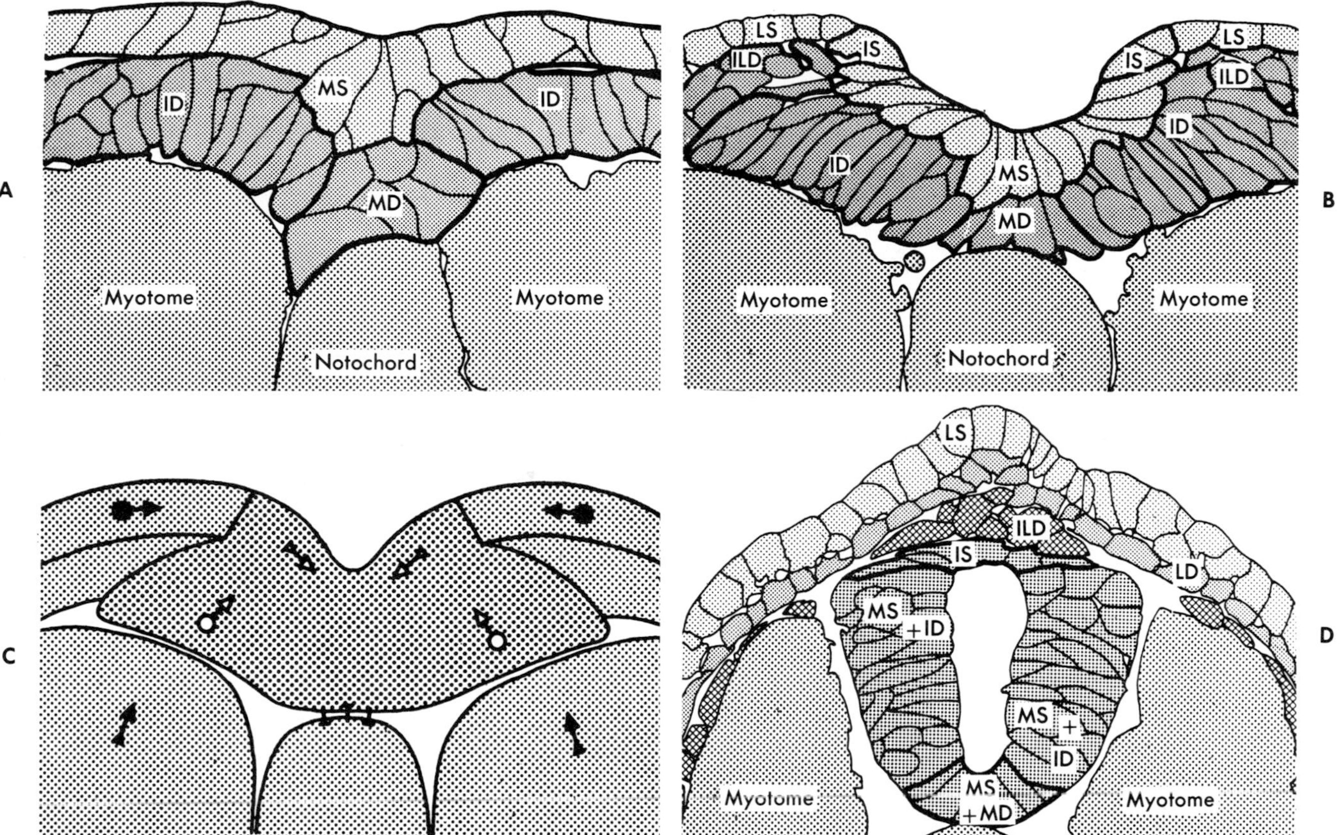

Fig. 9-4. Neurulation in *Xenopus laevis* (African clawed toad). **A,** Diagram of a transverse section through the neural plate showing its superficial and deep layers and underlying mesodermal structures. *MS,* Median superficial ectoderm; *MD* and *ID,* median and intermediate deep ectoderm, respectively. **B,** Diagram of a transverse section through the neural folds. Note the presence of bottle-shaped cells in the *MS* region where the neural groove is forming. *IS* and *LS,* Intermediate and lateral superficial ectoderm, respectively; *ILD,* intermediolateral deep ectoderm. Other abbreviations as in **A. C,** Diagram indicating the possible sources of mechanical force affecting the progress of neurulation. Intrinsic forces within the neural plate cells lead to apical contraction of the *MS* zone (empty double arrows) and cellular elongation of the *ID* zones (empty circled arrows). Extrinsic forces are provided by elongation of myotome cells (solid double arrows), medial convergence of epidermal cells (solid squared arrows), and the attachment of the notochord to the neural plate. **D,** Diagram of a transverse section through the early neural tube. The floor (*MS* and *MD*) and the roof (*IS*) of the neural tube are now definitely unilayered. The early neural crest (*ILD*) overlies the neural tube. *LD,* Lateral deep ectoderm. (After Schroeder, 1970.)

these changes, epidermal ectoderm that is lateral to the neural plate begins to migrate medially, aiding in the closure of the neural tube by pushing the neural folds together (Fig. 9-4, *A* to *C*). During this time the notochord, which is firmly attached to the neural plate, elongates and opposes any longitudinal shortening of the plate during infolding. The neural folds forming from the narrow regions of the plate fuse in an anteroposterior direction, with the most cranial and caudal folds fusing last. This results in the formation of the neural tube (Fig. 9-4, *D*).

Numerous approaches have been used to examine whether the neuroepithelium during neural tube formation already consists of germinal and differentiating cells or whether the population is still undetermined. Through the use of mitotic inhibitors, such as colchicine or vincristine sulfate, and the DNA synthesis marker, tritiated thymidine, it was found that all cells in the wall of the neural groove appeared capable of undergoing DNA synthesis and mitosis.[39,59] These cells form a pseudostratified epithelium and are connected to each other by terminal bars in the inner or juxtaluminal zone

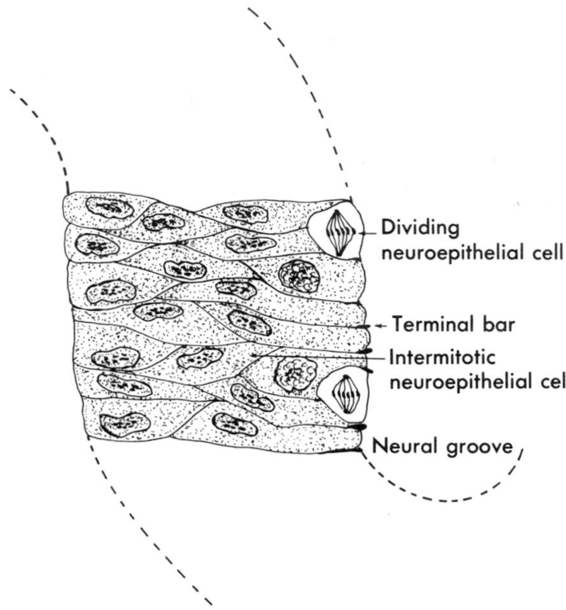

Fig. 9-5. Diagram of a transverse section through the wall of the neural groove of a chick embryo (see text). (After Langman, 1968.)

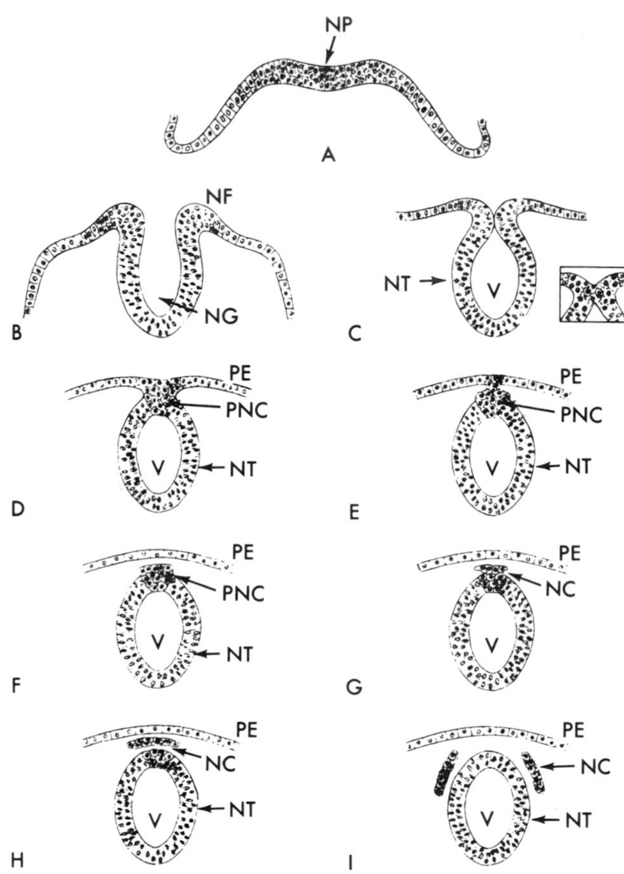

Fig. 9-6. Development of the neural tube and crest in the hindbrain of the chick embryo. The presumptive neural crest (*PNC*) is seen as a wedge-shaped mass of cells in the roof of the neural tube (*NT*) in **D, E,** and **F.** *NC,* Neural crest; *NG,* neural groove; *NF,* neural fold; *PE,* presumptive epidermis; *V,* ventricle. (After DiVirgilio and others, 1967.)

(Fig. 9-5). The interphase cells are wedge-shaped, with the nuclei located in the broader portion near the external limiting membrane. A slender cytoplasmic portion extends to the inner surface of the forming tube. It is in this state that the cells undergo DNA synthesis. Very soon after DNA synthesis has occurred, the cell nucleus moves toward the inner or luminal surface, accompanied by contraction of the cytoplasm toward the terminal bars. At the beginning of metaphase the whole cell appears to be at the inner surface, but it is actually still attached to the external limiting membrane by a slender cytoplasmic thread. After mitosis the daughter nuclei move away from the inner surface, and again the cell assumes a wedge shape. During neurulation all daughter cells remain attached by terminal bars to the inner surface, and no signs of neuronal or glial differentiation are seen.

Light microscopic studies of the fusion process in chick embryos indicate that differentiation and alteration of the cellular patterns occur soon after fusion.[14] At the area of fusion of the folds there is a loss of the radially arranged pattern of cells seen in the rest of the tube. The cells in this region then enter a very active mitotic period. Eventually a wedge-shaped mass of cells is seen to extend dorsally and become continuous with the superficial ectoderm, with the base against the ectoderm and the apex extending ventrally into the fused neural folds. The superficial ectoderm then separates from the neural tube, and soon the cells in the upper part of the wedge separate from the tube. These cells form the neural crest (Fig. 9-6).

MITOTIC BEHAVIOR AND STRUCTURE OF THE EARLY NEURAL TUBE

Soon after the fusion of the neural folds, certain structural changes occur in the wall of the neural tube, other than those resulting in formation of the neural crest. Initially the wall of the neural tube consists of a *ventricular zone* (also called the matrix, or medulloepithelial, layer), the original pseudo-

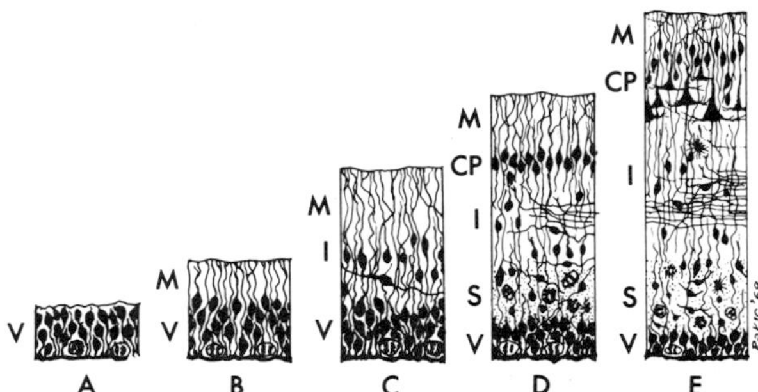

Fig. 9-7. Diagram of five stages in the development of the CNS (see text). *CP*, Cortical plate; *I*, intermediate zone; *M*, marginal zone; *S*, subventricular zone; *V*, ventricular zone. (From The Boulder Committee: Embryonic vertebrate central nervous system: revised terminology, Anat. Rec. **166**:257, 1970.)

stratified columnar neuroepithelium of the neural plate and folds (Fig. 9-7, *A*). These cells demonstrate the same mitotic behavior as that described for the cells in the neural folds.* A new region, the *marginal zone,* soon appears as a cell-sparse layer composed of the outermost cytoplasmic parts of the ventricular cells (Fig. 9-7, *B*). Nuclei of ventricular cells are not seen to enter this cytoplasmic zone. Examination of the basal region of the neural tube wall at this time reveals a new layer of cells forming between the ventricular and marginal zones; this layer has been designated as the *intermediate zone* (Fig. 9-7, *C*). These cells are characterized by a large round nucleus with pale nucleoplasm and a highly basophilic nucleous. They are no longer connected by terminal bars to the other ventricular cells. In addition they are different from the ventricular cells in that they are postmitotic cells, no longer showing incorporation of tritiated thymidine. The manner in which these cells are released from the ventricular surface is unknown, but it has been suggested that they represent daughter cells formed from a dividing cell whose mitotic spindle is perpendicular to the ventricular surface. Such mitotic figures have been seen, and a daughter cell formed from a division in that plane would not be in a position to form terminal bars. Thus, it would be free to migrate away from the ventricular surface.[38]

These changes in the basal region of the neural tube are accompanied by a decrease in the number of proliferating cells as compared with the alar region. This would appear to be a manifestation of the pattern first established during neural induction. For example, in the spinal cord somatic motor neuroblasts are primarily derived from cells of the intermediate zone of the basal region, with the initial stimulus for their formation coming from notochordal mesoderm. Somatic sensory neurons, on the other hand, are formed by cells of the intermediate zone of the alar region, which are derived from neuroepithelium stimulated by lateral mesoderm. Localization of sensory and motor differentiation tendencies is, in fact, already established in the appropriate areas of the neural plate long before overt differentiation occurs. This has been demonstrated in amphibians by explanting various areas of the neural plate and comparing the morphology and function of the differentiated explant with the area of defect in the operated embryo after brain differentiation.[12]

The translation of two-dimensional patterns laid down in the neural plate into the three-dimensional patterns of the neural tube requires localized migration and differentiation. This process is aided by the terminal bar type of attachment present at the ventricular surface. The basic radial arrangement of cells in the ventricular wall is due in great part to the forces created by the terminal bars. This primary radial structure imposes a secondary radial orientation upon neuroblasts during their migration to the intermediate zone and beyond. This ultimately influences the direction the axons of primary motor neurons take during their penetration of the neural tube wall. Since cell migration is not randomly oriented, cells of a given type remain close together, facilitating their eventual aggregation into columns and nuclei. Also, since terminal bars prevent all but released cells from changing position, stimuli from localized interactions within the ventricular zone or from outside the neural tube are capable of acting on specific groups of cells for long periods of time.[59]

Localized increases in mitotic activity seem to precede all localized migrations and changes in the structure of the neural tube. Differences in the mitotic activity of cells in the alar and basal regions in the early neural tube appear to be partially due to mitotic inhibition by the notochord and mitotic stimulation by the somites. However, as the neural tube grows in thickness, these influences on the mitotic behavior of the ventricular cells most likely decrease. Other possible controlling factors, such as changes in the CSF or production of growth regulators by postmitotic migrating and differentiating cells, then must be considered.

After the initial wave of cell migration that re-

*See references 1, 7, 21, 38, 39, and 59.

sults in the formation of the intermediate zone, secondary rearrangement of cells occurs within this zone. In some regions, such as the anterior horn (somatic motor column) of the spinal cord, the intermediate zone remains relatively simple; however, in the cerebrum and cerebellum cell bodies migrate or are displaced outward through it. This initially results in the formation of a *cortical plate* between the marginal and intermediate zones (Fig. 9-7, *D*). In the cerebrum, neurons derived from the cortical plate will form the deepest layer of the complex laminated cortex. Each more superficial layer is formed by a series of sequential cell migrations passing through the newly formed deeper layers. During the period of cortical plate formation, afferent axons from sensory neurons outside the neural tube enter the intermediate zone of the spinal cord, as do efferent axons from differentiating cortical plate neurons.*

In addition to the ventricular zone, secondary regions of proliferation develop in mammalian embryos in the latter third of gestation. This occurs somewhat earlier in lower vertebrates[1,7,38] Initially a layer of cells forms at the junction of the ventricular and intermediate zones; this new layer is called the *subventricular zone* (Fig. 9-7, *D* and *E*). It is composed of small round or oval cells that do not exhibit the interkinetic nuclear movements seen in ventricular cells. In the cerebrum this zone becomes quite prominent, with maximum proliferation and outward migratory activity reached after birth. In the cerebellum the subventricular zone expands to form the rhombic lip at the lateral margins of the fourth ventricle (Fig. 9-8). Cells in this region form a secondary proliferative zone, the *external granular layer,* which eventually is found in a subpial position over the surface of the cerebellar cortex. In mammals proliferation in this region begins at the time of birth, but it starts considerably earlier in lower vertebrates and is followed by cell migration into the deeper regions of the cortex.

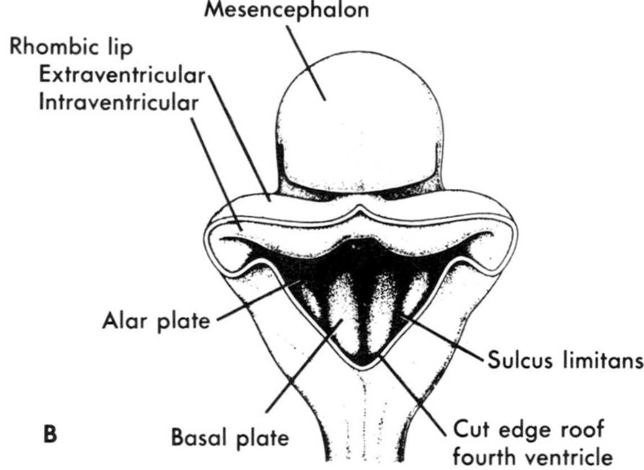

Fig. 9-8. Diagram showing a dorsal view of the early development of the rhombic lip and fourth ventricle in the human embryo. **A,** Six weeks after gestation; **B,** eight weeks after gestation. (From Langman, J. In Bourne, G. H., editor: The structure and function of nervous tissue, vol. I, New York, 1968, Academic Press, Inc.)

While the changes in cell proliferation and migration just described are occurring within the wall of the neural tube, the total structure of the neural tube is undergoing extensive changes. Soon after its formation, three segments develop in the future brain region. These segments appear as expansions related to the three vesicles that are the cavities that define the forebrain, midbrain, and hindbrain (Fig. 9-9). The forebrain becomes the *telencephalon* and *diencephalon,* the midbrain (*mesencephalon*) continues undivided, and the hindbrain becomes the *metencephalon* (pons and cerebellum) and *myelencephalon* (medulla). These divisions become more prominent with the development of flexures, or bends, in the neural tube. The flexures are produced by unequal growth of the nervous tissue and the marginal tissue attached to it. The *cervical flexure* produces a posterior convexity between the spinal cord and medulla. This is temporary and gradually disappears. The *cephalic flexure* occurs at the midbrain and turns the forebrain anteriorly and downward. The *pontine flexure* forms at the junction of the metencephalon and myelencephalon and eventually produces the belly of the pons (Fig. 9-9). The terminal

*See references 1, 7, 21, and 38.

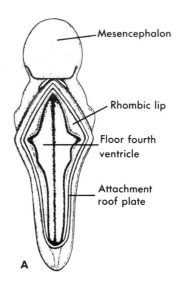

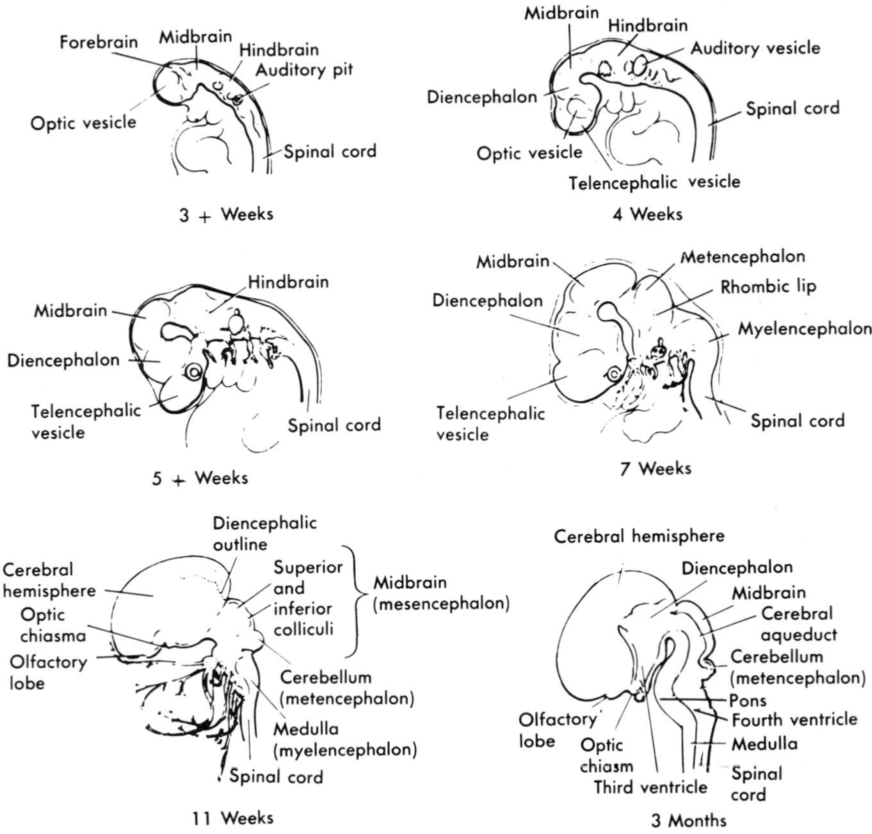

Fig. 9-9. Morphologic changes in the neural tube of early human embryo (see text). Side views in Fig. 7-5 are continuation to adult.

part of the forebrain becomes the inconspicuous *telencephalon medium,* and the paired cerebral hemispheres expand around it in all directions. The hemispheres separate into the *basal nuclei* (ganglia), which are composed of a medial and ventral nuclear mass, and a thin-walled surface mantle, or *pallium* (cortex). The olfactory cortex, which is represented in man as the *archipallium* and *paleopallium,* evolved earlier than the non-olfactory cortical mass, the *neopallium.* The olfactory cortical fields in each hemisphere are primarily connected by the *anterior commissure* and are composed of bundles of association fibers. The neopallium in man overgrows the rest of the brain and connects through the *corpus callosum* (Fig. 9-10). Optic vesicles and stalks, as well as auditory vesicles, arise as diverticula of the forebrain in very early embryos. The olfactory apparatus is relatively poorly preserved in man as a retention of olfactory lobe equivalents.

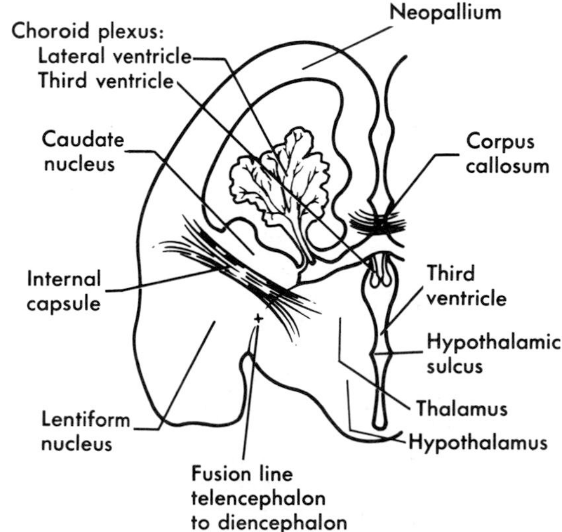

Fig. 9-10. Diagram of a frontal section through the telencephalon and diencephalon of a developing human brain.

The *diencephalon* develops as greatly thickened walls of the forebrain vesicle. Diverticula occur ventrally in the wall of the neural tube, forming the *infundibulum* and *posterior pituitary* gland, and dorsally, forming the *pineal body*. The diencephalon (thalamus) forms medial to the internal capsule and eventually is covered by pallium. The thalamus subdivides early into the *thalamus proper* and the *hypothalamus* (Fig. 9-10).

The *mesencephalon,* or midbrain, represents the most anterior segment subject to inductive action of the notochordal mesoderm. The midbrain remains a stalk-like conduit for tracts, primarily but also houses several important nuclei, including those of cranial nerves III and IV, and the tectum. In reptiles, birds, and mammals four swellings, the *corpora quadrigemina,* arise in the tectum (two in fish and amphibians) and are inordinately large in fetal life. They probably represent the highest centers of hearing and vision in many lower forms.

The *metencephalon* develops from masses of migrating cells that undergo further mitotic division within the external granular layer of the growing cerebellum. The pons includes the extending fibers to and from the midbrain and medulla, in addition to masses of cells that connect to the cerebellum after crossing. The pons is most highly developed in man. The cerebellum establishes a basic unit (afferents to cortex, and efferents from cortex to central cerebellar nuclei and thence to midbrain via brachium conjunctivum), which is compiled in varying complexity upon initial connections (primarily vestibular).[43] The *myelencephalon* is oriented around the rhomboid fossa, as is the metencephalon, and contains the inferior olive, an extremely conspicuous nucleus in man. This interrelates the basal nuclei and cerebellum in a manner similar to the linking of the cerebral cortex to the cerebellum by the pons. The distribution of nuclei in the hindbrain (and midbrain) occurs in relationship to the delineation of embryonic "plates," which is best defined in conjunction with the spinal cord.

The embryogenesis of the spinal cord is oriented around the formation of six plates. This pattern probably extends cranially only to the level of the midbrain (Fig. 9-11). A *roof plate* and a *floor plate* interconnect the two bulkier, lateral masses of the neural tube. The lateral masses are subdivided by the *sulcus limitans* into *alar* and *basal plates.* The afferent, or sensory, nuclei form within the alar plate; the efferent, or motor, nuclei arise within the basal plate. The general patterns in these nuclear groups at various levels are illustrated in Fig. 9-11. Since extending fibers conveying afferent impulses farther into the CNS arise in the alar plate, this component is the parent substance of much of the central structure (probably ninety percent).[15]

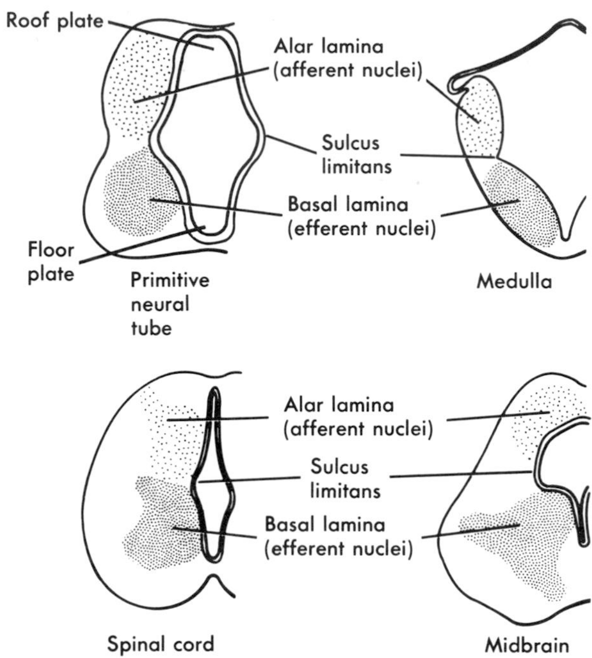

Fig. 9-11. Diagram showing the early development of the alar and basal laminae in the neural tube.

During morphogenesis of the neural tube wall, the ventricle formed by the fusion of the neural folds is also changing. In the developing forebrain the neural tube splits into two lateral ventricles within the cerebral hemispheres and forms a third ventricle in the diencephalon. These ventricles are interconnected by *interventricular foramina.* A fourth ventricle forms between the developing cerebellum and medulla oblongata. Anteriorly it is connected to the third ventricle by the *cerebral aqueduct* (aqueduct of Sylvius), which runs through the midbrain, and posteriorly it is continuous with the *central canal.* The central canal runs through the lower part of the medulla oblongata and throughout the length of the spinal cord (Fig. 9-12). All ventricles contain CSF secreted by a *choroid plexus* within each one. Each choroid plexus develops as blood vessels that invaginate both the overlying leptomeningeal membrane and the layer of primitive ependymal cells lining the vesicles. The complex of capillaries and

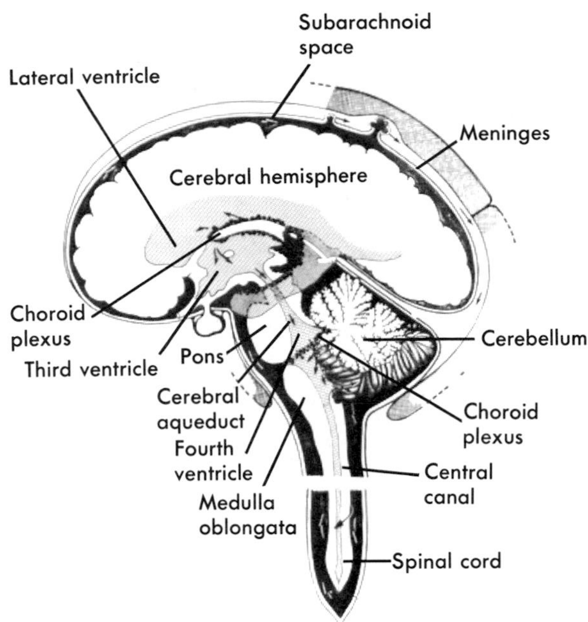

Fig. 9-12. Diagram showing the ventricular system and choroid plexus in the human brain.

ependyma becomes a highly folded membrane that bulges into the ventricular cavity. The plexus appears first in the fourth ventricle, next the third ventricle, and finally in the paired lateral ventricles, sites where there is intense proliferation of subventricular cells. The choroidal cells produce a rich protein fluid and are probably nutritive in function during the embryonic period.[35] In the human embryo the choroid attains its general adult makeup by the third month and retains the embryonic secretory features up to the seventh or eighth month. After this, the epithelium assumes the more cuboidal characteristics of the adult plexus. During the third month several holes, the lateral and median apertures, develop in the choroid plexus covering the fourth ventricle. This results in expulsion of the CSF into the primitive leptomeninges, which produces the subarachnoid space and establishes the adult pattern of production and absorption of CSF.

As previously mentioned, the developing brain is surrounded by a series of membranes, the *meninges.* They develop in the tissues formed between bone and the neural tube. The mesoderm nearest bone condenses into the *pachymeninx,* or *dura mater,* and that nearest the neural tissue forms the *leptomeninges,* or *arachnoid membrane* and the *pia mater.* Neural crest cells also contribute to the formation of these membranes. The meninges function as protective coverings, as support for the blood vessels that supply the brain and spinal cord, and as a medium for circulation of extraventricular CSF.

FORMATION OF THE PERIPHERAL NERVOUS SYSTEM

Two main elements contribute to the formation of the peripheral nervous system—the neural crest and the epidermal placodes. As indicated earlier, the neural crest is composed of cells derived from the lateral part of the neural plate. Soon after their formation, neural crest component cells begin to migrate from the dorsal part of the tube. By marking these cells during their formation with a suitable substance, such as tritiated thymidine, the progress of their migration can be followed to their ultimate destination. Other methods, such as removing regions of the neural folds before crest migration and placing them in either a neutral or nonneutral environment, allow determination of both potential and actual pathways for crest differentiation. This is revealed through examination of both the explant and donor embryos after further development. Using these methods on amphibian and avian embryos, it has been determined that trunk neural crest cells initially migrate in two streams. Cells in the dorsolateral stream come to lie mainly in the germative layer of the ectoderm and differentiate into *pigment cells.* A ventral stream of cells moves into the mesenchyme between the neural tube and the myotome. This stream becomes segmented into two groups, cells between somites and cells within the somites. The latter seem to migrate further ventrally (to the dorsal aorta). Except during segmentation, the initial direction of migration appears to be influenced by the neural tube, not by the mesenchyme. The ventrad stream gives rise to neurons and supportive cells in the *spinal sensory* and *sympathetic ganglia, chromaffin* cells in the adrenal medulla, *paraganglia, pigment* cells, some parts of the *meninges,* and some *Schwann* cells.[28,61] The migration of cranial neural crest cells (derived from posterior forebrain, midbrain, and hindbrain) is similar to that of the cells of the trunk crest. A small proportion of the cells migrate dorsolaterally to form *pigment* cells. The majority of cells migrate ventrad into the head mesenchyme. Some of these cells combine with the ectodermal placodes to form *sensory ganglia* of the head. These include the *root ganglia* of the facial (VII), glos-

Table 9-1. Summary of normal neural crest fates*

Nervous system				
Pigment cells	**Sensory tissue**	**Tissue of Autonomic system**	**Skeletal and connective tissue**	**Supportive tissue**
Trunk crest (including cervical crest)				
1. Melanophores 2. Xanthophores (erythrophores) 3. Iridophores (guanophores) in dermis, epidermis, and epidermal derivatives	1. Spinal ganglia 2. Some contribution to vagal (X) root ganglia	1. Sympathetic Superior cervical ganglion Prevertebral ganglia Paravertebral ganglia Adrenal medulla 2. Parasympathetic Remak's ganglion Pelvic plexus Visceral and enteric ganglia	1. Mesenchyme of dorsal fin in Amphibia	1. Some supportive cells Neuroglia (oligodendroglia) Schwann sheath cells Some contribution to meninges
Cranial crest				
1. Small, belated contribution	1. Trigeminal (V)† 2. Facial (VII) root 3. Glossopharyngeal (IX) root (superior ganglia) 4. Vagal (X) root (jugular ganglia)	1. Parasympathetic ganglia Ciliary Ethmoidal Sphenopalatine Submandibular Intrinsic ganglia of viscera	1. Visceral cartilages (except basibranchial 2) 2. Trabeculae cranii (anterior) 3. Contributes cells to posterior trabecula, basal plate, parachordal cartilages 4. Odontoblasts 5. Head mesenchyme (membrane bones)	1. Supportive cells†

*After Weston, J. A.: The migration and differentiation of neural crest cells, Adv. Morph. **8**:41, 1970.
†Also receives contribution from placodes in lateral ectoderm. Trunk ganglia of nerves VII, IX, and X derived from ectodermal epibranchial placodes. Some supporting cells of these ganglia presumably also derived from placodal ectoderm.

sopharyngeal (IX), and vagal (X) nerves. In addition, ectodermal placodes give rise to the *trunk ganglia* of the facial, glossopharyngeal, and vagal nerves, and contribute to organs of special sense (olfactory neuroepithelium, lens of the eye, and auditory vesicle). The cranial crest also contributes to the formation of the *parasympathetic ganglia* and much of the *visceral skeleton* of the head.[33,61] The derivatives of the cranial and trunk crests are summarized in Table 9-1.

HISTOGENESIS OF THE NERVOUS SYSTEM

The cells comprising nervous tissue can be grouped into the following four broad categories: *macroneurons, microneurons, neuroglia,* and *microglia.* All but the last originate in the proliferative zones of the neural tube or neural crest. Macroneurons are long-axoned nerve cells making up the afferent, relay, commissural, and efferent elements of the CNS and peripheral nervous system. Microneurons are moderately long-axoned, short-axoned, or anaxonic interneurons of the CNS. They are thought to function as integrating and modulatory cells in association with macroneurons. Their role in specific afferent-efferent pathways, unlike that of macroneurons, is apparently unspecified until quite late in development or after birth. This imparts a great deal of plasticity in the imprinting of neural circuits. Neuroglia are the supporting elements of nervous tissue. Glial elements of the CNS are composed of oligodendrocytes, astrocytes, and ependymal cells. In the peripheral nervous system glia equivalents are composed of Schwann cells, satellite cells, and capsule cells. In addition to their supportive function, some glial cells (Schwann cells and oligodendrocytes) form the myelin that insulates axons, and

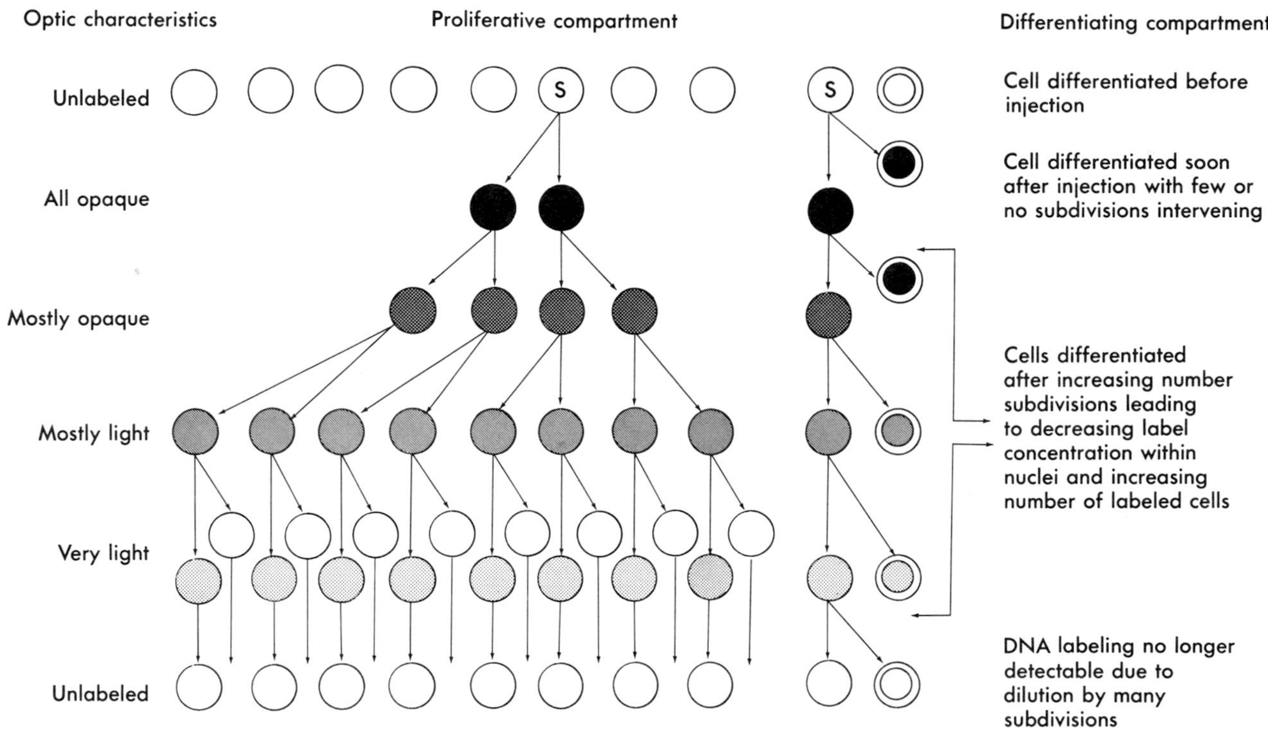

Fig. 9-13. Diagram of expected labeling characteristics of cells passing from the proliferative phase to the differentiative phase, after exposure to H^3 thymidine. (After Altman, 1969.)

all probably play an important role is establishing the necessary environment for sustained normal neural functions. Microglia are of mesenchymal origin and act as phagocytes under pathologic conditions.

Accurate determination of the cell cycle, time and area of origin, and migration pathways of neurons and glia has been made possible through the use of tritiated thymidine in cell marking. If the DNA of a dividing population is labeled with tritiated thymidine during a short pulse, those cells that cease dividing soon afterward will remain heavily labeled. Further cell division results in progressive dilution of the label in DNA, observed in an autoradiogram as a decrease in the number of silver grains over the nucleus. Thus, unlabeled cells are those that cease dividing before addition of the tritiated thymidine or those that continue to replicate until the label is no longer detectable (Fig. 9-13). Mammals are especially suited to this type of study, as unincorporated thymidine is catabolized by the liver within about thirty minutes after injection. Chick embryos, on the other hand, do not break down thymidine very quickly, so it is necessary to remove and then transplant the region to be pulse-labeled.[1,61]

Evaluation of nuclear labeling patterns during histogenesis indicates that only cells that appear undifferentiated replicate. These cells are found primarily in the ventricular zone, subventricular zone, and external granule cell layer. Some migrating, presumptive glial cells also continue to replicate. Overtly differentiated cells are never seen to incorporate tritiated thymidine, but the exact relationship between DNA synthesis, with accompanying replication, and early differentiation is unknown. Studies with a variety of other cell types, such as cartilage cells, suggest that a special type of DNA synthesis is a prerequisite for differentiation and may, in some cases, occur simultaneously with early synthesis of cell-specific products.[40]

The first cells to migrate away from the ventricular zone differentiate as macroneurons. As described earlier, in the spinal cord these cells are represented by efferent motor and afferent sensory neurons, which are generally derived from the basal and alar plates, respectively. This pattern is also repeated in the hindbrain. In the cerebellum the macroneurons are represented by Purkinje cells, Golgi cells, and neurons of the deep cerebellar nuclei. In the cerebrum macroneurons include the mitral cells of the olfactory bulb and the pyramidal cells of the hippocampus. In the peripheral nervous system, both sensory and autonomic neurons are included in this group.[1,2,61]

All microneurons except those of the spinal cord are probably derived from the subventricular zone or the external granule cell layer. In the spinal cord microneurons begin to differentiate from the ventricular zone.[7] Since the secondary germinal regions are not formed in mammals until birth, all microneurons of the brain are derived postnatally. Microneurons are not found in the peripheral nervous system.

The following three types of microneurons have been identified: (1) anaxonic neurons, such as some of the granule cells of the olfactory bulb and amacrine cells of the neural retina; (2) unmyelenated, short-axoned neurons, such as Golgi type II cells or stellate cells found in such regions as the neocortex; and (3) unmyelinated, long-axoned neurons, such as the granule cells of the cerebellar cortex and hippocampal dentate gyrus.[2]

Neuroglial cells of the CNS, with the exception of ependymal cells, are derived almost exclusively from the subventricular zone; a small number also come from the external granule cell layer.[1] Ependymal cells differentiate from the ventricular zone after all cell migration from it ceases. Thus, as with microneurons, gliogenesis in the mammalian spinal cord begins prenatally but is postnatal in all regions of the brain. Most glial cells in the peripheral nervous system are derived from neural crest cells, with some contribution of Schwann cells from the ventral neural tube.[61] The overall scheme of histogenesis is presented in Fig. 9-14.

Closer examination of histogenesis within the different classes of neurons in the CNS indicates that the migration and differentiation of different types of neurons within those classes are staggered in time. For example, in the spinal cord motor neurons begin to differentiate sooner than sensory neurons; in the mammalian cerebellar cortex basket cells are almost all differentiating by the time stellate and granule cells begin to differentiate.* In the peripheral nervous system this phenomenon is not evident, since cell migration to all derivatives occurs continually over a long period of time.

Are the factors that determine the time of migration, final destination, and differentiated state of all

*See references 1, 7, 38, and 59.

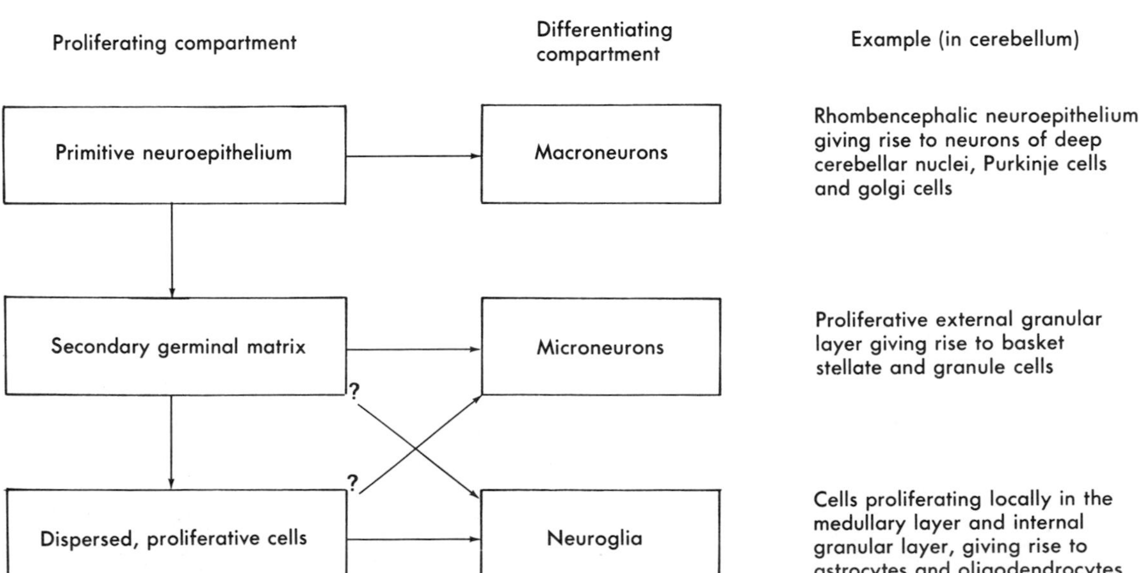

Fig. 9-14. Diagram showing the relationship of the three proliferative pools of the developing nervous system and the general classes of cells arising from them. (From Altman, J.: DNA metabolism and cell proliferation. In Lajtha, A., editor: Handbook of neurochemistry, vol. II, New York, 1969, Plenum Publishing Corporation.)

neural cells present within the cells prior to their migration, or do other interactions occurring during cell migration direct their fate? As discussed in an earlier section, the inductive process imparts both a regional and a functional pattern to the various areas of the neural plate. These factors would impart a special mosaic pattern in three dimensions within the neural tube. This would suggest that: (1) the fates of all the cells were predetermined so that subsequent division would result in the formation of clones of, say, pyramidal and Purkinje cells; (2) none of the germinal cell fates was predetermined; or (3) a combination of the two. Since no study has ever determined the regional and functional potentials of individual ventricular cells, it is difficult to choose between these possibilities. The very early differentiation of sensory and motor neurons in specific regions of the spinal cord suggests that predetermined clonal populations may be formed for these cells. In the neural crest, on the other hand, only general crest potentialities appear to be specified. Further differentiation appears to be influenced by interactions occurring during migration of these cells. Various studies indicate that the length of time a cell is in the neural crest before it migrates does not limit how it can differentiate.[61] This may also be true of the secondary germinal areas. However, until cell cloning techniques are utilized to study these problems, it will not be possible to define with any certainty either the state of individual germinal cells at any one time or the conditions that would promote a stable phenotype in the original germinal cell or its progeny.

CYTOGENESIS OF THE NERVOUS SYSTEM

Differentiation of any cell involves the attainment of those morphologic, chemical, and behavioral characteristics typical of its normal adult state. Since the attainment of these properties may occur at different rates and be interdependent, a proper description of the differentiation of neurons and glia should include mention of all of them.

Morphologic differentiation of nervous tissue, especially of neurons, has been investigated extensively in recent years with the aid of the electron microscope in an attempt to refine earlier light microscope studies.* *Neuroblasts* of the CNS and the peripheral nervous system progress from an apolar to a bipolar stage during their migration to the intermediate zone or prospective neural crest derivative (Figs. 9-15 and 9-16). These cells possess an ovoid nucleus containing dense nucleoplasm and a large nucleolus. Rough endoplasmic reticulum (RER) is well developed in the perinuclear cytoplasm, but Nissl complexes are missing. There are many mitochondria and free ribosomes, one or two Golgi complexes, and fine filaments and microtubules in the cytoplasm as well. One of the first changes seen in developing motor neurons of the spinal cord, for example, is the loss of physical connection with the luminal surface and formation of an *axon*. The axon contains filaments, microtubules, some mitochondria, small, smooth-surfaced vesicles, and a few free ribosomes (not seen in most mature axons). This description also holds for axons of other CNS and peripheral nervous system neurons. As development proceeds the cell body enlarges, and the nucleus becomes rounder. The nucleoplasm decreases in electron density, and the nucleolus becomes more prominent. This is accompanied by an increase in RER, the size of the Golgi complex, and the number of filaments and tubules. In many types of neurons there is an outgrowth of *dendrites,* which contain many filaments and most of the organelles found in the cytoplasm. Histochemically these changes are seen as an increase in cytoplasmic and nucleolar basophilia, and the appearance of an affinity for certain silver stains by filaments and microtubules. Later development of neurons is accompanied by organization of RER into parallel arrays called Nissl bodies. Free ribosomes form small clusters, often in a rosette pattern. There is further development of the axon and dendrites both in length and in number of branches. A number of separate Golgi complexes are now seen scattered throughout the cytoplasm and in the dendrites. The nucleus often becomes quite round and contains a very prominent nucleolus. Lysosomes also appear and increase in number, and in older, mature neurons lipofuscin pigment granules are seen.

Neurons communicate with each other through contacts, or synapses, involving their processes. The afferent process or axon, carries information away from a cell body and may communicate with other dendrites, cell bodies, or possibly axons. During the growth of an axon, its course and the contacts it makes play an essential role in the determination of specific neuronal circuits. Factors involved in the growth of axons have been studied both in vivo and in nerve cell culture (see Chapter 11). The axon begins as a *growth cone,* or conical thickening of protoplasm, that spreads out away from the

*See references 6, 13, 20, 22, 23, 43, 44, 46, 53, 55, 56, 57, and 60.

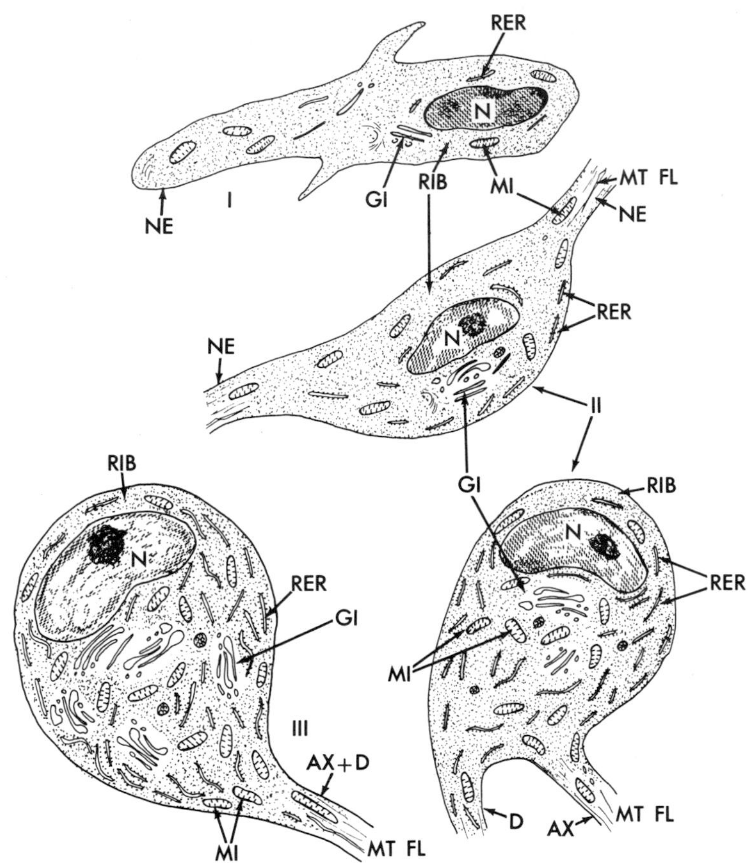

Fig. 9-15. Diagram illustrating the differentiation of dorsal root neuroblast from an embryonic rabbit. **I,** Migrating neuroblast with a single developing neurite (*NE*); **II,** transformation of a bipolar neuroblast from a spindle shape to a bell shape. In this latter stage, the ultrastructures of the two neurites differ with one resembling a dendrite (*D*), and the other an axon (*AX*). **III,** An immature neuron. The single process resulting from the fusion of the two neurites eventually comes to resemble an axon. *RER,* Rough endoplasmic reticulum; *G,* Golgi apparatus; *MI,* mitochondria; *MT FL,* microtubules and filaments; *RIB,* free ribosomes. (After Tennyson, 1965.)

cell body into prickly flanges or lamellar appendages.[8,13,56] At the ultrastructural level, the growth cone is seen to begin as a local accumulation of vesicles near the cell membrane of the neuroblast body, and it develops as a short, thick process containing many vesicles. As the process elongates, mitochondria, filaments, and microtubules begin to extend into it. The tip of the process is a swollen bulb that contains predominately membranous structures in the form of a loose reticulum, some mitochondria, and dense bodies.[8,56] Fine processes containing fine fibrillar material also extend from the main part of the growth cone. The initial outgrowth of the *neurite* (axon and growth cone) does not appear to require new protein synthesis but is dependent upon the assembly of microtubules or filaments from preformed protein subunits. This conclusion is based on experiments indicating that cycloheximide, a protein synthesis inhibitor, does not block neurite formation. On the other hand, treatment with colchicine or vinblastine sulfate leads to microtubule dissolution or precipitation, completely blocking their formation.[52] Continued growth of the newly formed neurite occurs at the growth cone by accretion of new surface materials.[8] These materials apparently are transported by axoplasmic flow to the point of assembly. This is inferred from experiments in which it has been shown that in mature neurons incubated with labeled colchicine, the colchicine will bind to microtubular protein in the cell body and be transported down the axon.[24] Since the growth cone membranes and

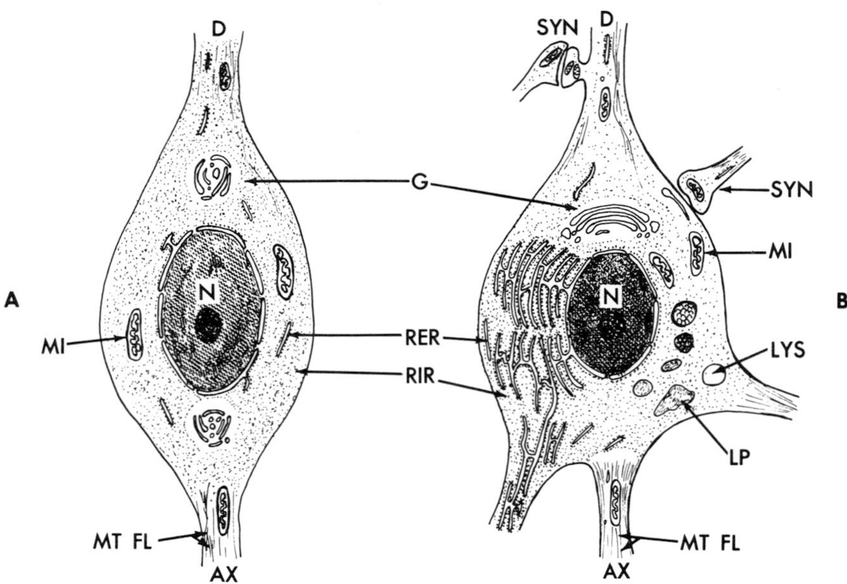

Fig. 9-16. A, Diagram of a bipolar neuroblast, and **B,** a mature multipolar neuron. *AX,* Axon; *D,* dendrite; *RER,* rough endoplasmic reticulum; *G,* Golgi apparatus; *LP,* lipofuscin granule; *LYS,* lysosome; *MI,* mitochondrion; *MT FL,* microtubules and filaments; RIB, free ribosomes; SYN, synapse. (After Wechsler and Meller, 1967.)

components are constantly being renewed, this might provide an extremely sensitive and dynamic mechanism for contact guidance through the environment. While neurite formation and initial elongation is independent of new protein synthesis, it is quite probable that extended growth of axons requires synthesis of new component proteins.

The initial direction of axon outgrowth appears to be determined to a great extent by the primary axis orientation of the migrating neuroblast. This is determined either by the orientation of the cells in the ventricular zone or by secondary clues, such as substrate affinity.[16,59] However, the factors that initially determine the point on a membrane at which a growth cone forms are still unknown.

The first sign of junctional interaction or synapsis between two neurons is the increase in thickness of both cell membranes at the point of contact. Soon afterward vesicles begin to appear near the membrane on the presynaptic or axonal side. Mitochondria also appear somewhat distal to the vesicles. An axodendritic and an axosomatic synapsis are illustrated in Fig. 9-16.

Morphologic studies of the early phases of glial cell differentiation indicate that there is very little difference between a glioblast and a neuroblast. The glioblast nucleus is somewhat more irregular, its nucleus and cytoplasm have a greater electron density, and there appear to be fewer ribosomes and endoplasmic reticulum profiles in its cytoplasm.[60] As differentiation proceeds the early astrocyte can be identified by its round nucleus of medium electron density, processes of low density that penetrate the *neuropil* (region of extreme neuronal fiber density), coming into close relation with neurons and blood vessels, and cytoplasmic fibrils and dense glycogen granules. Each oligodendrocyte possesses a nucleus in an eccentric position that contains regions of condensed chromatin and nucleoplasm of high density and a cytoplasm containing many ribosomes, few filaments, and well-developed RER. Ependymal cells differentiate from those ventricular cells remaining after potential neuroblasts and glioblasts have migrated. The first sign of differentiation is the appearance and proliferation of microvilli and cilia at the luminal surface from the apical process of the ventricular cell. This is accompanied by a shift of the Golgi apparatus to the cellular apex, where it enlarges. An increase in the number of mitochondria, smooth cytoplasmic vesicles, tubules, and pinocytotic vesicles is also seen. Both rough and smooth endoplasmic reticulum is seen in the apical process. The basal process differentiates much more slowly. It grows out and eventually makes contact with other glial cells, neurons, and subventricular blood vessels.[57,60]

The structural changes seen in neurons and glia, such as an increase in RER or an enlargement and multiplication of the Golgi complex, are usually a reflection of increased synthetic activity. For example, several examinations of the appearance of brain-specific antigens and protein (S-100) during differentiation have been made.[18,19] It was found that the antigens and protein accumulate in a fashion that parallels the increase in neuronal and glial differentiation. The beginning of accumulation also coincided with an increase in the enzyme glucose-6-phosphate dehydrogenase, which is important in providing ribose, through the pentose cycle, for RNA synthesis.[10] Synthesis of new RNA species at this time has in fact been demonstrated, using the technique of DNA-RNA hybridization.[32] When this new RNA is isolated and included in a cell-free protein synthesis system, it promotes the synthesis of an antigen immunologically identical to S-100 protein.[18] A similar differentiation of a biochemical pathway has been demonstrated in sympathetic neurons for catecholamine synthesis.[17,30]

Differentiation of physiologic[25,47,54] and behavioral[25,26,49] patterns also parallels morphologic and biochemical specialization. However, the limited scope of this chapter does not permit their discussions.*

*For discussion of the role of growth factors and hormones in neurogenesis see references 27 and 41, and for discussion of the involvement of peripheral and central connections see references 29, 31, and 36.

REFERENCES

1. Altman, J.: DNA metabolism and cell proliferation. In Lajtha, A., editor: Handbook of neurochemistry, vol. II, New York, 1969, Plenum Publishing Corporation.
2. Altman, J., Postnatal growth and differentiation of the mammalian brain, with implications for a morphological theory of memory. In Quarton, G. C., and others, editor: The neurosciences, New York, 1967, The Rockefeller University Press.
3. Baker, P. C., and Schroeder, T. E.: Cytoplasmic filaments and morphogenetic movements in the amphibian neural tube, Develop. Biol. **15**:432, 1967.
4. Barth, L. G., and Barth, L. J.: Competence and sequential induction in presumptive epidermis of normal and hybrid frog gastrulae, Physiol. Zool. **40**:97, 1967.
5. Barth, L. G., and Barth, L. J.: The role of sodium chloride in the process of induction by lithium chloride in the cells of the *Rana pipiens* gastrula, J. Embryol. Exp. Morph. **19**:387, 1968.
6. Bellairs, R.: The development of the nervous system in chick embryos, studied by electron microscopy, J. Embryol. Exp. Morph. **7**:94, 1959.
7. The Boulder Committee: Embryonic vertebrate central nervous system: revised terminology, Anat. Rec. **166**: 257, 1970.
8. Bray, D.: Surface movements during growth of single explanted neurons, Proc. Nat. Acad. Sci. U.S.A. **65**:905, 1970.
9. Burnside, M. B., and Jacobson, A. G.: Analysis of morphogenetic movements in the neural plate of the newt *Taricha torosa,* Develop. Biol. **18**:537, 1968.
10. Burt, A. M., and Wenger, B. S.: Glucose-6-phosphate dehydrogenase activity in the brain of the developing chick, Develop. Biol. **3**:84, 1961.
11. Corner, M. A.: Development of the brain in *Xenopus laevis* after removal of parts of the neural plate, J. Exp. Zool. **153**:301, 1963.
12. Corner, M. A.: Localization of capacities for functional development in the neural plate of *Xenopus laevis,* J. Com. Neurol. **123**:243, 1964.
13. DelCerro, M. P., and Snider, R. S.: Studies on the developing cerebellum. Ultrastructure of the growth cones, J. Comp. Neurol. **133**:341, 1968.
14. DiVirgilio, G., and others: Sequence of events in neural tube closure and the formation of neural crest in the chick embryo, Acta Anat. **68**:127, 1967.
15. Duncan, D., and Hild, W.: Histogenesis and cytogenesis of neural structures. In Minckler, J., editor: Pathology of the nervous system, vol. I, New York, 1968, McGraw-Hill Book Co.
16. Eccles, J. C.: Neurogenesis and morphogenesis in the cerebellar cortex, Proc. Nat. Acad. Sci. U.S.A. **66**:295, 1970.
17. Enemar, A., and others: Observations on the appearance of norepinephrine in the sympathetic nervous system of the chick embryo, Develop. Biol. **11**:268, 1965.
18. Friedman, H. P., and Wenger, B. S.: Accumulation of an organ specific protein during development of the embryonic chick brain, J. Embryol. Exp. Morph. **23**:289, 1970.
19. Friedman, H. P., and Wenger, B. S.: Adult brain antigens demonstrated in chick embryos by fractionated antisera, J. Embryol. Exp. Morph. **13**:35, 1965.
20. Fujita, H., and Fujita, S.: Electron microscopic studies on neuroblast differentiation in the central nervous system of domestic fowl, Z. Zellforsch. **60**:463, 1963.
21. Fujita, S.: Applications of light and electron microscopic autoradiography to the study of cytogenesis of the forebrain. In Hassler, R., and Stephan, H., editors: Evolution of the forebrain, phylogenesis and ontogenesis of the forebrain, Stuttgart, 1966, Georg Thiene Verlag.
22. Glees, P., and Sheppard, B. L.: Electron microscopic studies of the synapse in the developing chick spinal cord, Z. Zellforsch. **62**:356, 1964.
23. Glees, P., and Meller, K.: Morphology of neuroglia. In Bourne, G. H., editor: The structure and function of nervous tissue, vol. I, New York, 1968, Academic Press, Inc.
24. Grafstein, B., and others: Axona transport of neurotubule protein, Nature **227**:289, 1970.
25. Hamburger, V.: Origins of integrated behavior, Develop. Biol. Suppl. **2**:251, 1968.
26. Hamburger, V.: Some aspects to the embryology of behavior, Quart. Rev. Biol. **38**:342, 1963.
27. Hamburgh, M.: The role of thyroid and growth hormones in neurogenesis. In Moscona, A. A., and Monroy, A., editors: Current topics in developmental biology, New York, 1969, Academic Press, Inc.
28. Horstadius, S.: The neural crest, New York, 1950, Oxford University Press.
29. Hughes, A. F. W.: Aspects of neural ontogeny, London, 1968, Logos Press.
30. Ignarro, L. J., and Shideman, F. E.: Appearance and concentrations of catecholamines and their biosynthesis

in the embryonic and developing chick, J. Pharm. Exp. Ther. **159**:38, 1968.
31. Jacobson, M.: Development of specific neuronal connections, Science **163**:543, 1969.
32. Johnson, D. E., and others: Changes in functional classes of RNA in developing chick embryo brain, Proc. Fed. Amer. Soc. Exp. Biol. **28**:864, 1969.
33. Johnston, M. C.: A radioautographic study of the migration and fate of cranial neural crest cells in the chick embryo, Anat. Rec. **156**:143, 1966.
34. Kelly, R. O.: An electron microscope study of chordamesoderm association in gastrulae of a toad, *Xenopus laevis,* J. Exp. Zool. **172**:153, 1970.
35. Klosovskiy, B. N.: Hydrocephalus. In Minckler, J., editor: Pathology of the nervous system, vol. I, New York, 1968, McGraw-Hill Book Co.
36. Kollros, J. J.: Order and control of neurogenesis (as exemplified by the lateral motor column), Develop. Biol. Suppl. **2**:274, 1968.
37. Landesman, R.: Neural-mesodermal interactions subsequent to neural induction in *Ambystoma,* Develop. Biol. **16**:341, 1967.
38. Langman, J.: Histogenesis of the central nervous system. In Bourne, G. H., editor: The structure and function of nervous tissue, vol. I, New York, 1968, Academic Press, Inc.
39. Langman, J., and others: Behavior of neuroepithelial cells during closure of the neural tube, J. Comp. Neurol. **127**:399, 1966.
40. Lasher, R.: Studies on cellular proliferation and chondrogenesis. In Cameron, I. L., and others, editors: Developmental aspects of the cell cycle New York, 1970, Academic Press, Inc.
41. Levi-Montalcini, R., and Angeletti, P. U.: Nerve growth factor, Physiol. Rev. **48**:534, 1968.
42. Lyser, K. M.: Early differentiation of motor neuroblasts in the chick embryo as studied by electron microscopy, II. Microtubules and neurofilaments, Develop. Biol. **17**:117, 1968.
43. Meller, K., and others: The differentiation of endoplasmic reticulum in developing neurons of the chick spinal cord, Z. Zellforsch. **69**:189, 1966.
44. Mugnaini, E., and Forstronen, P. F.: Ultrastructural studies on the cerebellar histogenesis, I. Differentiation of granule cells and development of glomeruli in the chick embryo, Z. Zellforsch. **77**:115, 1967.
45. Nieuwkopp, P. D.: Problems of embryonic induction and pattern formation in amphibians and birds, Exp. Biol. Med. **1**:22, 1967.
46. Pannese, E.: Developmental changes of the endoplasmic reticulum and ribosomes in nerve cells of the spinal ganglia of the domestic fowl, J. Comp. Neurol. **132**:331, 1968.
47. Provine, R. R., and others: Electrical activity in the spinal cord of the chick embryo, *in situ,* Proc. Nat. Acad. Sci. U.S.A. **65**:508, 1970.
48. Rao, B. R.: The appearance and extension of neural differentiation tendencies in the neurectoderm of the early chick embryo, Wilhelm Roux' Archiv. **160**:187, 1968.
49. Riss, W.: Introduction to a general theory of spinal organization, Brain Behav. Evolut. **2**:51, 1969.
50. Saxen, L., and Toivonen, S.: Primary embryonic induction, London, 1962, Logos and Academic Press.
51. Schroeder, T. E.: Neurulation in *Xenopus laevis.* An analysis and model based upon light and electron microscopy, J. Embryol. Exp. Morph. **23**:427, 1970.
52. Seeds, N. W., and others: Regulation of axon formation by clonal lines of a neural tumor, Proc. Nat. Acad. Sci. U.S.A. **66**:160, 1970.
53. Shanta, T. R., and others: The morphology and cytology of neurons. In Bourne, G. H., editor: The structure and function of nervous tissue, New York, 1969, Academic Press, Inc.
54. Sharma, S. C., and others: Unit activity in the isolated spinal cord of chick embryo, *in situ,* Proc. Nat. Acad. Sci. U.S.A. **66**:40, 1970.
55. Tennyson, V. M.: Electron microscopic study of the developing neuroblast of the dorsal root ganglion of the rabbit embryo, J. Comp. Neurol. **124**:267, 1965.
56. Tennyson, V. M.: The fine structure of the axon and growth cone of the dorsal root neuroblast of the rabbit embryo, J. Cell Biol. **44**:62, 1970.
57. Tennyson, V. M., and Pappas, G. D.: An electron microscope study of ependymal cells of the fetal, early postnatal and adult rabbit, Z. Zellforsch. **56**:595, 1962.
58. Tiedeman, H.: Biochemical aspects of primary induction and determination. In Weber, R., editor: The biochemistry of animal development vol. II, New York, 1967, Academic Press, Inc.
59. Watterson, R. L.: Structure and mitotic behavior of the early neural tube. In DeHaan, R. L., and Ursprung, H., editors: Organogenesis, New York, 1965, Holt, Rinehart & Winston, Inc.
60. Wechsler, W., and Meller, K.: Electron microscopy of neuronal and glial differentiation in the developing brain of the chick, Prog. Brain Res. **26**:93, 1967.
61. Weston, J. A.: The migration and differentiation of neural crest cells, Advances Morph. **8**:41, 1970.

CHAPTER 10

TISSUES OF THE NERVOUS SYSTEM

JEFF MINCKLER

The elements within and surrounding the mature nervous system include notochordal remnants and bone and connective tissues (see Chapter 9).[19,38] The basic structures that are immediately pertinent to the makeup and function of the nervous system itself (meninges, vasculature, Schwann cells, microglia, neuroglia, ependyma, choroid plexus, neuron, neuropil, and the special related structures, including pituitary gland, pineal body, other neuroendocrine structures, CSF, and interstitial substance) remain to be discussed. In reviewing these it is necessary to touch upon the borderlands of physiology, chemistry, and physics, as well as the ultrastructure of these elements. The present chapter deals principally with the histologic and electron microscopic characteristics of the basic tissues, and ensuing chapters will arrange them into an overall functioning system complex. An overall interrelating histogenetic scheme is provided in Fig. 10-1. For discussion of histogenesis and cellular development see Chapter 9.

MENINGES

Both major segments of meningeal tissue (dura and leptomeninx) are made up of the same elements, *meningothelium* and *fibrous components* (Fig. 10-2). The meningothelial cells are flattened, mesothelium-like cells that line all meningeal spaces and cover the arachnoid trabeculae. *Arachnoid rests* are nests of epithelioid meningothelium that form thickenings along the arachnoid or are buried within the dura (Fig. 10-3). They are most frequently located along the dural sinuses and the dorsum of the spinal cord. These rests are sometimes regarded as the parent cells of meningeal tumors. By stimulation with carbon particles or blood pigment the meningothelium of the arachnoid reacts like fibroblasts of connective tissue and walls off the area of irritation. The dural cells also can act like fibroblasts and lay down collagen. The meningothelium of the pia is a more prominent reacting element to bacterial stimulation and will produce phagocytes. In general the differences in adaptive behavior on the part of meningothelium are regarded as topographic variations. There is some tendency to regard the meningothelium of the subdural space as basically different from that of the subarachnoid spaces. The two spaces do not communicate, and the subdural appears to connect, at least functionally, with lymphatics of the nose, throat, and nerve roots—this despite the fact that no definite lymphatics are known to exist in the meninges. If lymphatics exist at all, they appear to be confined to the trabecular structures. Under the electron microscope the dural meningothelium is seen to possess a dense nucleus, many RNA granules, a well-developed endoplasmic reticulum, and a compact cytoplasmic mass. By contrast, the subarachnoid meningothelium is hydropic or foamy and possesses a poorly developed endoplasmic reticulum and Golgi apparatus (in some species), numerous large mitochondria, and some cytoplasmic dense bodies, vesicles, and inclusions (Fig. 10-4).[28,37]

The fibrous components of the meninges are predominantly collagenous but contain some elastic fibers in the pia-arachnoid, very few in the dura. The collagen fibers are interlaced but are oriented prominently along tension lines in the dural folds. *Melanin-producing cells* are scattered regularly within the meninges and appear most prominently in the basal pia-arachnoid membranes of the brain and in the fissures of the spinal meninges, frequently in only the upper part of the cord. *Min-*

Central nervous system

Notochord
Chordal rests and nuclei pulposi
Vertebral column disks, cranium

Medulloepithelium
Ependymoepithelium
Medulloblast
Ependymoblast
Oligodendroblast
Spongioblast
Neuroblast (apolar)
Neuroblast (polar)
Astroblast
Ependyma
Oligodendroglia
Astrocyte
Neurocyte
Pituitary
Pineal
Nuclei satellite cells
Axons
Choroid plexus
Microglia
White matter interfascicular supporting cells (myelin cover)

Neural crest
Migrant cells
Neuroblast
Neurocyte
Capsule cells
Dorsal root ganglia
Neuroblast
Neurocyte
Supporting cells
Capsule cells
Sheath cells
Autonomic ganglia
Other peripheral neurogenic cells
1. Adrenal
2. Chromaffin
3. Melanoblast
4. Special endings
Peripheral nerves
Epineurium
Perineurium
Endoneurium
Mesoderm

Pia
Arachnoid
Leptomeninx
Pachymeninx
Bone
Vasculature
Mesoderm
Neuroskeletal intertissue

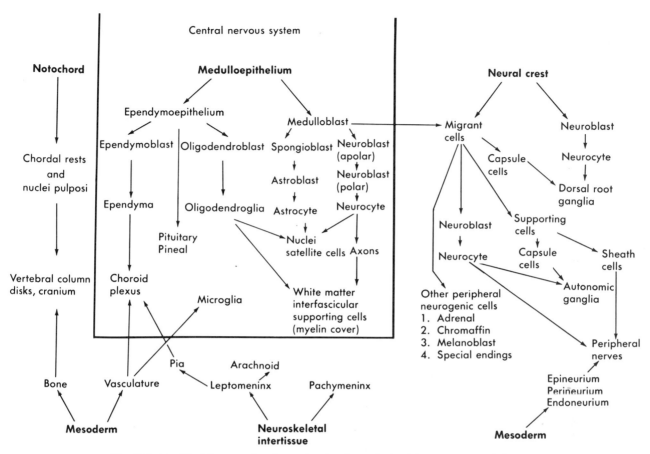

Fig. 10-1. Possible histogenetic scheme showing interrelationship among neural tissues.

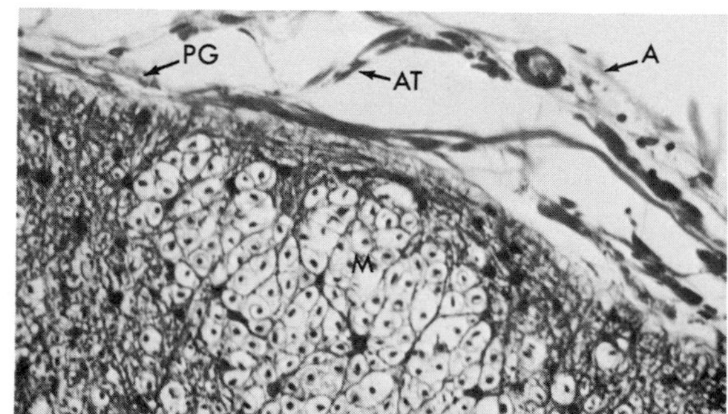

Fig. 10-2. Elements and relationships of parts of leptomeninges. *A,* Arachnoid; *AT,* arachnoid trabecula; *PG,* pia-glial membrane; *M,* myelinated fibers.

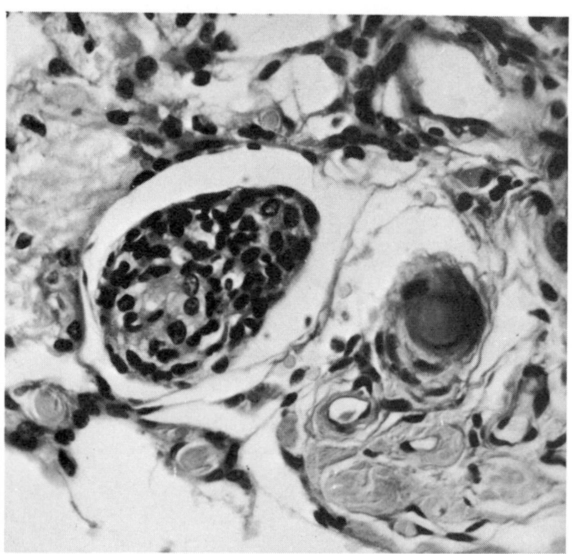

Fig. 10-3. Arachnoid rest.

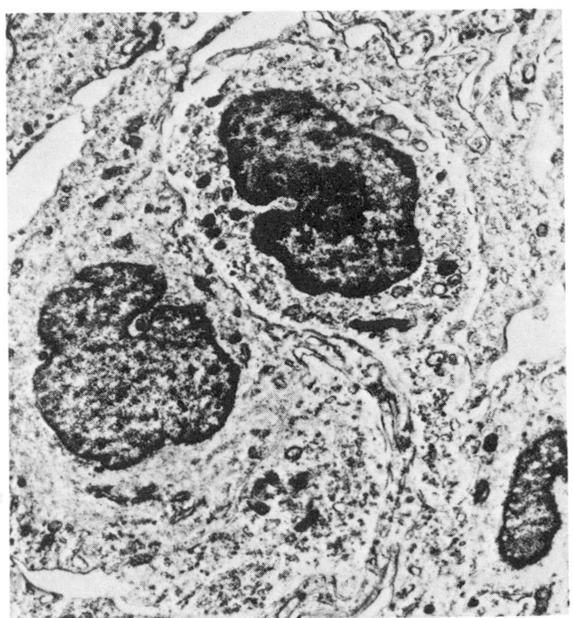

Fig. 10-4. Meningothelial cells in electron micrograph. (From Minckler, J. In Anderson, W. A. D., editor: Pathology, ed. 5, St. Louis, 1966, The C. V. Mosby Co. Courtesy Sarah Luse.)

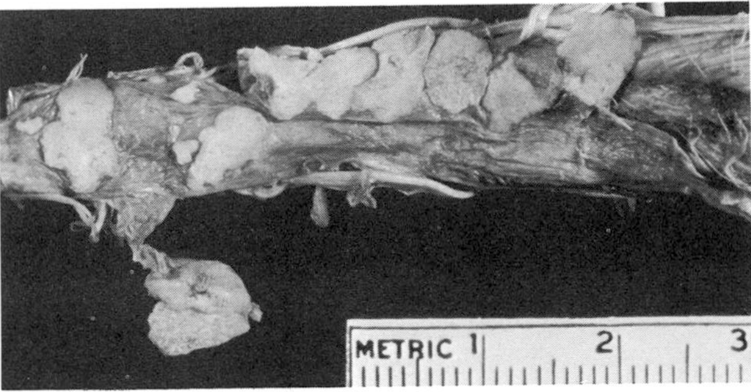

Fig. 10-5. Arachnoid placques, lumbar cord. (From Minckler, J. In Anderson, W. A. D.: editor: Pathology, ed. 5, St. Louis, 1966, The C. V. Mosby Co.)

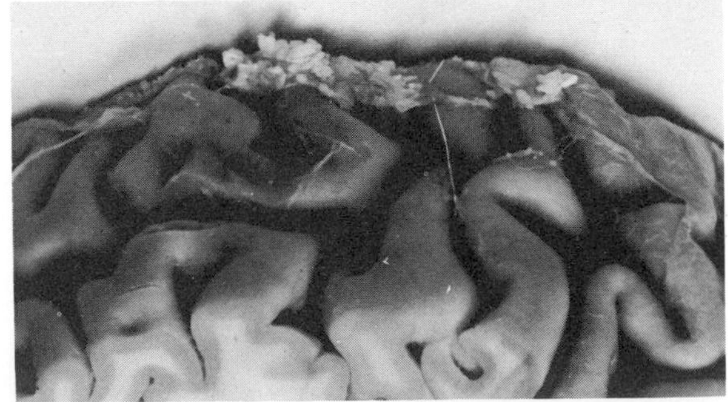

Fig. 10-6. Arachnoid granulations (Pacchionian bodies) pulled away from overlying venous sinus.

eralization of the meninges is common, particularly the deposit of calcium. This occurs along the falx of the dura and in the arachnoid membrane of the dorsum of the lumbar segments (*arachnoid plaques*) (Fig. 10-5).[37]

Arachnoid granulations (Pacchionian) are the exit pathways for CSF to enter the dural venous sinuses from the subarachnoid space. A similar structural complex effects the same purpose around most of the intracranial venous sinuses and near the exit of nerves where dura and arachnoid are fused. The term *granulations* applies to the gross villous invaginations that stand out prominently along the vertex as the dura is peeled away or that project into the lateral lacunae after reflecting their roofs (Fig. 10-6). The exact mechanism of operation remains controversial. One view is that the projecting arachnoid acquires valve-like tubes that open through the dura mater and sinus endothelium to empty CSF whenever fluid pressure is greater than venous sinus pressure.[43] The more common view is that the granulations retain a covering of dural membrane and sinus endothelium, which are attenuated to permit unidirectional fluid migration subject to somewhat the same membrane

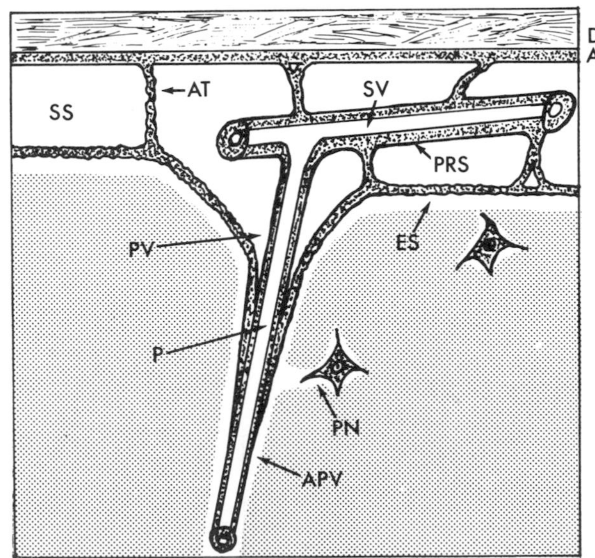

Fig. 10-7. Meningovascular relationships at brain surface. *D,* Dura mater; *A,* arachnoid; *AT,* arachnoid trabecula; *SS,* subarachnoid space; *SV,* subarachnoid vessel; *P,* penetrating cerebral vessel; *PG,* pia-glial membrane; *PV,* perivascular space, disappearing by coalescence of pia-glial membrane with perivascular reticular sheath (*PRS*); *PN,* artifactual perineuronal space; *APV,* artifactual perivascular space; *ES,* epispinal artifactual space of His.

barrier restrictions as in the ingress mechanism for production of CSF (Fig. 3-16). The arachnoid granulations possess whorled arachnoid cell rests and frequently will display calcified, laminated hyaline bodies (*psammoma bodies*) (Fig. 10-3).

The histogenetic pathway of meningeal tissue has excited interest for years and still remains unsettled. As mentioned previously, each layer possesses distinctive capability in reactions to stimulation, and there are slight structural differences. Whether these differences represent more than adaptations from the same parent tissue remains unsettled. Mesoderm vs. neuroectoderm originating tissue has dominated the contest. Opinions include: (1) all meninges are ectodermal; (2) all are mesodermal; (3) the tissues are mixed ectodermal (pia-arachnoid) and mesodermal (dura); and (4) they are mixed ectodermal (inner pia-arachnoid only) and mesodermal (arachnoid and dura).[12,37] The controversy is avoided (not settled) by labeling the primordial tissue as *neuroskeletal intertissue,* from which all meningeal structures differentiate (Figs. 10-1 and 10-7).

VASCULATURE

The vessels of the CNS possess unique features in the anatomy of both the vessels themselves and of the perivascular wrappings. *Arteries,* like other vessels, are made up of intima, media, and adventitia. The penetrating cerebral vessels are seldom more than 0.5 mm. in diameter. The endothelial lining is single-layered and is supported by an internal elastic lamina that is free of lamellations and fenestrations and that diminishes in thickness with age. The media of all cerebral arterial walls is relatively thin compared to that of extracerebral vessels. The smooth muscles are disposed circularly and have from five to twenty layers. In vessels less than 70 μ in diameter the media is principally collagen.[3] No external elastic lamina exists. The adventitia amounts to a few collagenous fibers intervening between muscle and a reticular perivascular sheath. There is a gradual reduction in size to arterioles, which arbitrarily are those vessels less than 100 μ in diameter. The smallest arterioles amount to a single layer of smooth muscle overlying endothelial cells. In both arterioles and arteries the adventitia abuts against vascular feet of glial origin (principally astrocytic). Each component of this apposition retains a separating membrane (outer and inner laminae of a reticular membrane) that interposes between the glial extremities and the thin adventitia (Figs. 10-7 to 10-9).

The *capillaries* amount to an endothelial tube with the nuclei oriented to the long axis of the vessels. In studies using electron microscopy (EM) the nuclei frequently are observed to bulge into the lumen. The edges of adjoining cells overlap slightly. The cytoplasm contains vesicles that may be part of the transport mechanism by pinocytosis. The outer aspect of the capillary wall is surrounded by perivascular feet of glial cells that account for some eighty-five percent of the capillary surface area (Fig. 10-9). Some microglial cells and neurons also lie adjacent to the capillaries. An external lamina (basement membrane) is apparent in electron micrographs of capillaries; it fuses with the external lamina of adjacent glial cells to obliterate the perivascular reticular space in the depths of the vascular bed associated with capillaries.

The *cerebral veins,* like the arteries, possess thinner walls than comparable vessels elsewhere. Smooth muscle is absent in all but the largest veins, and there is little elastic tissue. There are no valves in cerebral veins.

The nature of the *perivascular wrappings* of intracerebral vessels has been clarified with the advent of EM. Vessels traversing the subarachnoid space possess a wrapping that is a fine reticular membrane of arachnoid origin. An outer lamina of reticular membrane is added by the pial layer as the CNS is penetrated (Figs. 10-7 through 10-10).

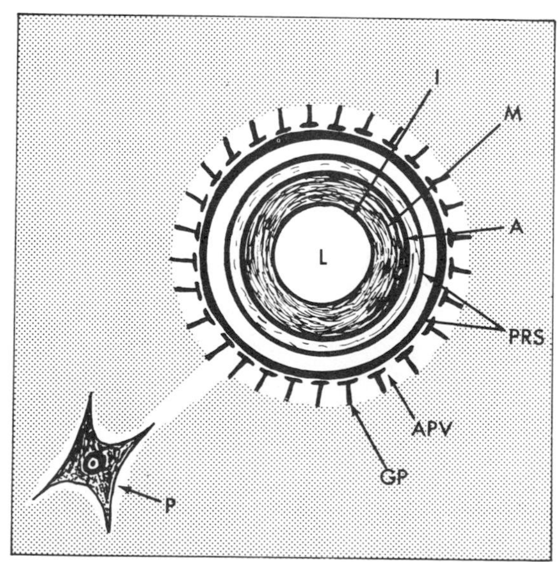

Fig. 10-8. Detail of perineuronal and perivascular spaces. *L,* Lumen; *I,* intima; *M,* media; *A,* adventitia; *PRS,* perivascular reticular sheath (space); *GP,* glial processes projecting into shrinkage space; perineuronal space (*P*), artifactual perivascular space (*APV*).

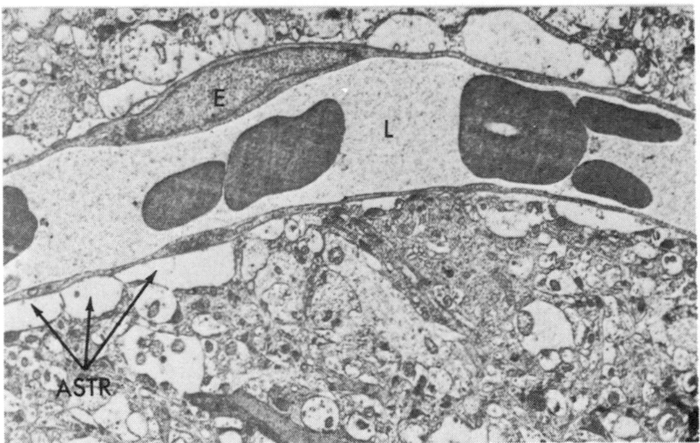

Fig. 10-9. Electron micrograph showing perivascular relationships of cells. *ASTR,* Astroctyes; *E,* endothelial cell projecting into lumen (*L*). Note absence of demonstrable interstitial space. (After Woollam, D. H. M., and Millen, J. W. In Minckler, J., editor: Pathology of the nervous system, vol. I, New York, 1968, McGraw-Hill Book Co.)

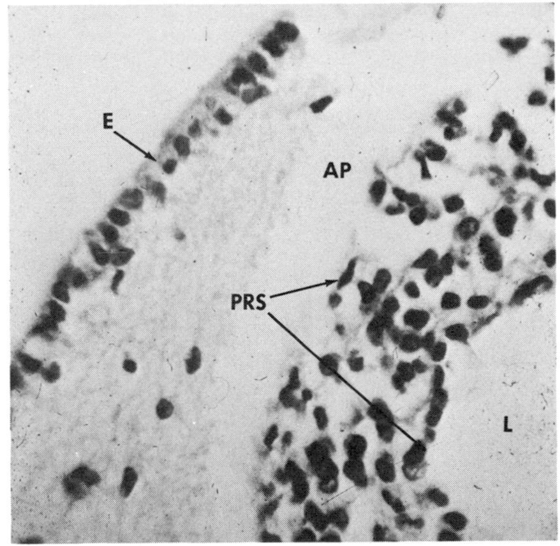

Fig. 10-10. Resting cellular cuff (normal) showing perivascular reticular sheath (*PRS*) with surrounding artifactual perivascular space (*AP*). *L,* Lumen; *E,* ependyma.

This provides the true reticular perivascular sheath, made up of an inner layer continuous with the arachnoid reticular layer and an outer layer continuous with the pial external lamina (Virchow-Robin space). The limbs of the reticular perivascular sheath fuse to obliterate the space around the deeper vessels. The degree of penetration of the sheath is not known but extends to precapillaries in some parts of the white matter. The space thus becomes a blind diverticulum of the subarachnoid space and represents the Virchow-Robin space of neurohistology. Two additional artifactual perivascular spaces exist: (1) a potential cleft between the adventitia and the inner layer of the reticular sheath, and (2) the artifactual space (of Held or His), which is produced as a shrinkage cleft in histologic preparations between the outer reticular sheath and the neuropil. This space is continuous with the artifactual perineuronal space and the shrinkage defect called the epispinal space of His (Figs. 10-7 and 10-12).[46]

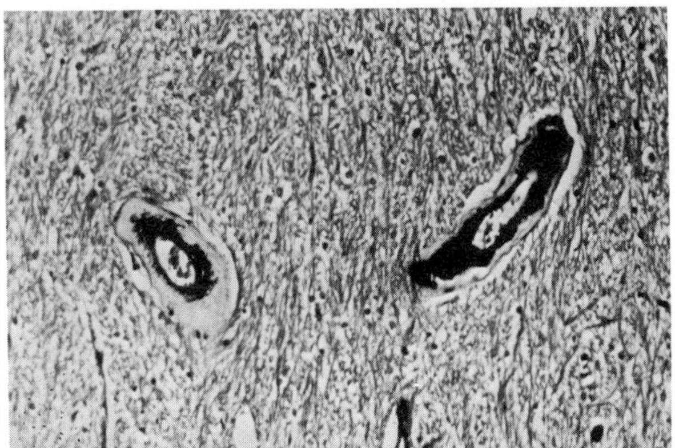

Fig. 10-11. Pseudocalcium deposits in cerebral vessels.

The reticular perivascular space accommodates reacting cells in many diseases to produce *perivascular cuffing.* In nonpathologic circumstances that are poorly understood the vessels of the paraventricular area display *perivascular resting cells,* which seem to portend no disease process (Fig. 10-10).[18] Another common structural variation in vessels is the mineralization (or pseudomineralization) of vessels in the basal nuclei by early middle age (Fig. 10-11).

SCHWANN CELLS

The normal histogenetic pathway of the Schwann cell remains in doubt after more than one hundred years of speculation and experimentation. However, a tremendous amount of information exists about the behavioral aspects of the cell, and the sources have been dramatically diverse. Experimental embryology,[15] tissue culture,[27] physiologic studies, degeneration-regeneration studies,[1] and electron microscopic studies[6,24] have displayed beyond question what these remarkable cells can do when subject to various stimulations. It seems certain that they can arise in the embryo from migrant cells of either medulloepithelial or neural crest origin, de-

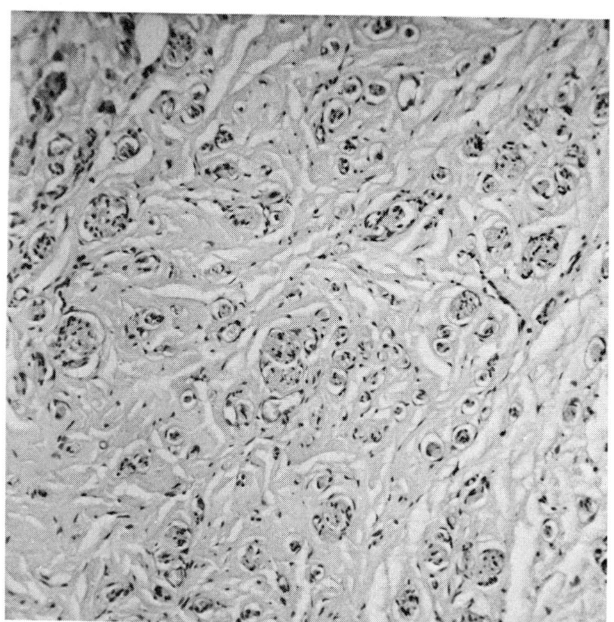

Fig. 10-12. Hyperplasia of Schwann cells (nuclear clusters) around regrowing nerves in injured peripheral nerve.

pendent upon the experimental manipulation applied and the interpretation. It is assumed that capsule and sheath cells of the distalmost ganglia (such as the mural visceral autonomic) have the same origin, but some have argued for mesodermal derivation in these locations.[6]

Both in the embryo and in responding to regrowth in nerves, Schwann elements exhibit the self-regulatory population control devices of emergency cell responses. With maturation to the point of engulfing nerve fibers experimentally, they seem to cut off their own cell supply.[1] This is of course subject to interpretation. The Schwann cells appear to be stimulated to multiply by the degeneration of nerve fibers, myelinated or not, and in proportion quantitatively to the number of fibers in the nerve before degeneration. Schwann cells in tissue culture exhibit a pulsatile action at eight-minute intervals. The significance of the pulsing, if it occurs in vivo as it does in vitro, is unknown.

To summarize this histogenetic pathway briefly, the Schwann cells appear to be derived in the embryo from migrant cells of neuroepithelial origin, either from the neural crest or medulloepithelium. Second, in the mature peripheral system, the Schwann cells can be derived by multiplication of preexisting Schwann cells in the neural complex stimulated (Fig. 10-12).

Myelin

Because peripheral *myelin* is now known to be part and parcel of the Schwann cell membrane, a discussion of this sheath of peripheral nerves becomes part of the Schwann cell review. By definition, myelin is a stainable material surrounding peripheral nerves of larger dimension (axis-cylinders over 1.5 μ) and imparting to the nerves a characteristic white appearance in the fresh state. This is in contrast to nerves that appear gray in the fresh state and display no myelin on special staining. Since the myelin sheath represents Schwann cell membrane, and since all peripheral fibers have Schwann wrappings of some sort, the distinguishing definition of a myelinated fiber must be rephrased somewhat. A myelinated nerve thus becomes one in which the Schwann membrane wrapping is of sufficient density and size to accept myelin stains. By contrast, an unmyelinated nerve is one in which the Schwann wrapping is either shared or arranged in such a manner as to fail to stain with myelin procedures. The points of difference become critical in assessing disease processes in the nervous system that are characterized by poor myelin formation or by myelin dissolution after it has been established.*

Since an electron microscopic demonstration in 1954,[13] myelin sheaths of peripheral nerves have been recognized as spirally wrapped, continuous sheets of Schwann cell membrane into which an axis-cylinder has been enfolded (Fig. 10-13). The axis-cylinder is suspended immediately by apposing folds of membrane, the *inner mesaxon;* the area of penetration along the membrane surface forms the bilaminar *outer mesaxon* (Fig. 10-14). The mechanism of the enfolding remains unsolved and may represent a rotation of the Schwann cell around the axis, a rotation of the axis within the cell, or a fusion of cell membrane derivatives (vesicles or tubes) within the Schwann cytoplasm. However it is laid down, each Schwann cell houses a segment of myelinated axis-cylinder as an *internodal section* between the *nodes of Ranvier* (Fig. 10-17). The nodes thus terminate the continuity of the Schwann membrane at either extremity of an *elongate Schwann cylinder.* The manner of termination of Schwann membrane at the node of Ranvier is such that the outer wrappings overlap the inner (Fig. 10-17). The unmyelinated node is the structure from which axis-branchings occur. An external lamina, or basement membrane, which is continuous with the membrane over the Schwann cells, crosses the nodes. Apart from this basement mem-

*See references 24, 30, 31, and 44.

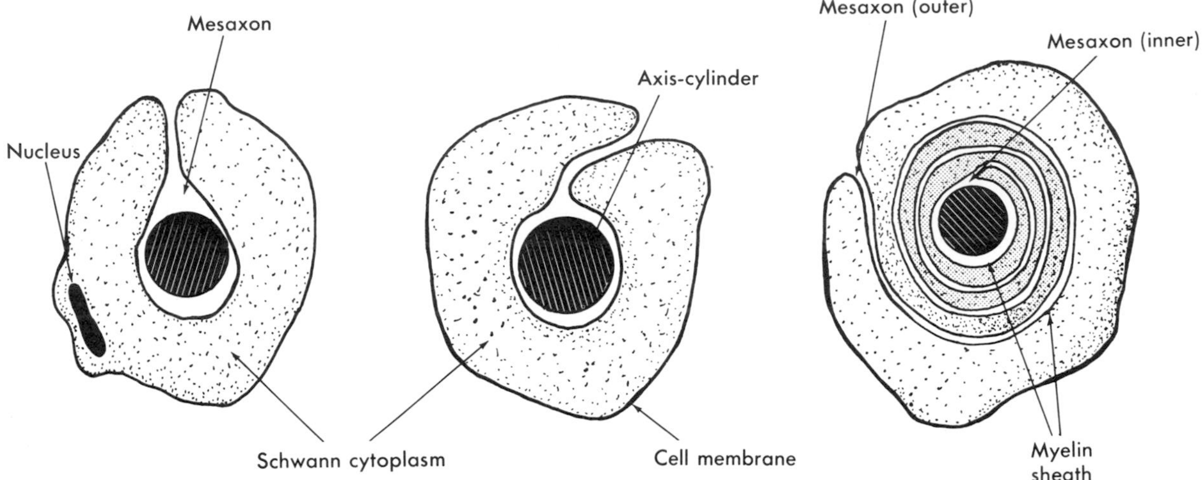

Fig. 10-13. Schwann cell membrane wrapping to form myelin sheath of peripheral nerve.

Fig. 10-14. Electron micrographs of myelin sheaths. **A,** Mesaxon *(MES)* of Schwann membrane *(SM)*, leading to laminated myelin; *S*, Schwann cell cytoplasm. (×60,000.) **B,** Spiral lamination of myelin *(M)* around central axon *(AX)*. (×38,500.) **C,** Major dense (period) lines *(P)* in myelin sheath, separated by intraperiod lines *(I)*. (×450,000.) (From Hager, H., and Wolman, M. In Minckler, J., editor: Pathology of the nervous system, vol. I, New York, 1968, The McGraw-Hill Book Co.)

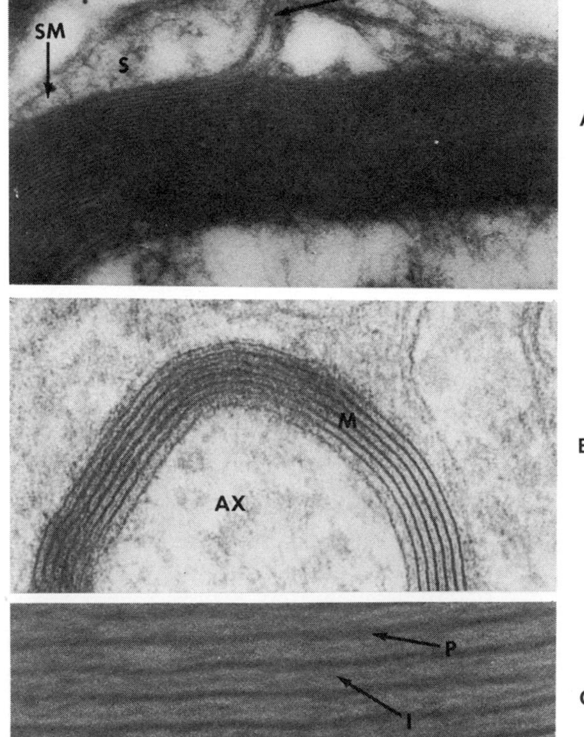

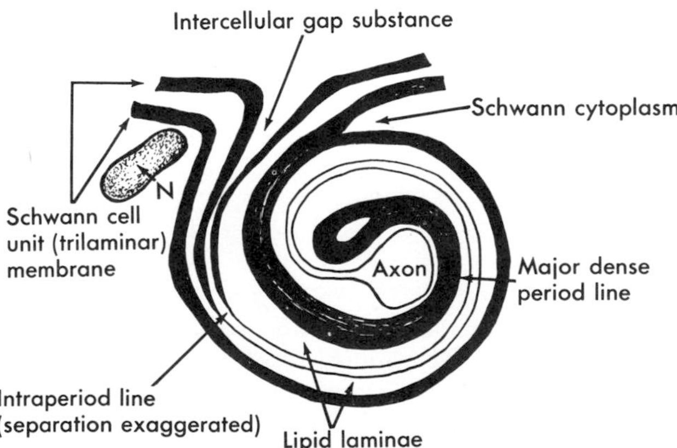

Fig. 10-15. Presumed mechanism of formation of periodicity. Intraperiod line formed by fusion of external protein laminae of unit membrane. Major dense period lines formed from apposition of inner protein membranes. Lipid layers thus border the intraperiod line.

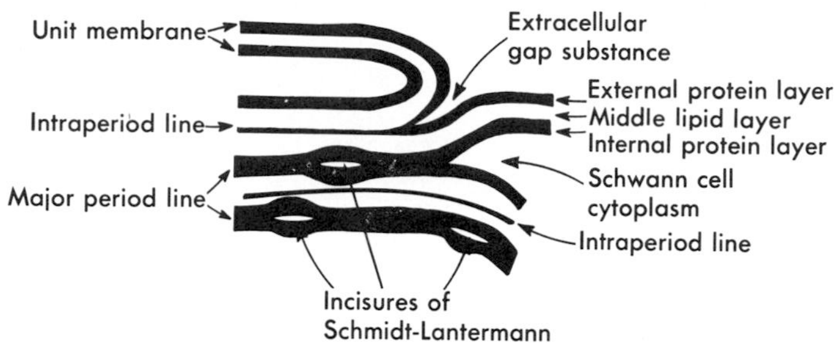

Fig. 10-16. Clefts appearing within the inner laminar fusion form Schmidt-Lantermann incisures, which are continuous with Schwann cell cytoplasm.

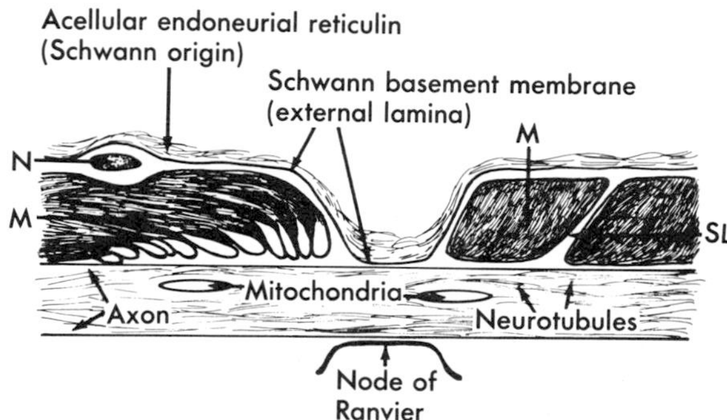

Fig. 10-17. Longitudinal schematic drawing through node of Ranvier. Note Schwann cell external lamina (basement membrane), bridging node overlying axon. On the left, the myelin termination at the node is the laminated pattern, as seen in EM. On the right are light microscopic characteristics, with inclusion of a Schmidt-Lantermann cleft *(SL)*. *M,* Myelin layer; *N,* nucleus of Schwann cell.

brane, the node of Ranvier represents bare axis-cylinder, covered only by interdigitating extensions of Schwann cell membranes (Figs. 10-14 to 10-18).

The myelin layers possess many distinctive features in electron micrographs. An electron-dense concentric line reappears approximately every 120 Å in the cross section of the myelin mass. This imparts a *periodicity* of spacing that is characteristic of myelin (Fig. 10-15). The major dense lines are presumed to arise from the apposition of the inner layers of the trilaminar unit membrane as they make a circumferential turn. The outer lamina is joined at the point of invagination by the adjacent outer lamina (Fig. 10-14 and 10-15). These fused laminae become compressed as a fine *intraperiodic line,* which is carried in circumferential pattern between two layers of the middle lipid lamina of unit membrane origin (Fig. 10-19). This composite at high magnification EM characterizes myelin as *major dense lines* recurring at a periodicity of 150 Å, with a narrow *intraperiodic line* in the center of the light zone.

Schmidt-Lantermann incisures, or *Lantermann clefts,* appear as funnel-shaped fissures along the myelin sheaths of peripheral nerves (not central) (Figs. 10-16 and 10-17). Their explanation remains something of a mystery, but their existence is confirmed in EM. With this technique the clefts appear as an oblique row of separations of the Schwann cell membranes by splitting of the major dense lines.[44] According to Robertson they represent shearing defects marking a helical channel that interrelates the periaxonal space with Schwann cell cytoplasm.[33] They may have a role in the metabolic transport systems of the myelin sheath.

In paraffin-embedded material and under the light microscope, myelin residue presents a faint network pattern that has been designated *neurokeratin.* Although these fine strands are evident only in extracted material, they orient in a radial pattern and provide basic suggestions regarding the molecular makeup of myelin. At the molecular level myelin appears to be represented by layers of lipid between layers of protein not unlike cell membranes elsewhere, but with remarkably complex linkages and chemistry (Fig. 10-18).[44] These items figure prominently in the physiologic capabilities of the membrane (see Chapter 12).

Capsule cells (satellite)

The Schwann cells provide the capsular coverings for peripheral ganglion cells in cranial, spinal, and autonomic ganglia (Fig. 10-19). Some of these ganglion cells are myelinated, at least in experimental animals.[34] In these ganglia (ciliary, vestibular, and cochlear) the myelin may be formed in a loose pattern of strands rather than the compact layers of peripheral nerves. It is probable that more than one Schwann capsule cell contributes myelin

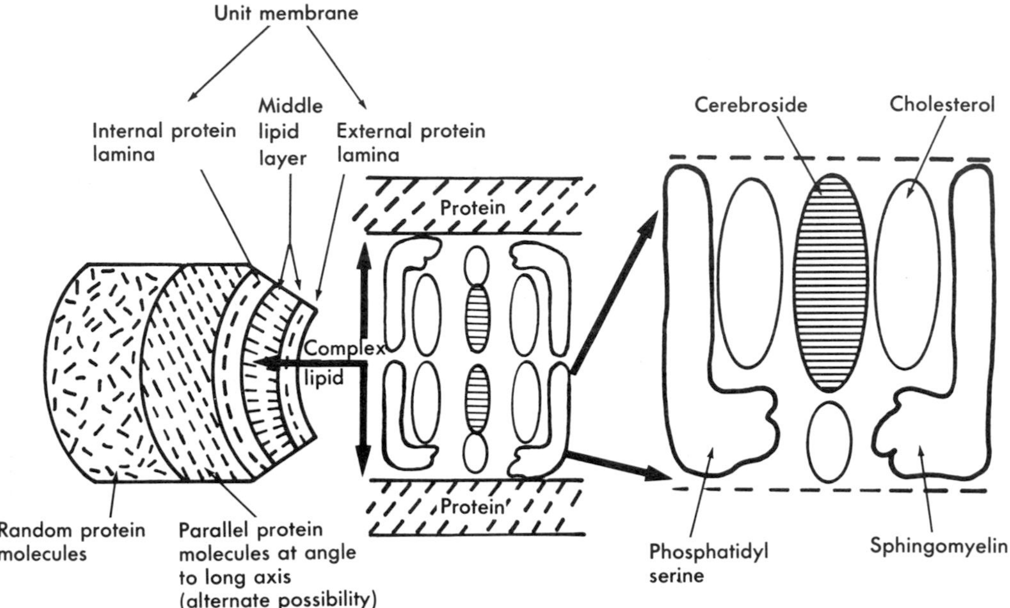

Fig. 10-18. Diagram of possible molecular configurations within the protein and complex lipid laminae of myelin. (After Wolman, M., and Austin, J. In Minckler, J., editor: Pathology of the nervous system, vol. I, New York, 1968, McGraw-Hill Book Co.)

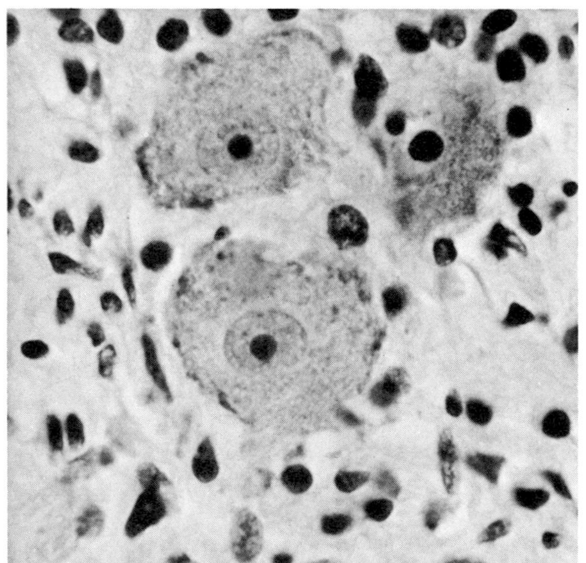

Fig. 10-19. Capsule cells oriented around autonomic ganglion cells.

to a neuron. The exact arrangement of myelin deposits around ganglion cells is not established. From cell to cell, the sheath is discontinuous and from cell to axon it is interrupted by a node. The basement membrane of the capsule cells, as of Schwann cells elsewhere, persists in the ganglia and separates the cell from its surroundings. This same external (basement) membrane persists as characteristic of Schwann cells in unmyelinated ganglia. Here the capsule cell membrane is flattened as a wrapping and is continuous with the myelin membrane spreading along the axon. The capsular Schwann cell membrane junctions sometimes overlap as applied to the ganglion cell surface.

Sheath cells

The Schwann cells that provide the covering for nerve fibers do so in a pattern that may be unmyelinated as well as myelinated. In unmyelinated fibers the nerve filaments within the cells are frequently multiple. Often the fibers will possess their own mesaxon; in other instances they indent the Schwann capsule only, and sometimes they share a mesaxon.[8] In all cases the external lamina or basement membrane of the Schwann cell bridges the indentation that in effect separates the fibers from the extracellular microenvironment. The multiple use of Schwann cells by nerve fibers

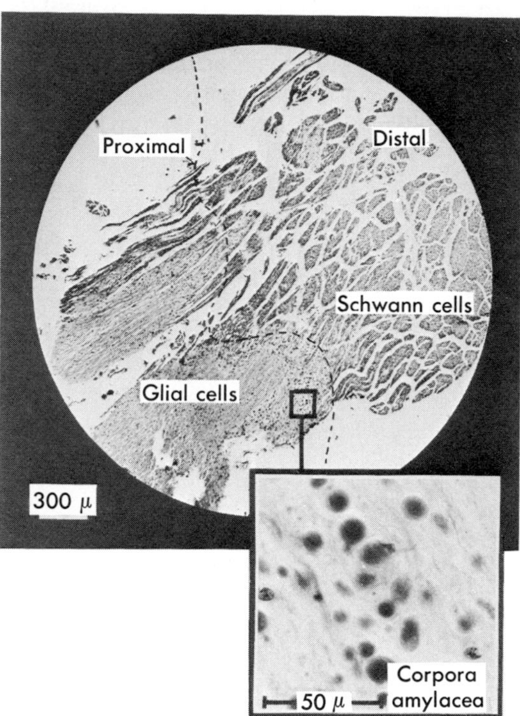

Fig. 10-20. Glio-Schwannian junction of cranial nerve VIII (broken line). Note corpora amylacea marking the demarcation zone. Schwann cells are distal, glial cells proximal. Note subdivisions of peripheral part into fascicles by perineurium. (Courtesy Dr. Max Powers.)

is best exemplified in the embryo, where large numbers of nerve filaments occupy the same cell. With multiplication of the Schwann cells the structure eventually separates one axon to one Schwann cell in a segment. Variations of the fiber-to-sheath relationship are displayed in the olfactory nerve, in Auerbach's plexus,[32] and in the pineal.[29] The common structural relationship of the Schwann sheath cell and a myelinated fiber is illustrated in Fig. 10-17.

Along the nerve roots of each cranial and spinal nerve the *glio-Schwannian junction* (*Obersteiner-Redlich zone*) marks the point where glial covering of the nerve changes to a covering by Schwann cells (Fig. 10-20). The junction is quite distal in cranial nerves (at the internal auditory meatus in nerve VIII) and more proximal in spinal nerves. Glio-Schwannian junctions also occur well within the substance of the spinal cord.[11] In the adult the junction is identified by a row of corpora amylacea on the glial side. Half of a node of Ranvier occurs on the Schwannian side of the junction with glial type myelination proximally. *Reich granules* (pi or protagon granules) are metachromatic, irregular, frequently comma-shaped granules that appear in the perinuclear zone of Schwann cells of myelinated axons stained with nile-blue sulfate in frozen sections. They also appear in electron micrographs. Reich granules increase in number with age, and their function is unknown.[24]

Nerve endings

Evidence has been compiled to suggest that Schwann cells enter into the formation of complex sensory endings, such as Meissner and Pacinian corpuscles.[24] The evidence arises from the demonstration of basement membrane typical of Schwann cells, of pinocytotic vesicles that are consistent in pattern with those of Schwann cells, and from the occurrence of *fibrous, long-spacing collagen,* which occurs both in peripheral nerves and in Schwann cell tumors.[24] The Schwann cell also enters into the structure of the neuromuscular junction.[6] (For details of sensory and motor endings in connection with specific systems see Chapters 16 to 22.)

Connective tissue relationships

In the overall structure of a peripheral nerve, the Schwann cell becomes interrelated with mesodermal elements that provide fibrous coverings for the nerve. The outermost wrapping, the *epineurium,* is distinguished by a loose fibrous character, by inclusion of blood vessels and small nerves, and by a cellular makeup principally of fibroblasts. The tissue covers the nerve itself and hence is an outer covering, often for many fascicles. The derivation is mesodermal, and the structure contains lymphatics. The epineurium can be stripped grossly from the nerve, with little reliability attending an expected cleavage plane.

The *perineurium* is the distinctive, compact, circumferentially oriented, fibrous layer surrounding fascicles of a gross nerve (Fig. 10-20). Septa extend from the perineurium to subdivide the fascicles as they branch away from the parent nerve. Lymph spaces continue into perineurium from larger channels in epineurium with which the perineurium gradually blends. On the inner aspect of this wrapping there appears to be a rather distinctive flattened, endothelial-like or mesothelial limiting membrane,[6] which separates perineurium from endoneurium. There is general agreement that perineurium is mesodermal. It contains fibroblasts, vasculature with endothelium, and pericytes (histiocytes) of mesodermal origin. The parallel of this tissue to meningeal wrappings has been advanced,

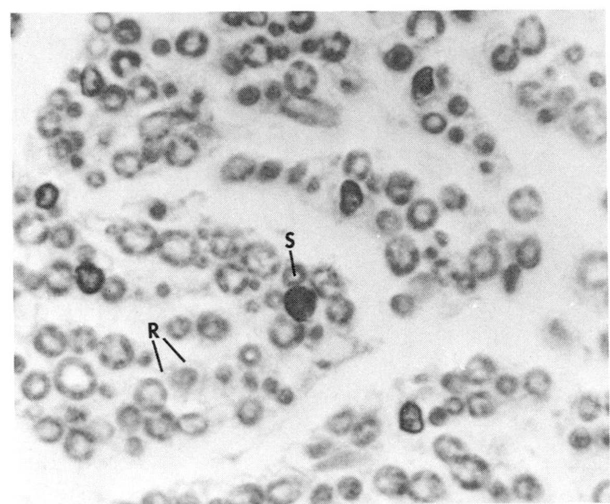

Fig. 10-21. Peripheral nerve with Schwann cells (*S*). Note almost cell-free fine fibrillar material (*R*) (Schwann reticulin?), related to each fiber as endoneurium.

and there are proponents of a neuroectodermal origin of this tissue. No indifferent term (such as neuroskeletal intertissue for meninges) exists to define a noncommittal origin for nerve coverings. The preponderance of evidence, and certainly of opinion, favors a mesodermal origin for perineurium. This structure thus becomes by definition a boundary tissue between the epineurium and the endoneurium and remains uncommitted as to origin.

The *endoneurium* is represented by the fine, almost acellular connective tissue of both reticulin and collagen types that embraces the individual nerve fibers (Fig. 10-21). No decisive separation has been established to part this material from the Schwann cell. The usual view however is that the endoneurium is a mesodermal derivative that is an added covering within the perineurial limits apart from Schwann cells. Electron microscopic study however seems to relate this material specifically to Schwann cells. In addition, fibroblasts are not in evidence within the perineurial covering. Cell counts reveal that eighty-five percent of the intraperineurial cells are related to fine nerve filaments and hence are identifiable as Schwannian in character.[6] Of the remaining fifteen percent, ten percent are endothelial cells from vasculature, and five percent are unidentified as to origin (fibroblasts?, histiocytes?). The ability of Schwann cells to produce reticulin in vitro is well established.[27] The cells also seem able to produce, or in some way condition, the production of collagen. In abnormal Schwann cells (such as Schwannomas), one of the distinguishing features is the production of fibrous, long-spacing collagen.[24] As mentioned previously, the Schwann cells possess a distinctive external lamina, or basement membrane. This membrane may seat strands of collagen within its substance in varying depths. This presumably means that the collagen forerunner (protocollagen) penetrates the Schwann membrane and is subsequently converted to mature fibrillar collagen, which is somehow governed by the Schwann cell.

In summary, the endoneurium is regarded as neuroectodermal in origin and is derived from Schwann cells. The cells are capable of producing reticulin and of governing the production of collagen. Schwann cells represent almost the entire cell population of subperineurial tissues.[6]

Degeneration and regeneration

The Schwann cells have provided the traditional cellular center in inquiries regarding degeneration and regeneration of peripheral nerves. More recently, with the recognition that myelin is a part of the Schwann cell, this element has become a major focus of attention in the pathology of dysmyelination and demyelination as disease processes.* The justification for brief mention of this information in an introductory text of neuroanatomy lies in the evidences of cellular origins and relationships apparent from the studies of Schwann cells as they react to injury. The alterations in degeneration occasioned by severing the axon of peripheral myelinated nerve is termed *Wallerian degeneration* (Fig. 14-2). The part of the nerve separated from its perikaryon, or parent cell body, undergoes dissolution attended by fragmentation and eventual disappearance by digestion of the axis-cylinder. Meanwhile the Schwann cells exhibit globular fragmentation of their myelin component, which becomes incorporated as ovoids within the cytoplasm. The cells align themselves in rows (Büngner's bands), divide mitotically under some circumstances, and enlarge. Collagen is produced, probably by the Schwann cells themselves. With regrowth of the nerves from the proximal stumps, the filaments are engulfed by the Schwann cells to reestablish the invaginating type of intracellular seating of the fibers. In unmyelinated fibers the axis-cylinders fragment and are extruded. The process is slower in unmyelinated fibers than in those that are myelinated. An extensive literature has developed pertaining to degeneration of peripheral

*See references 2, 30, 31, and 44.

nerves.* The regenerative hyperplasia of Schwann cells seems to be related to the volume of fibers available before destruction. Hence, the reaction to injury is markedly different in different nerves. This has great importance in repair predictability.[25,36,45]

MICROGLIA

Microglia (mesoglia) are probably the reticuloendothelial cellular representatives in the CNS. The separation of this group of cells from the neuroglia was effected by del Rio Hortega, but many biologic characteristics of microglia remain unknown. The origin seems to be mesodermal and reticuloendothelial. The cells enter the CNS in the circumnatal period from pia-arachnoid, where it lies in apposition to white matter (cerebral peduncles, tela choroidea). Under a light microscope and with routine staining the cells present only their nuclear characteristics, which vary from rounded to comma to elongate shapes (Fig. 10-22). These are regarded as representing resting phases of the cells, during which they may be related by apparent contact with vessels, nerve cells, or even glia. With silver staining technique (Hortega's silver carbonate) the cells are seen to possess abundant short processes (Fig. 10-23). Microglia are known to present themselves in three additional forms—as *motile forms,* as *rod cells,* and as *phagocytic forms* (*fat-granule* or *gitter cells*). The motile form is distinguished by cytoplasmic pseudopods seen only with silver staining. Rod cells represent a pathologic form that implies an inflammatory process. Such cells are particularly abundant, for example, in the cerebral cortex in syphilis of the nervous system. Fat-granule cells, as the name suggests, are lipid-

*For review see Chapter 14 and references 16, 21, 24, and 44.

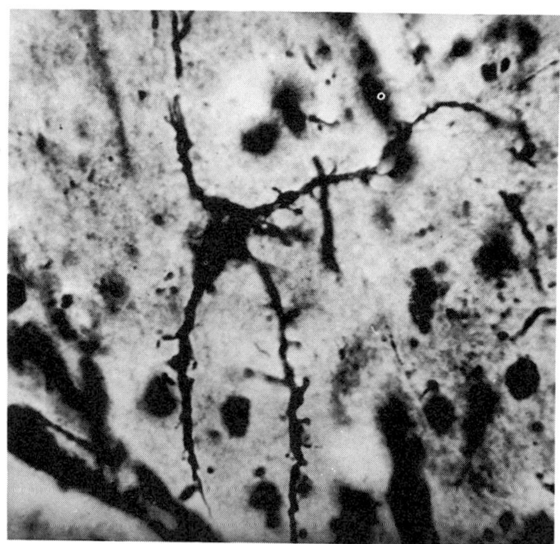

Fig. 10-23. Microglia, metallic stain.

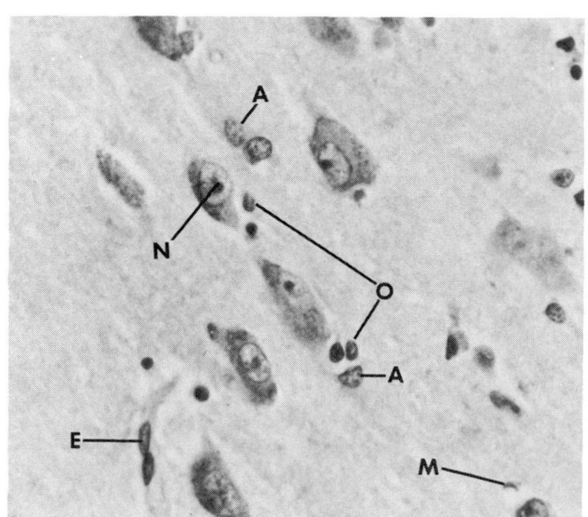

Fig. 10-22. Nuclear differential features in low-power H & E section. *N,* Neuron nucleus; *A,* astrocyte nucleus; *O,* oligodendroglial nucleus; *E,* endothelial nucleus; *M,* microglial nucleus.

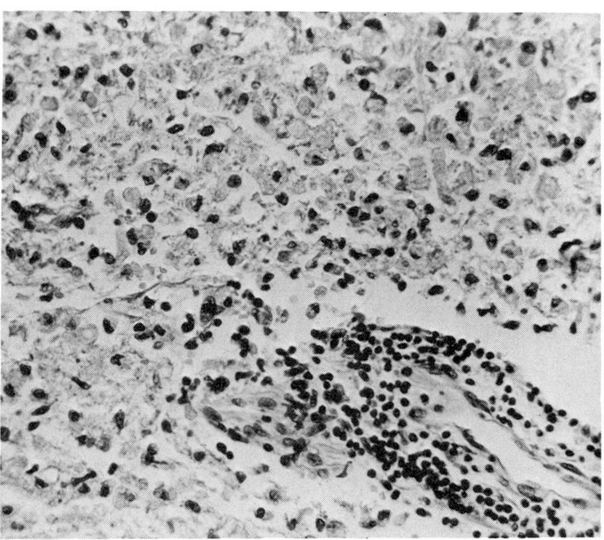

Fig. 10-24. "Gitter" (fat granule or macrophage) form of microglia.

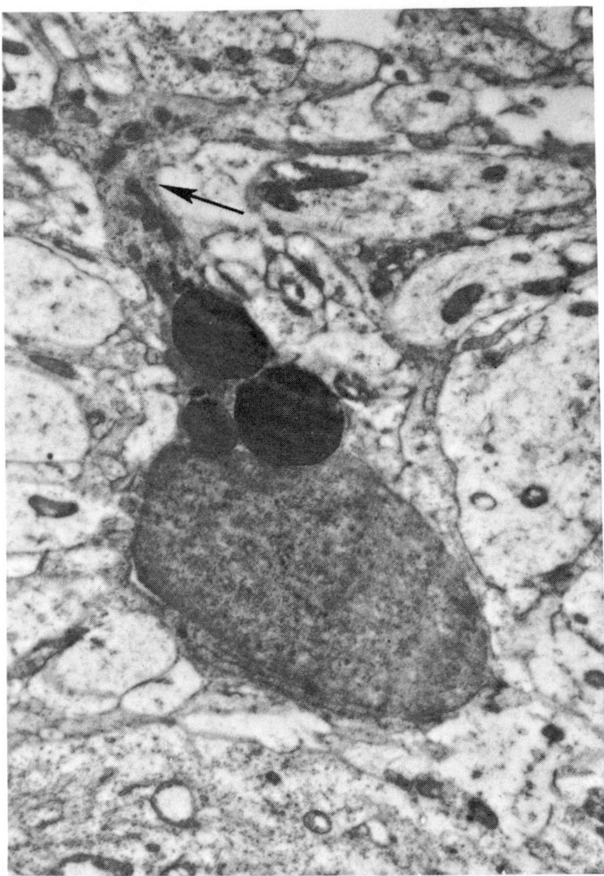

Fig. 10-25. Electron micrograph of microglial cell showing lipid inclusions and elongate process (arrow). (From Luse, S. In Minckler, J., editor: Pathology of the nervous system, vol. I, New York, 1968, McGraw-Hill Book Co.)

laden, rounded elements with the nucleus pressed to one side. They represent the phagocytic phase of the microglia and respond as reacting elements when CNS tissue is destroyed and lipid is released as a breakdown product (Fig. 10-24).

In electron micrographs the microglia possess projecting processes that extend between other cellular elements, a presumed reflection of the motile capability of these cells. They exhibit few mitochondria and a scanty Golgi complex and are extremely electron-dense (Fig. 10-25). Compiled evidence from all sources does not completely settle the origin of gitter cells, which can be mobilized rapidly in pathologic or experimental destructive lesions. Radioisotopic tagging has located them as derivatives of leukocytes, which is helpful in explaining their mobilization in such large numbers. While in the CNS they retain remarkable motility and divide by mitosis. In many respects they behave like transiently settled histiocytes of connective tissue capable of calling upon the hemic system for recruits if necessary.

NEUROGLIA

The neuroglia are traditionally regarded as the supporting members (*glia,* glue) of the neural family of cells. Recent developments impart to these cells, however, a rather more exciting existence than mere support. On structural and functional grounds the neuroglia are subdivided into *astrocytes* (star cells) and *oligodendrocytes* (cells with few processes). In routine preparations, such as with hematoxylin and eosin or toluidin blue, only the nuclei show, and it is customary to separate the two types of cells on the basis of nuclear configuration and staining properties (Fig. 10-22). Astrocytes exhibit a pale, vesicular, ovoid nucleus, while oligodendrocytes have a smaller, rounded, dark-staining nucleus. Quantitative estimates usually leave about ten to twenty percent of a glial cell population uncommitted as to type on the basis of routine preparations.[20] The *glial index* has some value in relating the number of glial cells to the number of nerve cells in a CNS nucleus. The ratio varies greatly, but averages from five to seven glial cells per nerve cell in most nuclei. In general, astrocytes are the dominant glial cell in gray matter, and oligodendrocytes are predominant in white matter. Oligodendroglia are however most numerous around both nerve cells and blood vessels in gray matter (*satellites*). With metallic stains both types of cells exhibit small granular deposits along their cytoplasmic substance (*gliosomes*). These are recognized as mitochondria under the electron microscope.

Astrocytes exist normally in two structurally different forms, *protoplasmic* and *fibrous.* The protoplasmic forms are fewer than the fibrous and appear throughout the gray matter. They attach to vessel walls by one or more processes known as *sucker feet* (Fig. 10-26). These extend in multiples to several vessels and have extensions beyond the vessel walls. Both by metallic staining and by EM the protoplasmic astrocyte exhibits meagre perinuclear cytoplasm and enormous numbers of thin, elongate, projecting cytoplasmic processes. These blend with the neuropil in thin, undulating, membranous extensions that relate to vessels, other astrocytes, and nerve cells. It is estimated that astrocytic processes account for forty to sixty percent of the total exposed cellular surface area in the neuropil. The proportion of vessel surface covered by

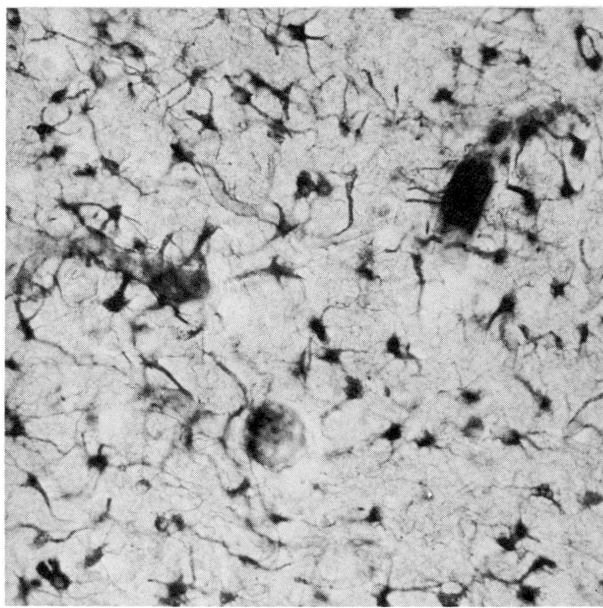

Fig. 10-26. Astrocytes with sucker-feet attachments to blood vessels.

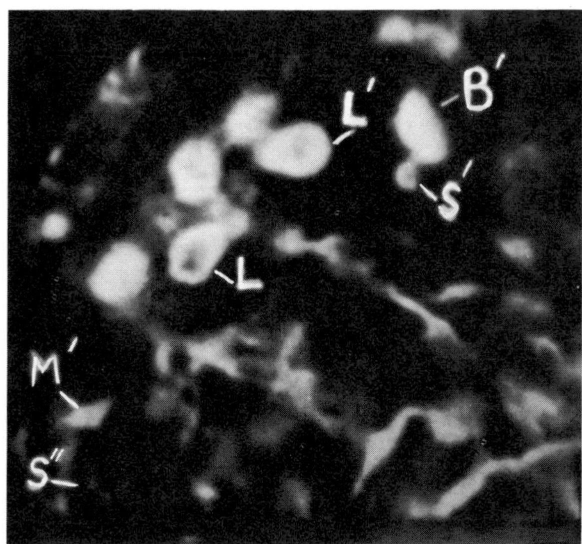

Fig. 10-27. Boutons in negative print to show density on cell surfaces. Letters refer to structural variations in silver preparations.

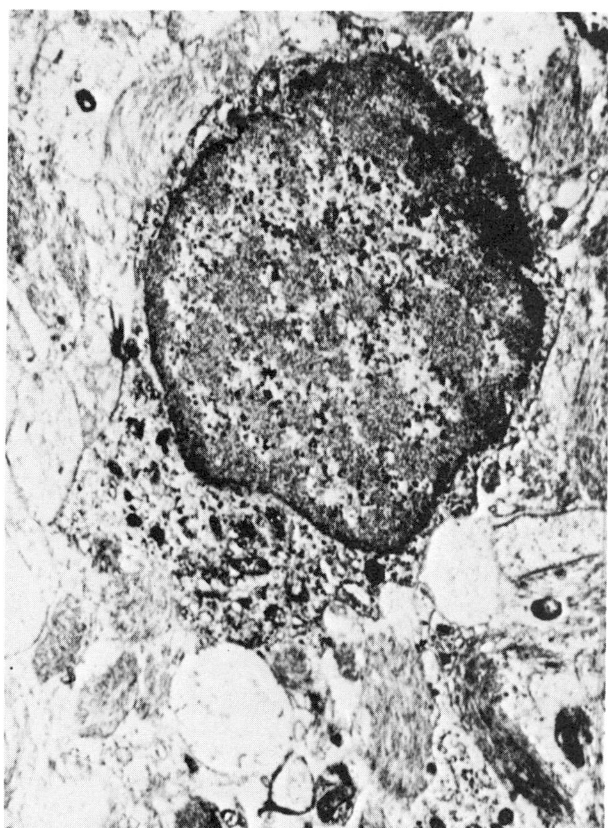

Fig. 10-28. Electron micrograph of astrocyte from astrocytic tumor (optic nerve glioma), showing character and density of processes. (From Minckler, J. In Anderson, W. A. D., editor: Pathology, ed. 5, St. Louis, 1966, The C. V. Mosby Co. Courtesy Sarah Luse.)

astrocytic extensions is considerable but variable. The same is true of astrocytic processes that come into relationship with neuronal surfaces. Of the perineuronal satellites, astrocytes are least important numerically in terms of their nuclei surrounding the nerve cell body. Their processes however cover a substantial surface area of the nerve cells and may provide a source of metabolic exchanges with the perikaryon and nerve processes.[17] Silver stains suggest that about fifty percent of nerve cell surface area may be engaged in bouton contact with other neurons (Fig. 10-27). Phase contrast would suggest somewhat the same occupancy by boutons. The remainder of the surface involves contact with glial processes, principally astrocytic, and with capillaries and occasional microglia (Fig. 14-6). It is possible to rearrange these proportions experimentally,[21] and possibly expansion and contraction of these contact points occur as physiologic excursions (also probably pathologically). The crowded surface relationships are undoubtedly influenced considerably in tissue hydration, wherein the astrocytic processes swell.

Protoplasmic astrocytes become fibrous by producing gliofibrils, the basic earmark of the astrocyte. Protoplasmic astrocytes are devoid of fibrils, in contrast to the other form, *fibrous astrocytes,* which are characterized by inclusion of gliofibrils and are the abundant member of the astrocyte family. With routine stains the two forms cannot be distinguished. With metallic stains the fibrous form is seen to possess fewer and thicker processes than the protoplasmic astrocytes. Fibrous astrocytes possess perinuclear cytoplasm that contains delicate fibrils, as do the branching processes. These cells concentrate in the subpial zone, the white matter, and the thalamus. As reactive cells, astrocytes form glial scars by deposition of gliofibrils and round up in plump forms called *gemistocytes* (fat astrocytes).

Electron microscopic characteristics of astrocytes are essentially the same for both fibrous and protoplasmic types, with the exception of inclusion of intracytoplasmic bundles of gliofibrils in the fibrous type. One outstanding feature is the widespread distribution of astrocytic processes in the neuropil. These possess lipochrome pigments, the nature of which is not established. The nuclei of astrocytes are large, pale, vesicular, and irregular in electron micrographs, as in histologic preparations (Fig. 10-28).

Oligodendrocytes (oligodendroglia, oligoglia, oligocytes) occur as *satellites to nerve cells* in gray matter, as *satellites to vessels* in both gray and white matter, and as *interfascicular supporting cells* in white matter (Fig. 10-29). They are the only glial structures, for example, in the corpus callosum, a purely "white" structure. The processes do not stain in routine preparations, and are relatively

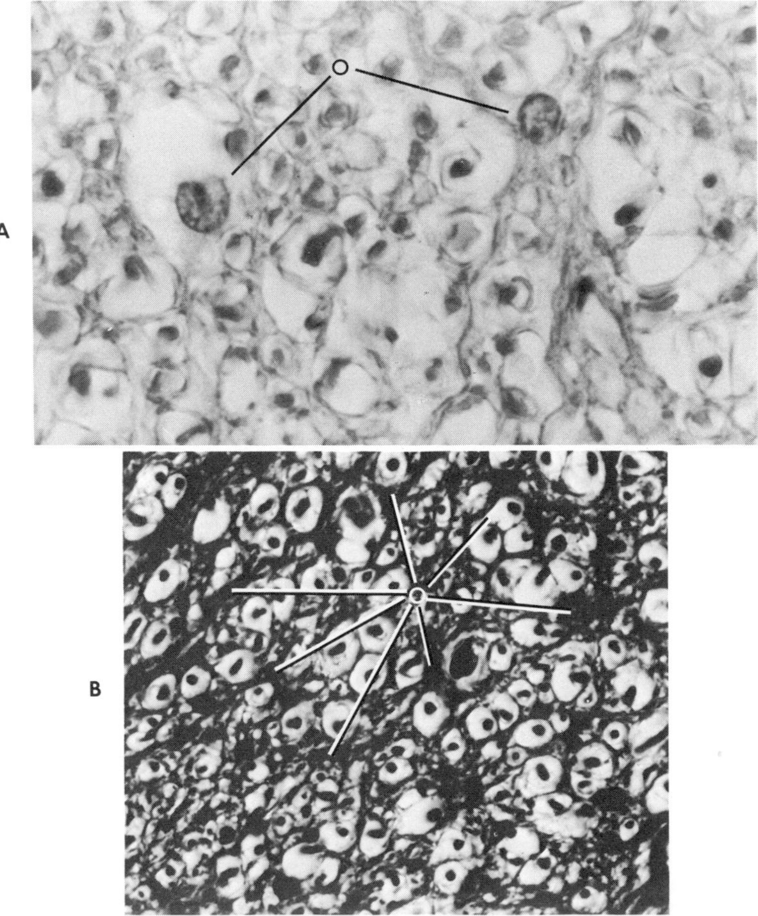

Fig. 10-29. A, Oligodendroglia (*O*) in proximal peripheral nerve (VIII) in H & E; **B,** in white column of cord with metallic stain. Note density with respect to number of fibers.

few in metallic impregnations (Fig. 10-22). It is common for oligodendroglial cells to swell in routine preparations of autopsy material. This swelling presents a halo effect about the dark-stained nucleus. Oligodendroglia are the most numerous neural cellular components in the CNS. They number about 70,000 per cu. mm. and represent more than fifty percent of glial elements in most nuclear areas and up to one hundred percent in some white areas. They extend into the roots of all nerves and provide the myelin wrapping for the nerve fibers outward as far as the glio-Schwannian junction (Obersteiner-Redlich zone) (Fig. 10-20). In a peripheral position they number approximately forty-four percent of the number of Schwann cells for the same volume of nerve. Their electron micrographic characteristics are subject to some variation, although they usually present an electron-dense nucleus with pale cytoplasm in which the ribonucleoprotein is dispersed (Fig. 10-30). This distinguishes them from astroyctes. At the time of myelination the cytoplasm is filled with microvesicles. In tissue cultures oligodendrocytes exhibit pulsatile action.[22]

Central myelin. It seems clear that central myelin is formed by wrappings of oligodendroglial cell membranes. The manner of formation and the relationship of the oligodendrocyte to the axis-cylinder is somewhat different from the pattern of peripheral myelin as developed from the Schwann cell membranes. Each oligodendroglial cell is associated with several or many axis-cylinders (Fig. 10-30). This is accomplished by pedunculated processes extending from the cell body, which expand distally into broad, flat membranes that are shaped like a paddle. The expanded parts provide the internodal myelin wrapping of the nerve fibers (Fig. 10-31). EM has established beyond question the existence of the nodes of Ranvier, which are bare areas of central nerve fibers equivalent to those of the peripheral system. Mesaxons in central myelin are multiple, and frequently numerous axons are incorporated in oligoglial walls by invagination (Fig. 10-31). The mechanisms of forming the myelin wrapping of central fibers is not clearly established.[9,30] The process may come about by rotation of the glial membrane around the axis, by fusion of membrane vesicles, or by rotation of the axon itself. Oligoglial membrane is also applied to vessels and to neuronal perikarya from the satellite relationship. Oligodendrocytes provide a fluid reservoir in their cytoplasmic mass and possibly in the folds of their cell membranes. The myelin of oligodendroglial origin is devoid of Lantermann incisures.

CNS degeneration and regeneration of myelin. The degenerating sequence in the CNS, insofar as myelin is concerned, when an axon is cut is very different from that in peripheral nerves. The nerve fiber distal to the damage will fragment and disappear by autolysis. The oligodendroglia also disappear, and the area of injury is filled with swarms

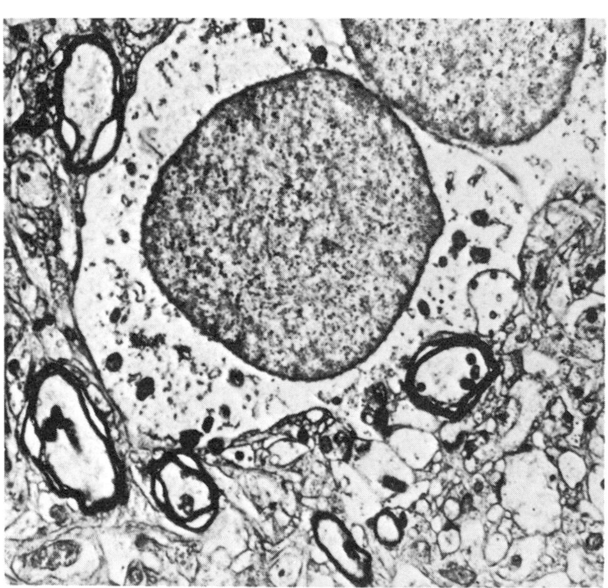

Fig. 10-30. Electron micrograph of oligodendroglial cell. Note multiple related, thinly myelinated axons.

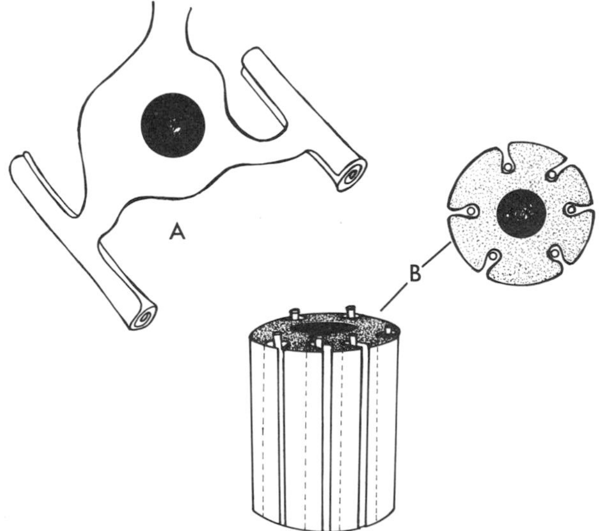

Fig. 10-31. Drawing of presumed relationship of heavy myelinated fibers, **A,** and nonmyelinated fibers, **B,** to oligodendroglia.

of microglia, which scavenge the cellular debris. There is frequently an abortive effort at regrowth by the neuron, but the growing tip encounters principally glial fibrils, which form a scar. Oligodendroglia are not mobilized and do not engulf the regrowing filaments in a manner paralleling the Schwann cell behavior. As a consequence, regrowth to physiologic recovery does not occur in destruction of CNS tissue (Figs. 14-3 and 14-4).[26]

Origin of neuroglia. A general histogenetic scheme for all neural components is shown in Fig. 10-1. As might be expected, the developmental sequence in the formation of the glia is controversial. While astrocytes and oligodendroglia are almost invariably presented together as the glial elements, it is apparent from the foregoing pages that the two are strikingly different in structure and function. This difference appears early in the embryonic neuroepithelium with the appearance of oligodendroglia delayed and concurring, as might be expected, with the onset of myelination. Astrocytes develop from a sequence of cellular differentiations arising in elongate cells that pull away from attachment to the lumen surface of the medullary tube. These are *spongioblasts,* which differentiate further by attaching to vessels and pia, the former supplying the sucker-foot process. This establishes the *astroblast,* which is the immediate stage before the *astrocyte* (Fig. 10-1). This series of developmental stages is recapitulated in the tumors of astrocytic origin and seems generally accepted among histologists. Glial fibrils appear in the circumnatal period. Spongioblasts are apparent in the early embryo, and differentiation to recognizable astrocytes is apparent by the fourth month.

The means of division of astrocytes remains unsettled. There is little question that they increase in number during reactions related to glial scarring. Mitoses have been observed,[23] but usually there is a striking lack of mitotic activity in these cells. This has forced the suggestion of amitotic division as part of the biologic capability of these cells. Because astrocytes are the least responsive cells in the CNS apart from nerve cells, it is possible that the increased number is more apparent than real in their density related to scars.

Oligodendroglia are not apparent as differentiated forms in the early embryo. In late embryonic life they appear as migrant forms taking up interfascicular and satellite positions related to both vessels and neurons. The immature forms are called *oligodendroblasts.* It is possible that they are derived from spongioblasts as needed for myelination, although at the time of their occurrence for myelination spongioblasts are little in evidence. Kernohan has suggested a closer relationship to ependyma for oligodendroglia on the basis of concurrence of tumors of these cellular types (Fig. 10-1) (see Chapter 9).[3]

EPENDYMA

The lining of the ventricular system and its interrelating ducts is made up an epithelial glial cellular

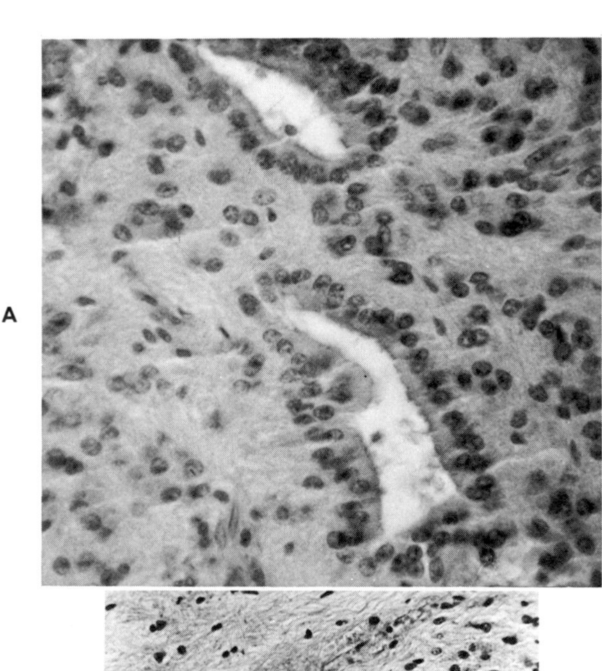

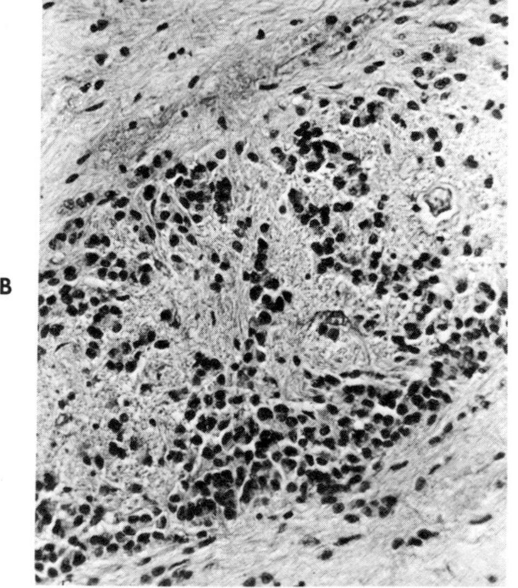

Fig. 10-32. A, Ependymal inclusions over white matter showing cilia and blepharoplasts. **B,** Ependymal hyperplasia (normal) with obliteration of central canal. (From Minckler, J. In Anderson, W. A. D., editor: Pathology, ed. 5, St. Louis, 1966, The C. V. Mosby Co.)

layer called *ependyma* (Fig. 10-10). Where lining covers white matter the cells are flattened, with nuclei widely spaced. By contrast, the ependyma overlying gray matter is cuboidal or columnar, with the nuclei close together. Hyperplasia of ependymal cells in the lower cord of adults contributes to normal obliteration of the central canal (Fig. 10-32, *B*). Even in the adult the ependyma sometimes retains *cilia,* particularly in fresh material. *Blepharoplasts* (Fig. 10-32, *A*) are remnants of cilia (basal bodies) that are retained in the cell after the cilia are lost. Ependyma is tied to the underlying brain substance through a subependymal *glial fiber layer* in which the fibers generally parallel the surface. The fiber layer arises in the underlying *subependymal cell layer* made up of fibrous astrocytes and transitional cells, which are probably ependymal in origin.[40] The subependymal zone is largely avascular. EM reveals a surface brush border (cuticle) made up of short microvilli as well as projecting cilia, with the typical nine pairs of filaments disposed peripherally around a central pair (Fig. 10-33). A zonula occludens occurs near the terminal bar area of adjacent ependymal cells, and zonula adhaerens plaques are common (Fig. 8-3).

Tennyson and Pappas[40] have classified the ependymal cells as *flattened, cubic or cylindric,* and *pseudostratified or multilayered.* The flattened type characteristically is applied to white matter. The cells have few cilia and microvilli. The cell borders have prominent interdigitations. Such areas are almost devoid of subependymal fibers and cell layers. The cubic and cylindric forms cover gray matter. The cell boundaries are straight, and processes extend from the basal surface into the subependymal fibrous layer. Pseudostratified and multilayered ependyma is rare in the adult (near the taenia choroidea, in the lateral recess of the fourth ventricle, in the aqueduct, and in part of the floor of the third and fourth ventricles). The multilayered pattern is typical however of embryo and newborn ventricular linings. A cell of special interest is the *tanycyte,* a stretched-out ependymal element of some species (rabbit, mouse) that occurs in multilayered linings. The tanycyte contains distended cisterns of endoplasmic reticulum and probably serves as an agent for transmitting substances from CSF to subependymal vessels. The staining characteristics permit these cells to be confused with neuroblasts. In migrant form in a subependymal position they resemble oligodendroblasts, which indeed they might be. Another cellular variant in the ependymal layer is the ependymal astrocyte, which sometimes is subependymal in position.

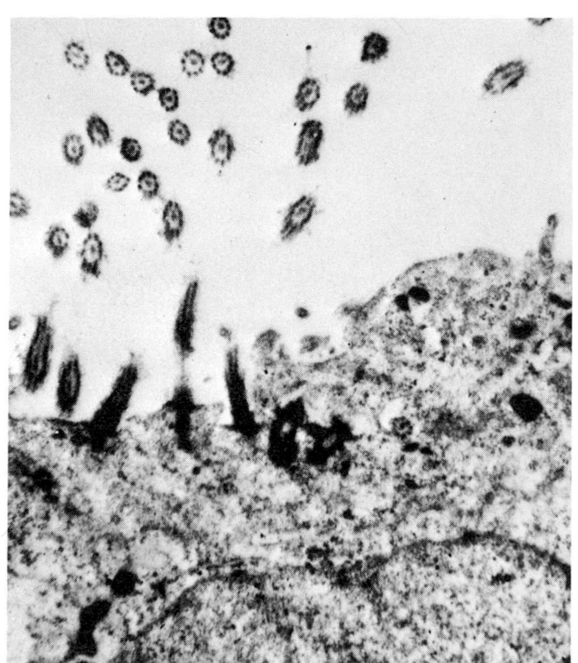

Fig. 10-33. Electron micrograph of ependymal cell with cilia and blepharoplasts.

Two special ependymal areas merit special note: *subcommissural organ* and *area postrema.* The subcommissural organ is an area of specialized ependyma underlying the posterior commissure in many animals. It appears in the human fetus but disappears circumnatally. The specialized cells connect by processes to blood vessels. In some forms the structure elaborates a secretion that forms a fiber extending into the aqueduct (*Reissner's fiber*). The subcommissural organ may take part in salt and water metabolism.[40] In the area postrema (the posterior limiting ridge of the fourth ventricle, adjacent to the ala cinerea) the ependymal zone is distinguished by inclusion of sinusoid vessels that transfer usually nondispersable substances into the parenchyma.

Because the ependyma represents the most epithelial-like substance of the nervous tissues and delimits fluid-filled cavities, it has special importance in its side-to-side junctions. These are both *tight junctions* (zonula occludens) and *intermediate junctions* (zonula adhaerens). The tight junctions occur near the terminal bar area with zonula occludens adjacent, often on both sides (Fig. 8-3). Intraventricular injected particulate material (ferritin) does not penetrate the intercellular gap beyond the zonula occludens, which is therefore regarded as a watertight seal. The limiting functions pertaining to exchanges of fluids and solutes through ependyma vary with the structural character of the membrane.

CHOROID PLEXUS

The choroid plexus represents a combination of ependyma-like epithelium, vascular tufts, and pia-arachnoid arranged in branched, villous processes (Fig. 10-34). The plexuses invaginate the ventricles in the patterns with gross configurations as outlined in Chapter 3 for lateral, third, and fourth ventricular cavities. The core carries arteriovenous anastomoses that bear on the control of the blood supply to the capillary networks underlying the epithelium. The blood supply to the choroid of the lateral ventricle is through the choroidal arteries (anterior and posterior), which anastomose freely. The choroid of the third ventricle is supplied by the posterior choroidal artery, and that of the fourth ventricle by a branch from the posterior inferior cerebellar arteries. Drainage is via the internal cerebral veins for the lateral and third ventricular choroid plexuses, and through the posterior median vein for the fourth ventricular plexus. Innervation is known to arise in cervical sympathetic ganglia and extends to the plexuses via carotid branches. These nerves undoubtedly go to vessel walls. Other nerves of possible vagal nuclear origin and from nucleus ambiguus (Benedikt's thirteenth nerve), may supply connective tissue and even the epithelium.[40]

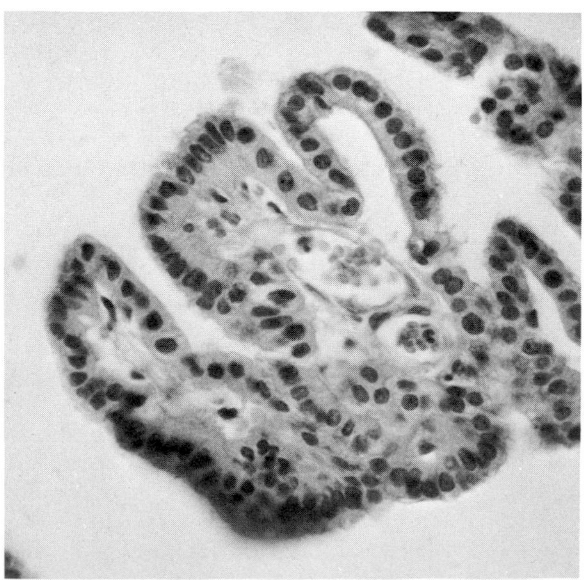

Fig. 10-34. Choroid plexus.

Choroid arises in the embryo in a thin *choroid epithelial lamina.* Richly vascularized pia-arachnoid becomes associated with this lamina in forming the *tela choroidea,* which expands into the ventricles as the choroidal tufts. They form first during the second fetal month in the fourth ventricle, followed by their appearance in the lateral ventricles, and then the third. The plexus epithelium is at first pseudostratified and limited to a simple fold of the neural tube (in the six-week-old embryo). At eight weeks the growth is exuberant, and the plexuses fill the ventricles. The size of the choroid gradually decreases in proportion to the size of the ventricles. The final proportion is reached in the fourth month as the cells begin to resemble the adult form. Glycogen is specially abundant in early choroid epithelium (before the fourth month) and is thought to play a nutritive role as a source of glucose in the fetal nervous system. Glycogen is still present in volume in the newborn.[40] It disappears in the adult.

Histology

The cuboidal adult cells of choroid epithelium possess the prominent surface folding of secreting epithelia. These occur as apical microvilli, which produce a brush border. Fetal cells have far less complex surfaces (Fig. 10-35). Cilia are present and attach to blepharoplasts that lie adjacent to the brush border. The role of the cilia in fluid movements is unknown but probably is a factor to be considered.[22] The lateral borders and interfaces between cells are quite straight toward the surface and more interdigitated toward the base. In the terminal bar region there is a tight junction (zonula occludens), which produces membrane fusion density at that point and obstructs passage of large molecules in the intercellular gap (Fig. 10-35). The gaps in the areas of interdigitation concentrate transport enzymes and no doubt play a significant role in the fluid production of the choroid plexus. The basal area of choroid is only slightly folded and lies adjacent to a basement membrane of approximately 1,000 Å thickness.[40] The cells possess rounded vesicular nuclei that contain one or more nucleoli.

The choroid cells often appear vacuolated under the light microscope. The vacuoles probably represent artifactual gaps induced by solvents in preparation. The cytoplasm is stuffed with pinocytotic vesicles, droplets, organelles, granules, and pigments. Pinocytotic vesicles are numerous and undoubtedly play a significant role in fluid transport in choroid cells. Electron micrographs display *mitochondria,* which are presumed to provide the energy for transport activity. *Ribonucleoprotein* exists as particles of about 150 Å, some of which attach to endoplasmic reticulum. This unit membrane is relatively sparse in choroid cells, as might be expected where secretory activity is directed mainly to water rather than protein. A *Golgi complex* exists in a supranuclear position. Its function in the choroid is not known. Dense bodies (*microbodies*) occur in the choroid as membrane-bound ovals with electron-dense granules in them. Some exhibit inclusion of microvesicles (*multivesicular bodies*). Both microbodies and multivesicular bodies appear experimentally to segregate foreign particles. They are regarded as *lysosomes.* Pigment granules and lipid droplets also occur in choroid epithelium (Fig. 10-35). The pia-arachnoid of the choroidal core is loosely arranged and commonly is represented by only a few collagen strands in the small villi. Usually reticulin, a few macrophages, and fibrocytes can be discerned in the cores of bulkier villi. Arterioles are not distinctive among intracerebral vessels and are relatively thin-walled. Veins exhibit marked distention and are especially cavernous in the plexus of the confluent part of the lateral ventricles (*glomus*) (Figs. 3-3 and 4-19). The selective transport characteristics of the vascular bed, the epithelium, and basement membrane probably contribute to the blood-CSF barrier phenomenon.

NEURON

The *neuron,* or *nerve cell,* is the conductive cellular unit making up the neural parenchyma. Perhaps more than any other cell, neurons are

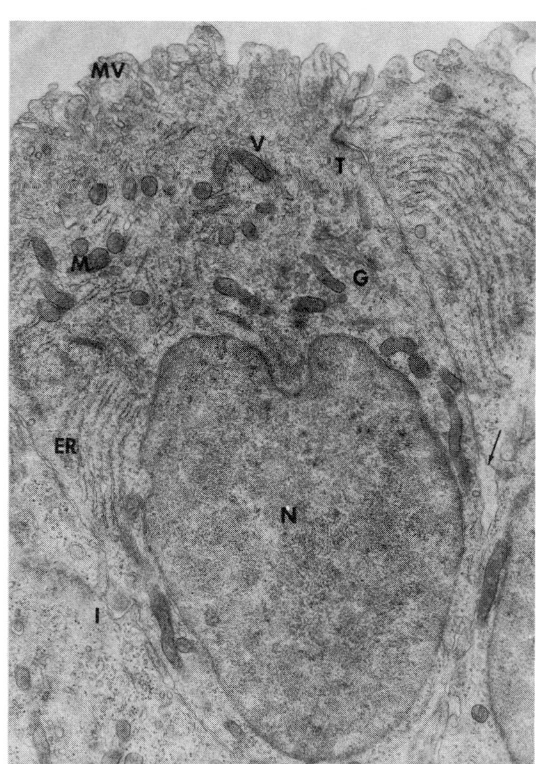

Fig. 10-35. Electron micrograph of choroid cell (from rabbit embryo). *N,* Nucleus; *MV,* microvilli; *T,* terminal bar junction; *M,* mitochondria; *G,* Golgi complex; *ER,* endoplasmic reticulum; *V,* vesicles; *I,* infolding, or interdigitation; arrow, cleft of fine, flocculent materials in intercellular gap substance. (From Tennyson, V. M., and Pappas, G. D. In Minckler, J., editor: Pathology of the nervous system, vol. I, New York, 1968, McGraw-Hill Book Co.)

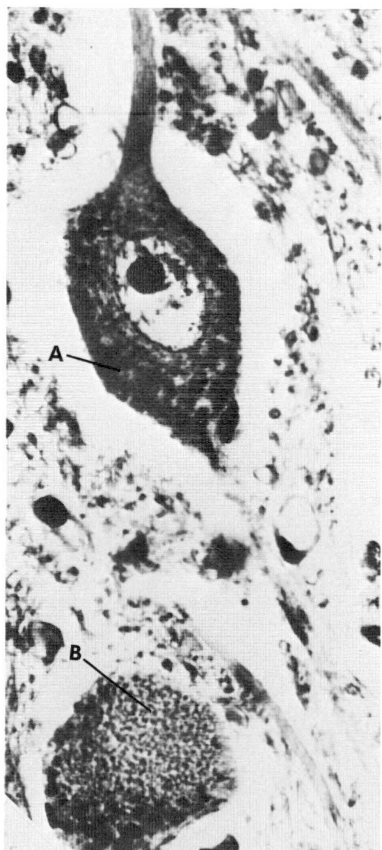

Fig. 10-36. Neurons showing coarse Nissl clumping, **A,** and inclusion of lipofuscin, **B.** (H & E.)

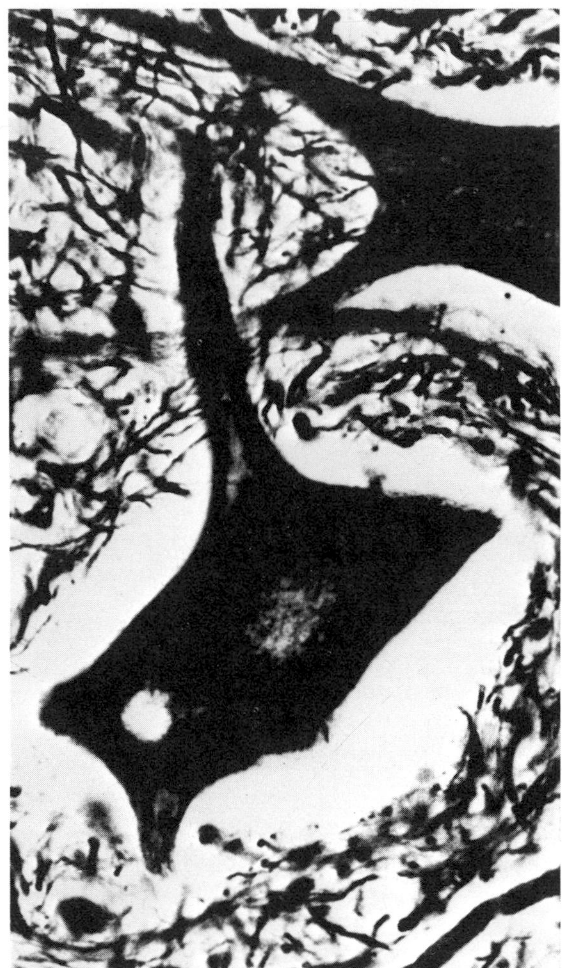

Fig. 10-37. Silver stained neurons and neuropil. Perineuronal spaces are artifactual.

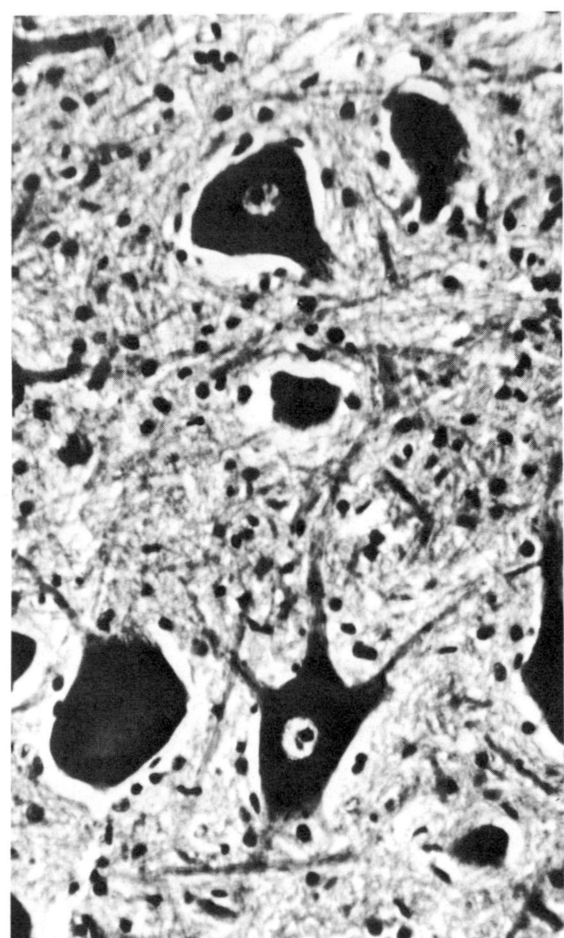

Fig. 10-38. Prototype large, multipolar neurons in anterior spinal nucleus. (H & E.)

enormously varied in size (from a few microns to more than two meters) and in shape (single processes to dozens of varying thickness). Each neuron is made up of four components that subserve rather specific functions: *cell body* (perikaryon), *dendrites* (dendritic zone), *axon* (axis-cylinders), and *terminals* (axonic telodendria) (Fig. 1-4).

Cell body

The *cell body,* or *perikaryon,* is the trophic center of the entire cell. In it there are a nucleus and its membrane, a large nucleolus within the nucleus, and cytoplasmic organoids of many types, which govern cellular activity. Chromidial clumps (Nissl substance) are common in the cytoplasm. The above features, seen with hematoxylin and eosin and Nissl stains, characterize nerve cells and distinguish them from the other elements in the nervous tissues (Fig. 10-36). Metallic impregnations display fibrils within the perikaryon, which also serves to distinguish the cells under the light microscope (Fig. 10-37). The cell bodies vary from a few microns in diameter (microneurons, such as granule cells in the cerebellum) to a hundred or more microns in maximum dimension (Betz cells in cerebral cortex, and final-common-path neurons in the spinal cord). The cell body may be placed along the axon, close to the dendritic zone, or offset from the axon (Fig. 1-4). In cells possessing a body close to the dendritic zone the usual configuration is multibranched, with numerous dendrites projecting from the cell surface. This *multipolar* pattern typifies the central neuronal silhouette in the CNS (Figs. 10-38 and 10-39). When the cell bodies are some distance

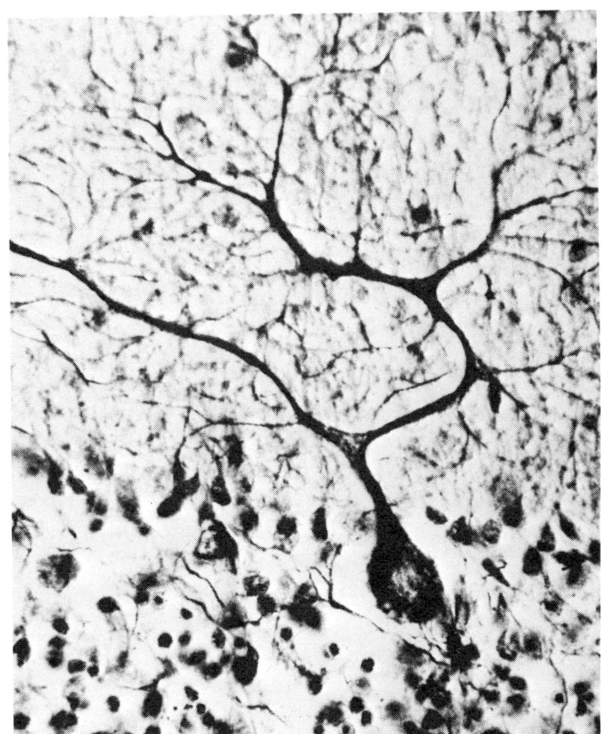

Fig. 10-39. Dendritic pattern of Purkinje cell.

along the axon, they interrupt the contour as thick fusiform enlargements, known as *bipolar* cells (Fig. 1-4). This configuration characterizes the ganglion cells of the cochlear and vestibular nerves. In other sensory ganglion cells and in the mesencephalic nucleus of cranial nerve V the cell bodies are offset from the axon and attach to it by a single fiber. This forms the *unipolar* cell (Fig. 1-4). A substantial number of variations that do not fit any of these types occur. Olfactory neurons utilize the cell body extremity itself as a chemoreceptor. Bipolar retinal cells are anaxonic, and amacrine cells of the retina possess cell bodies that are partially offset (see Chapters 17 and 20). Polarity in the cells arises by virtue of reception of the nervous impulse at one side (toward the dendritic zone) and emission of the impulse toward the axon. In cells such as bipolar and unipolar cells the limb of the neuron between dendritic zone and cell body can be very long. It is still referred to as axon or axis-cylinder, although the direction of the impulse is toward the cell body.

Cell membranes of neurons in electron micrographs display *subsurface cisterns,* whose functions are uncertain, but they may play a part in impulse generation. The membrane itself has three layers of 25Å each, two electron-dense laminae separated by a lighter central zone (the unit membrane). *Endoplasmic reticulum* exists in both granular and smooth forms. *Ribosomes* are both free in the matrix and attached to endoplasmic reticulum as *ribonucleoprotein granules* (RNP) (Fig. 8-6). The RNP and endoplasmic reticulum provide the clumped material that stains as Nissl substance (Fig. 10-36). This chromidial substance in the cytoplasm of nerve cells varies in appearance and density from CNS nucleus to nucleus. It is most prominent in the large motoneurons, and in this location it is most reliable in displaying *chromatolysis.* This is a dispersion, peripheralization, and disappearance of Nissl substance in a cell body after section of its axon (Fig. 14-1). Chromatolysis is of experimental value in detecting the parent cell of a severed axon and has been enormously helpful in locating nuclei of origin (see Chapter 14).[5] The *Golgi apparatus* is made up of smooth endoplasmic reticulum in the form of vesicles and flattened cisterns. The cytoplasmic membrane systems are related to protein secretion and storage, neurosecretions, and enzyme activity.[35]

Mitochondria within neuronal cytoplasm are small and round to oval, with delicate cristae. By contrast they are elongate in axons and dendrites. Mitochondria are recognized as energy-generating agents through their production of oxidative enzymes. *Neurofilaments* (neurofibrils) can be demonstrated within cell bodies by metallic staining. They appear to increase in density with age and under stimulation with alumina gel. EM establishes their existence beyond question, not only in the perikaryon but also in axons and dendrites. A relationship of neurofibrils to microtubules has been suggested.[21] The function of these filaments remains obscure. *Microtubules* occur in the perikaryon as well as in the axon. They may be formed from neurofibrils and probably take part in transport and fluid movement. *Multivesicular bodies* occur in the cytoplasm. Their function is unknown. *Centrioles* have been identified in neuroblasts and in nerve cells of lower forms.[39] Since mature neurons in the adult are permanently, wholly postmitotic, it is not surprising that centrioles are inapparent. *Lysosomes* are pigment bodies that appear to be closely related to, or identical to, lipofuscin. The material accumulates with age. Lysosomes appear to house hydrolytic enzymes, which participate in intracellular digestion and contribute to lysis of the content of phagosomes. It is probable that lysosomes act as organelles in young forms and that part of their constituents become inclusions with age.

Numerous *inclusions* are identifiable in nerve cell body cytoplasm. *Glycogen* occurs as particulate masses of from 200 to 400 Å. The inclusions are PAS positive under the light microscope. *Pigment* inclusions (*neuromelanin*) occur in the cells of substantia nigra and locus caeruleus. The chemical nature of this cerebral melanin-like pigment remains unknown. Metabolic activity related to it is altered in some diseases, such as Parkinson's and Wilson's diseases. *Lipofuscin* has been mentioned in connection with lysosomes, and the two are somehow closely related. The pigment appears in nerve cells in early middle age and accumulates with time. It is yellow-brown in hematoxylin and eosin preparations and frequently distends the cytoplasmic mass (Fig. 10-36). The physiologic effect, if any, is not known. Many inclusions in the form of vacuoles, fragments, crystals, laminated bodies, lipids, filaments, and virus particles appear within the cytoplasm in pathologic circumstances.[23]

The *nucleus* of the neuron is housed in the nuclear membrane, or envelope. This displays pores at which nucleoplasm and cytoplasm appear to be confluent. Some pores possess a single-layered cover, the diaphragm. In general the chromatin of the neuronal nucleus is slightly clumped, but great variation occurs depending on size and location. In cells with abundant Nissl substance the nucleolus tends to be large, and at the same time the nuclear limiting membrane. The nucleus of mature neurons apparently functions only as the protein template (DNA) and the nucleolus as some sort of carrier in transferring DNA makeup to protein synthesis in the cytoplasm (RNA) (see Chapter 8). The usual nuclear function of chromosomal orientation and division in the reproductive cycle is absent. The last of the dividing cells in the neuronal family is the neuroblast, and its production generally ceases by the time of birth.

The perikaryon thus must be regarded as the metabolic center of the cell in the adult and the center of growth for its processes in the embryo. The transport mechanisms of its membranes, whether by diffusion or active, are poorly understood. The role of the perikaryon in impulse generation, transfer, and maintenance is probably minimal or nonexistent. The weight of cell body importance as a trophic center is implicit in the overall cell death resulting from destruction of the perikaryon. The cell body undoubtedly governs regrowth following destruction of its processes (see Chapter 9).

Dendritic zone

The *dendritic zone* is functionally the receptive field of the neuron. The individual *dendrites* are processes that project from the cell body or axon and taper into fibrillar terminations. They also possess stubby branches, the *dendritic spines*. By definition the dendritic processess and zone represent the field that receives impulses from other neurons and transmits impulses toward the cell body. This definition applies for most neurons of the CNS. However, in many peripheral cells (such as sensory ganglion cells) the receiving limb or dendritic zone of the cell is decidedly remote from the body, and the impulse is already aggregated into the axonic conducting mechanism before the cell body is reached. This isolates perikaryon from the impulse-conducting and generating mechanism. On structural grounds this elongate fiber (frequently several feet) carrying impulses toward the cell body represents an axon from which the cell body is offset. The point at which the diverse dendritic branches are assembled into a single fiber is the start of the axonic zone (Fig. 1-4).

Dendrites, as ramifying extensions of cell bodies, account for more than eighty percent of the total cell surface (amounting to more than 50,000 square microns) in the larger cells of the spinal cord. This percentage varies to less than thirty percent in some small internuncial cells. Of the total surface, from

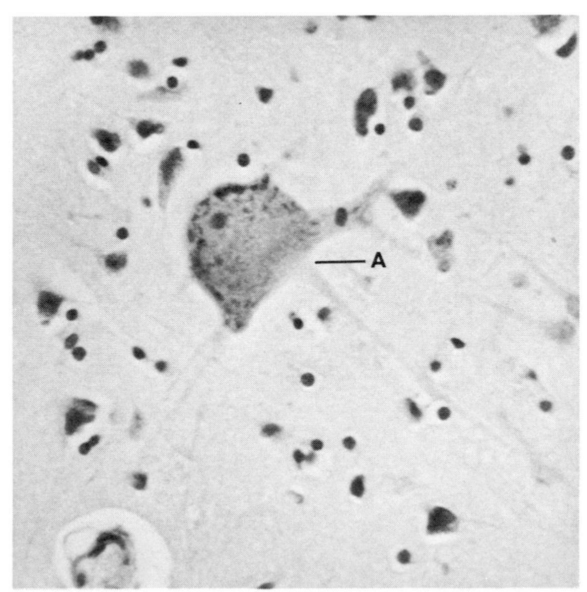

Fig. 10-40. Betz cell. Note clear axon hillock (*A*). (H & E ×500.)

twenty-five to fifty-five percent is engaged in synaptic contact, and in this the dendrites play the greatest quantitative role. Dendrites contain RNP granules, although Nissl substance is not conspicuous beyond a few microns distant from the cell body. Mitochondria are few, although they do exist, and those present seem to be structurally different from mitochondria in the perikaryon and axon. The characterizing feature of the dendrite in electron micrographs is the neurotubule. The tubules are longitudinally oriented and appear as vesicles in cross section with diameters of 200Å. Neurofibrils are also demonstrable in dendrites.[23]

The structural configurations of dendrites are remarkably diverse (Fig. 10-36 to 10-43). The various types of receptors that serve as dendritic zones in environmental contact are reviewed in Chapters 16 to 20. The types of receptors related to other neurons by synapses include every conceivable pattern of ramification and density. The common variants include the following patterns. (1) Motoneurons (Fig. 10-38) possess dendrites in which the processes are tapering and branching in all planes. (2) Those of Clark's column have a thick base and are club-shaped, with the cell body representing the knob. (3) The dendrites of the large cortical neurons project long distances from the pyramidal apex and possess numerous spines (Fig. 10-40). (4) Those of internuncial, or connecting, neurons are stellate in pattern. Purkinje cells display remarkably widespread arborization in a single plane oriented across the folia (Fig. 10-39). These variations are adapted to the receptive requirements of the interneuronal patterns involved. (For structural details see Chapters 21 and 22.)

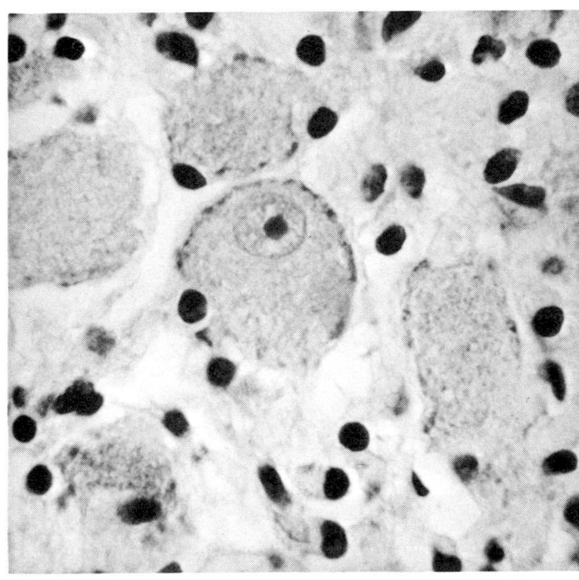

Fig. 10-42. Sympathetic ganglion cell. (H & E ×1,250.)

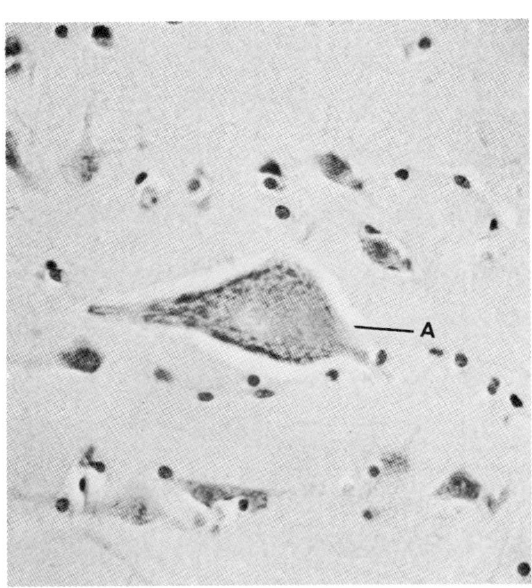

Fig. 10-41. External pyramidal cell of area 4. Note axon (*A*) arising from dendrite root. (H & E ×320.)

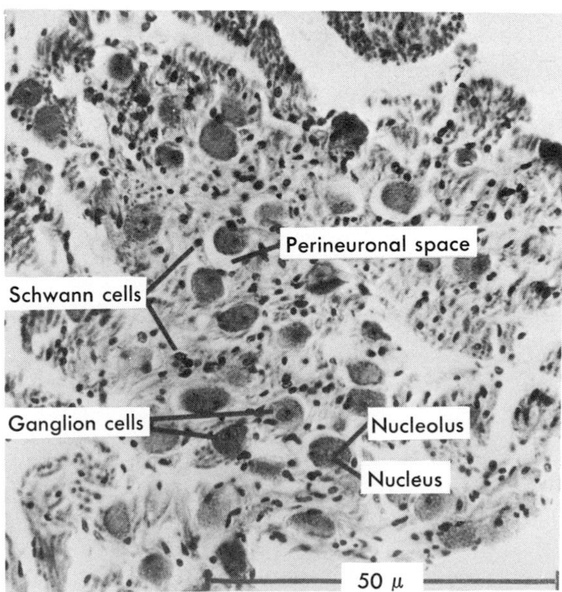

Fig. 10-43. Sensory ganglion cells (nerve VIII). Note that axons of bipolar cells do not show in H & E section.

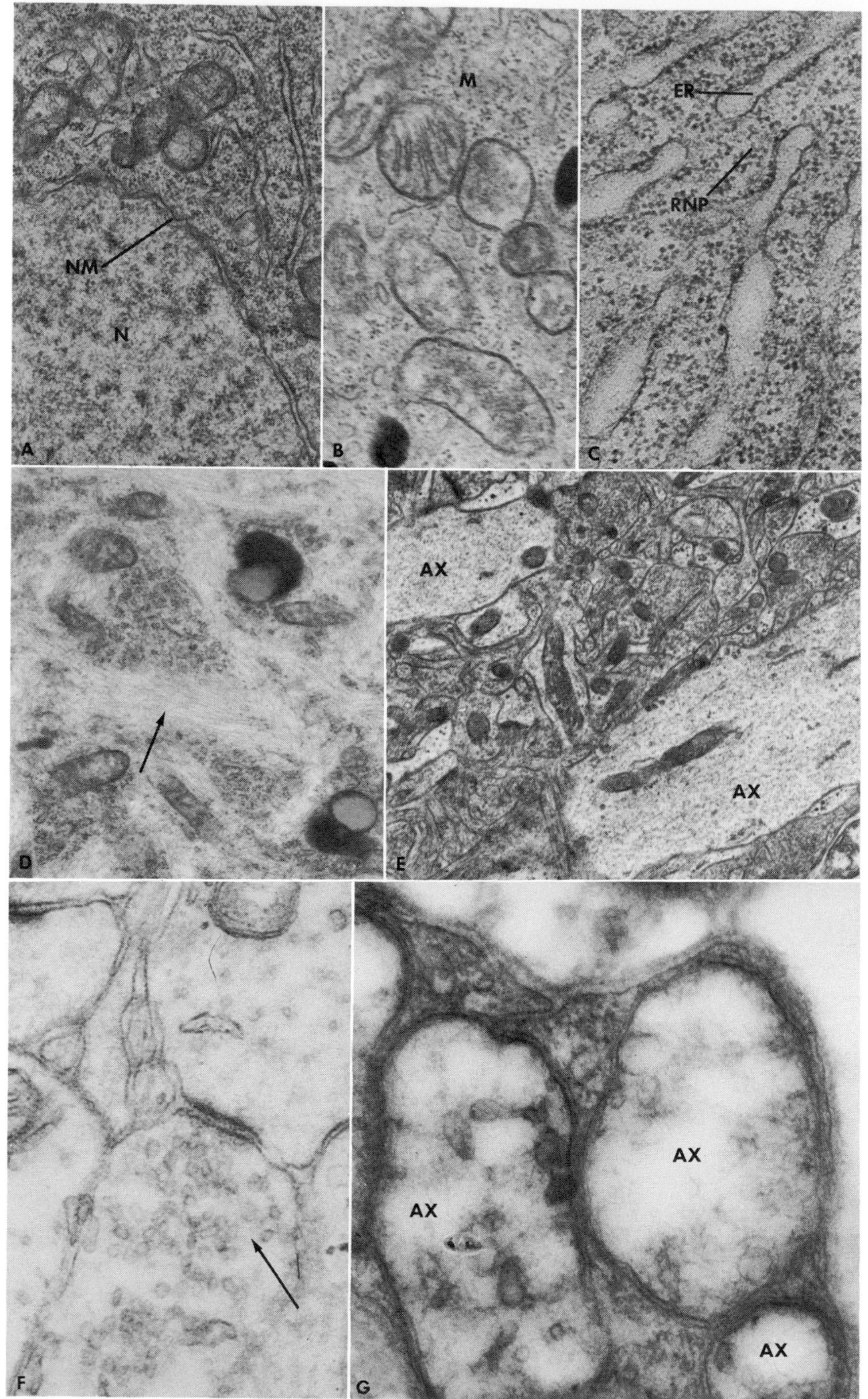

Fig. 10-44. Electron micrographs of neurons. **A,** Nucleus (*N*); trilaminar nuclear membrane (*NM*); **B,** mitochondria; **C,** endoplasmic reticulum (*ER*) and RNP granules; **D,** neurofibrils in cytoplasm; **E,** axons of varying size in neuropil; **F,** bouton terminals; **G,** axis-cylinders (unmyelinated in multiples within a Schwann cell). (Composite from Luse, S., and Hager, H. In Minckler, J., editor: Pathology of the nervous system, vol. I, New York, 1968, McGraw-Hill Book Co.)

The dendritic zone is functionally oriented to stimulus reception, with the stimuli arriving from other neurons by various means (see Chapter 14).[14] This type of input is *synaptic,* in contrast to *receptor* input, which is impressed by various stimuli (such as heat, radiation, mechanical stimulation) through environmental contact. In either case the input mechanism operates as a transducer by which the energy applied to the dendritic zone is converted to an electropotential relating to the dendritic zone membrane. This generates the nerve impulse to follow in the axon. The dendritic zone thus functions not only as a stimulus-receiving area, but also in electrogenesis of the axonic impulse. The electrogenetic phenomenon in the receptive zone in response to the various excitants is graded in proportion to the character and quantity of the stimulus. Stimulation of the dendritic zone therefore does not necessarily produce an axonic impulse. Such stimulation can in fact even inhibit the axonic response (see Chapters 13 and 15).[14]

Axon

The *axon* is a single process of the neuron, which conducts the nervous impulse away from the dendritic zone. In the synaptic neurons of the CNS the common arrangement is an elongate extension arising from the cell body and branching at varying distances from its origin. In the sensory neurons of receptor type the axon begins at the point of assembly of the dendritic processes into a single strand. The related perikaryon may be inserted in the axonic course, as in nerve VIII ganglia (bipolar), or it may be offset from the course, as in general sensory neurons (unipolar) (Fig. 1-4). The axon is of uniform diameter and is related to an oligodendroglial covering in the CNS and to a Schwann cell covering in the peripheral system. The distal extremity of the axon ordinarily subdivides into branches leading to nerve terminals (*telodendria*), which end in relationship to other nerve cells (Fig. 1-4). In final-common-path neurons the terminals are represented by special endings in muscles or glands (see Chapter 22).

The axon possesses a surface membrane (axolemma), which is continuous with the plasma membrane of the parent cell body. The central substance is the axoplasm, which is continuous with the cytoplasm of the nerve cell. The attachment to the cell body is however usually quite narrow and bases on the pale pyramidal structure, the axon hillock (Fig. 10-40). Occasionally the hillock arises from a dendritic root (Fig. 10-41). The hillock and axon are seen under the light microscope to be free of Nissl substance (ribosomes in electron micrographs), in contrast to dendritic roots. The axon contains elongate mitochondria, which are distinctive, and both neurotubules and neurofilaments (Fig. 10-44). The filaments vary from 70 to 100 Å, and the tubules from 200 to 300 Å, in diameter. Some vesicles occur in the axoplasm. These may be derived from the tubular systems. The interrelationships among filaments, tubules, and vesicles are not yet established with certainty. It is possible that the filaments enter into the structural makeup of the tubules. The neurotubules may participate in axoplasmic flow and give rise to vesicles, particularly near the terminals.[21,42] The axoplasm displays a movement (axoplasmic flow) that may account for transport from the trophic center in the perikaryon to the terminals of the branching axon. There is opposing flow of particulate material along the axon; this implies exchange transport along the axis-cylinder.[17]

The relationship of axons to myelin sheaths has been reviewed for both central and peripheral nerves. As stated previously, branching collaterals arise at the nodes of Ranvier in both central and peripheral situations. The covering of the axon hillock is by basal membrane, in the same way as covering at the nodes. The base of the axon has been described as the *initial segment* by Bodian[4] and represents the position where the *all-or-none* or

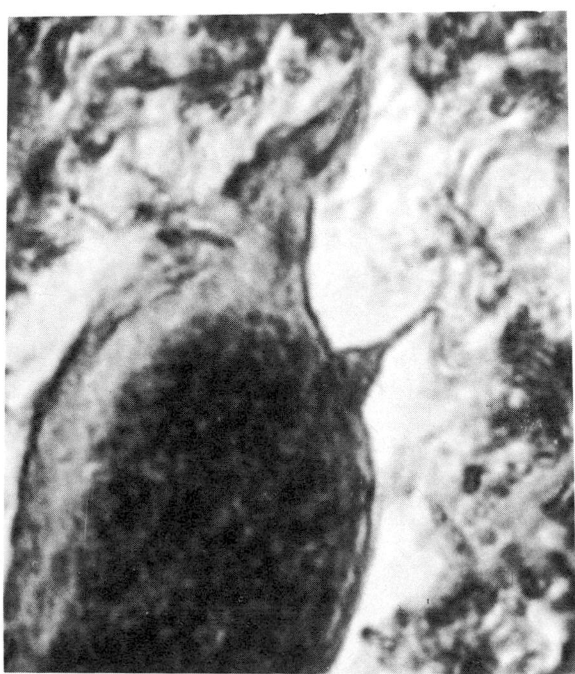

Fig. 10-45. Bouton on cell membrane. Cajal block silver.

spike potential is initiated as the neural impulse. The remainder of the axon constitutes the *conducting* part, in which the self-propagating action potential is carried to the nerve terminals (see Chapter 15).[4]

Nerve terminals

The nerve *terminals* (*axonic telodendria*) represent the terminal arborizations of the axon. They fall into the following three general categories: (1) those ending in neuronal synapses, (2) those ending in muscle or glands as specific stimulating structures, and (3) those elaborating neurohumoral substances that affect distant cells (neurohormones). (For a review of the latter two types of terminals see Chapter 22.)

The synaptic type endings occur both centrally and in peripheral ganglia. The connecting patterns at the synapse are dependent upon the location of the contiguous contact points and are designated by this arrangement. *Axodendritic* synapses are those with contiguity between axon terminals and dendrites. *Asosomatic* junctions occur between axon terminals and cell body (Fig. 10-45). *Axoaxonic* junctions are those formed when an axon terminal abuts against another axon. This last type is probably inhibitory in function (Fig. 10-46).

The synaptic terminals related to a single cell number from a few individual endings to several thousand, dependent upon the size of the cell, the diversity of its feeding circuits, and the function it subserves (Fig. 10-46). The great structural variations apparent with the light microscope (Fig. 10-28) have become meaningless in the face of greater clarity rendered by the electron microscope. The commonest ending in the CNS is the *bouton* (button, knob, endfoot) (Fig. 10-4, *A*). These may be terminal or occur as expanded contact plates (en passant) along the course of a terminal filament. The bouton is distinguished in electron micrographs by the general shape of a distended knob containing *synaptic vesicles* (microvesicles), a density of *mitochondria,* and an electron-dense thickened membrane (*presynaptic membrane*), which is a plaque on the presynaptic side of the *synaptic cleft* (Fig. 10-44). Bodian has ascribed excitatory or inhibitory functions to synapses, dependent upon the character and size of the synaptic vesicles.[4] It is probable that the synaptic vesicles contain a transmitter substance that is liberated into the synaptic cleft through the presynaptic membrane at the time a neural impulse reaches the bouton (Fig. 10-46). It is presumed that this transmitter substance (when excitatory) stimulates the *post-*

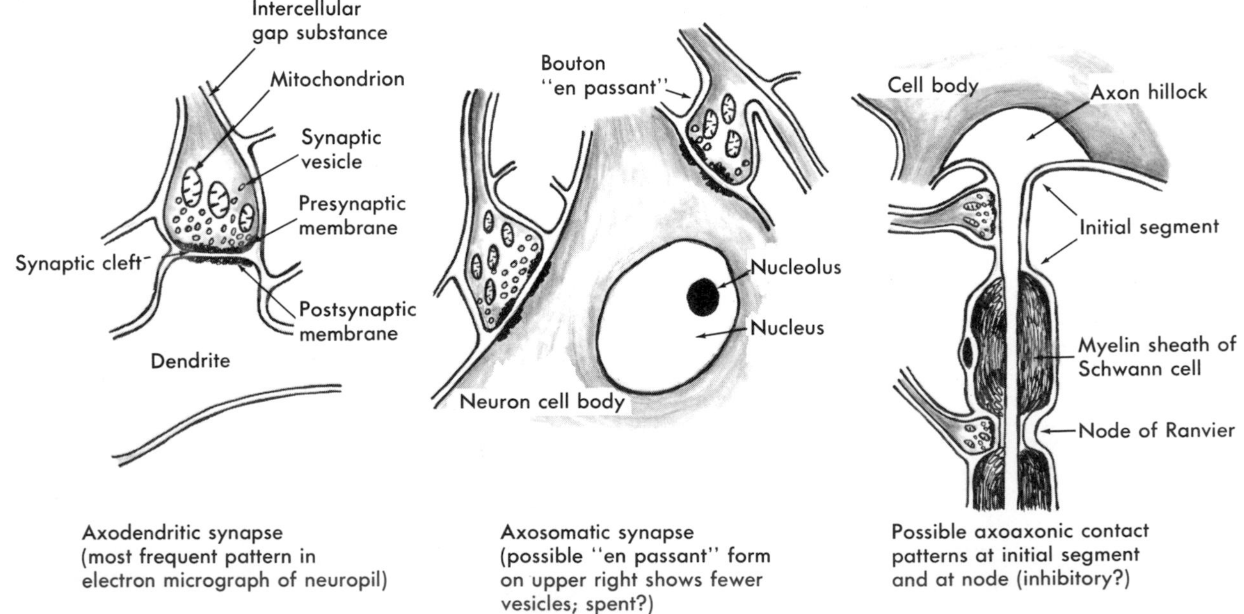

Fig. 10-46. Types and locations of nerve terminals (boutons), and change in structure with physiologic activity.

synaptic membrane with a response that contributes to the electrogenesis of the ensuing neuronal discharge in the nerve contacted.*

NEUROPIL

The *neuropil* is the unbelievably intricate and complex interlacing and interdigitating mass of glial fibers, dendrites, axons, and vessels of gray matter (nuclei) apart from the cell bodies themselves. Estimates suggest that the neuropil accounts for about 94 percent of nuclear tissue volume.[20] It is almost impossible to identify each of the components with a light microscope (Fig. 10-37) except with special stains that display individual cellular entities usually alone with background unstained. Dendrites can be detected in electron micrographs by their microtubules (Fig. 10-44); axons by their elongate mitochondria, neurofilaments, and neurotubules; and glial structures by their fibrils and cytoplasmic characteristics. Of particular interest in the neuropil is the intercellular space or gap substance, which has been established by EM in no greater volume than four to seven percent of the total gray matter.

NEUROENDOCRINE TISSUES

The CNS exerts a direct influence on the pituitary gland and secondarily some degree of regulatory action on the hypophyseal target organs. This is accomplished by release of neurohumoral substances in the hypothalamus and their transport to the pituitary (see Chapter 22).

CEREBROSPINAL FLUID (CSF)

The anatomy of the ventriculomeningeal spaces and the choroid plexus is reviewed in Chapter 3 and later in this book. The fluid itself and its basic biology are now discussed to place CSF in its proper perspective as a functioning tissue of the nervous system. Quantitative features are reviewed on p. 139; in summary they represent some 140 ml. total volume in the adult, with 35 ml. of this within the ventricles. Homeostasis is exceedingly important and is accomplished through free circulation, which depends upon formation, movement, and absorption.

Bulk *production* of CSF amounts to 50 to 100 ml./day in a healthy individual and may be greatly increased in rate under pathologic circumstances. The choroid plexus is credited with the major role in production. Input into the ventricles is presumed to exceed absorption, which accounts for the outward flow of the fluid. The mechanism of CSF production remains controversial. The choroid plexus, with about 100 million cells and 150 to 300 sq. cm. of surface area, is structurally set up in a pattern consistent with a secretory organ, a dialyzing system, an absorbing device, and an organ suited to rapid bidirectional transport. Experimentally the choroid can both secrete and absorb, and it can do both simultaneously. Probably it must be concluded that various components of CSF are elaborated and exchanged by various means. For example, water moves bidirectionally through choroid plexus with ease but also does so through other limiting compartment membranes (ependyma, vessel walls, arachnoid lining, and perineuronal sheaths). Electrolytes and proteins exhibit graded exchange rates and move in and out of CSF most rapidly within the ventricles. It is known that sodium and proteins are moved by active transport rather than by diffusion. While the question of production of CSF remains unsettled, current opinion favors active secretion of electrolytes and proteins by the choroid plexus, with water added from choroid and other sources by diffusion to make up the bulk. Ultrafiltration is probably relatively unimportant as part of the mechanism.*

The *flow* of CSF arises from the inequity between production and absorption. The flow pattern seems quite certainly to be from lateral to third ventricles via interventricular foramina, thence through the cerebral aqueduct and fourth ventricle to the subarachnoid spaces via the apertures of Luschka and Magendie. The intraventricular flow may be influenced by cardiac pulse excursions in the choroidal vessels. Circulation in the subarachnoid space is remote from the choroid pulse, and the number of arterial excursions falls to forty percent of those in the ventricles. Nonetheless, subarachnoid flow is undoubtedly related to cardiac action as well as to respiratory excursion, strain with glottic closure, and posture. After entering the cisterna magna the CSF pathway is either into the spinal subarachnoid space or upward via the cisterns, principally Sylvian, to the arachnoid granulations along the dural sinuses of the vertex.

While some fluid is *absorbed* en route (in vessels, neural spaces, arachnoid membranes), the principal bulk is moved to the Pacchionian bodies of the

*For the neurophysiology of impulse transfer, excitation, and inhibition, see Chapter 15 and references 4 and 14.

*For extended review of CSF formation and experimental manipulation with physiologic and nonphysiologic substances see references 5 and 22.

Table 10-1. Composition of normal CSF

Constituent	Average value	
Total leukocytes	1.8	per cu. mm.
Lymphocytes	79	percent
Monocytes	17	percent
Other	4	percent
Total protein	28.2	mg./100 ml.
Albumin	62	percent
Globulins		
Alpha-1	5	percent
Alpha-2	5	percent
Beta	9	percent
Tau-beta	6	percent
Gamma	10	percent
Others (prealbumin protein-coh)	3	percent
Glucose (including nonglucose reducing substance)	61	mg./100 ml.
Total phospholipids	0.38	mg./100 ml.
Cephalins	0.10	mg./100 ml.
Lecithins	0.18	mg./100 ml.
Sphingomyelin	0.10	mg./100 ml.
Nonphosphorus sphingolipids	0.08	mg./100 ml.
Total cholesterol	0.40	mg./100 ml.
Free	33	percent
Neutral fat	0.42	mg./100 ml.
Total lipid	1.25	mg./100 ml.
Total base	155	mEq./liter
Sodium	141	mEq./liter
Potassium	3.3	mEq./liter
Calcium	2.5	mEq./liter
Magnesium	2.4	mEq./liter
Chloride	124	mEq./liter
Bicarbonate	21	mEq./liter
Carbon dioxide tension	46	mm. Hg.
pH	7.32	
Ammonia	6.4	μ gm./100 ml.
Nonprotein nitrogen	19	mg. N/100 ml.
Urea	6.4	μ gm. N/100 ml.
Uric acid	0.6	mg. N/100 ml.
Creatinine	4.0	mg. N/100 ml.
Amino acids	2.2	mg. N/100 ml.
Vitamin C	3.7	mg./100 ml.
Iron	38	μ gm./100 ml.
Copper	12.5	μ gm./100 ml.
Total solids	1.0	gm./liter
Specific gravity	1.008	

Enzymes—amylase, oxidase, lipase present in traces. Glycolytic enzymes not present.
Hormones—pituitary hormones can be identified.
Immunologic substances—bacteriolysins, antitoxins, precipitins, agglutinins, complement are not normally present.

cerebral dura and their spinal equivalents at the nerve root outlets. The normal range of CSF pressure in the lateral recumbent position is from 117 to 183 mm. of spinal fluid.

The composition of CSF is summarized in Table 10-1. Its function in the embryo may be nutritive, but this function appears to be unimportant in the adult except possibly for avascular areas of ependyma and pia-arachnoid. The principal function of CSF in the adult seems to be protection.

INTERSTITIAL SUBSTANCE

With the advent of electron microscopic examination of the CNS the idea of fluid compartmentation has had to be revised. The intercellular gap substance is estimated as less than seven percent of total tissue volume. Fluids therefore appear to be taken up in neural tissues in an intracellular compartment, a point of great importance in fluid exchanges.

REFERENCES

1. Abercrombie, M., and Santler, J. E.: An analysis of growth in nuclear population during Wallerian degeneration, J. Cell Comp. Physiol. **50**:429, 1957.
2. Austin, J.: Globoid leukodystrophy. In Minckler, J., editor: Pathology of the nervous system, vol. I, New York, 1968, McGraw-Hill Book Co.
3. Baker, A. B.: Structure of the small cerebral arteries and their changes with age, Amer. J. Pathol. **13**:453, 1937.
4. Bodian, D.: The generalized vertebrate neuron, Science **137**:323, 1962.
5. Bowsher, D.: Experimental anatomic pathology. In Minckler, J., editor: Pathology of the nervous system, vol. I, New York, 1968, McGraw-Hill Book Co.
6. Causey, G.: The cell of Schwann, Edinburgh, 1960, E. & S. Livingstone.
7. Dawson, H.: Physiology of the ocular and cerebrospinal fluids, Boston, 1956, Little, Brown, and Co.
8. DeLorenzo, A. J.: The fine structure of synapses in the ciliary ganglion of the chick, J. Biophys. Biochem. Cytol. **7**:31, 1960.
9. DeRobertis, E.: Morphogenesis of the retinal rods. An electron microscope study, J. Biophys. Biochem. Cytol. **2**:209, 1956.
10. DeRobertis, E., and Gerschenfeld, H. M.: Submicroscopic morphology and function of glial cells, Int. Rev. Neurobiol. **3**:1, 1961.
11. Duncan, D., and Hild, W.: Histogenesis and cytogenesis of neural structures. In Minckler, J., editor: Pathology of the nervous system, vol. I, New York, 1968, McGraw-Hill Book Co.
12. Flexner, L. B.: The development of the meninges in Amphibia: a study of normal and experimental animals, Contrib. Embryol. **20**:31, 1929.
13. Geren, B. B.: The formation from the Schwann cell surface of myelin in the peripheral nerves of chick embryos, Exp. Cell Res. **7**:558, 1954.
14. Grundfest, H.: Pathophysiologic mechanisms in neural transmission. In Minckler, J., editor: Pathology of the nervous system, vol. I New York, 1968, McGraw-Hill Book Co.
15. Horstadus, S.: The neural crest, New York, 1950, Oxford University Press.
16. Hughes, J. T.: Trauma to peripheral nerves. In Minckler, J., editor: Pathology of the nervous system, vol. II, New York, 1970, McGraw-Hill Book Co.
17. Hyden, H.: The neuron, New York, 1967, American Publishing Co., Inc. Elsevier.

18. Innes, J. R. M., and Saunders, L. Z.: Comparative neuropathy, New York, 1962, Academic Press, Inc.
19. Jacobson, S. A.: Skeletogenic affections. In Minckler, J., editor: Pathology of the nervous system, vol. II, New York, 1970, McGraw-Hill Book Co.
20. Jaeger, M., Crace, R. and Minckler, J.: Quantitative study of the medial geniculate body, Thesis, University of Denver, 1968.
21. Kreutzberg, G. W.: Neural degeneration and regeneration. In Minckler, J., editor: Pathology of the nervous system, vol. II, New York, 1970, McGraw-Hill Book Co.
22. Lumsden, C. E., and Pomerat, C. M.: Normal oligodendrocytes in tissue culture. A preliminary report on the pulsatile glial cells in tissue cultures from the corpus callosum of the normal adult rat brain, Exp. Cell Res. **2**:103, 1951.
23. Luse, S. A.: The neuron. In Minckler, J., editor: Pathology of the nervous system, vol. I, New York, 1968, McGraw-Hill Book Co.
24. Luse, S. A.: The Schwann cell. In Minckler, J., editor: Pathology of the nervous system, vol. I, New York, 1968, McGraw-Hill Book Co.
25. Lyons, W. R., and Woodhall, B.: Atlas of peripheral nerve injuries, Philadelphia, 1949, W. B. Saunders Co.
26. McCouch, G. P.: Degeneration and regeneration in the central nervous system. In Minckler, J., editor: Pathology of the nervous system, vol. I New York, 1968, McGraw-Hill Book Co.
27. Murray, M. R., and Stout, A. P.: Demonstration of the formation of reticulin by Schwannian tumor cells in vitro, Amer. J. Path. **18**:585, 1942.
28. Nelson, E., Blinzinger, K., and Hager, H.: An electron microscopic study of bacterial meningitis, I. Experimental alterations in the leptomeninges and subarachnoid space, Arch. Neurol. **6**:390, 1962.
29. Pellegrino de Iraldi, A., Zieher, L. M., and DeRobertis, E.: Ultrastructure and pharmacological studies of nerve endings in the pineal organ, Prog. Brain Res. **10**:389, 1965.
30. Peters, G.: Multiple sclerosis. In Minckler, J., editor: Pathology of the nervous system, vol. I, New York, 1968, McGraw-Hill Book Co.
31. Poser, C. M.: Diseases of the myelin sheath. In Minckler, J., editor: Pathology of the nervous system, vol. I, New York, 1968, McGraw-Hill Book Co.
32. Richardson, K. C.: Electron microscopic observations on Auerbach's plexus in the rabbit with special references to the problem of smooth muscle innervation, Amer. J. Anat. **103**:99, 1958.
33. Robertson, J. D.: In Locke, M., editor Cellular membranes in development, New York, 1964, Academic Press, Inc.
34. Rosenbluth, J., and Palay, S. L.: The fine structure of nerve cell bodies and their myelin sheaths in the eighth nerve ganglion of the goldfish, J. Biophys. Biochem. Cytol. **9**:853, 1961.
35. Scharrer, E., and Brown, S.: Neurosecretion, XIII. The formation of neurosecretory granules in the earthworm, Zumbricus terrestris L., Z. Zellforsch. **54**:530, 1961.
36. Seddon, H. J., editor: Peripheral nerve injuries, London, 1954, Her Majesty's Stationery Office.
37. Slager, U. T.: The meninges. In Minckler, J., editor: Pathology of the nervous system, vol. I, New York, 1968. McGraw-Hill Book Co.
38. Steegman, A. T.: Notochordal tissue and its development and reactions. In Minckler, J., editor: Pathology of the nervous system, vol. I, New York, 1968, McGraw-Hill Book Co.
39. Taxi, J.: Electron microscopy of sympathetic ganglia in mammals, Comp. Rend. Acad. Sci. **245**:564, 1957.
40. Tennyson, V. M., and Pappas, G. D.: Choroid plexus. In Minckler, J., editor: Pathology of the nervous system, vol. I, New York, 1968, McGraw-Hill Book Co.
41. Tennyson, V. M., and Pappas, G. D.: Ependyma. In Minckler, J., editor: Pathology of the nervous system, vol. I, New York, 1968, McGraw-Hill Book Co.
42. Weiss, P.: In Kety, S., and Elkes, editors: Regional neurochemistry, New York, 1961, Pergamon Press, Inc.
43. Welch, K., and Pollay, M.: Perfusion of particles through arachnoid villi of the monkey, Amer. J. Physiol. **201**: 651, 1961.
44. Wolman, M.: Myelin structure, ultrastructure and degeneration. In Minckler, J., editor: Pathology of the nervous system, vol. I, New York, 1968, McGraw-Hill Book Co.
45. Woodhall, B., and Beebe, G. W.: Peripheral nerve regeneration, Washington, D. C., 1956, U. S. Government Printing Office.
46. Woollam, D. H. M., and Millen, J. W.: Vascular tissues in the central nervous system. In Minckler, J., editor: Pathology of the nervous system, vol. I, New York, 1968, McGraw-Hill Book Co.

CHAPTER **11**

TISSUE CULTURE

ROBERT LASHER

The term *tissue culture* generally encompasses the methods involved in the study of organs, tissues, and cells in an artificial environment outside of the animal for more than twenty-four hours. An *organ culture* involves the growth or maintenance of an organ, its primordia, or its parts under conditions that may allow differentiation (includes the parameters of morphology, behavior, function, and biochemistry) and the continuance of normal cell relationships and functions. In *tissue culture* parts of tissues are maintained or grown in vitro under conditions that may allow or promote differentiation but do not necessarily preserve the original architecture. *Cell culture* requires that tissues be dissociated into their component parts (cells), which are subsequently grown in vitro. Under suitable conditions, single cells may grow into colonies (*clones*), which may possess some of the characteristics of an organized tissue. The present chapter concerns methods and applications of these three types of "tissue culture" in the study of neurons and glia.[45,49]

METHODS

The choice between organ, tissue, or cell culture will be dictated to a great extent by the goals of the experimenter. Each mode of culture has its own special conditions, including the means of tissue removal and preparation, the culture medium, the substrate, the culture vessel, and the atmospheric conditions.[59]

Organ culture requires that regions of the CNS and peripheral nervous system be removed from the organism with minimal disturbance to the tissue organization. To achieve this, whole regions, such as the cerebellum or a sensory ganglion, are removed rapidly under sterile conditions. If the organ is small enough, it can be cultured whole; otherwise, it is cut into smaller pieces. In general, the ideal size of the explant should not exceed 1 cu. mm., in order to allow adequate diffusion of gases, nutrients, and wastes.

The process of removal and preparation is quite traumatic, especially to the neurons. Axons are cut, and connection with the blood vascular system is lost, resulting in immediate anoxia, anemia, and physical damage to a large number of cells. This leads to a number of degenerative changes in the first few days of culture. These changes include demyelination, cytoplasmic vacuolation and granulation, nuclear pyknosis, and characteristics of chromatolytic reaction in neurons. It usually takes about five days for the initial shock phase to pass; the time required is based on metabolic criteria. The normal Nissl pattern lost during chromatolysis requires almost three weeks for redevelopment.[45,49] To some extent, both prenatal and postnatal neurons from all sources including man appear to be able to regenerate cut processes.

During the course of dissection, the meninges are usually removed as well as possible to minimize contamination with endothelial and mesenchymal cells. While the outgrowth of these cell types appears to be inhibited for the most part in organotypic cultures,[45,49] they often become the dominant elements in dispersed tissue and cell cultures.

Methods for further dispersal of neural tissue into fragments or single cells depends to some extent on tissue age and origin. As indicated in Chapter 9, the ventricular cells forming the neural tube and later lining the neurocoele are held together by terminal bar junctions that form very strong connections. Partial dissociation can be achieved by repeated gentle pipetting of the tissue in a balanced saline or other suitable medium using a wide bore pipette. Brain tissue from chick embryos and newborn rats prepared in this manner differentiate and survives for several months under suitable conditions.[39]

Single cells can be isolated for cell culture and cloning purposes by allowing larger clumps and small aggregates of tissue to settle out or by putting this suspension through several layers of Nitex monofilament screen cloth. The mesh size of the Nitex cloth to be used depends on the smallest diameter of the aggregates to be removed. Mechanical dissociation of chick embryo and rat brain has also been achieved by placing small pieces of the material in a Nitex nylon bag (of 202 μ mesh), immersing the bag in a suitable medium, and gently stroking it with a glass rod. Single cells and small clumps of viable cells are released into the medium.[85] These mechanical techniques are most suitable for cultures of embryonic brain, in which the number of connections is small, and the amount of intercellular mucopolysaccharide ground substance produced by glial cells is minimal. For dissociation of cells in an older brain, a combination of enzymatic (trypsin) and mechanical treatments has been used, but physical damage to the cells is quite extensive.[57,68]

Dissociation of sensory and sympathetic ganglia has been achieved by both mechanical and enzymatic means. The connective tissue capsule of a ganglion can be broken either by freehand dissection[29] or weakened (or dissociated) through the use of enzymes such as trypsin, collagenase, or pronase.[39,72,83] After enzyme treatment dissociation is usually completed by gentle agitation or pipetting, preferably in a medium containing serum. Neurons are quite sensitive to proteolytic enzymes, and the presence of serum during final dissociation helps neutralize the effects of any residual enzymes. When used properly, a combination of enzymatic and mechanical methods of dissociation permits isolation of large numbers of neurons possessing processes up to several hundred microns long with little contamination by connective tissue elements (Fig. 11-1, *A*).

Once the desired tissues or cells have been obtained, they must be placed in an environment that promotes their recovery and enables them to differentiate for a length of time sufficient to achieve the goals of the experiment. Early studies of nerve cells in culture utilized either a medium composed of physiologic saline based upon the ionic composition of blood plasma, or a natural medium, such as lymph. For studying avian and mammalian tissues, the saline was usually supplemented with glucose and buffers.[88] These media proved to be sufficient to allow organ function, such as heartbeat, for several hours and maintenance of tissue for several days, or longer in exceptional cases. Chick embryo sympathetic nerve tissue was maintained in saline for up to twelve days, amphibian embryo cells were found to be capable of surviving for several weeks or longer in saline. These latter cells contain a large supply of yolk protein, which is catabolized to supply nutrients for survival and growth. Natural biologic media were also used for tissue culture. Murray reports that the first nerve cultures were composed of pieces of amphibian neural tube in a drop of lymph, which was clotted on a coverslip.[49] The coverslip was inverted and sealed with paraffin over a depression ground out of a glass slide. A hanging drop of saline has also been used in place of clotted lymph (Fig. 11-2, *A*). However, the clotted lymph has the advantage of providing a three-dimensional matrix facilitating firm attachment of the tissue and outgrowth of cells and neurites against the force of gravity. More recently, natural media composed of mixtures of blood plasma and embryo extract (homogenate of nine- to ten-day-old chick embryos in saline) have been used in place of lymph for avian and mammalian tissues, in an effort to supply needed nutrients. When embryo extract and plasma are mixed, a clot is formed, permitting the use of the depression slide for these tissues as well.

Since the early 1900's the technique of organ culture of nerve tissue has had several important modifications. The single coverslip–depression slide technique is adequate for short-term cultures, but it is poorly adapted to repeated feeding of the culture. Murray and Stout adapted the Maximow double coverslip method (Fig. 11-2, *B*) to the culture of nerve tissues.[50] In this method the tissue is clotted in plasma on a small coverslip that has been previously placed over a drop of saline on a larger, sterile coverslip. The surface tension of the saline holds the two coverslips together. The larger coverslips is then inverted and sealed to a depression slide. The culture is fed by opening the assembly, dipping the small coverslip in saline to wash the culture and rewet the glass, and adding a drop of liquid feeding solution (a mixture of balanced saline, serum, and embryo extract). The coverslips are reassembled and sealed for further culture. Through experience it has been found that a lying drop culture offered more optimal conditions than a hanging drop culture for gas diffusion, draining of wastes, and refeeding. Organotypic cultures of nerve tissue have been main-

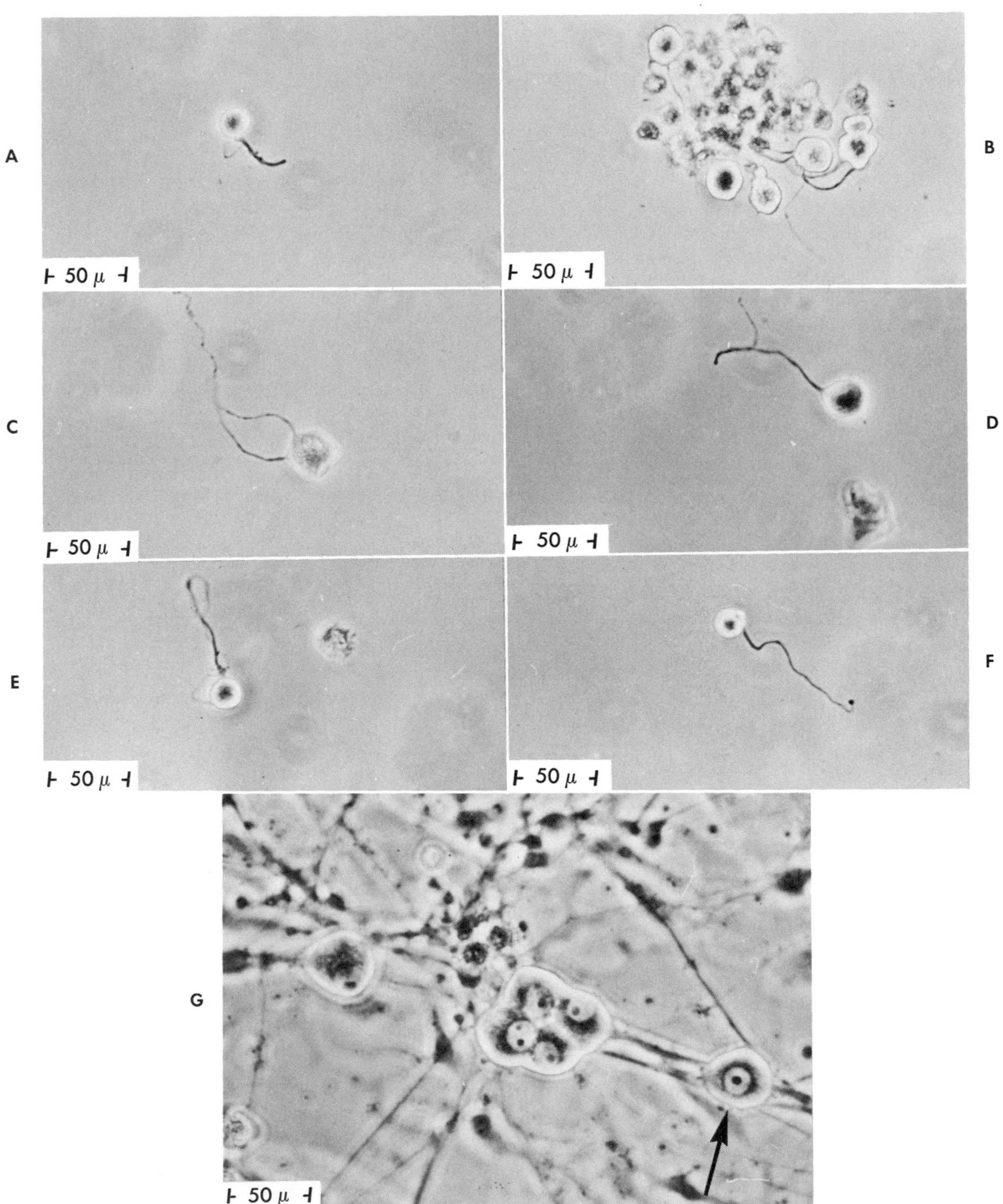

Fig. 11-1. A-F, Dissociated ten-day chick embryo sensory ganglion neurons from a partially dispersed pellet. (Phase contrast.) **G,** Same neurons twelve days in culture. Nucleus becomes more centralized with maturation *(arrow)* and becomes surrounded by nissl substance (phase-dense). (Phase contrast.)

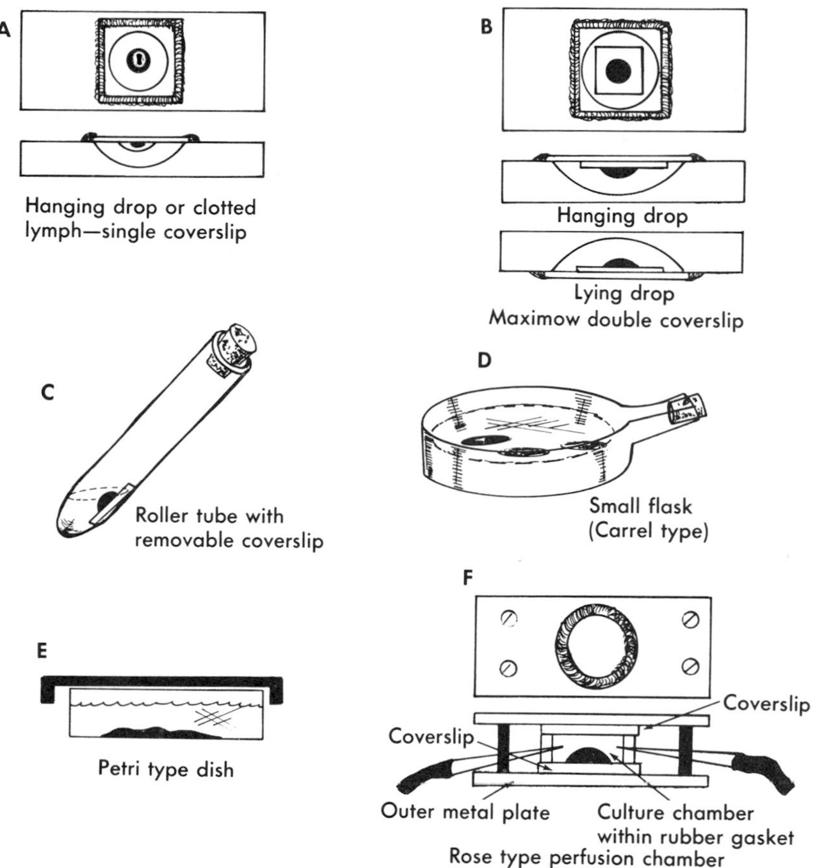

Fig. 11-2. A-F, Types of chambers utilized in culture of neural tissues and cells.

tained in good condition for six months or longer using this method.

Other important modifications involve the development of more suitable culture media and substrates. For example, it has been found that human cord or placental serum is superior to adult serum for survival and differentiation of mammalian CNS tissues. Also an increased glucose content (approximately 600 mg./100 ml.) was found to be optimal, especially for myelin formation. While these medium modifications have permitted better survival and differentiation, the plasma clot has proved to be a poor substrate for some types of tissues. Chick embryo ganglia, for example, possess enzymes that liquefy the plasma clot, necessitating patching every few days. Bornstein modified the Maximow method by substituting a layer of reconstituted rat-tail collagen for the plasma clot. This has proved to be a suitable substrate for many types of neural tissues with the Maximow technique, and has permitted the use of a variety of liquid media.

Other sources of variability in Maximow cultures have been found to be associated with differences in the composition of the serum and other medium constituents, the type of glass coverslips used, the pH of the medium, and the temperature of the incubator. Serum has been found to vary with the diet and health of the donor. Some types of glass are toxic. Optimal pH is between 6.8 and 7.1, and optimal temperature is about 36° C., especially for myelin formation.

A variety of culture vessels other than the Maximow assembly have also been used for organotypic nerve cell culture. They include test tubes (with or without coverslips), small flasks or dishes, and several types of perfusion chambers (Fig. 11-2, *C* to *F*). In all cases the explant is anchored to the substrate with a plasma clot or is allowed to attach to a collagen film. The media used are liquids that contain salts and are designed to equilibrate either with air or other gases (such as five percent CO_2 in air), and other supplements, such as glucose and serum.

Organotypic cultures have the advantage of maintaining the original tissue structure to a great extent. This aids in the identification of cell types and allows direct comparison with in vivo counterparts. However, due to the multilayering of cells, there is limited accessibility to individual cells and their processes. This is a disadvantage both in conducting electrophysiologic studies and in quantitating data. Tissue or cell cultures of partially or completely dissociated neurons and glia are more advantageous for these purposes. However, in the preparation of these cultures normal functional relationships are lost (although they may be partially regained during culture), and morphologic identification of specific types of neurons and glia is often difficult. Tissue and cell cultures are most easily done in small flasks or plastic tissue culture dishes using collagen, gelatin, or the plastic itself as a substrate. Most recent studies have utilized relatively defined media supplemented with serum and occasionally extra glucose, hormones, embryo extract, brain extract, or nerve growth factor.

IDENTIFICATION OF NEURAL CELL TYPES

Positive identification of neurons and glial cells in culture generally requires consideration of morphology, behavior, physiology, and biochemistry. In embryonic tissues the differences between neurons and glia are less sharply defined, as are the differences between neural cells and mesenchymal or endothelial elements. Therefore, as many criteria as possible must be considered before a decision is made.

Neurons

Most types of neurons are nonmigratory. The main exception is sympathetic neurons, which in explants of ganglia often migrate out along nerve processes and in dissociated cultures tend to aggregate into small groups. Neurons in newly set-up organotypic cultures of CNS tissues may appear to migrate, but this movement is brought about by the overall spreading of the explant.

Cell division is not a common characteristic of neurons. However, mitoses are occasionally seen in migratory sympathetic neurons[45,50] and in ganglia after treatment with compounds such as deuterium oxide[51] and nerve growth factor.[42]

Neuron morphology is related to the state of differentiation, area of origin, and types of interactions with other neurons. Neurons from sensory ganglia are easily recognized by their relatively large size (20 to 40 μ in diameter), rounded cell bodies containing dense cytoplasm, large round nuclei each with clear nucleoplasm and one or two prominent nucleoli (Fig. 11-1, *B*). In addition, they are pseudounipolar when mature, although occasionally a bipolar or tripolar neuron may be observed. Sympathetic neurons are somewhat smaller than sensory neurons and are multipolar; otherwise they have a similar appearance. Neurons from the CNS are less rounded than ganglionic neurons and are multipolar, with one axon and several or many dendrites (Fig. 11-3). Neuronal processes have membranous expansions only at the front of a growth cone, while glial cells produce membranous expansions from the perikaryon as well as from the stems and tips of processes.[54] After fixation, a selective affinity for silver by neurofibrils in the neuronal processes and by the cell body can be demonstrated, using the methods

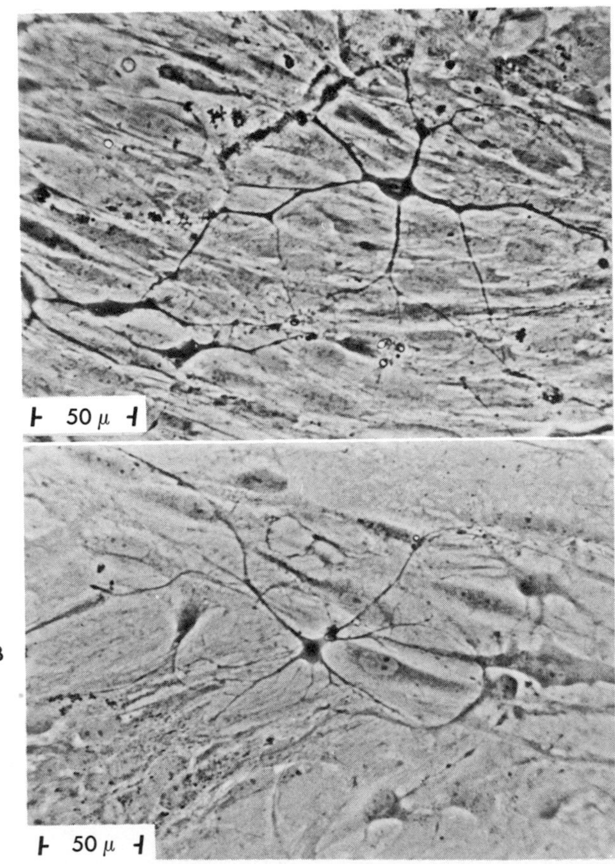

Fig. 11-3. A, **Multipolar neuron from four-day rat brainstem,** partially dissociated. Thirty days in culture. (Phase contrast.) **B,** Multipolar neuron from four-day rat cerebrum, partially dissociated. Thirty days in culture. (Phase contrast.)

of Bodian and Holmes. However, silver staining can be quite variable both within and between cultures. In general, staining is much more reliable in explants than in thinly spread cultures.

Functional activity can also be used to identify and characterize neurons. Membrane potentials, evoked potentials, and spontaneous activity of single neurons can be measured by electrophysiologic means, and are characteristic for different types of cells. The electrical activity of a tissue or group of tissues can also give much information about the degree of synaptic interaction between neurons. The ability of a neuron to function as a sensory or motor unit is another identifying characteristic. This may be seen, for example, by the development of a functional neuromuscular synapse in a mixed culture of spinal cord cells and skeletal muscle.[15,23]

Late-maturing sensory ganglion neurons during part of their life, and most sympathetic neurons during all of their life, require nerve growth factor for survival and maturation in culture. Neurons from the CNS and all types of glial cells have no such requirement.[42]

Biochemical characteristics can be used to identify neuronal types in certain cases. For example, sympathetic neurons and neurons from certain regions of the brain produce catecholamines (such as dopamine and norepinephrine), which can be identified by their characteristic fluorescence after treatment with paraformaldehyde vapor.[69]

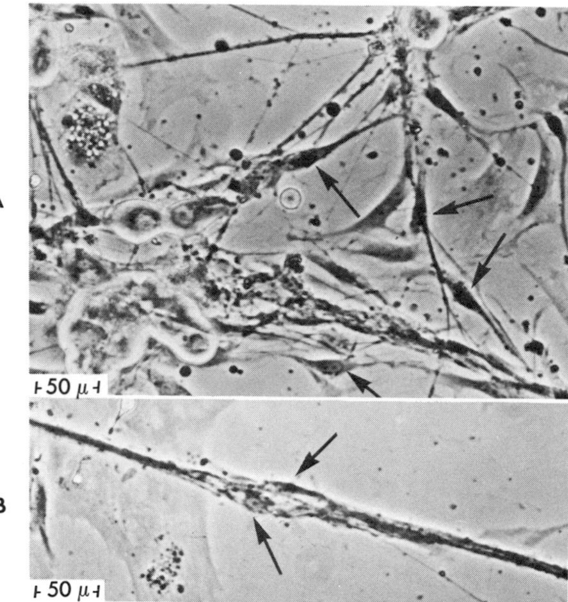

Fig. 11-4. A, Schwann cells *(arrows)* along and near fibers. (Phase contrast.) **B,** Schwann cells *(arrow)* associated with nerve fiber bundle from twelve-day culture of ten-day chick embryo sensory ganglion neurons. (Phase contrast.)

Neuroglia

Like neurons, most types of glial cells show little migratory behavior in culture. The exceptions are oligodendrocytes and Schwann cells, which are respectively the myelin-forming cells in the CNS and peripheral nervous system. In cultures of embryonic sensory ganglia, a Schwann cell can be seen to migrate to a nerve fiber, attach and spread itself out along the fiber, and eventually wrap itself around the fiber to become part of the myelin sheath (Fig. 11-4, *B*).

There have been many conflicting reports about the ability of glial cells in culture to divide. There is no doubt that Schwann cells from embryonic and postnatal animals and oligodendrocytes can reproduce mitotically in culture.[45] However, cells having the characteristics of mature astrocytes apparently do not divide mitotically in organotypic cultures. There are several reports of cell lines derived from dissociated brain tissue that have some astrocyte-like characteristics.[64,65,84] However, glial origin was not definitely established. Identification of different types of glial cells by their morphologic characteristics is often very difficult. Cell morphology is often transitory and rarely corresponds exactly with the pictures obtained from preparations of tissue taken directly from brain. The composition of the culture medium, temperature, age and health of the donor, and other variables can affect cell morphology. In general, an astrocyte possesses a large perikaryon (30 to 50 μ in diameter) containing a round or oval nucleus (10 to 15 μ in diameter). Sometimes astrocyte nuclei are morphologically indistinguishable from neuronal nuclei. Protoplasmic astrocytes can usually be distinguished from fibrous astrocytes by the number and degree of branching of their processes. Both types are stellate, giving off processes in all directions. Fibrous astrocytes possess from ten to twenty or more thin processes, which show little branching and are often quite long. Protoplasmic astrocyte processes are not quite as numerous and frequently possess secondary and tertiary branching (Fig. 11-5, *A* and *B*). Many types of transitional forms are also seen. Membranous expansions of both the perikaryon and processes are quite common.

In oligodendrocytes the nucleus occupies most of the perikaryon (10 μ in diameter) and is quite dense. There are generally two to four processes,

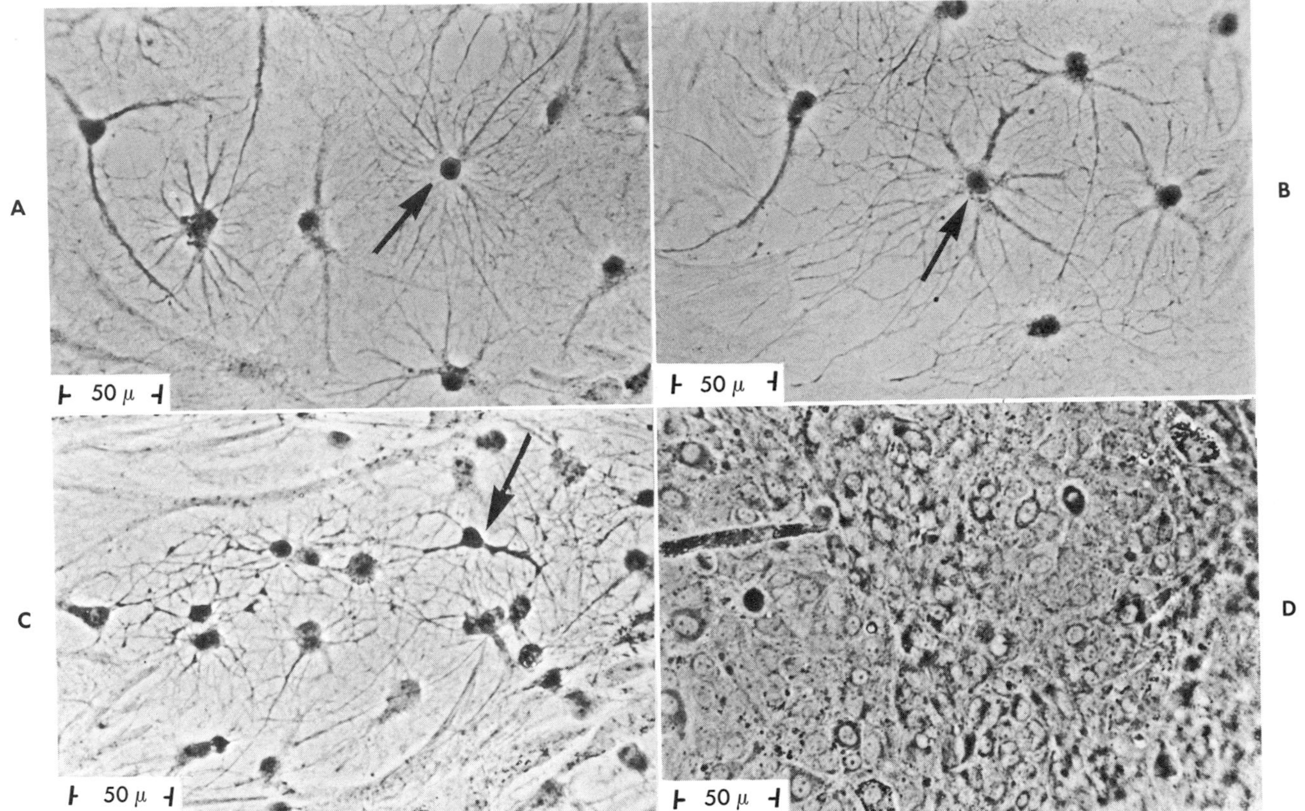

Fig. 11-5. A, Fibrous type astrocyte *(arrow)* in thirty-day culture of partially dissociated four-day rat cerebrum. (Phase contrast.) **B,** Protoplasmic type astrocyte *(arrow)* in thirty-day culture of partially dissociated rat cerebrum. (Phase contrast.) **C,** Oligodendrocytes *(arrow)* in thirty-day culture of partially dissociated four-day rat cerebrum. (Phase contrast.) **D,** Ciliated ependymal cells in epithelial membrane from thirty-day culture of four-day rat cerebrum. (Phase contrast.)

which are highly branched, and which lack the conical swelling seen in astrocytes at the point of origin the cell body (Fig. 11-5, *C*). Dark lumps composed of focal aggregations of mitochondria are often seen within the processes of both oligodendrocytes and astrocytes. Many oligodendrocytes demonstrate a rhythmic pulsatile movement with a periodicity of about five minutes. There is a contractile period lasting about two minutes, during which there is a decrease in the volume of the perikaryon and a swelling of the processes in the proximal region. A period of dilation then occurs, lasting about three minutes.[56]

Schwann cells are fusiform and contain an oval nucleus and dense cytoplasm (Fig. 11-4, *A*). They demonstrate rhythmic pulsations similar to those seen in oligodendrocytes,[45] and they are highly phagocytic and migratory in nature. Embryonic Schwann cells reproduce mitotically and can be cloned in clones. In clones they tend to link together in chains.[39]

Cultures of cerebrum, cerebellum, and spinal cord often contain ependymal cells derived from the wall of the ventricles or central canal. They form either epithelial-type membranes (where the cells are tightly packed) (Fig. 11-5, *D*) or organoid structures.[54,66] The organoid structures may consist of rosettes (circular rows) of cells having the appearance of a cross section through a ventricle. Cells in both types of formations are often ciliated, with the cilia present on the free surface of the membrane or oriented inward in the sectioned vesicle-type structure. Choroid plexus cells also form a ciliated epithelium and may demonstrate apocrine activity. [45]

After fixation, glial cells can be demonstrated by selective methods to possess an affinity for silver,[70,82] but they may also stain with methods selective for neurofibrils. In the latter case, silver deposits only on the surface of glial processes and is not found in the cytoplasm.[54]

Glial cells possess certain electrophysiologic characteristics that may help differentiate them from neurons. Like neurons, they have high resting potentials, but unlike neurons they are electrically inexcitable.[37,80,87] However, many neurons in culture are also incapable of being excited. The reason for this is often unclear, but one instance in which it occurs is when neurons and glia are electrically coupled.[87] Glial cells also possess a selective permeability to the potassium ion[37] and respond to an electrical stimulus with a graded, long-lasting depolarization.[87] The applicability of these characteristics to all types of glial cells is uncertain, since astrocytes have been the primary subject for the studies cited.

The brain-specific protein S-100 is thought to be mainly derived from glial cells.[12] When neural tissue is stained with S-100 antibody coupled with fluorescein, glial cell cytoplasm and neuronal nuclei fluoresce.[32] Use of this technique with cultured neural tissue provides information on both the location and functional state of glial cells.

APPLICATIONS

For tissue culture to be an effective aid in studies relating to development and function of neural tissues and cells, the method used must provide an environment that maintains them in a morphologic and functional state as close as possible to that present in situ over a similar period of time. Failure of the culture to do so makes meaningful interpretation of data very difficult. For this reason, much work has been involved in validating experimental methods. Present organotypic culture techniques are capable of permitting development and maintenance of myelinated axons, dendrites, normal Nissl patterns, other cytoplasmic structures such as neurofibrils and intranuclear rodlets, functional synaptic junctions, normal enzymatic and metabolic activities, normal cell morphology and function, and nearly normal neuronal organization.*

Organotypic cultures possessing these characteristics have in turn served as model systems for the study of myelination and demyelinating diseases; factors affecting differentiation, such as nerve growth factor, various types of embryo extracts, hormones, and nutritional and physical factors; effects of anoxia, drugs, and irradiation; mechanism of neurite outgrowth and fasciculation; axoplasmic transport; neuronal-glial interaction; and development of neuronal-neuronal and neuronal-muscle synapses.*

Tissue and cell cultures have been used to advantage to study mechanisms of neurite outgrowth, axoplasmic transport, growth and characteristics of normal and malignant glial cells and neurons, effects of nerve growth factor, nucleus-cytoplasmic interaction in neuronal-nonneuronal heterokaryons, formation of neuromuscular synapses, and many other areas.†

*See references 8-10, 16-18, 21, 25, 28, 36, 41, 42, 45, 48, 49, 75, 79, 89, and 90.

*See references 2, 3, 6, 13, 17, 18, 24-28, 30, 33, 34, 36, 38, 42, 45-47, 49, 52, 53, 58, 60, 61, 63, 67, 83, 86, 90, and 91.

†See references 5, 7, 11, 14, 19, 20, 23, 29, 31, 39, 40, 43, 44, 55, 62, 64, 65, 71-74, 76-78, 81, 84, 85, 91, and 92.

REFERENCES

1. Amaldi, P.: Incorporation of RNA and protein precursors into embryonic nerve cells of *Periplaneta americana* cultured in vitro, Brain Res. **21**:305, 1970.
2. Amaldi, P., and Rusca, G.: Autoradiographic study of RNA in nerve fibers of embryonic sensory ganglia cultured in vitro under NGF stimulation, J. Neurochem. **17**:767, 1970.
3. Angeletti, P. U., Gandini-Attardi, D., and Toschi, G.: Metabolic aspects of the effect of nerve growth factor on sympathetic and sensory ganglia protein and ribonucleic acid synthesis, Biochim. Biophys. Acta **95**:111, 1965.
4. Augusti-Tocco, G., and Sato, G. H.: Establishment of functional clonal lives of neurons from mouse neuroblastoma, Proc. Nat. Acad. Sci. U.S.A. **64**:311, 1969.
5. Benda, P. J., Lightbody, J., and Sato, G.: Differentiated rat glial cell strain in tissue culture, Science **161**:370, 1968.
6. Bornstein, M. B., and Murrey, M. R.: Serial observations on pattern of growth, myelin formation maintenance and degeneration in cultures of newborn rat and kitten cerebellum, J. Biophys. Biochem. Cytol. **4**:499, 1958.
7. Boyde, A., James, D. W., and Tresman, R. L.: Outgrowth from chick embryo spinal cord in vitro, studied with the scanning electron microscope, Z. Zellforsch. **90**:1, 1968.
8. Bray, D.: Surface movements during the growth of single explanted neurons, Proc. Nat. Acad. Sci. U.S.A. **65**:905, 1970.
9. Bunge, M. B., Bunge, R. P., and Peterson, E. R.: A light and electron microscope study of long-term organized cultures of rat dorsal root ganglia, J. Cell Biol. **32**:439, 1967.
10. Burdman, J. A.: Uptake of (^{3}H) catecholamines by chick embryo sympathetic ganglia in tissue culture, J. Neurochem. **15**:1321, 1968.
11. Chen, J. S., and Levi-Montalcini, R.: Axonal growth from insect neurons in glia-free cultures, Proc. Nat. Acad. Sci. U.S.A. **66**:32, 1970.
12. Cicero, T. J., Cowan, W. M., and Moore, B. W.: The cellular localization of the two brain specific proteins, S-100 and 14-3-2, Brain Res. **18**:25, 1970.

13. Corner, M. A., and Crain, S. M.: Spontaneous contractions after differentiation in culture of presumptive neuromuscular tissues of the early frog embryo, Experientia **21**:422, 1965.
14. Cowell, L. A., and Weston, J. A.: An analysis of melanogenesis in cultured chick embryo spinal ganglia, Develop. Biol. **22**:670, 1970.
15. Crain, S. M.: Bioelectric interactions between cultured fetal rodent spinal cord and skeletal muscle after innervation in vitro, J. Exp. Zool. **173**:353, 1970.
16. Crain, S. M., and Peterson, E.: Complex bioelectric activity in organized tissue cultures of spinal cord (human, rat, and chick), J. Cell. Comp. Physiol. **64**:1, 1964.
17. Crain, S. M., Bornstein, M. B., and Peterson, E. R.: Maturation of cultured embryonic CNS tissues during chronic exposure to agents which prevent bioelectric activity, Brain Res. **8**:363, 1968.
18. Crain, S. M., Peterson, E. R., and Bornstein, M. B.: Formation of functional interneuronal connections between explants of various mammalian central nervous tissues during development in vitro. In Wolstenholme, G. E. W., and O'Connor, M., editors: Symposium on growth of the nervous system, London, 1968, J. and A. Churchill.
19. DiZerega, G., and Morrow, J.: The effect of nerve growth factor on dispersed neuronal-Hela keterokaryons, Exp. Neurol. **28**:206, 1970.
20. Dorfman, A., and Ho, P. L.: Synthesis of acid neucopolysaccharides by glial tumor cells in tissue culture, Proc. Nat. Acad. Sci. U. S. A. **66**:495, 1970.
21. England, J. M., and Goldstein, M. N.: The uptake and localization of catecholamines in chick embryo sympathetic neurons in tissue culture, J. Cell Sci. **4**:677, 1969.
22. Federoff, S.: Proposed usage of animal tissue culture terms, Exp. Cell Res. **46**:642, 1967.
23. Fischbach, G. D.: Synaptic potentials recorded in cell cultures of nerve and muscle, Science **169**:1331, 1970.
24. Grainger, F., and James, D. W.: Association of glial cells with the terminal parts of neurite bundles extending from chick spinal cord in vitro, Z. Zellforsch. **108**:93, 1970.
25. Guillery, R. W., Sobkowicz, H. M., and Scott, G. L.: Relationships between glial and neuronal elements in the development of long term cultures of the spinal cord of the fetal mouse, J. Comp. Neurol. **140**:1, 1970.
26. Hamburgh, M.: An analysis of the action of thyroid hormone on development based on in vivo and in vitro studies, Gen. Comp. Endocr. **10**:198, 1968.
27. Hendelman, W. J., and Booher, J.: Factors involved in the culturing of chick embryo dorsal root ganglia in the Rose Chamber, Texas Rep. Biol. Med. **24**:83, 1966.
28. Hild, W.: Cell types and neuronal connections in cultures of mammalian central nervous tissue, Z. Zellforsch. **69**:155, 1966.
29. Hillman, H., and Khalawan, S. A.: The growth of new processes from isolated dorsal and sympathetic cell bodies of rat and rabbit, Tissue and Cell **2**:249, 1970.
30. Hoffman, H.: Immunology of nerve growth factor (NGF). The effect of NGF antiserum on sensory ganglia in vitro., J. Embryol. Exp. Morph. **23**:273, 1970.
31. Hugosson, R., Källén, B., and Nilsson, O.: Neuroglia proliferation studied in tissue culture, Acta Neuropath. **11**:210, 1968.
32. Hydén, H., and McEwen, B.: A glial protein specific for the nervous system, Proc. Nat. Acad. Sci. U.S.A. **55**:354, 1966.
33. James, D. W., and Tresman, R. L.: An electron-microscopic study of the de novo formation of neuromuscular junctions in tissue culture, Z. Zellforsch. **100**:126, 1969.
34. James, D. W., and Tresman, R. L.: Synaptic profiles in the outgrowth from chick spinal cord in vitro, Z. Zellforsch. **101**:598, 1969.
35. Kim, S. U.: Cytochemical demonstration of "marker" enzymes in nerve cells cultured in vitro, Experientia **26**:292, 1970.
36. Kim, S. U.: Observations on cerebellar granule cells in tissue culture, Z. Zellforsch. **107**:454, 1970.
37. Kuffler, S. W., and Nicholls, J. G.: The physiology of neuroglia cells, Ergebn. Physiol. **57**:1, 1966.
38. Larrabee, M. G.: Metabolic effects of nerve impulses and nerve growth factor in sympathetic ganglia, Prog. Brain Res. **31**:95, 1969.
39. Lasher, R.: Unpublished data, 1970.
40. Lasher, R., Mathews, D., and Whitlock, D. G.: Axoplasmic transport in cultured chick embryo sensory neurons, J. Cell Biol. **47**:116a, 1970.
41. Lehrer, G. M., Bornstein, M. B., and Weiss, C.: Enzymes of carbohydrate metabolism in the rat cerebellum developing in situ and in vitro, Exp. Neurol. **27**:410, 1970.
42. Levi-Montalcini, R.: The nerve growth factor: its mode of action on sensory and sympathetic nerve cells, Harvey Lect. **60**:217, 1966.
43. Lightbody, J., and others: Biochemically differentiated clonal human glial cells in tissue culture, J. Neurobiol. **1**:411, 1970.
44. Lodin, Z., Booher, J., and Kasten, F. H.: Phase-contrast cinematographic study of dissociated neurons from embryonic chick dorsal root ganglia cultured in the Rose chamber, Exp. Cell Res. **60**:27, 1970.
45. Lumsden, C. E.: Nervous tissue in culture. In Bourne, G. H., editor: The structure and function of nervous tissue, vol. I New York, 1968, Academic Press, Inc.
46. Manuelidis, L., and Bornstein, M.: ^{125}I- labelled thyroid hormones in cultured mammalian nerve tissue, Z. Zellforsch. **106**:189, 1970.
47. Masurovsky, E. B., Bunge, M. B., and Bunge, R. P.: Cytological studies of organotypic cultures of rat dorsal ganglia following X-irradiation in vitro, II. Changes in Schwann cells, myelin sheaths, and nerve fibers, J. Cell Biol. **32**:497, 1967.
48. Masurovsky, E. B., Benitez, H. H., and Kim, S. U.: Origin, development, and nature of intranuclear rodlets and associated bodies in chicken sympathetic neurons, J. Cell Biol. **44**:172, 1970.
49. Murray, M. R.: Nervous tissues in vitro. In Willmer, E. N., editor: Cells and tissues in culture, vol. II, New York, 1965, Academic Press, Inc.
50. Murray, M. R., and Stout, A. P.: Adult human sympathetic ganglion cells cultivated in vitro, Amer. J. Anat. **80**:225, 1947.
51. Murray, M. R., and Benitez, H. H.: Denterium oxide: direct action on sympathetic ganglion isolated in culture, Science **155**:1021, 1967.
52. Nakai, J.: Studies on the mechanism determining the course of nerve fibers in tissue culture, II. The mechanism of fasciculation, Z. Zellforsch. **52**:427, 1960.
53. Nakai, J.: The development of neuromuscular junctions in cultures of chicken embryo tissues, J. Exp. Zool. **170**:85, 1969.
54. Nakai, J., and Okamoto, M.: Identification of neuroglia cells in tissue culture. In Nakai, J., editor: Morphology

of neuroglia, Springfield, Illinois, 1963, Charles C Thomas, Publisher.

55. Nakajima, S.: Selectivity in fasciculation of nerve fibers in vitro, J. Comp. Neurol. **125:**193, 1965.
56. Nakazawa, T.: Biological response of oligodendrocyte and astrocyte in tissue culture. In Nakai, J., editor: Morphology of neuroglia, Springfield, Illinois, 1963, Charles C Thomas, Publisher.
57. Norton, W. T., and Poduslo, S. E.: Neuronal soma and whole neuroglia of rat brain: a new isolation technique, Science **167:**1144, 1970.
58. Olenev, S. N.: Doses and action of pharmacological agents on growth of neuroblasts in culture, Neurosci. Trans. **12:**111, 1969.
59. Paul, J.: Cell and tissue culture, ed. 4, Baltimore, 1970, The Williams & Wilkins Co.
60. Peterson, E. R., and Murray, M. R.: Modification of development in isolated dorsal root ganglia by nutritional and physical factors, Develop. Biol. **2:**461, 1960.
61. Peterson, E. R., and Crain, S. M.: Innervation in cultures of fetal rodent skeletal muscle by organotypic explants of spinal cord from different animals, Z. Zellforsch. **106:**1, 1970.
62. Pfeiffer, S. E., and others: Synthesis by a clonal line of rat glial cells of a protein unique to the nervous system, J. Cell. Comp. Physiol. **75:**329, 1970.
63. Pomerat, C. M.: Observations on newborn rat dorsal root ganglia in vitro following gamma irradiation. In Haley, J., and Snider, R. S., editors: Response of the nervous system to ionizing radiation, Boston, 1964, Little, Brown and Company.
64. Pontén, J., and Macintyre, E. H.: Long term culture of normal and neoplastic human glia, Acta Path. Microbiol. Scand. **74:**465, 1968.
65. Pontén, J., Westermark, B., and Hugosson R.: Regulation of proliferation and movement of human glia-like cells in culture, Exp. Cell Res. **58:**393, 1969.
66. Pyl'dvere, K. I.: Growth and transformation of embryonic ependyma in tissue culture, Neurosci. Trans. **12:** 102, 1969.
67. Raine, C. S., and Bornstein M. B.: Experimental allergic encephalomyelitis: A light and electron microscope study of remyelination and "sclerosis" in vitro, J. Neuropath. Exp. Neurol. **24:**552, 1970.
68. Rose, S. P. R.: Neurons and glia: separation techniques and biochemical interrelationships. In Lajtha, A., editor: Handbook of neurochemistry, vol. II, New York, 1969, Plenum Publishing Corporation.
69. Sano, Y., Odake, G., and Yonezawa, T.: Fluorescence microscopic observations of catecholamines in cultures of the sympathetic chains, Z. Zellforsch. **80:**345, 1967.
70. Scharenberg, K., and Liss, L.: Neuroectodermal tumors of the central and peripheral nervous system, Baltimore, 1969, The Williams & Wilkins Co.
71. Schubert, D., Humphreys, S., and Baroni, C.: In vitro differentiation of a mouse neuroblastoma, Proc. Nat. Acad. Sci. U.S.A. **64:**316, 1969.
72. Scott, B. S., Engelbert, V. E., and Fisher, K. C.: Morphological and electrophysiological characteristics of dissociated chick embryonic spinal ganglion cells in culture, Exp. Neurol. **23:**230, 1969.
73. Scott, B. S., and Fisher K. C.: Potassium concentration and number of neurons in cultures of dissociated ganglia, Exp. Neurol. **27:**16, 1970.
74. Seeds, N. W., and others: Regulation of axon formation by clonal lines of a neural tumor, Proc. Nat. Acad. Sci. U.S.A. **66:**160, 1970.
75. Seil, F. J., and Herndon, R. M.: Cerebellar granule cells in vitro, J. Cell Biol. **45:**212, 1970.
76. Sensenbrenner, M., and others: Autoradiographic study of RNA synthesis in isolated cells in culture from chick embryo spinal ganglia, Z. Zellforsch. **106:**615, 1970.
77. Shein, H. M.: Neoplastic transformation of hamster astrocytes and choroid plexus cells in culture by polyoma virus, J. Neuropath. Exp. Neurol. **24:**70, 1970.
78. Shimada, Y., Fischman, D. A., and Moscona, A. A.: The development of nerve-muscle junctions in monolayer cultures of embryonic spinal cords and skeletal muscle cells, J. Cell Biol. **45:**382, 1969.
79. Sobkowicz, H. M., Guillery, R. W., and Bornstein, M. B.: Neuronal organization in long term cultures of the spinal cord of the fetal mouse, J. Comp. Neurol. **132:** 365, 1968.
80. Trachtenberg, M. C., and Pollen, D. A.: Neuroglia: biophysical properties and physiologic function, Science **167:**1248, 1970.
81. Ciesielski-Treska, J., Hermetet, J. C., and Mandel, P.: Histochemical studies of isolated neurons in culture from chick embryo spinal ganglia, Histochemie **23:**36, 1970.
82. Tsujiyama, Y.: Normal and pathological figures of neuroglia strained with Tsujiyama's methods. In Nakai, J., editor: Morphology of neuroglia, Springfield, Illinois, 1963, Charles C. Thomas, Publisher.
83. Utakoji, T., and Hsu, T. C.: Nucleic acids and protein synthesis of isolated cells from chick embryonic spinal ganglia in culture, J. Exp. Zool. **158:**181, 1965.
84. Varons, S., and others: A cell line from trypsinized adult rabbit brain tissue, Z. Zellforsch. **59:**35, 1963.
85. Varon, S., and Raiborn, C. W.: Dissociation, fractionation, and culture of embryonic brain cells, Brain Res. **12:**180, 1969.
86. Veneroni, G., and Murray, M. R.: Formation de novo and development of neuromuscular junctions in vitro, J. Embryol. Exp. Morph. **21:**369, 1969.
87. Walker, F. D., and Hild, W. J.: Neuroglia electrically coupled to neurons, Science **165:**602, 1969.
88. Waymouth, C.: Osmolality of mammalian blood and of media for culture of mammalian cells, In vitro, **6:**109, 1970.
89. Winkler, G. F., and Wolf, M. K.: The development and maintenance of myelinated tissue cultures of rat trieminal ganglion, Amer. J. Anat. **119:**179, 1966.
90. Wolf, M. K.: Differentiation of neuronal types and synapses in myelinating cultures of mouse cerebellum, J. Cell Biol. **22:**259, 1964.
91. Yamada, K. M., Spooner, B. S., and Wessels, N. K.: Axon growth: roles of microfilaments and microtubules, Proc. Nat. Acad. Sci. U.S.A. **66:**1206, 1970.
92. Zagan, I. S., Lasher, R., and Stone, G. E.: Some preliminary light and electron microscope observations on colcemid and vinblastine sulphate-treated glioblastoma, J. Cell Biol. **47:**234a, 1970.

PART III Functional neuroscience

CHAPTER 12

NEUROCHEMISTRY

HAROLD B. ANSTALL

This chapter is concerned with some aspects of the chemistry of the nervous system. The first to be discussed is analytic neurochemistry, which reviews the basic chemical components of this complex tissue. The remaining parts deal with physiologic chemistry and interrelate some of the more important chemical systems with the functioning of the neural complex.

ANALYTIC NEUROCHEMISTRY

A gross analysis of the brain shows that it is composed of about seventy to eighty percent water, about one percent carbohydrate, about eight percent protein, ten to twelve percent lipid, about two percent simple diffusible organic substances, and about one percent inorganic salts.

The percentage of water corresponds fairly closely with that in other cellular tissues. In contrast with other tissues, most of the fluid in the tissue of the CNS is intracellular and thus primarily in the grey matter, as it is distributed in both neurons and glial cells. There appears to be very little interstitial fluid in the nervous system.

Solid substances account for relatively little of the total brain mass. Of these, simple diffusible materials, the organic solutes, and simple inorganic salts, account for only about two percent of the total mass. Of the other solids, protein and lipid together comprise up to twenty percent of the brain mass, with lipids predominating over protein. Protein is located within the cellular substance. The lipid components are varied and comprise several classes of compounds, which have been the subject of intensive study.

Brain lipids

The lipids that occur in the CNS are listed in the following outline:

I. Neutral fats (triglycerides)
II. Phospholipids
  A. Lecithins
  B. Phosphatidylethanolamines
  C. Cephalins (phosphatidylserines)
  D. Acetylphosphatides
  E. Phosphatidylinositides
III. Sphingolipids
IV. Steroids

Lecithins. Lecithins are phosphatidyl esters of glycerol in which a phosphatide acid is esterified with the hydroxyl group of choline. Hydrolysis yields glycerol, fatty acid, choline, and phosphate (see Fig. 12-1).

Phosphatidylethanolamines. Phosphatidylethanolamines are phospholipids in which ethanolamine replaces choline.

Cephalins. Cephalins, or *phosphatidylserines,* have the amino-acid serine in place of choline or ethanolamine. The name *cephalin* was originally given to a lipid fraction that is insoluble in alcohol, is isolated from homogenized brain, and contains both phosphatidylethanolamines and phosphatidylserines. The term has since become limited to use in referring to phosphatidylserines. The fatty acids, depicted in Fig. 12-1 as R_1 and R_2, are chiefly oleic and stearic acids. More variation is found amoung lecithins, where in addition to oleic and stearic acids, palmitic, linoleic, and arachidonic acids are also found. In general, lecithins found in the brain contain one unsaturated and one saturated fatty acid moiety, usually with a chain length greater than twenty carbon atoms.

Acetylphosphatides. Acetylphosphatides are very similar to phosphatidylserines. They have been shown to contain two long-chain alkyl components, one present in simple ester linkage, and the other in an unsaturated vinyl-ether linkage. The acetalphosphatides are also called *plasmalogens.* In the plasmalogens of the CNS, ethanolamine is the prominent base, although examples with both choline and serine are known.

Because of the configuration of the linkage to the secondary alcohol group of the glycerol moiety, these substances have some aldehydic properties. The aldehydes corresponding to stearic and palmitic acids have been obtained from acetylphosphatides obtained from brain in crystalline form.

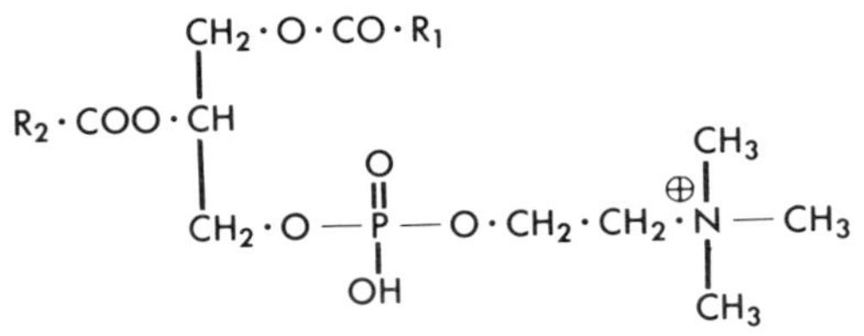

α–LECITHIN

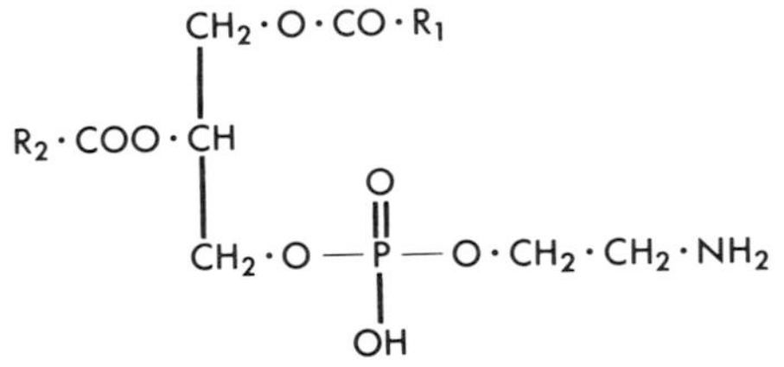

α–PHOSPHATIDYLETHANOLAMINE

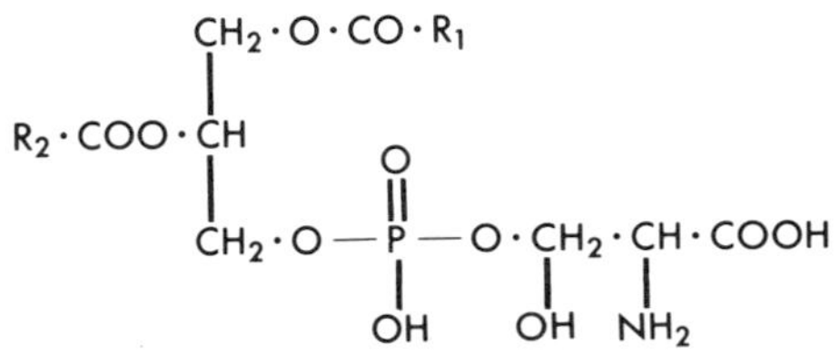

PHOSPHATIDYLSERINE

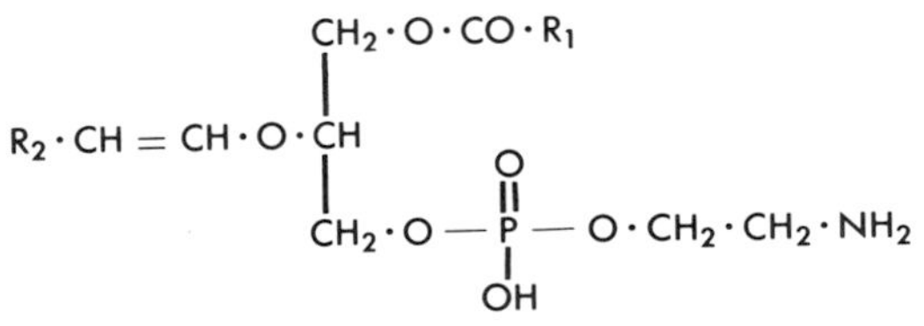

α–ETHANOLAMINE PLASMALOGEN

Fig. 12-1. Important phospholipids.

Phosphatidylinositides. Small amounts of *phosphatidylinositides* have been recovered from brain material, although these phospholipids are much more abundant in heart and liver and among plant tissues. In these substances, the organic base is inositol. It is probable however that phosphatidylinositides occur in the nervous system as a component of complex polymers. Other forms may be found, such as the (di)-α-phosphatidylinositol, in which two phosphate groups are esterified in the inositol ring at the meta-position (see Fig. 12-2).

Sphingolipids. Sphingolipids derive their name from a long-chain organic base described by Thudichum.[22a] The structure of the organic base was determined relatively recently, and the information regarding this has been well summarized.[4] It is 2-amino-4-octadecene-1,3-diol. It occurs naturally as D(+)*erythro*-1,3-dihydroxy-2-amino-4-*trans*-octadecene:

$$\overset{}{CH_3}\cdot(CH_2)_{12}\cdot\overset{5}{C}H{=}\overset{4}{C}H\cdot\underset{OH}{\overset{3}{C}H}\cdot\underset{NH_2}{\overset{2}{C}H}\cdot\overset{1}{C}H_2OH$$

The term *erythro* defines the positions of the substituent groups on the second and third carbon atoms, and *D* refers to the steric configuration of the asymmetric carbon atom at position 2. Saturated forms, in which the double bond between atoms 4 and 5 is lost, are known.[21] Other forms, in which chainlengths of twenty carbon atoms occur, have been described.[20] Sphingolipids contain as their

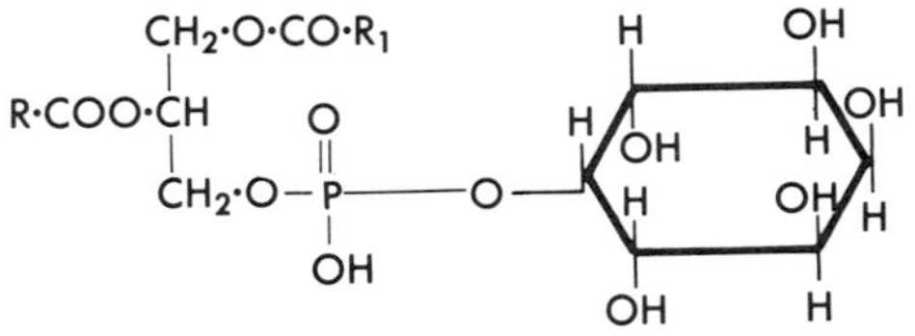

Phosphatidylinositide

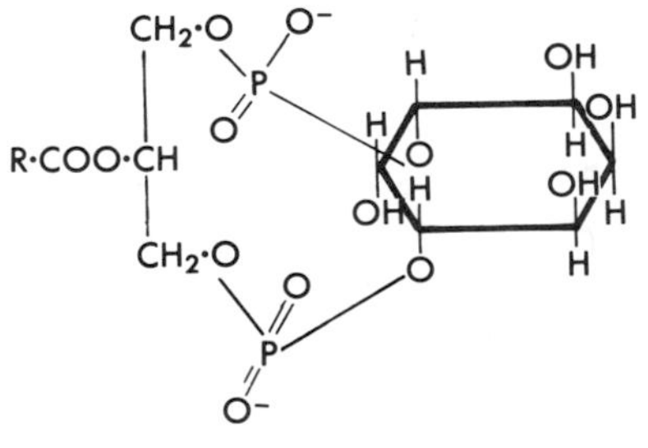

(DI)—α-Phosphatidylinositol

Fig. 12-2. Phosphatidylinositides.

basic unit an N-acetyl derivative of sphingosine, in which a long-chain fatty acid is attached to the amino group of the parent base at position 2, by means of an amide bond. Such a compound is called a *ceramide*. The sphingolipids have been variously classified. A rough division can be made between those with a substituent fatty acid of eighteen carbon atoms in length, found in gangliosides, and those with longer chains, occuring in cerebrosides and sphingomyelins.

More detailed classification is based on the nature of substituents on the primary alcohol group at position 1. In the ceramide hexosides, which include gangliosides and cerebrosides, a hexose is linked to this group as a glycoside; in the sphingomyelins the hexose is esterified with phosphorylcholine. Examples of these ceramide hexosides are cerebrosides, cerebroside sulfatides, ceramide di- and trihexosides, and gangliosides. Cerebrosides are composed of sphingosine, a hexose (glucose or galactose), and a 22- or 24-carbon acid. Cerebroside sulfatides (cerebron sulfonic acid) contain sphingosine, galactose, sulfate, and a 22- or 24-carbon acid. Ceramide di- and trihexosides are hexosides in which two or three sugars or amino-sugars are linked to position 1 of sphingosine. Gangliosides are ceramide trihexosides in which one or more hexose substituents are replaced by N-acetyl neuraminic (sialic) acid. One ganglioside is as follows:

sphingosine-glucose-GalNAc-galactose-NANA

in which GalNAc is N-acetyl galactosamine, and NANA is N-acetyl neuraminic acid.

These substances were orginally found in the brain of a patient with Tay-Sachs disease. Similar substances, variously called *strandins* or *proteolipids,* were later described.[7,19] Gangliosides in solution form complex micelle-like structures with a molecular weight of about 200,000, and in nature they are almost certainly bound to protein. They occur in neurons as a component of lysosomes. Activation of lysosomal enzymes may be concerned with disruption of molecular associations between ganglioside-protein complexes and the lysosomal enzymes themselves.

Sphingomyelins are phosphate-containing sphingolipids in which a molecule of phosphorylcholine is esterically linked to the primary alcohol group of N-acetyl sphingosine, as follows:

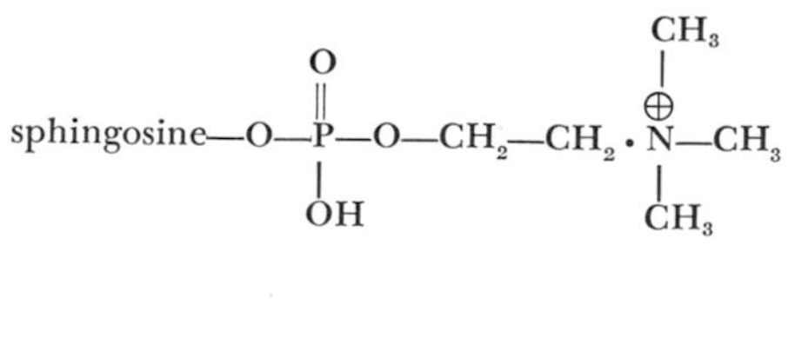

$$\text{sphingosine—O—}\overset{\displaystyle O}{\overset{\|}{\underset{\displaystyle OH}{\underset{|}{P}}}}\text{—O—}CH_2\text{—}CH_2\cdot\overset{\displaystyle CH_3}{\overset{|}{\underset{\displaystyle CH_3}{\underset{|}{\overset{\oplus}{N}}}}}\text{—}CH_3$$

In addition, the sphingomyelin contains a 10- to 24-carbon fatty acid.

The association of the polar groups of lipid phosphatides and protein at biologic interfaces, such as cell membranes and membranes of intracellular organelles, is of considerable importance. The varied composition of the phosphatides undoubtedly confers many peculiar properties on such interfaces, although the precise function of any one of them is not known. Little is known of the function of sphingomyelin in particular. It is distributed throughout the body in all tissues and is particularly well represented in such tissues as white matter, which has an abundance of myelin sheaths. The sphingomyelins of nervous tissue differ from those of other tissues, such as red cells or liver cells, in having fatty acids with longer chain-lengths (from 22 to 24 carbons). Those sphingomyelins elaborated within the cytoplasm of liver and other parenchymal cells have chain-lengths of from 16 to 18 carbons. It is advantageous to speak of *short-chain* (cytoplasmic) spingomyelins and *long-chain* (membrane-type) sphingomyelins.

Steroids. Cholesterol and its esters (steroids) are represented in nervous tissue, as in other tissues; they are found as components of cell membranes.

Lipid turnover in the nervous system is low.* Cerebral lipids are little affected by starvation, and tracer studies indicate relatively little metabolic exchange. Lipid distribution between white matter (myelin sheaths) and gray matter (neurons and glia) shows a preponderance of sphingolipids, cerebrosides, and phosphatides in the white matter. This distribution is expected, as these substances are major components of myelin.

Myelin is a highly complex material made up of various lipids, proteins, and polysaccharides. It has a well-defined geometric structure. The lipids found in myelin have already been discussed; they include cholesterol, various sphingolipids, simple phosphatidic lipids (lecithins, cephalins, plasmologens), and phosphatidinositols.

There are several protein components in myelin, and at least one is antigenic and has been used to produce allergic encephalomyelitis in other species. Myelin also contains complex glycaminoglycans.

Special optical studies using polarized light suggest that the myelin sheath is comprised of radially arranged lipid layers, with additional protein laminae situated between them. The precise ar-

*For a discussion of various aspects of synthesis and degradation of brain lipids see reference 7, and for a review of cerebral lipidoses see references 8, 9, and 16.

rangement of protein molecules within their respective layers is not entirely known.

Because the distribution within myelin of cholesterol, phospholipid, and sphingolipid is in the ratio of 2:2:1, there may be two phospholipid-protein and two cholesterol-protein units for each sphingolipid-protein unit.[6] A protein component may be linked to a mucopolysaccharide by a sphingolipid bridge.[23] It is likely that calcium and magnesium ions play a significant role in stabilizing the structure of the myelin sheath.

Certain differences are noted between the myelin of nerves of the CNS and that of peripheral nerves. This is probably related more to internal binding and stability than to qualitative composition, since the cerebroside of peripheral nerve myelin cannot be extracted by lipid solvents, whereas that of the CNS is readily leached out. There are presumably significant differences in the manner of internal linkage of cerebrosides in the two locations.

Proteins

The physiologic behavior of proteins is related to their tertiary and quaternary structure, and to the distribution and location of charged surface groups. Such spiral configurations are of importance in the provision of specific receptor sites for many substances of varied physiologic functions (such as neurosecretory products). At present, little is known of this area. Evidence connects cerebral proteins with such higher functions as learning, information storage, and recall,[22] although their physiologic role is not currently understood.

Cerebral enzymes and overall metabolism

A number of enzymes systems appear to be peculiar to the CNS. Many others have widespread distribution in other tissues but are of paramount importance to the metabolism of the brain. These enzymes are for convenience considered under three major, though artificial, divisions of metabolism.

Carbohydrate metabolism. Glucose provides the principal energy source for the brain.[18] The main pathway for degradation of glucose is the Embden-Meyerhof glycolytic sequence. The pyruvate formed is largely oxidized aerobically through the Krebs tricarboxylic cycle. All of the enzymes concerned in these two cycles are of major importance in the normal basic function of the brain.

The aerobic glycolytic pathway (hexose-monophosphate shunt), though found in the brain, quantitatively plays little part in the utilization of glucose by that tissue. Its main significance may be the production of pentoses, which are later incorporated into nuclei acids and adenine-nicotinamide coenzymes.

Protein metabolism. As previously mentioned, little is known regarding overall protein metabolism in the brain. Uptake of amino acids by active transport at the blood-brain barrier has been demonstrated. Total protein turnover appears to be rather slow, but exchange of free amino acids is rapid. Thus, a marked difference is seen between the rate of incorporation of labeled amino acids into cerebral protein and exchange across the blood-brain barrier. Large discrepancies occur between the concentration of amino acids in the blood and the size of the amino acid pool within the brain. To what extent the demand for a particular amino acid affects its rate of transport is not known. However, the evidence showing how rapidly free amino acids can be exchanged suggests that it is probably of little consequence.

Actual measurements of protein turnover in the CNS are difficult, but they have yielded some interesting information. Turnover appears to be most rapid in the cerebral cortex and slowest in the spinal cord. It is likely that the rate of turnover is similar for both glial cells and neurons. This is in accordance with observations of proteases within the cell bodies of both neurons and glia in the cortex, distributed almost evenly between the two kinds of cells. It is possible that these enzymes are concerned in protein breakdown in the cortical cells. Information regarding the site of protein formation in the brain is scanty. That glial cells may actively synthesize proteins is well known, but to what extent neurons are able to do so is unclear. Certain enzymes, such as cholinesterase, are believed to be synthesized in the neuronal cell body and then transported intracellularly to the axon, but it is possible that such proteins may be primary products of glial cells rather than neurons. The intimate relationship of glial cells to neurons may actually permit exchanges of materials between such cells; in this case there is a truly symbiotic relationship. This question is not yet resolved with regard to protein.

Lipid metabolism. The brain is able to utilize long-chain fatty acids to some extent as a source of energy. In general, such sequences play little part in the overall economy of the tissue. Of far greater importance is the synthesis of the more complex lipids, which are significant for the structure of biologic membranes and the myelin sheath. The nature of these has previously been considered.

Enzyme systems of peculiar importance in the brain

Cholinesterase. This enzyme, widely distributed in nervous tissue of all animals, shows a high degree of specificity for acetylcholine. Similar enzymes occur in muscle cells and erythrocytes, but they seem to be largely absent from other parenchymatous tissue. Under the influence of cholinesterase, the hydrolysis of acetylcholine proceeds very rapidly. The enzyme displays maximal activity near the surface membrane of neurons and only very low activity in axoplasm. The hydrolysis of acetylcholine by cholinesterase at the membrane surface allows repolarization of the membrane. Other, nonspecific cholinesterases occur in neuroglial cells.

Cholinesterase is inhibited competitively by physostigmine and its analogues, and noncompetitively by organophosphorus compounds. This inhibition can be at least partially reversed by pyridine-2-aldoscime methiodide (PAM), which displaces the phosphoryl group of the inhibitor from the enzyme. This produces an acetylated enzyme complex that is directly hydrolyzed by water to give acetate and free enzyme.

Choline-acetylase. This enzyme has been obtained from nervous tissue of many species and is able to regenerate acetylcholine, as follows

$$\text{CoA} + \text{acetate} + \text{ATP} \longrightarrow \text{acetyl-CoA} + \text{AMP} + 2\text{Pi}.$$
$$\text{acetly-CoA} + \text{choline} \rightarrow \text{acetylcholine} + \text{CoA}$$

A molecule of ATP supplies the energy for the reaction. It is not surprising to find an enzyme capable of regenerating acetylcholine after its breakdown by cholinesterase. The distribution of the enzyme in the nervous system parallels that of cholinesterase, which in turn is most highly active in areas where the acetylcholine levels are high.

γ-Aminobutyric acid (GABA). This substance is of physiologic significance only in the nervous system. It is formed from the decarboxylation of glutamate. It occurs in the brain and spinal cord, but it not present in peripheral nerves.

The enzymes associated principally with this system are glutamate decarboxylase and GABA-α-oxoglutarate aminotransferase. GABA is formed in two stages—first the transamination of α-oxoglutarate to glutamate, followed by the decarboxylation of glutamate of GABA.

GABA appears to act by counteraction of facilitative impulses, which is achieved by limiting the degree of polarization of a neuron to a potential only slightly above that of the resting state.

Monoamine oxidase (MAO). This oxidative enzyme catalyzes reactions converting monoamines to the corresponding aldehyde. In these reactions hydrogen peroxide is liberated. The aldehyde produced is then generally oxidized to the corresponding carboxy-acid by the enzyme aldehyde dehydrogenase, with NAD^+ as coenzyme. The highest level of MAO activity is found in such regions as the hypothalamic nuclei that have low cholinesterase activity.

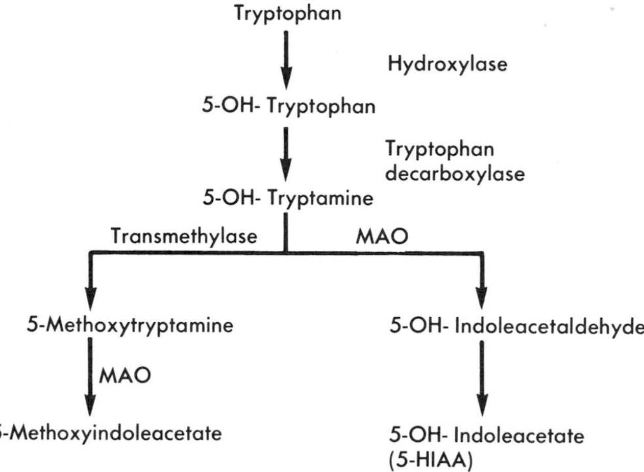

Fig. 12-3. The 5-OH-indole pathway of tryptophan degradation.

MAO activity in the nervous system is concerned with the breakdown of three amines that are active as neurotransmitters—epinephrine, norepinephrine, and 5-hydroxytryrptamine (5-HT, serotonin). Susceptible amine groups must be located at accessible sites at the ends of chains; those otherwise located are spared or affected only very slowly.

Tryptophan decarboxylase. Tryptophan is important in the brain as the precursor of 5-HT (serotonin), a neurochrome of great importance in several aspects of cerebral function. The pathway is indicated in Fig. 12-3.

Neurotransmitters and neurosecretion

It is becoming more and more apparent that the function and organization of the nervous system are dependent upon biochemical interactions. The advances in the understanding of neural function are chiefly due to recent progress in technology that permits quantitative microanalysis of the biochemistry of single nerve cells with a very small degree of error.[10]

Neurosecretion and synaptic transmission. Neurosecretion implies the elaboration of substances of definite chemical composition and having the properties of a secretory product. The cells concerned with neurosecretion exhibit the features of both nerve cells and secretory cells. Secretory products are identifiable histologically by the presence of stainable granules and functionally by the exhibition of hormone-like activity.

Such materials are formed in the perikaryon and are subsequently transmitted to the ends of the cell by axoplasmic flow. During this transfer the secretory granules have been observed to increase in size. The release of the materials is chiefly at the axonal endings of the cells. The axonal endings have been shown to possess synaptic vesicles, which upon excitement release the secretory products.

The role of neurosecretory substances in impulse transmission is well known. Studies of the autonomic nervous system and of the neuromuscular junctions of skeletal muscle have resulted in the conventional classification of autonomic junctions and effector endings as either adrenergic or cholinergic, depending upon the chemical mediator liberated.

Investigation of chemical neurosecretions and synaptic transmitters is extremely difficult because of the technical difficulties invovled and the complex organization of the CNS. However, as a result of numerous painstaking studies, a number of substances are now believed to meet the criteria for classification as central neurotransmitters. These substances are discussed in the following paragraphs.

Acetylcholine. Areas that respond to direct administration of acetylcholine are said to be cholinoceptive. There are several such regions in the CNS, including the caudate nucleus, the ventral basal thalamus, the lateral geniculate body, and the Renshaw cells of the anterior horn of the spinal cord. In such areas application of acetylcholine excites the postsynaptic structures for the same duration as the excitement resulting from presynaptic stimulation, and the same inhibitors counteract these identical effects. Additional cholinoceptive areas are now known to include the pyramidal cells of the auditory, visual, and somatic sensory areas of the cortex, the supraoptic nucleus, and certain cells in the posteromedial part of the thalamus.[13] One major difficulty in interpreting the results of these studies is the fact that varying dosages of acetylcholine produce different results; results depend upon the level of excitation of the particular structure being examined.

Norepinephrine and serotonin (*5-HT*). As mentioned previously, serotonin in nervous tissue originates from tryptophan. The catecholamines, dopamine, norepinephrine, and epinephrine are derived from phenylalanine, as shown in Fig. 12-4.

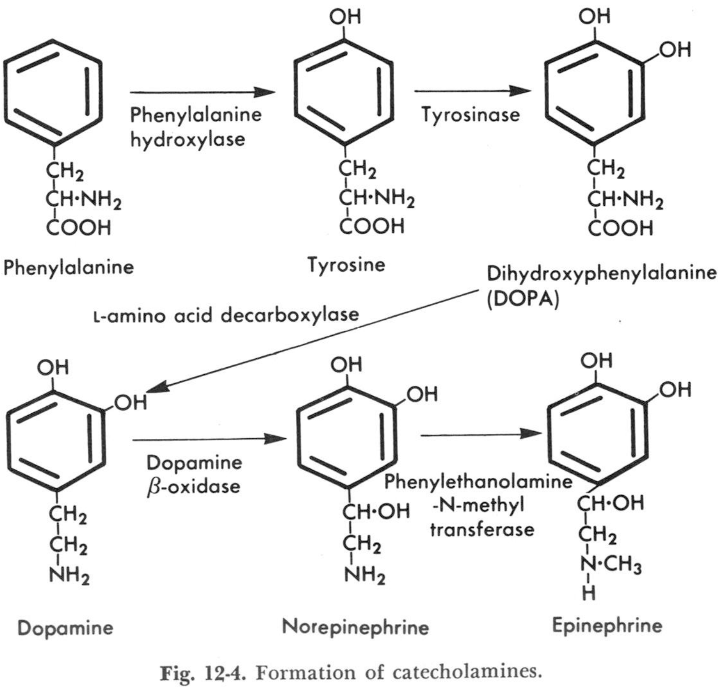

Fig. 12-4. Formation of catecholamines.

The catabolism of the catecholamines is summarized in Fig. 12-5. The decarboxylation of dihydroxyphenyl alanine (DOPA) to dopamine is performed by the enzyme l-amino acid decarboxylase. This substance, like monoamine oxidase (MAO), is an enzyme of wide application. It is this same enzyme that catalyzes the decarboxylation of 5-hydroxytryptophan, converting it to serotonin. Inhibition of this enzyme by analogues of DOPA is well known, and one such analogue, α-methyl-DOPA, has been used clinically to block this metabolic pathway in the treatment of hypertension. In the nervous system the metabolic pathway proceeds as far as norepinephrine. Conversion of this to epinephrine is probably confined to the adrenal medulla, and the enzyme catalyzing this step, phenylethanolamine-N-methyl transferase, has been found only in this tissue.

Monoamine oxidase catalyzes the oxidative deamination of epinephrine and norepinephrine with the formation of 3, 6 dihydroxymandelic acid, which is methylated at the 3-hydroxy to 3-methoxy-4-hydroxymandelic acid (vanillic mandelic acid, VMA) by catechol-O-methyl transferase. VMA, with metanephrine and normetanephrine, has no physiologic activity. Metanephrine and normetanephrine are formed by methylation at the 3-position of epinephrine and norepinephrine, respectively. The same methyl transferase catalyzes the reactions. Each of these terminal products of catecholamine catabolim may be in part conjugated with glucuronic acid or sulfate and excreted.

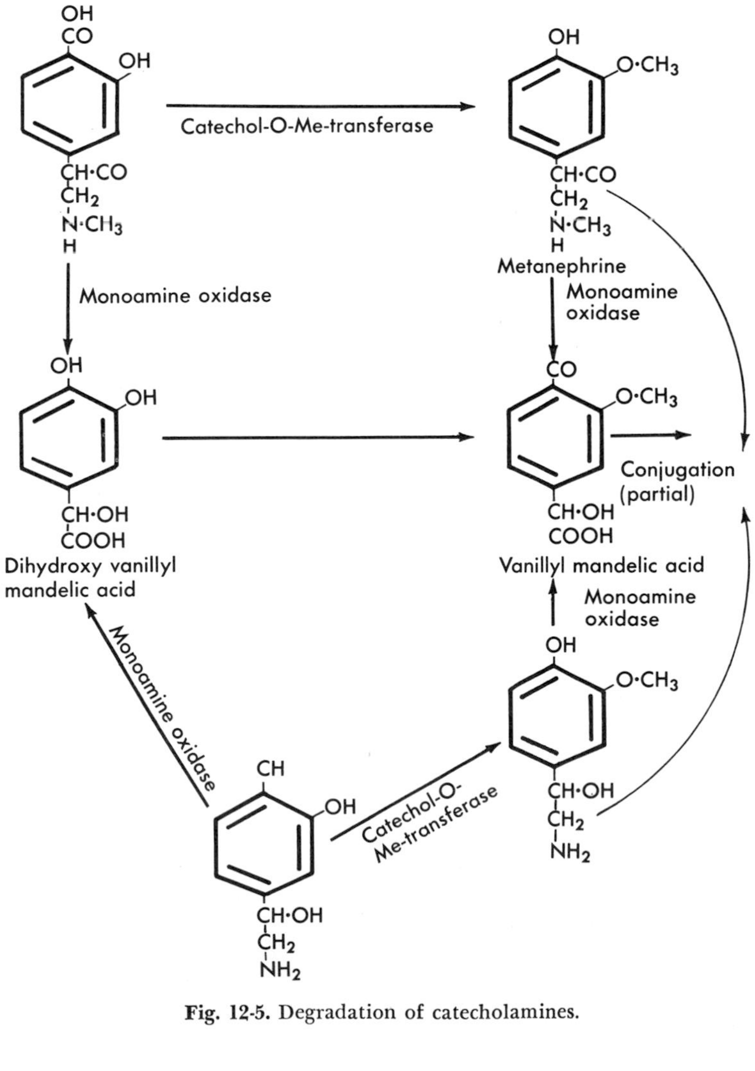

Catechol-O-Me-transferase
Metanephrine
Monoamine oxidase
Monoamine oxidase
Conjugation (partial)
Dihydroxy vanillyl mandelic acid
Vanillyl mandelic acid
Monoamine oxidase
Monoamine oxidase
Catechol-O-Me-transferase

Fig. 12-5. Degradation of catecholamines.

Serotonin and norepinephrine levels in the brain are both significantly reduced by reserpine, which produces a tranquilizing effect. However, if levels of both amines are artifically increased by blockage of monoamine oxidase, mood elevation and augmented activity results.[2,17] Local treatment of the limbic system and hypothalamus of the rat causes avid feeding, while acetylcholine causes drinking. On the other hand, injection of typhoid vaccine into the ventricular system produces fever. The fever can be prevented by the use of agents that block the effects of serotonin. Serotonin itself, when administered in this way, may also produce a febrile response.

Observation of the neurosecretory amines at their intracellular locations is now possible by use of a fluorescent technique.[3] This technique shows the amines to be located within neurosecretory neurons and associated with the granules that are transported axonally to the synaptic endings of these cells.

Dopamine

The formation of dopamine has previously been described. It is broken down by the routes shown in Fig. 12-6. High levels of dopamine are found within the putamen, the caudate nucleus, and in certain nerve endings related to the median eminence of the hypothalamus. Lower concentrations are found within the hypothalamus itself and in the substantia nigra. In these areas dopamine-β-oxidase, responsible for converting dopamine to norepinephrine, is absent. It is interesting that in persons with Parkinson's disease the corpus striatum, an area normally rich in dopamine, is depleted of this substance to levels less than fifty percent of normal. Such findings form the basis for the therapeutic administration of L-DOPA to patients with Parkinson's disease. It seems therefore that dopamine is intimately concerned with the function of the extrapyramidal system. Its presence in the synaptic terminals of secretory neurons in this system is good evidence that it functions as a synaptic transmitter.

Another material, *substance P,* has been located in the brain and is distributed in relatively high concentrations in several areas. However, it shows the unevenness of distribution that would be expected of a neurotransmitter. Thus, high concentrations are found in the dorsal roots of the spinal

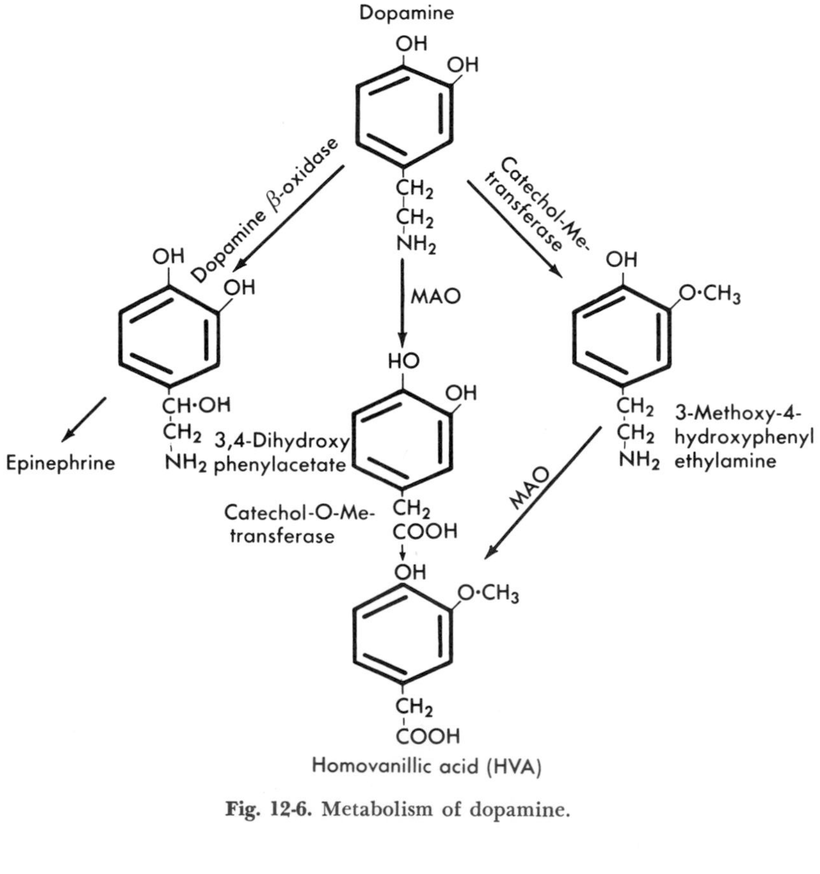

Fig. 12-6. Metabolism of dopamine.

nerves, in the main sensory tracts of the posterior columns of the spinal cord, in the substantia nigra of the brainstem, in the hypothalamus, and in the area postrema. It is a basic polypeptide of relatively low molecular weight (1600). Gross analysis yields thirteen anino acids, but sequential studies are not yet completed. Little or nothing is known of its metabolism.[12] It seems likely that substance P's role is that of a synaptic mediator at the central endings of main sensory tracts (pressure, touch, and vibration sense) in the cord, and it presumably may serve the same functions in the other areas where it is present in high concentration.

γ-Aminobutyric acid (GABA). The metabolism of this substance is shown in Fig. 12-7. Its intimate relationship with Krebs cycle intermediates is observed, as well as its association with three enzymes (transamination steps and glutamate decarboxylation) dependent upon pyridoxal coenzymes. GABA occurs only in the nervous system and is related to regulation of brain excitability. Thus, pyridoxal deficiency, causing interference with the formation of GABA, may result in convulsions. The intracellular location of GABA is as yet uncertain, but it is more likely found in glial elements than in neurons. It may function as an alternate substrate for oxidative cerebral metabolism. Its effects on cell membranes is largely nonspecific.

Histamine

Histamine is formed from histidine and is actively synthesized in the brain. Its formation is particularly marked in the hypothalamus, while its occurrence elsewhere in the nervous system is sparse (with the possible exception of autonomic ganglia). Its synthesis from histidine proceeds by decarboxylation (by l-amino-acid decarboxylase). It is subsequently converted to methylated iminazole derivatives, as illustrated in Fig. 12-8.

Histamine is unevenly distributed in the nervous system, and the distribution of histidine decarboxylase, the enzyme catalyzing its formation, closely parallels its occurrence. Its role as a synaptic transmitter is not understood, as the available data is too sparse to allow a definite pronouncement.

PSYCHOPHARMACOLOGIC EFFECTS

Much of our knowledge of the biochemistry of the brain results from the detailed study of the mechanism of action of psychopharmachologic drugs. Many substances have been synthesized that are able to produce profound effects upon the behavior and state of mind of an individual, and such substances have achieved something of a revolution in the management of many mental disorders. The study of their biochemical effects has

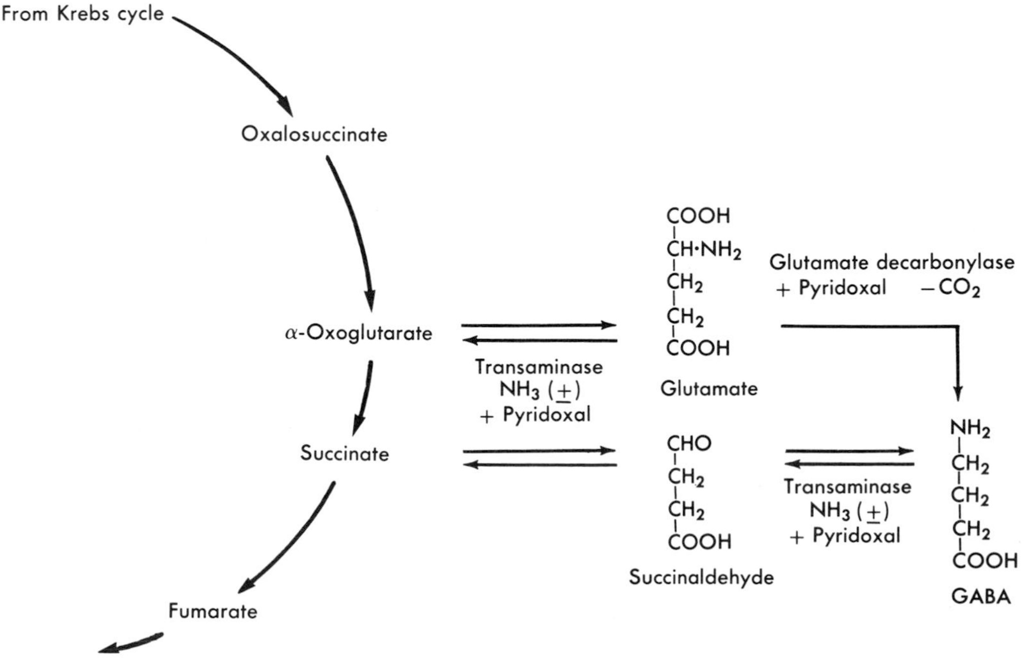

Fig. 12-7. Formation and fate of GABA from Krebs cycle intermediates.

brought more understanding of some of the functions of the transmitter amines.

The Rauwolfia alkaloids

The principal alkaloid produced by the Indian shrub *Rauwolfia serpentina* is reserpine, whose structure is shown in Fig. 12-9. Activity depends upon the presence of the 3, 4, 5-trimethoxybenzoyl component. Several related substances and analogues are also effective, such as deserpidine, rescinnamine, and syrosingopine (Fig. 12-10).

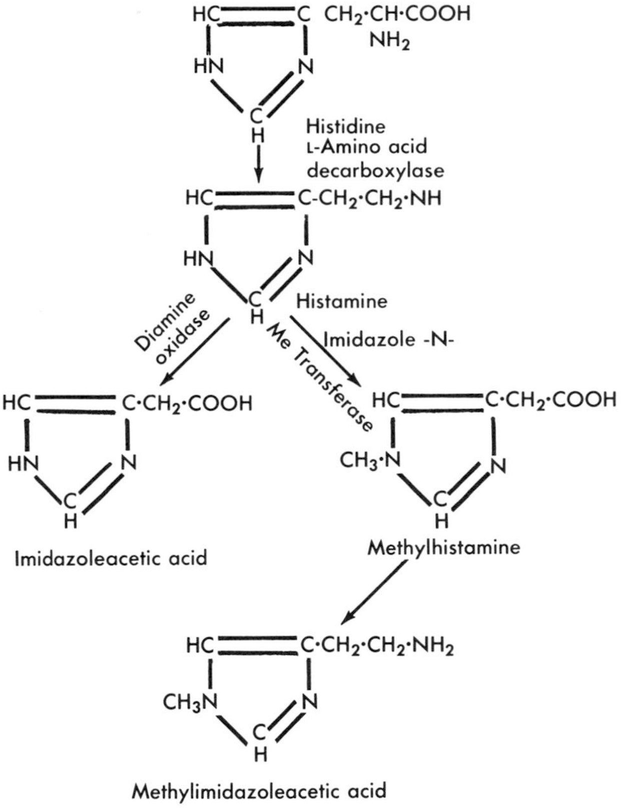

The most conspicuous effects of this group of alkaloids is the release of the transmitter amines, dopamine, norepinephrine, and serotonin. Continued administration of these compounds depletes the brain of all three amines. Various theories have been proposed relating the observed behavioral effects to the effect of the compound on each of these amines.

Some evidence is summarized here.

1. Since reserpine liberates serotonin, it was believed that the sedation it induces is due to the slow, continued release of serotonin in pharmacologically active amounts. However, pretreatment with monoamine oxidase inhibitors and subsequent administration of reserpine causes stimulation rather than sedation. Perhaps the prevention of breakdown of serotonin by the MAO inhibitors leads to the release of large enough amounts of serotonin to induce a paradoxic stimulation of synapses. This hypothesis is unproven. However, it is interesting to observe that during sleep the serotonin level of the brain rises while that of catecholamines decreases, and that during motor activity the serotonin level falls. It seems likely that some change in the balance between these two amines may account for the observed effects of reserpine.

Another intriguing phenomenon recently observed is the effect of reserpine on oligodendroglia. These cells in tissue culture exhibit rhythmic pulsations, which in the brain may be concerned with the distribution of fluid and metabolites. Reserpine markedly augments these pulsations, and this may significantly affect cerebral metabolism.[24]

2. Large doses of reserpine cause a marked depletion of norepinephrine in the brain, and the sedation observed is the opposite of the effects

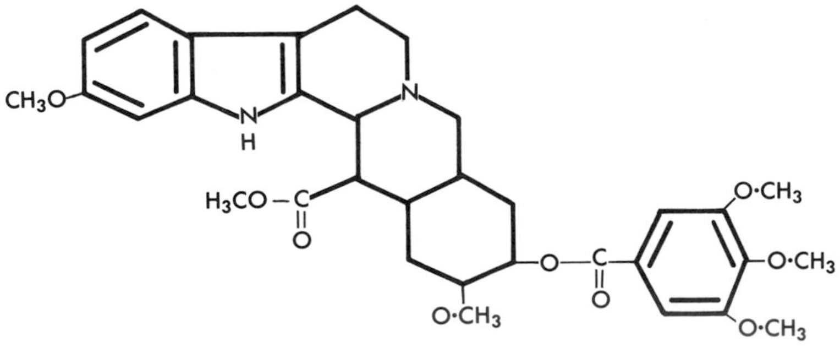

Fig. 12-8. Histidine and histamine metabolism.

Fig. 12-9. Reserpine.

of central sympathetic stimulation induced by such substances as picrotoxin, nicotine, and morphine. The administration of MAO inhibitors produces similar stimulant effects, which can be correlated with *increases* in the norepinephrine content of the brain. It seems possible that the sedative effects of reserpine are related to this depletion of catecholamines in the sympathetic centers; their function is thereby inhibited. Depletion of catecholamines could also account for some of the parasympathetic effects produced by the drug. The theory is inadequate in some respects, for it is known that certain agents like picrotoxin, which cause central sympathetic stimulation, also cause a significant reduction of catecholamines in the hypothalamus. Yet reserpine, which also causes such depletion, invariably produces sedation. After prolonged treatment with reserpine, the central sympathetic centers still function normally, despite almost complete depletion of norepinephrine.

3. Reserpine has been observed to diminish the dopamine content of the brain. As mentioned previously, this amine is distributed in high concentration in the extrapyramidal system. Prolonged treatment with reserpine has been shown to produce a parkinson-like state. Parkinson's disease is similarly associated with depletion of dopamine in the extrapyramidal system. Effect of reserpine on the extrapyramidal system is therefore important. At present, all areas of reserpine activity are considered important, and it is not yet possible to interpret the total reserpine effect in terms of the depletion of one particular amine. It is most likely that the observed effects are the complex

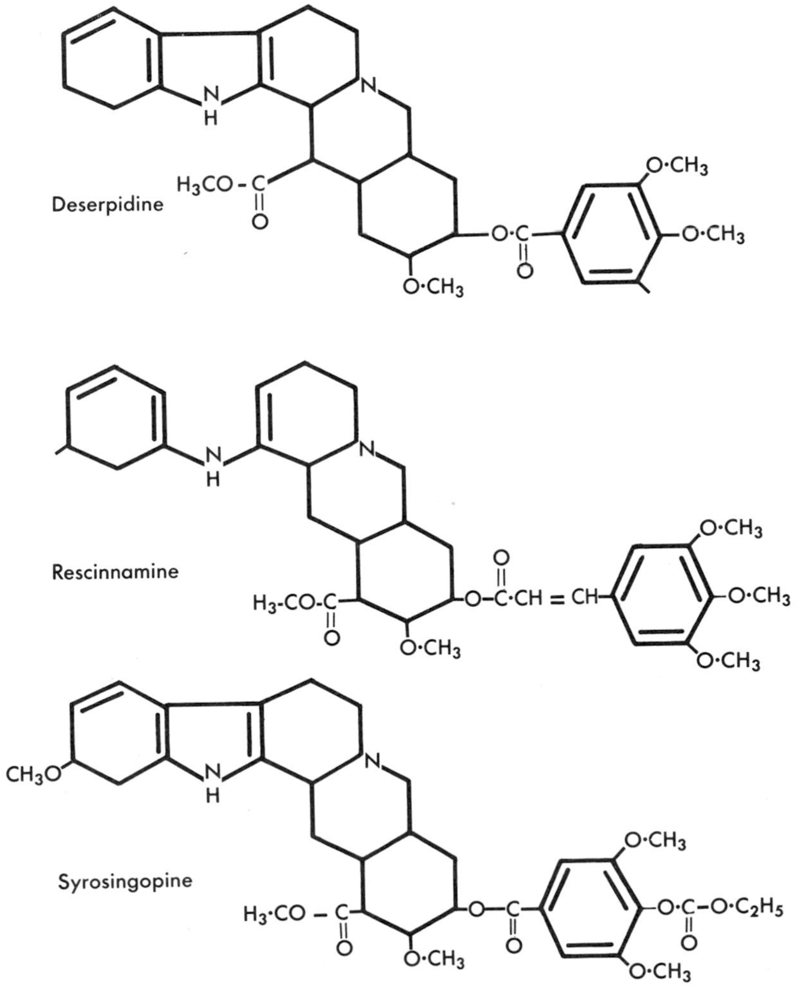

Fig. 12-10. Rauwolfia alkaloids related to reserpine.

result of amine depletion in a variety of cerebral centers, although the coordinated function of these centers is presently unknown.

The effects of reserpine in the CNS appear to be largely synaptic. Amine depletion is probably due to inhibition of uptake and binding of the transmitter amines at the postsynaptic membrane.

The phenothiazine compounds

Phenothiazine has the following structure:

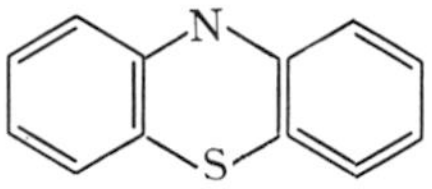

A variety of derivatives of this substance are now available as tranquilizing agents. The first to be introduced was chlorpromazine, which appeared in 1950. Central activity of phenothiazines is largely concerned with substitution at the 2-position of the nucleus and at the nitrogen *bridge*. Some prominent, active phenothiazines are shown in Fig. 12-11.

The phenothiazines are potent, surface-active substances. Their central effects are complex and multiple.

1. They inhibit a number of enzyme systems in which flavin adenine dinucleotide (FAD) is the coenzyme. As a result of this inhibition, respiration is decreased, and oxidative phosphorylation is uncoupled. Similar effects have been demonstrated with phenothiazines and phenazines in vitro using liver cell mitochondria.[1] However, these observations were made with in vitro systems and under nonphysiologic circumstances. The familiar pharmacologic effects are much more likely to be due to the relation of phenothiazines to the neurotransmitters than to less specific biochemical effects that may be observed only at drug concentrations that clinically would be toxic.

2. Phenothiazines prevent or retard liberation of acetylcholine, probably by a stabilizing effect in the membranes of synaptic vesicles of acetylcholine-containing endings.

3. Phenothiazines do not affect the concentration of norepinephrine, dopamine, and serotonin in the brain. They antagonize the effect of the MAO inhibitor, iproniazid, and prevent the elevation of norepinephrine induced by this drug. However, they are unable to prevent a concomitant rise in the dopamine level. They are also able to prevent the depletion of serotonin usually observed after reserpine treatment.

4. From electrophysiologic studies these agents appear to exert much of their effect on the reticular formation, the hypothalamus, and the extra-

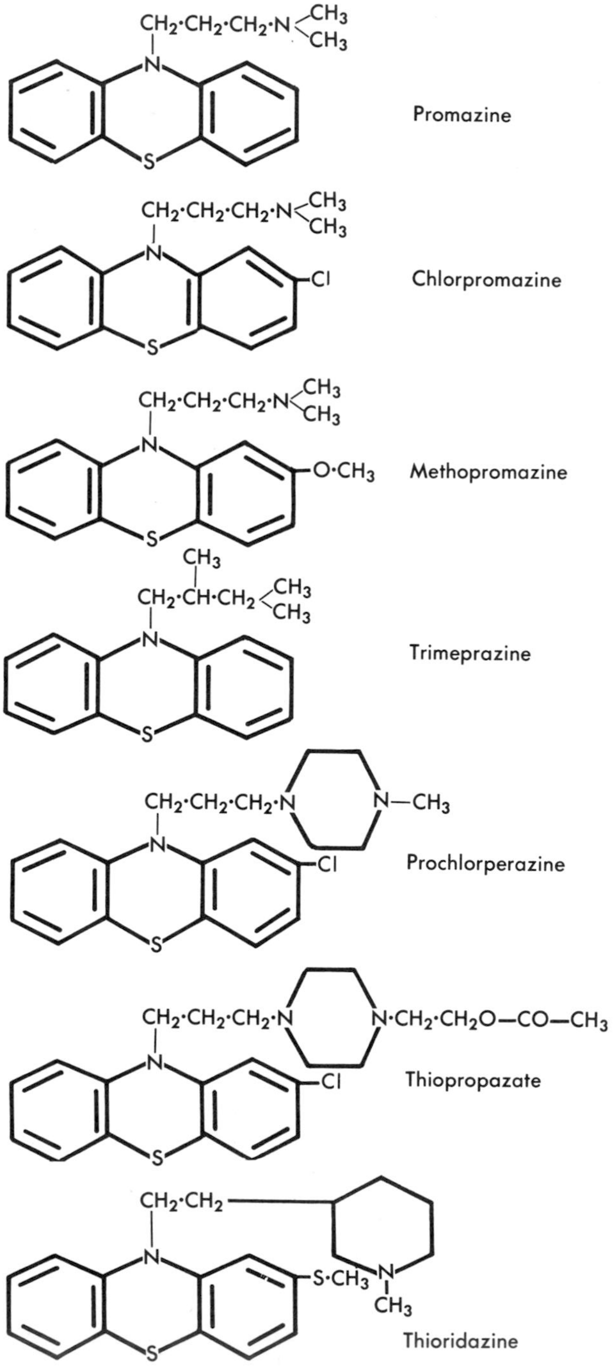

Promazine

Chlorpromazine

Methopromazine

Trimeprazine

Prochlorperazine

Thiopropazate

Thioridazine

Fig. 12-11. Some important phenothiazines.

pyramidal system. These regions are variously rich in either catecholamine, dopamine, or serotonin. There is close correlation between the distribution of these amines and the sites of action (as electrophysiologically demonstrated) of the phenothiazines.

The occurrence of parkinsonism as a consequence of treatment with phenothiazines is interesting, as it also occurs with reserpine (antagonists of phenothiazines). It is probably due to interference by phenothiazines with the uptake of newly formed amines into specific storage sites. Himwich and Rinaldi have observed that large doses of chlorpromazines induce significant increases in the electrical activity of the ascending reticular system in the rabbit. Extension of this activity to the descending reticular system also seems to occur. This extension results in uncoordinated entrapyramidal activity that leads to parkinson-like states. Selective destruction of specific regions such as the substantia nigra or reticular formation can also induce parkinsonism. These two areas are identical with those shown to respectively contain dopaminergic secretory neurons and noradrenergic secretory neurons, so that selective interference with their function by phenothiazines could readily lead to parkinsonism. The occurrence of mild parkinsonian symptoms is often regarded as a measure of effective dosage. Withdrawal of the drug allows the parkinsonian state to revert to normal.

Phenothiazines produce a subjective state of transquility. Motor activity is generally reduced, and inquiring or exploratory behavior is retarded. Hostility and aggressiveness are notably reduced. With larger amounts a marked sedative effect is observed, and with yet greater doses there is profound central depression.

Monoamine oxidase (MAO) inhibitors

These compounds are widely used in treatment by psychiatrists because of their profound antidepressant effects.[25]

Several types of chemicals can act as MAO inhibitors. These include hydrazine derivatives containing the group configuration R_1-NH-NH-R_2, where R_1 and R_2 can be varied, but for activity at least one contains an alkyl residue. The group includes hydrazine derivatives, such as benzylhydrazine, and hydrazides, such as iproniazid, nialamide (2-benzyl carbamyl ethyl hydrazid isoniotinic acids), and isocarboxazide. The alkaloids harmine and harmaline are also MAO inhibitors, as are certain indolyl alkylamines such as methyl tryptamine. Certain other amines, such as paraline (N-methyl-N-2-propynylbenzylamine) and 2-phenylcyclopropylamine, are also effective.

MAO inhibitors produce the following specific effects.

1. They augment the action of both endogenous and exogenous monoamines.
2. They increase the concentration of monoamines in the brain and elsewhere.
3. They antagonize reserpine by preventing amine release.
4. They have a marked antidepressant effect.
5. They inhibit certain peripheral effects, including a hypotensive action.

Most experimental evidence links their antidepressant action to their inhibition of monoamine oxidase and consequent elevation of cerebral monoamine levels.

Thymoleptic agents

These are valuable antidepressant drugs that are not concerned with MAO inhibition. They include such compounds as the iminodibenzyls (such as impiramine), the iminostilbenes, and the dibenzodiazepines and dibenzocycloheptatrienes. Many of these agents have marked antihistaminic effects, which may be of central significance in the CNS; some also appear to potentiate the effects of norepinephrine. Their central effects may be due to their providing increased availability of norepinephrine at certain vital sites. Unlike phenothiazines, they antagonize the central depressant effects of reserpine and its analogues.

REFERENCES

1. Anstall, H. B., Ahearn, M. J., and Jardine, J. H.: The effects of phenazinium and phenothiazine upon mitochondrial metabolism, Biochem. Pharmacol. **16**:561, 1967. 1967.
2. Brodie, B. B., Maichel, R. P., and Weslermann, E. G.: In Kety, S. S., and Elhes, J., editors: Regional neurochemistry, Oxford, 1961, Pergamon Press, Inc.
3. Carlson, A., and Hillarp, N-A.: A histochemical localization of the cellular level of hypothalamic noradrenaline, Acta Physiol. Scand., **56**:385, 1962b.
4. Carter, H. E.: Sphingolipids. In Chemistry of the lipids as related to atherosclerosis, Springfield, Illinois, 1958, Charles C Thomas, Publisher.
5. Elliot, K. A. C., Page, I., and Gvaslet, J. H.: Neurochemistry, Springfield, Illinois, 1962, Charles C Thomas, Publisher.
6. Finean, J. B.: In Richter, D., editor: Metabolism of the central nervous system, London, 1957, Pergamon Press, Inc.
7. Folch-Pi, J., and Lees, M.: Studies on the brain ganglioside strandin in normal brain and in Tay-Sach's disease, J. A. M. A. Dis. Child. **97**:730, 1959.
8. Frederickson, D. S.: Sphingomyelin lipidosis-Niemann-Pick disease. In Stanbury, J. B., Wyngaarden, J. B., and

Frederickson, D. S., editors: The metabolic basis of inherited disease, New York, 1966, McGraw-Hill Book Co.

9. Frederickson, D. S., and Trams, F. G.: Ganglioside lipidosis-Tay Sach's disease. In Stanbury, J. B., Wyngaarder, J. B., and Frederickson, D. S., editors: Metabolic basis of inherited disease, New York, 1966, McGraw-Hill Book Co.
10. Giacobini, E.: Chemical studies on individual neurons. In Ephenpreis, S., and Solnitzky, O. C., editors: Neuroscience research, vol. I, New York, 1968, Academic Press, Inc.
11. Grenell, R. G.: Neurochemistry. In Minckler, J. editor: Pathology of the nervous system, vol. I, New York, 1968, McGraw-Hill Book Co.
12. Haefely, W., and Huerlimann, A.: Substance P, a highly active naturally occuring polypeptide, Experientia **18:** 297, 1962.
13. Hernandez-Péon, R.: Central neuro-humoral transmission in sleep and wakefulness, Progr. Brain Res. **18:**96, 1965.
14. Holtz, P.: Role of L-dopa decarboxylase in the biosynthesis of calecholamines in nervous tissue and the adrenal medulla, Pharmacol. Rev. **11:**317, 1959.
15. McIlwain, H.: In Biochemistry and the central nervous system, Boston, 1959, Little, Brown and Co.
16. Moser, H. W., and Lees, M.: Sulfatide lipidosis. In Biochemistry and the central nervous system, Boston, 1959, Little, Brown and Co.
17. Poschel, B. P., and Ninteman, F. W.: Norepinephrine: a possible excitatory neuro-hormone of the reward system, Life Sci. **10:**782, 1963.
18. Rogers, R. L.: Carbohydrate metabolism in the nervous system. In Minckler, J., Pathology of the nervous system, vol. I, New York, 1968, McGraw-Hill Book Co.
19. Rosenberg, A., and Chargaff, E.: A study of a mucolipid from ox brain, J. Biol. Chem. **230:**1031, 1958.
20. Sambasivarao, K., and McCluer, R. H.: Characterization of the long chain bases in gangliosides, Fed. Proc. **22:**300, 1963.
21. Sweeley, C. C., and Moscatelli, E. A.: Qualitative microanalysis and estimation of sphingolipid bases, J. Lipid Res. **1:**40, 1959.

22a. Thudichum, J. L. W.: Die chemische Konstitution des Gjehirns des Measchen und der Tiere, Tübingen, 1901, Tirang Pieteyeker.

22. Waelsch, H.: The biochemistry of the developing nervous system, New York, 1956, Academic Press, Inc.
23. Wolman, M., and Hestrin-Lerner, S.: A histochemical contribution to the study of the molecular morphology of myelin sheath, J. Neurochem. **5:**114, 1960.
24. Wooley, D. W., and Shaw, E.: Evidence for the participation of serotonin in mental processes, Ann. N. Y. Acad. Sci. **66:**649, 1957.
25. Zirkle, C. L., and Kaiser, C.: Monoamine oxidase inhibitors. In Gordon, M., editor: Psychopharmacologic agents, vol. I, New York, 1964, Academic Press, Inc.

CHAPTER 13

ELECTROPHYSIOLOGY

LaVAR G. BEST

The purpose of this chapter is to introduce the student to the electrophysiology of nervous tissue as a part of the larger bioelectric phenomenon.

FUNDAMENTALS OF BIOELECTRICITY

The living biologic organism is a chemical battery. In some species of fish the voltage developed (up to 500 v) is sufficient to produce a stunning shock. The capability of relatively massive electric discharge displays the presence of electric potential at the biologic cell level. The presence of so-called *animal electricity* was noted by experimenters soon after Galvani's work on the effect of electricity on the muscles of frogs. He demonstrated that an electric current applied to the excised leg muscle of the frog would cause the muscle to twitch. This demonstration is perhaps the first experiment in electrophysiology.

An early demonstration of animal electricity was performed by preparing two frog nerve-muscle specimens. The nerve from one of the preparations was placed against the cut surface of the muscle in the other preparation. When this was done, the muscle in the first preparation would twitch. The reason for this is now known to be the electric potential of about 70 mv. between the cut and the normal surfaces of the nerve-muscle preparation. This electric potential created within the preparation acts the same on a nerve as an externally electric potential. Thus, when the nerve was placed on the cut muscle tissue, it was activated in a way that permitted the nerve to excite the muscle to which it was attached.

The action in this nerve-muscle preparation is the result of the electric potential that exists between the inside and outside of a muscle or nerve fiber. Production and maintenance of this potential between the outside and the inside of a nerve cell, its conduction along the fiber, and its transmission to other cells has been the object of intensive experimentation among electrophysiologists, neurophysiologists, and neurochemists. Some of these findings, as they apply to the general notions of neurobiology, are reviewed in the following paragraphs.

Membrane potential

If the junction of two solutions of different ionic composition is separated by a membrane, the diffusion potential is restricted, and a resting potential exists between the two solutions. The permeability of the membrane to ion flow determines the extent to which the potential remains constant. A cell membrane of 50 to 100 Å thickness surrounding the cytoplasm of a nerve or muscle cell provides a restrictive barrier between two different electrolyte pools. This is the basis of the −70 mv. potential between the inside and outside of the cell. With a nerve cell at rest it may be observed that, of the several ions present both inside and outside the cell, potassium (K^+) and sodium (Na^+) probably account for most of the transmembrane potential. Potassium ions are twenty times more concentrated within the cell than they are outside the cell. Sodium ions, by contrast, are ten times more concentrated outside the cell than within the cell. The cell membrane shows selective permeability to these two ions and maintains this imbalance of potential.

This steady-state potential imbalance, or *resting potential,* may be calculated quantitatively by a modification of Goldman's constant field equation, as follows:

$$E = \frac{RT}{zF} \ln \frac{P_K (K_i) + P_{Na} (Na_i) + P_{Cl} (Cl_o)}{P_K (K_o) + P_{Na} (Na_o) + P_{Cl} (Cl_i)}$$

where R = universal gas constant
T = absolute temperature
F = *Faraday* (electric charge per gram equivalent of univalent ions)
P = permeability (relative)
i = intracellular concentration
o = extra cellular concentration

Substituting the appropriate values as calculated by McLennan[9] into the formula, a value of −72.5 mv. is obtained. This is in agreement with the average of −70 mv. commonly given.

The equilibrium potential at the membrane for either the K+ or Na+ concentration may be calculated by the Nernst equation:

$$E_K = 0.058 \log \frac{(K_i)}{(K_o)}, \text{ and}$$

$$E_{Na} = 0.058 \log \frac{(Na_i)}{(Na_o)}$$

Using a 20:1 ratio of potassium concentration as an average, the calcuated equilibrium potential is −75 mv. Assuming at 10:1 average ratio of sodium concentration, the calculated equilibrium potential is 58 mv. Because the equilibrium potential at the membrane is not the same as the resting potential, an active transport has been postulated to maintain the K+ concentration within the cell and prevent the infusion of Na+ into the cell.

This imbalance becomes important when the nerve changes from the resting state to the active state, as shown by the appearance of the action potential. When a nerve becomes active its cell membrane becomes so highly permeable to an inward flow of Na+ that the concentration of Na+ within the cell becomes several times larger than the K+ concentration. This influx results in a reversal of the cell potential value, with the inside of the cell becoming as much as 40 to 50 mv. positive. In going from the resting potential, of −70 mv. to a measured +50mv., a total potential change of 125 mv. may be accomplished. At the peak of the action potential the maximum permeability to Na+ is reached, and thereafter the influx of Na+ starts to decline. At the same time that Na+ reaches its peak concentration, the membrane becomes permeable to K+, and the resulting efflux of K+ begins to return the membrane potential to its resting value. Once this action potential has been elicited, it transmits a unidirectional orthodromic mode throughout the length of the nerve fiber.

After the action potential has passed, the Na+ and K+ influx and efflux are probably reversed by metabolic processes in the nerve, in order to bring the membrane potential back to its resting state. One theory is that this stabilization comes about by Na+ expulsion, which is one notion of active sodium transport. An intracellular carrier enzyme that is an electron acceptor is presumed to exist. This combination permits attachment of the Na+, which is carried in this manner to the cell membrane. Here this carrier complex dissociates, with the Na+ moving to the outside of the membrane. A membrane-carrier enzyme captures the electron attached to the intracellular enzyme, which then returns to an intracellular position. The membrane carrier then loses its electron to the intracellular carrier, which traps a sodium ion and repeats the process again. Some measure of balance occurs by a slow drift of Na+ from outside to inside the membrane. This drift is governed by the concentration gradients between the inside and outside membrane surfaces. Potassium ions move across the membrane much more easily than sodium and display a continuing drift from inside to outside. Just how the Na+ and K+ overcomes the electrostatic gradient to reestablish the normal −70 mv. potential is unknown. The metabolic drive must be directed prin-

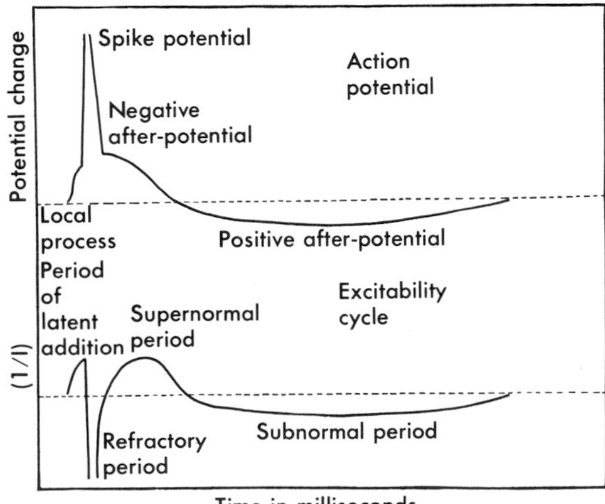

Fig. 13-1. The action potential and excitability cycle of a typical nerve fiber. For diagrammatic purposes the duration of the first two phases of each curve has been exaggerated. The spike potential is the action potential and corresponds to the refractory period. (From Physiological psychology, ed. 3, by Morgan, C. T., and Stillar, E. Copyright 1965 by McGraw-Hill Book Co. Used with permission of McGraw-Hill Book Co.)

cipally to Na+ to work against a potential of 130 mv.[4,8]

Coincident with the metabolic activity to restore the nerve fiber to its resting potential is the refractory period of the nerve. Classically the refractory period is divided into two divisions. First there is the absolute refractory period, during which the nerve is incapable of firing regardless of stimulus intensity, and then follows the relative refractory period, during which the nerve can fire again in response to a stimulus of above average intensity. The total refractory time period is somewhat variable with the absolute period, lasting one or two msec., and the relative period, extending for several msec. beyond the absolute (Fig. 13-1).

During the refractory period the influx of Na+ has been stopped, but the K+ efflux is very active. This condition means that the membrane potential drops below the normal resting level, prohibiting the development of another action potential. With the passing of time the membrane potential rises to the resting level, and the nerve fiber then passes out of its refractory state and is once again ready to fire.

Conduction

A nerve impulse is the conduction of the action potential through the length of the nerve fiber. The action potential, as mentioned previously, is initiated by the influx of Na+ into the nerve cytoplasm. As the influx of Na+ occurs there is an inward flow of electric current to the interior of the nerve fiber, which is called the *sink*. Adjacent to this sink area there is an area of outward flow of electric current, the *source*. The current emitting from the source upsets the resting potential of the nerve fiber just ahead of the source current. Upset of the resting potential in turn increases the Na+ permeability at this new area, resulting in an influx of Na+. The influx of Na+ causes the development of a new active site, or sink. The action potential (*spike*) is thus propagated along the nerve fiber, as shown in Fig. 13-2. This propagation is an all-or-none situation; if the threshold level for triggering an action potential has been reached, the propagated potential is immediately brought up to full strength and travels the whole length of the axon without any decrease in amplitude. Stimulus intensities above the minimum for firing do not result in a larger propagated impulse, but rather the impulse remains at the proper level. The all-or-none feature does not apply in the dendritic zone.

The speed at which the nerve impulse travels along the axon is in proportion to the diameter of the nerve fiber. The larger the diameter of the fiber the greater the speed of conduction of the impulse. In the mammalian neural system the most rapid rates of propagation occur in the large myelinated fibers. Here the myelinated axon propagates the action potential not by a smooth sequential sink-source advance, but by jumping from node to node.[6] This *saltatory* method of neural propagation in myelinated fibers results in a speed-up rate of propagation without a corresponding increase in axon diameter.

The movement of the impulse into and along the central pathways is invariably dependent upon additive assistance by other neuronal activities. The conductive systems are basically organized into complexes of short, interconnecting links and long pathways, which subserve only the *lemniscal systems*.

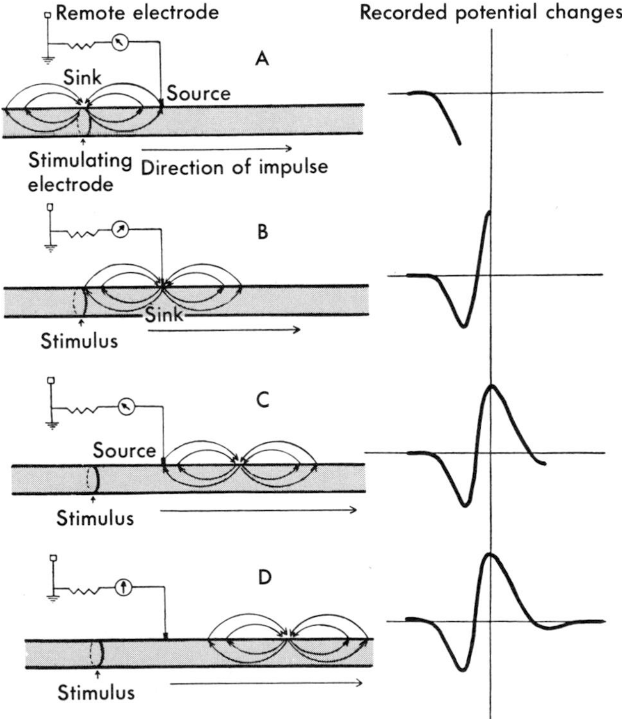

Fig. 13-2. Schematic diagram of the passage of an impulse along a nerve in a conducting medium. The exploring electrode is on the surface of the nerve; the second electrode on inactive tissue has the properties of an electrolytic conductor. The resultant excursions of the recording instrument are shown on the right. (From Brazier, M. A. B.: The electrical activity of the nervous system, New York, 1960, The MacMillan Co.)

Synapse

The means by which the nerve impulse is transmitted across the neural synapse has traditionally been considered either electrical or chemical. For several decades debate centered on all synapses as electrical or all synapses as chemical. As knowledge about synapses and their functioning has accumulated, it has become evident that both types of synapse exist. In some situations a particular synapse may transmit both electrically and chemically.

The chemical synapse is the most common synapse in man and has received the most study.[4] This type of synapse is essentially composed of a presynaptic ending separated from a postsynaptic ending by a cleft of approximately 200 Å. The presynaptic ending, or synaptic knob, typically contains a large number of synaptic vesicles. These vesicles apparently release a transmitter substance when triggered by the arrival of an action potential. The major transmitter substance is acetylcholine. This transmitter substance in turn diffuses through the synaptic cleft, depolarizing the subsynaptic membrane and initiating an action potential in the postsynaptic nerve fiber. The action potential is delayed by about 1 or 2 msec. as it traverses the synapse.

Before the action potential in the postsynaptic nerve fiber is triggered, there is an intervening potential called the *postsynaptic potential.* This potential may be either excitatory (E) or inhibitory (I). The excitatory postsynaptic potential (EPSP) has a rising phase of about 0.5 msec., then falls off rapidly in about 1 msec. However, it persists for several more milliseconds. The EPSP may be strong enough in a single discharge to trigger an action potential, or the EPSP may summate in space and time to achieve the necessary voltage to trigger the action potential. Several individual nerve endings converging on one postsynaptic membrane may summate, or several subthreshold events over time may summate.

The inhibitory postsynaptic potential (IPSP) is nearly a mirror image of the EPSP. Peak voltage is in the opposite direction, and duration is approximately the same, with the exception that the IPSP does not hold its minimal voltage as long as the EPSP.

> The essential difference between an excitatory (E) and inhibitory (I) action on the postsynaptic membrane can be stated in very simple terms: the E effect causes a depolarization; the membrane potential is driven to, or beyond, the threshold level at which action potentials (and/or contractions) arise. The I effect causes the membrane potential to be stabilized at (or move toward) a subthreshold level at which no active response (spike or contraction) can arise. Both effects are produced by an increase of ionic permeability; the difference lies in the particular "ionic gates" that are being operated by the excitatory and inhibitory transmitter action.*

The different ionic gates are an increase in permeability to Na^+ for EPSP and an increase in permeability to K^+ for IPSP.

The electrical synapse has two characteristics that are different from the chemical synapse. The most obvious difference is the shorter transmission time of about 0.1 msec.; the second difference is the possibility of transmission reversal in the electrical synapse.

Using microelectrode techniques it has been shown that the action potential at the electrical synapse postsynaptic fiber begins to develop almost concurrently with the arrival of presynaptic action potential at the synapse. This is evidence of an electrical spread of depolarization directly across the synapse. There is some evidence that the synaptic cleft in electrical transmitting synapse is much reduced in size, or there may be no cleft whatsoever.[1] This finding would be compatible with the flow of depolarization through the synapse.

Another type of synapse is the neuromuscular synapse, or motor end-plate. The structural anatomy of the end-plate has been well described, especially since the development of the electron microscope (see Chapter 22). The efferent nerve fiber divides at its terminal into several branches, with each branch lying in a depression on the muscle cell surface. The underlying muscle cell in turn is invaginated into secondary clefts. At the axon terminal there is again an abundance of synaptic vesicles and a cleft of from 500 to 700 Å between the nerve tissue and muscle tissue. Release of the neurohumoral transmitter (acetylcholine) brings about a depolarization of the end-plate, with a subsequent depolarization of the muscle surface membrane.

The method of release of acetylcholine at the neuromuscular junction is characterized by random release of quantified amounts of transmitter substance in the "resting" junction. These random releases result in small depolarizations in the subsynaptic muscle fiber region; the measured potential is about 0.5 mv. in amplitude.[5] It is now concluded that these miniature end-plate potentials do not constitute the muscle end-plate action potential, but when a nerve impulse arrives at this structure several hundred of these end-plate potentials

*Katz, B.: Nerve, muscle, and synapse, New York, 1966, McGraw-Hill Book Co., p. 147.

are synchronized to produce the full end-plate potential.

Full details on how the action potential at the cell membrane activates the contracting protein filaments (myosin and actin) in the muscle fiber are not presently known. Evidently the electric activity is led from the cell surface into the contractile mechanism by some sort of pathway.[6] At this point chemical reactions involving calcium ions and adenosine triphosphate (ATP) trigger the contracting mechanism.

Sense receptors

The various senses of the body have their distinctive end-organs; however, once the end-organ has been excited the conduction of the message through the nervous system is accomplished by the common and familiar action potential of a nerve fiber.

The transduction of the external stimulus energy to a nerve action potential is accomplished in several ways peculiar to the type of end-organ structure. An example of mechanical transduction is found in the Pacinian corpuscle. This pressure-sensitive end-organ evokes a graded potential, proportional to the amplitude and rate of mechanical distortion being applied to the end-organ. These graded potentials are summated until a critical level is reached. At this point the all-or-nothing action potential is triggered in the axon.

Smell and taste depend upon a chemical interaction at the end-organ. The olfactory cells are apparently excited by direct contact with inhaled particles dissolved in the moisture provided by the nose. The four basic taste qualities—salt, sour, bitter, and sweet—are perceived chemically at the so-called *taste buds* of the tongue. There are several exceptions to each condition, but generally it is believed that the hydrogen ion of an acid elicits sour taste, and the anion (for example, the Cl ion of a chloride) elicits salt taste. Sweet and bitter are even more confused, with little chemical constancy apparent, and no simple statement of chemical property can be made.

The visual end-organ is also chemical. The two receptor cell types, cones and rods, contain the photosensitive substances iodopsin and rhodopsin. The breakdown of these substances by light waves causes the generation of a retinal action potential in a manner not yet understood.

The auditory sense end-organ is a mechanoelectric transducer. An electric potential exists between the endolymph of the scala media, polarized at +80 mv., and the intracellular polarization of the hair cell at −60 mv. A variable resistance between the two polarizations is found at the cuticular surface layer of the hair cell; the bending of the hair in the hair cell is the active force in the variable resistance. Changes in the resistance modulates the flow of current through the hair cell. This current flow in turn modulates the liberation of acetylcholine, which then triggers the action potential in the afferent nerve ending.

THE ELECTROENCEPHALOGRAM

The information presently available regarding the electrical activity within a single excited neuron is not complete, nor is interneuronal electrophysiology well settled even in its basic mechanisms. It would appear however that enough knowledge has been developed to allow the use of neuroelectric potentials in the practical and experimental investigations of the neural system in man and animals.

One application of neuroelectric principles has been in the study of the function of the cerebral cortex. Of the several possible electrophysiologic approaches to the study of cerebral function, the most commonly known is the electroencephalogram (EEG). In 1929 Berger reported recording ongoing potentials from the human brain; the technique used he called an *elektrenkephalogram*. His report triggered a rapid development of the field of the EEG. Specialties soon developed. Some investigators addressed themselves to clinical application, while others pursued a basic research approach.

The EEG is characterized by several different rhythms of electric potentials, which may be somewhat localized to specific areas of the skull. The most outstanding of these rhythms is the alpha rhythm (Fig. 13-3). This rhythm has a frequency of eight to thirteen cycles per second. It is most prominent in the occipital area and to a slightly less degree in the parietal area, and is desynchronized by visual activity or alert attention. Beta rhythms have a frequency range of eighteen to thirty cycles per second and are frequently found over the frontal lobes. Delta rhythms of three to five cycles per second and theta rhythms of six to eight cycles per second are most often seen in stages of sleep or narcosis.

The site of origin of these rhythms is still not completely determined. The cortical structures that appear to be possible sources are the dendrites of the pyramidal cells. Some researchers caution against the use of the noninformative term *dendritic potentials*.[11] It has not been shown precisely which of the neuron potentials account for the brain waves or if all potentials are to some degree

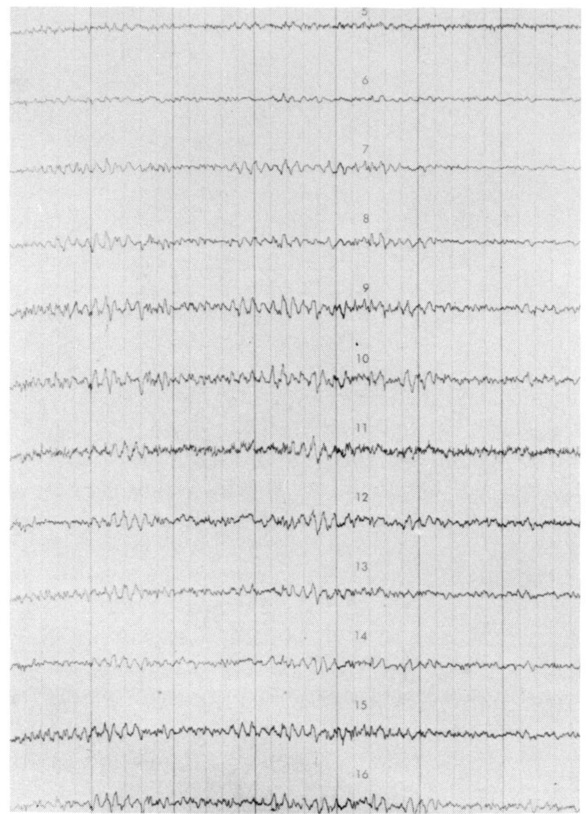

Fig. 13-3. Segment of a clinical EEG. Tracings 5, 6, 7, and 8 are from the parietal area; tracings 9 and 10 from the occipital area; tracings 11 and 12 from the frontal area; tracings 13, 14, 15, and 16 from the temporal area. Even numbers are from the right hemisphere, and odd numbers are from the left hemisphere.

responsible for the macrorhythms. The dendrites are uniformly radially oriented. They may possess thousands of terminal sites and make contact with thousands of other cells. There may in addition be axodendritic synapses between these apical dendrites and the collateral fibers of the tract from the thalamic reticular formation as the tract courses to the cortex.[2] This synapse would then provide a method of modulating the output of the pyramidal cells by the activity of the thalamic reticular formation. This proposed neural system would be compatible with research findings demonstrating that stimulation of thalamic nuclei can modulate both alpha-like activity and the spike and dome rhythm seen in petit mal epilepsy.

Deviations from the so-called normal rhythms of the brain have been interpreted by the clinical technician as evidence of different brain pathologies. The *spikes* appearing in the rhythm of patients with epilepsy present a classic example. Tumors of the brain may be detected by the presence of aberrant rhythms, and gross localization may also be determined by comparing the tracings from multiple electrode sites on the scalp. There are commonly sixteen electrode sites used, eight over each hemisphere with sampling from the frontal, parietal, temporal, and occipital lobe areas.

The underlying basis for the rhythm in the brain, what interrelationships exist between the various divisions of the higher CNS, and what the EEG might reveal in regard to such functions as memory, intelligence, and emotion are the primary interests of the EEG researcher.

EVOKED POTENTIALS

One component of the EEG that has recently been used both in research and in clinical application is the evoked potential. It was observed many years ago that a sensory stimulus such as a noise or flash of light elicits a change in the ongoing EEG. This change, the *cortical evoked potential,* could be a momentary change in the ongoing frequency rate, an increase or decrease in the amplitude of the tracing, and combinations of both frequency and amplitude changes. These evoked potentials were difficult to observe in the raw ongoing EEG tracing, and their usefulness in electrophysiology was not fully explored until the development of the electronic computer.

Averaged evoked potentials

Electronic computers are programmed to enhance the evoked potential so that it can be easily distinguished from the background EEG activity. A commonly used computer is the *summing,* or *averaging* device. This limited-use computer enhances the evoked potential by summing a series of time-locked segments of the EEG that are assumed to contain the evoked potential. The time-locking consists of opening the storage unit of the computer simultaneously with the starting of the stimulus. The EEG signal at that moment and for a period of time following the stimulus is stored in the memory of the computer. The stimulus is repeated several times, with the EEG signal sampled after each stimulus and added algebraically to the previously stored sum of signals. The negative and positive charges of the evoked potential are locked in time by the storage of the computer, and thus are added in a constant negative or positive direction with each successive stimulus presentation. The background EEG activity that is not triggered by the stimulus and therefore not consistently synchronized with the computer storage is randomly positive or negative at any particular moment in time. When added successively the background EEG signals will equal zero.

The technique of averaged evoked potential measurement has made possible new means of investigation. For example, the technique permits the use of awake human beings as subjects. This in turn permits investigation into the various parameters of the sensory-evoked potential coincident with the human variables of intelligence, emotion, and other psychologic states. These data, as they accumulate, should provide a great deal of information concerning the CNS.

Some interesting findings have already been reported. One study indicates that averaged evoked responses to spoken words recorded from the left temporal area may precede the evoked potential from the right temporal area when the words are understood. This sequence does not hold for potentials stimulated by words of a foreign language.[12]

Another application of the averaged evoked potential technique of EEG analysis is in determining threshold levels to sensory stimulation, particularly auditory stimuli. The procedure generally is as follows: the evoked potential is picked up by a unipolar electrode arranged with the active electrode placed on the scalp at the vertex, the indifferent electrode on one earlobe, and the ground electrode on the other earlobe. The evoked responses to a series of tones are added in the summing computer, and the summed response is read on an x-y graphic plotter. The summed evoked response to a tone is shown in Fig. 13-4. Determination of hearing threshold can be made by reducing the intensity of the tone until a response (evoked potential) is no longer apparent after summing a series of tone-locked EEG segments at that particular tone intensity. By using tones of varying frequencies presented to the right and left ear, a plot of the hearing threshold can be made. Evaluation of hearing threshold in infants, older children, and adults who could not or would not respond to conventional hearing test procedures has been possible by the use of this procedure.

Evoked potentials measured on the cortex

Measuring cortical potentials from the scalp has the disadvantages of substantially reduced intensity and loss of fine localization of site of origin. A cortical surface area of at least 2.5 by 2.5 cm. is necessary to evoke a potential visible on the EEG.[3] Evoked potentials measured at the surface of the cortex or deep into the cortex itself avoid these difficulties.

Utilizing the localization of site of origin of the evoked potential measured on the surface of the cortex, a plotting of the cortical localization of responses to specific stimuli can be made. A map of the localization of primary responses to auditory, visual, and somatic stimuli in the cat is shown in Fig. 13-5.

One method used in developing this type of plot is as follows. Using the cat as the experimental animal, the subject is anesthetized with pentobarbital. The scalp is then cut in the midline and reflected laterally, and the bony skull cap is cut off. The dura mater covering the cerebral cortex is then removed. The exposed cortex is kept moist by application of warm Ringer solution.

The electrode to be used in recording the evoked potentials is inserted into a stereotaxic instrument, and the tip of the electrode is gently but firmly placed in contact with the surface of the cortex. The head of the animal is also fixed in the stereo-

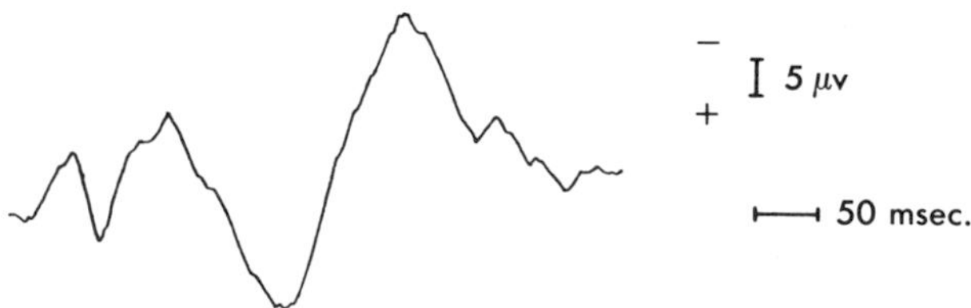

Fig. 13-4. Summed evoked response to a pure tone. The auditory stimulus was a 1K Hz. tone at an intensity of twenty-five decibels above threshold. Twenty stimulus-responses were summed for the potential illustrated.

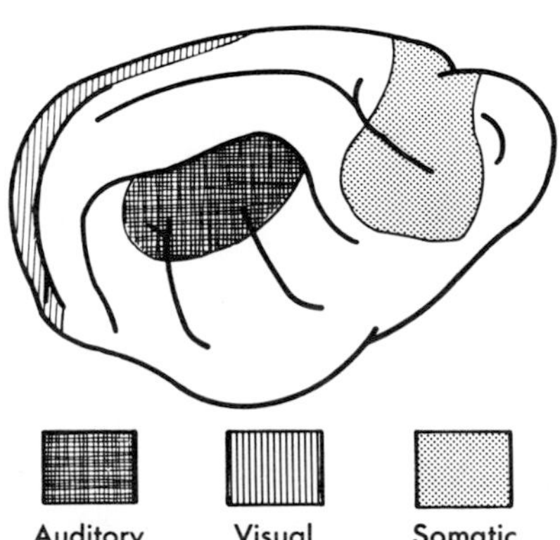

Fig. 13-5. Map of the projection areas of the cerebral cortex of the cat.

taxic device. The electrodes may be ball-tipped silver or stainless steel wire, or Ag-AgCl wick electrodes may be used. The stimulus to be used, (a click or tone for auditory measure, light flash for visual measure, or electric shock for somatic measure) is presented to the animal. The evoked cortical potential from the electrode site is then fed into an amplifier. Here the 300 to 400 μv. potential is amplified to raise the potential to a value compatible with the summing computer input—approximately 0.5 volts. Repeated stimuli are given, and the subsequent responses are stored in the computer. The enhanced evoked potential is then produced visually on an oscilloscope where it can be photographed, or the potential is read out on a graphic recorder.

The location on the cortex of the points to be studied are planned in advance by the use of a grid overlay. An oversize diagram of the exposed brain surface is drawn, and the points to be plotted are shown on the diagram. The points are generally in the form of a grid, with the points separated by a few millimeters. These plotted points are located on the cortex. The electrode is sequentially moved to each of the points, and the evoked response is recorded. The written potentials are then pasted on the appropriate spots of the diagram, resulting in a map of the evoked potentials found in that particular area of the brain for the particular stimulus used (Fig. 13-6).

Subcortical evoked potentials

Stereotaxic apparatus and the corresponding atlas of coordinate points provides a means whereby evoked potentials from centers in the auditory, visual and somatic pathways below the level of the cerebral cortex may be studied. For example, evoked potentials from the medial geniculate, inferior colliculus, and superior olivary nuclei in the auditory pathway can be obtained in this manner. Stereotaxic atlases showing the coordinates for subcortical neural centers are available for several species of animals, including cat, monkey, and rat. These atlases allow close approximation of the desired structure. However, optimum results require some probing of the area around the coordinate point for maximum response, and the position of the electrode must be verified at the end of the experiment by histologic examination.

Potentials measured at these subcortical centers are characteristically diphasic, as they are first positive and then negative. The response has a duration of from 10 to 30 msec. The obvious significance of these potentials is in determining whether a particular neural center is or is not involved in the transmission of a particular sensory input to the brain.

The detection of these evoked potentials are also valuable in plotting the sequence of neural centers in the various pathways. As the nerve impulse passes through the several nuclei with their synaptic junctions, the latency of the action potential increases so that the action potential at the cortex is several milliseconds later than the action potential at the brainstem level, for example. The sequence in which the nuclei become involved can be determined by the increasing time lag of the evoked potential at the various nuclei. This dynamic plotting of sensory pathways, coupled with anatomic plotting using techniques of nerve degeneration, will possibly provide a much clearer description of the sensory pathways from end-organ to cerebral cortex.

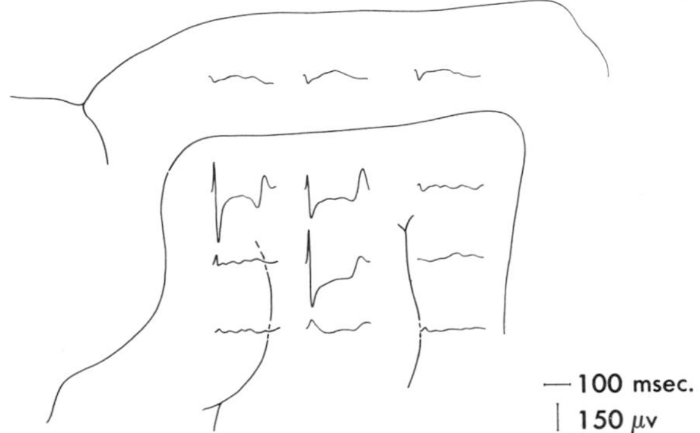

Fig. 13-6. Topographic plot of primary responses to auditory stimuli in the cerebral cortex of the cat. Area shown is the ectosylvian and suprasylvian gyri. Positivity of the active electrode is upward.

Intracellular potentials

Much of the knowledge presently available regarding nerve fiber conduction, neural synapse transfer, and neural-muscular end-plate transfer was gained by the use of intracellular electrodes. The electrodes, measuring no more than 1 μ in tip diameter, can be inserted into nerve fibers or nerve cells. In recording the potential from within a nerve cell, a −70 mv. potential should be recorded as the microelectrode penetrates the cell membrane into the soma. Once inside the cell the microelectrode enables the recording of an action spike when the cell is orthodromically stimulated by the appropriate neuron. The action spike has a duration of about 1 msec. and an amplitude of approximately 100 mv. (from −70 mv. to +30 mv).

INSTRUMENTATION

The electrical voltages that the electrophysiologist works with are extremely small, often in the range of 50 to 100 mv., and require amplification of several thousand times. However, it is not a simple matter of amplifying the desired signal from the electrode, as *noise* is also amplified. Noise is electrical energy from areas adjacent to the electrode site, electrical potentials floating free in the laboratory, or electrical interference noise generated by the amplifying equipment itself. This problem of noise must be solved in order to obtain accurate experimental results. Solving the problem entails good grounding procedure, use of specialized low-noise amplifiers, and most of all knowledge of electricity and electronic instrumentation.

Amplifiers

The necessary characteristics of a suitable biologic amplifier are summarized in the following sections from Bureš, Petran, and Zacher.

Input circuits

The following are the most important requirements:
(1) The input circuit must not affect the studied subtrate. It is especially important that it not take up too much energy nor supply energy to the subtrate.
(2) The input circuit must pass on impulses without distortion, i.e., the output amplitude must be exactly proportional to the input amplitude. This means that no frequency components must be suppressed or accentuated and no voltage not corresponding to the input voltage must be transmitted. For details see below.
(3) The input circuit must amplify the energy of the input signal. In some cases this is achieved by the output impulse having a considerably larger amplitude than the input impulse. At other times the amplitude remains practically unchanged or even decreases, but the output resistance is much smaller than the input resistance. Since power is e^2/R, power is also amplified in this case.

The first two requirements can be fulfilled only in part and the corresponding compromise must be considered for each case separately.

Middle stages

Requirements are somewhat less strict:
(1) Undistorted transmission (see above).
(2) The greatest possible amplification (usually voltage amplification).

The output (power) stage

(1) Must have necessary amplification (of voltage or power).
(2) Must compensate for the distortion occurring in the recording system.*

The types of amplifiers commonly used are A.C. single-ended, resistance-capacitance coupled amplifiers, balanced or push-pull A.C. amplifiers, and direct coupled (or D.C.) amplifiers. Each type has advantages and disadvantages for different measures of electrophysiologic activity.

Electrodes

Electrodes used to conduct the bioelectric potential to the wire circuitry are of several types. Macroelectrodes used for surface potential measurements such as the EEG are most commonly metal discs or needles. Stainless steel, silver, and nickel are the metals most frequently used. They are relatively inexpensive, easily obtainable, and of low resistance values. However, they are not desirable for chronic implant experimentation due to possible tissue reaction, and they are not the best electrode to use for measuring direct current potentials. A nonpolarizing electrode suitable for direct current measurement is the Ag-AgCl electrode, which is a silver electrode with a thin-coating layer of AgCl fused on its surface.

Microelectrodes comprise the second major category of electrodes. These electrodes are used for measuring electrical potentials within the tissue. For example, membrane potential or the action potential within a synapse can be measured using the microelectrode. The capillary microelectrode is formed from a glass tube drawn out at one end to a tip diameter of less than 1 μ. The electrode is a salt solution that fills the capillary glass tube.

Oscilloscopes

After the electrode has picked up the electrical potential, and the amplifier has brought the potential to a workable voltage, the voltage must be visualized and measured. The instrument most commonly used to accomplish this is the oscilloscope. On the screen of the oscilloscope the wave form of the potential can be seen. Amplitude of the potential is measured by the vertical value and time function of the potential by the horizontal value. Dual- or multiple-trace scopes make it possible to simultaneously view neural events

*Bureš, J. M., Petran, M., and Zacher, J.: Electrophysiological methods in biological research, New York, 1967, Academic Press, Inc., p. 131.

from several different sites. A polaroid-type camera attached to the screen of the oscilloscope may be used to make a permanent record of the potential as it appears.

Computers

The use of special purpose computers has been previously mentioned. These devices, which have the ability to detect small neural signals in a background of relatively much larger noises, have become an important instrument in the electrophysiology laboratory.

In addition to the limited-use *summary computer,* the general purpose computer is used more and more as a research tool. Storage of on-line electrophysiologic data on multichannel FM tape for later computer analysis is a profitable research technique. Analysis of multiple stimulus-response combinations and development of testing of neural models are further possibilities for study using a computer.

REFERENCES

1. Bennett, M. V. L., and others: Electrotonic junctions between teleost spinal neurones: electrophysiology and ultra structure, Science **141**:262, 1963.
2. Brazier, M. A. B.: The electrical activity of the nervous system, New York, 1960, The Macmillan Company.
3. Cooper, R., and others: Comparison of subcortical, cortical and scalp activity using chronically indwelling electrodes in man, Electroenceph. Clin. Neurophysiol. **18**:217, 1965.
4. Eccles, J.: The physiology of synapses, Berlin, 1964, Springer Verlag.
5. Fatt, P., and Katz, B.: Spontaneous sub-threshold activity at motor nerve endings, J. Physiol. (London) **117**:109, 1952.
6. Huxley, A. F., and Stampfli, R.: Evidence for saltatory conduction in peripheral myelinated nerve fibers, J. Physiol. (London) **108**:315, 1949.
7. Huxley, A. F., and Taylor, R. E.: Local activation of striated muscle fibres, J. Physiol. (London) **144**:426, 1958.
8. Katz, B.: Nerve, muscle and synapse, New York, 1966, McGraw-Hill Book Co.
9. McLennan, H.: Synaptic transmission, Philadelphia, 1970, W. B. Saunders Co.
10. Morgan, C. T., and Stellar, E.: Physiological psychology, New York, 1950, McGraw-Hill Book Co.
11. Petsche, H.: The physiologic bases of the pathologic electroencephalogram. In Minckler, J., editor: Pathology of the nervous system, vol. I, New York, 1968, McGraw-Hill Book Co.
12. Walter, D. O., and Brazier, M. A. B.: Advances in EEG analysis, Electroenceph. Clin. Neurophysiol. Supp. #27, 1969.

CHAPTER 14

EXPERIMENTAL NEUROBIOLOGY

RONALD COWDEN

Neurobiology represents an effort to understand the total function of the nervous system. Some of the most important information in this field has been derived from combining behavioral, anatomic, electrophysiologic, and neurochemical approaches.

DEGENERATION-REGENERATION REACTIONS

In vertebrates, and particularly in mammals, differentiated nerve cells do not have the ability to divide. For this reason the loss of neurons, for whatever cause, results in loss of an irreplaceable unit. In many cases adjacent or similar cells can take over the function of a lost cell, but neuron loss permanently diminishes the overall capacity of the system. A considerable proportion of the cytoplasm of a neuron lies outside the cell body proper in the form of the axonal and dendritic processes, which in humans may extend a distance of several feet. While neurons do not have the ability to replace themselves by division of either a preexisting neuron or a neuronal precursor, they do possess a considerable capacity for re-formation of cut or damaged processes. Regrowth of these processes, rather than formation of new cells, is implied by the term *nerve regeneration.**

For a nerve process to re-form, several conditions must be met. The cell body itself, often some distance from the site of damage, must be healthy and intact. In addition, a free pathway allowing the passage of the new nerve process must be available. Fibroblasts and other connective tissue elements will proliferate or infiltrate rapidly at a site of injury and inflammation. Therefore, particular steps must be taken to minimize trauma, which could lead to an inflammatory lesion blocking the outgrowth of new processes. If the channel remains clear, new processes will form and eventually reinnervate the target organ or site. In such cases however it is improbable that all of the original function of a severed nerve and regeneration of all fibers will be attained.

*See references 6, 10, 12, 14, and 15.

Chromatolysis

As might be expected, section of a distal process sets off a chain of events in the cell body of the neuron. The most dramatic of these is a condition referred to as chromatolysis, in which the neuronal cytoplasm loses a good deal of its capacity to stain with basic dyes (Fig. 14-1). At the biochemical and ultrastructural level this represents a disorganization of rough endoplasmic reticulum (aggregated in some cells in the form of Nissl substance) and a loss of ribosomes, including ribosomal RNA, which is responsible for binding basic dye in the cytoplasm. This disorganization may take two to seven days to occur. After sealing the cut processes it becomes necessary for the neuron to reestablish its capacity to support protein synthesis. This is accomplished through the synthesis of new ribosomes and their subsequent reorganization in the nerve cell cytoplasm. The nucleolus is the nuclear organelle in which precursors of ^{R}RNA are formed. After several days the nucleolus consequently begins to increase in size. The nucleus also enlarges and assumes an eccentric position in the cell body. The pattern obtained in both histochemical and autoradiographic studies is consistent with that of a cell rapidly synthesizing RNA and protein. As regeneration nears completion (possibly taking years), the nucleolus and nucleus decrease in size. Both protein and RNA levels in the neuronal cytoplasm achieve near normal values. Repair

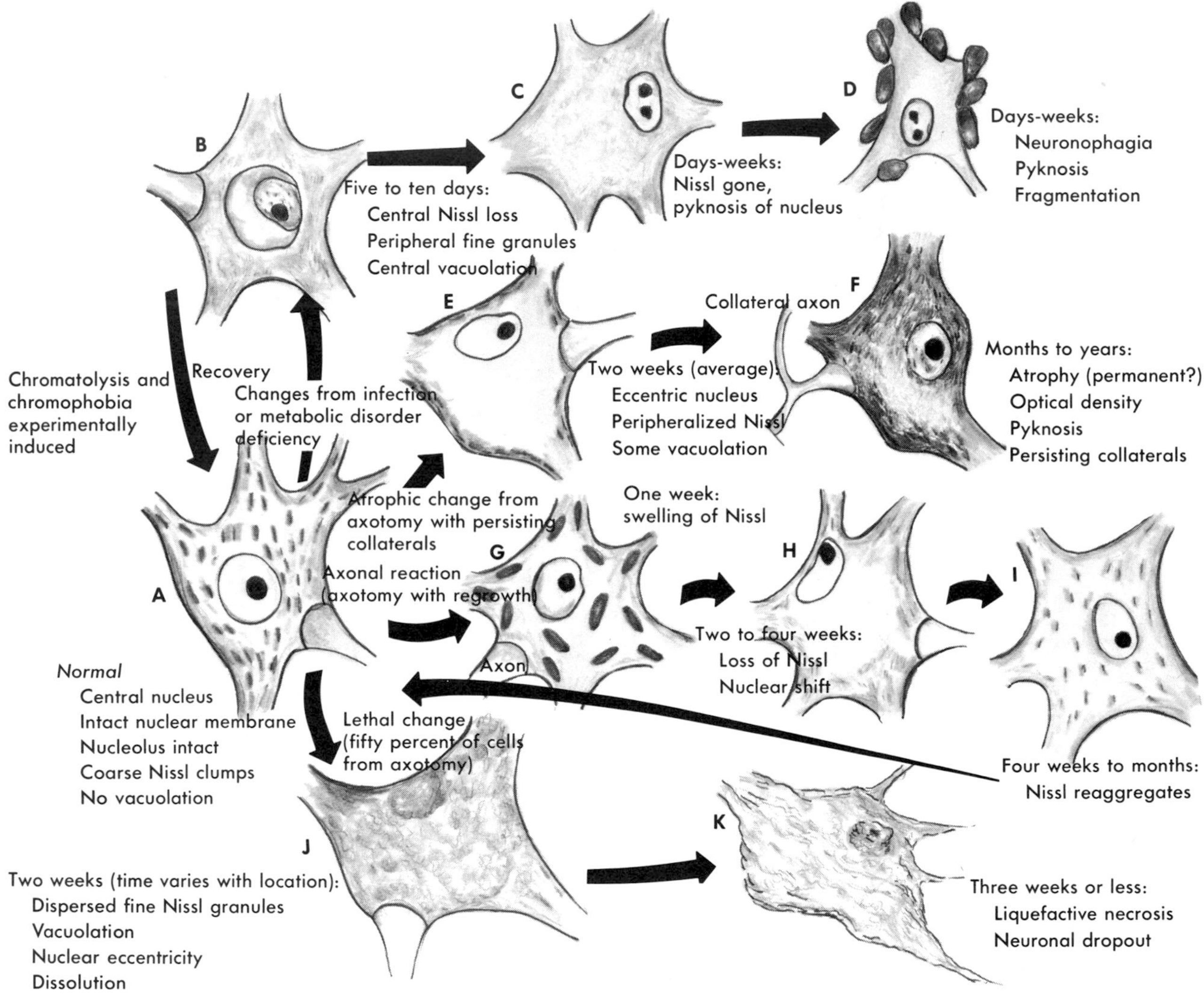

Fig. 14-1. Chromatolysis and chromophobia of neuron. *A-B-C-D* is sequence occurring from infective or metabolic experimental disruption. Reversion to normal can occur from *B*. *A-E-F* is sequence from axotomy when collateral axonic branches seem to sustain the atrophic terminal product permanently. *A-G-H-I* is the common sequence in axotomy when regrowth of the peripheral fibers takes place. Complete restitution occurs from *I* back to *A* for complete normality of the source cell. *A-J-K* is the sequence through chromatolysis to liquefactive necrosis (ghost cell) to "dropout." This probably occurs in half the cells axotomized.

of a nerve leading from severed dorsal root ganglia in a cat requires over one hundred days. A good deal of information concerning regeneration of neurons in mammals has been derived from experimental work on laboratory animals, particularly cats, rats, and monkeys. Hydén has found certain species of fish to be useful, as they possess particularly large nerve cell bodies.[6] Cumulative experience from war wounds of peripheral nerves has been the main source of information regarding human nerve regeneration.[12,15]

Wallerian degeneration

Degeneration occurs in cut processes. In the case of peripheral myelinated nerves, the investing myelin sheath degenerates distal to the site of injury and proximal to it for some distance (Fig. 14-2, *A* and *B*). Since myelin is composed of lipoprotein material, its degeneration leads to an accumulation of lipid droplets along the path of the nerve tract. These droplets are later removed by phagocytic macrophages. The Schwann cells, which produce the myelin sheaths, are neuroectodermal

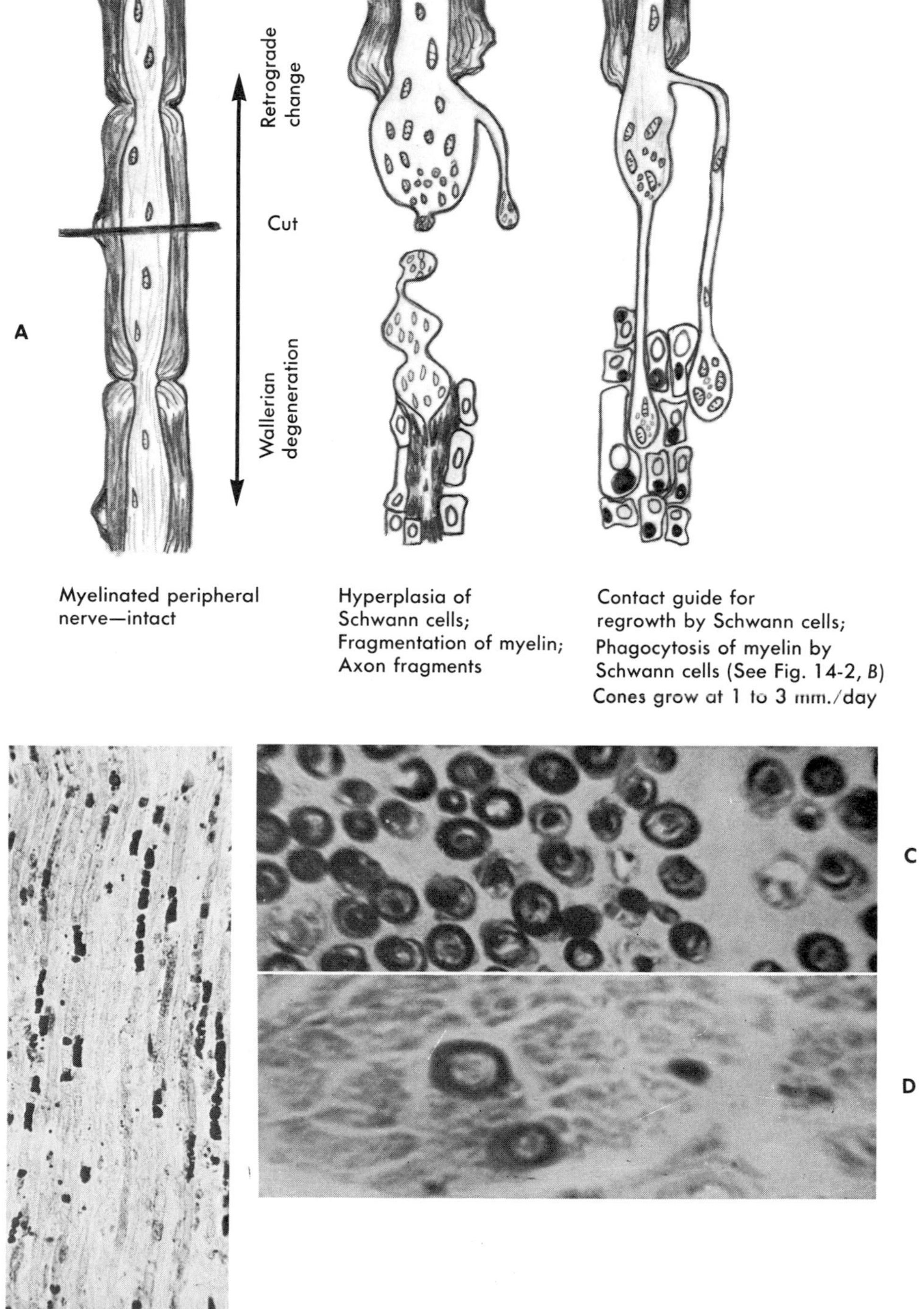

Fig. 14-2. A, Sequential stages in Wallerian degeneration with start of regrowth. At left is drawing at time of cut. Center shows beginning regrowth buds from proximal stump, hyperplasia of Schwann cells, and phagocytosis of myelin in distal stump. Right shows "contact guidance" for regrowth and further Schwann cell reaction; **B,** photomicrograph of Wallerian degeneration in peripheral nerve showing fragmentation and phagocytosis of myelin, hyperplasia of Schwann cells; **C** and **D,** demyelination in peripheral nerve. (From Minckler, J. In Anderson, W. A. D., editor: Pathology, ed. 5, St. Louis, 1966, The C. V. Mosby Co.)

derivations and display considerable capacity for both transformation into macrophages and for proliferation. As a peripheral nerve process re-forms, the Schwann cells proliferate and reinvest the growing neuron (Fig. 14-2, *C* and *D*). New side branches form from the nerve at the nodes.[13]

Central demyelination

Degeneration is quite different in the CNS. There the myelin sheaths are provided by neuroglial elements, the oligodendroglial cells, which like the neurons themselves are of ectodermal origin. They appear to have a very restricted regenerative capacity. As a result, nerves transected in the CNS do not re-form, The neuron proper attempts regrowth of processes, but the myelin sheath investment permanently degenerates. This degenerated pathway has provided one of the oldest and most productive experimental neurologic techniques, the tracing of degenerated nerve tracts within the CNS (Figs. 14-3 to 14-5).[12]

In tract-tracing experiments a small cut is made along a particular pathway, and the animal is allowed to live for a considerable period of time. When the animal dies or is killed, the CNS is sectioned and stained by a technique such as the Marchi stain for demonstrating degenerated pathways. Most information concerning the ramifications and connections of nerve processes from a nerve cell body (or more properly a *group* of cell bodies) has been obtained in this manner. It was discovered that the process of degeneration is considerably accelerated in newborn animals; therefore, the most profitable experiments of this sort are often performed on neonatal animals.

CNS macrophages

As might be expected, inflammatory processes differ in the peripheral and central nervous systems. In the peripheral nervous system, the connective tissue derivatives are chiefly concerned. As mentioned previously, if a nerve is to re-form along its original pathway, it is important to reduce the chances of a granuloma forming at the site of injury. Such a formation would impede the outgrowth of new processes. In such instances the nerve processes make some attempt to grow, but their path is deflected, and after a bit of disor-

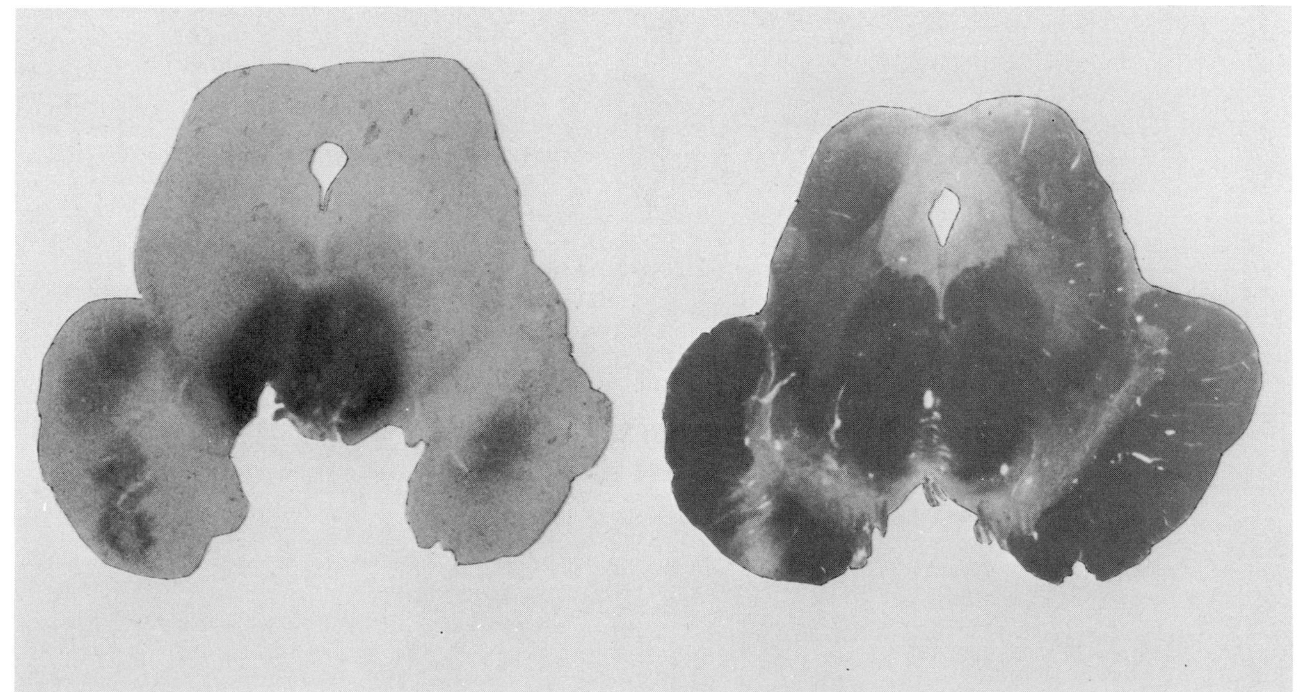

Fig. 14-3. Central demyelination through basis pedunculi from extirpation of area 6. **A,** Marchi preparation; **B,** Weigert preparation. Note matching overlay of peduncular lesions, which is a requirement of validity of the degenerating tract.

ganized wandering in the area, outgrowth ceases.[12,15] This is partially because the regrowing nerve experiences a trophic influence exerted by the target site.[14] This phenomenon is not clearly understood, but in its absence growth ceases. The CNS does

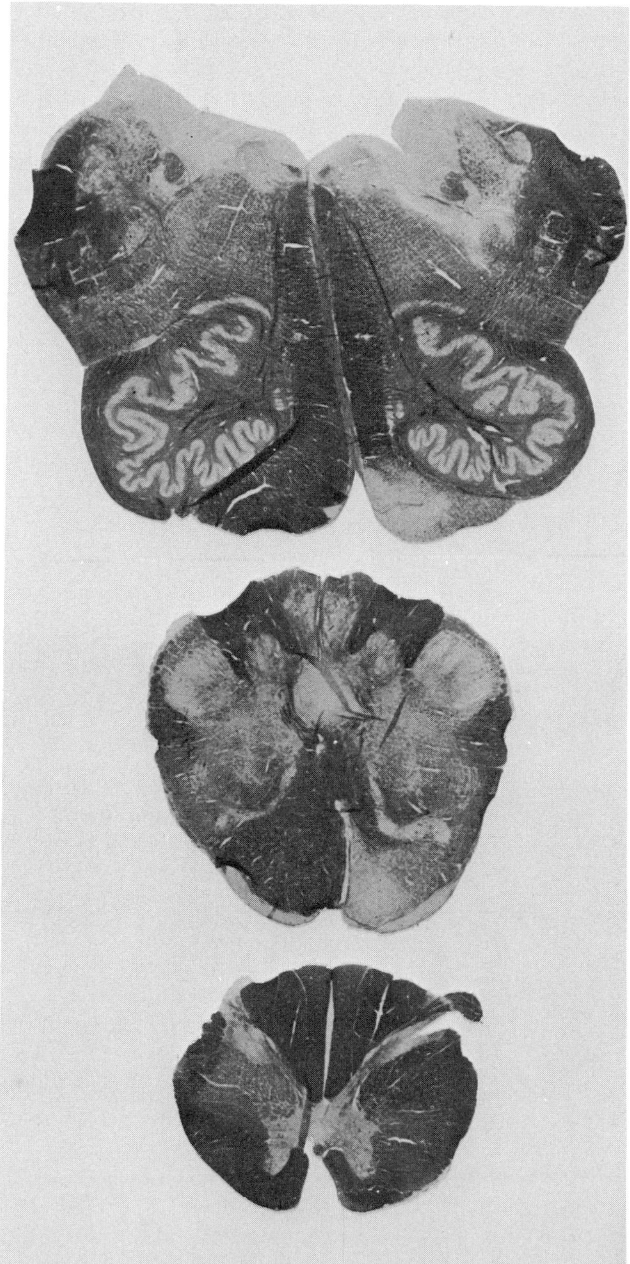

Fig. 14-4. Continuation of demyelinated corticospinal tract through pyramid to lateral corticospinal area of opposite side in upper cord. (Weigert preparation.)

not possess the elaborate connective tissue defense mechanism of the peripheral system. In fact, the principal inflammatory cell type of the CNS is the microglial cell, whose role and origin suggest that it is homologous to macrophages. Even so the number of microglial cells, which is not excessive, prohibits the massive accumulations of inflammatory cells that occur outside of the CNS. In persistent lesions a type of cell, the *gitter cell,* appears. It seems improbable that gitter cells are entirely derived from microglia, because they are more numerous than either the number of these cells or the number their rate of division would produce. It seems more probable that these cells arise through hematogenous transport and are produced from the general reticuloendothelial reservoir of macrophagic elements. In any event gitter cells possess a very distinct morphology. The cells are spherical, and the nucleus is usually compressed to one side and does not contain a nucleolus that can be seen with a light microscope. The cytoplasm usually contains a single large droplet of glycolipid material, but the cells may fill with small droplets that appear granular (fat granules) (Fig. 14-6).

Experimental deficiency degeneration

In addition to the purely experimental manipulation of the nervous system, focal or locatized degeneration of peripheral nerves may occur (Fig. 14-1). In other instances the process is manipulated by nutritional deficiencies. These focal demyelinations are the same as those termed *Wallerian degeneration.* The pattern followed is similar to that seen in a transected nerve. Following the initial degeneration, both the neuronal processes and investing Schwann cells attempt to restore the nerve, which degenerates distal to the site of injury. As in regeneration of a transected nerve, this process is frustrated if an inflammatory lesion develops at the site of injury or along the path of an injured nerve. And as in transection experiments, restoration of the neuronal processes does not occur in the CNS because of its inability to produce new myelinating oligodendroglia.[12,14,15]

Transneuronal degeneration

Although it is less useful experimentally than direct neuronal effects, transneuronal degeneration is studied as a manipulative procedure (Fig. 14-1). If the axonal process emanating from a particular neuron is interrupted, the process leading from that cell body degenerates, and the nerve cells and their processes with which it forms a chain of synaptic connections are also structurally altered. For example, if the optic nerve is severed on one side, degeneration subsequently occurs in alternating layers in the related lateral geniculate bodies and in the visual pathways. This factor has made it possible to detect the receiving cells in the synaptic chain and to trace the pathways of innervation that follow. Although they are tedious, transneuronal alterations combined with electrophysiologic records remain principal experimental techniques for relating distant neuronal pools.

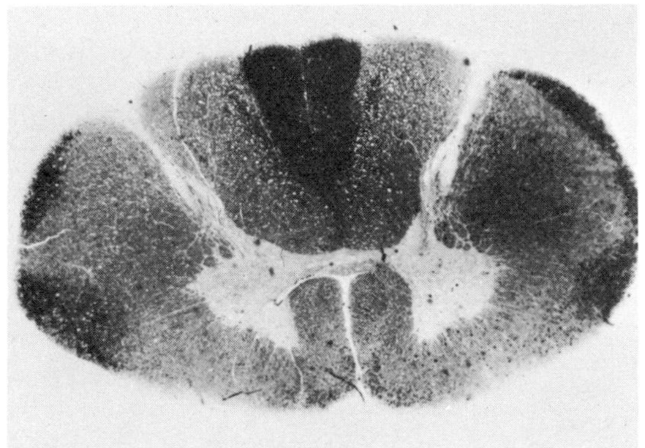

Fig. 14-5. Demyelination of ascending type in cervical cord from transection of low thoracic cord. Note definition of ascending pathways. (Marchi preparation.)

Bouton degeneration

The nerve endings, the end-feet processes called *boutons terminaux,* also displays changes in transected or degenerating nerves that have been subjected to a considerable amount of experimental manipulation and investigation. In degeneration, when viewed with silver staining and under a light microscope, they display swelling, vacuolation, and finally fragmentation (Fig. 14-7). A distinguishing characteristic is their increased ability to reduce silver. Thus, a considerable amount of experimentation has been carried out using silver staining methods.[2] Because the terminal processes are rather small (up to 1.4 μ in diameter), the resolution offered by ultrastructure techniques is advantageous in detecting swelling or vacuolation (Fig. 14-8),[4] although the sampling problem is severe.

Experimental regeneration

Within the continuum of organisms, the regenerative capacity of the nervous system of mammals is comparatively restricted (Fig. 14-1). Planaria and some annelids have the capacity to completely regenerate the nervous system. After study of these phenomena for over fifty years, the cytology

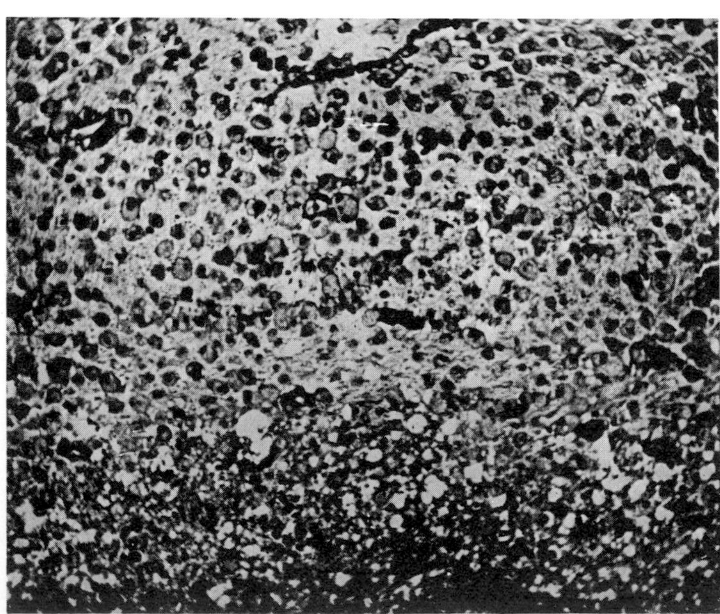

Fig. 14-6. Gitter (fat granule) cells representing phagocytes taking up degenerating myelin in CNS. (From Minckler, J. In Anderson, W. A. D., editor: Pathology, ed. 5, St. Louis, 1966, The C. V. Mosby Co.) (H & E.)

of lineage and the patterns of cell differentiation are still obscure. However, it is quite clear that new cells proliferate, and an entire CNS can be re-formed. In some planarians the whole process takes about three days. Within the vertebrates, amphibians display a considerable capacity for regeneration. They form new limbs if these are cut off, and they have displayed considerable capacity for neural regeneration. It has been repeatedly demonstrated that whole eyes can be removed and reimplanted. After several months, a new optic nerve grows out from the retina and establishes a connection with the CNS, restoring visual function to the eye. It has also been demonstrated that the pigmented retina can give rise to the neural retina if the latter is removed. The nerves also play a major role in regeneration of extremities in amphibians. If a limb stump of a salamander is denervated, no regeneration will occur. Substances emanating from the nerves are primary factors in organizing the regeneration blastema. In frogs and toads, which do not normally regenerate lost limbs, regeneration of the front limbs can be effected by diverting the nerves of the hind limb into the front limb. Followng section the front limbs regenerate.

TISSUE CULTURE

The techniques of tissue culture, combined with protracted visual observation of nerve cells in culture, have been quite useful. From such techniques it is possible not only to demonstrate the movement of material in nerve processes, but to gain some knowledge of both the rate of movement and of conditions that would accelerate or retard outgrowth of nerve processes.[7] The trophic influence of target structures can also be determined in this manner. It is now possible, for instance, to set up spatially separate cultures of heart myoblasts and neuroblasts. As the myoblasts mature into heart muscle cells, they gain the ability to contract. However, the contractions are disorganized until maturing nerve cells send processes into this mass and innervate the muscle cells. Though this nerve-muscle interaction, the contractions of the heart-muscle preparation becomes synchronized.

GROWTH FACTOR

Another example of use of a combination of techniques involves the study of *nerve growth factor,* a substance originally extracted from one of the salivary glands of the rat. This substance caused neurons in treated embryos to become substantially enlarged.[8] From ultrastructural studies it was established that nerve growth factor promotes proliferation of the neurofibrillar system, which is in turn composed of microtubules, the same fundamental structures that form the mitotic spindle, muscle fibrils, and cilia or flagella. The same effects were encountered when water in the tissue culture medium was replaced with *heavy water* (water made of two atomic weight hydrogen, D_2O). The alkaloid colchicine and its synthetic derivatives, known to inhibit microtubule formation, has an inhibitory effect, as might be expected.

MICROSCOPY

A combination of phase contrast, interference contrast, and differential interference contrast optical systems has also been usefully employed to examine neuronal function. It has been possible, for instance, to demonstrate the endoplasmic reticulum of living vertebrate and invertebrate neurons by carefully dissecting out the cell bodies and placing them in an osmotically balanced solution of appropriate refractive index. The interference contrast optical method has also been used to study changes in solid concentration in a blue

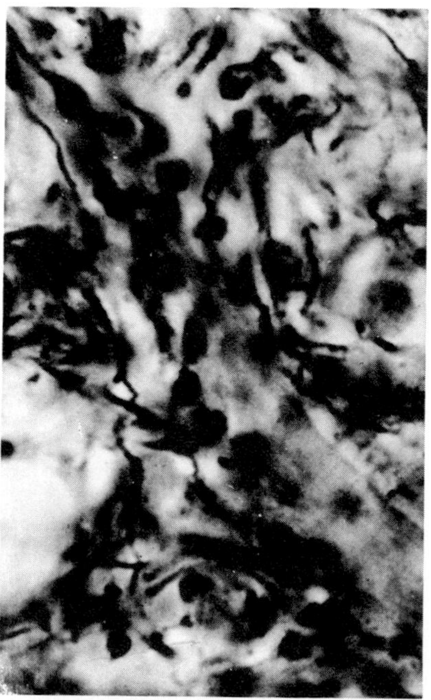

Fig. 14-7. Degenerating boutons (axodendritic) in nucleus dorsalis of human spinal cord. Silver stain and light optics display increased argyrophilia, fragmentation of bouton and telodendria. (From Minckler, J. In Anderson, W. A. D., editor: Pathology, ed. 5, St. Louis, 1966, The C. V. Mosby Co.)

crab stretch-receptor axon under varying conditions of external ionic concentration. In addition, it has been possible to examine electrical activity at the same time.

AUTORADIOGRAPHY

A considerable amount of information has been gained from the use of radioactive tracer techniques and sophisticated methods of ultramicrochemistry and cytochemistry. It is possible with the use of radioactive amino acids to determine rates of protein synthesis in whole sections of the nervous system by extraction techniques and in single cells by autoradiography. In the latter method a photographic emulsion is placed over a histologic section and allowed to expose in the dark for several days. The film is then developed and the slide processed through a stain as usual. Because the gelatin emulsion is transparent, sites of radioactive detonations show up as reduced silver grains overlying the cell or structure that incorporated the radioactive material. This can be turned into semiquantitative data by counting the number of reduced silver grains per unit area. Radioactive precursors of nucleic acids, carbohydrates, and lipids may also be used. They are useful for determining rates and distributions of metabolism, and through pulse-chase experiments they may also give some indication of the sequence of events. In a typical experiment several animals might be injected with a radioactive precursor. After a brief interval the first is killed and the tissues subjected to autoradiographic analysis. Analysis might show exclusive or near exclusive localization of radioactivity in glial cells surrounding neurons. Subsequent stages might show progressive movement from glia

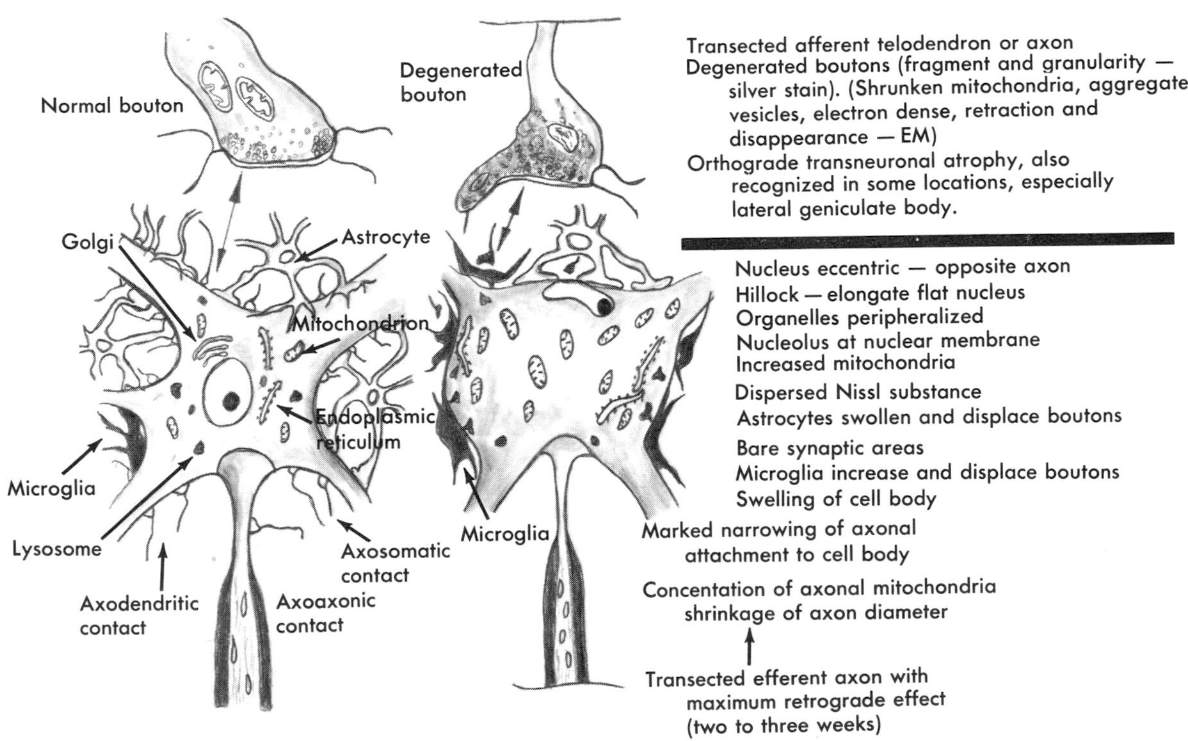

Fig. 14-8. Degeneration at synapse. Left shows normal representation, including boutons, astrocytic processes, few microglia, normal sized axon, and usual distribution of organelles. Right shows orthograde effect of axonic or telodendrial section as changes in bouton. Transneuronal effect varies with connections but may produce atrophy (for example, of connecting cell in lateral geniculate body). Cellular effect of retrograde origin is shown in withdrawal of boutons, covering of synaptic surface by swollen astrocytic processes and increased microglia, peripheralization of organelles (and Nissl substance), loss of Nissl stainability, eccentricity and flattening of nucleus, movement of nucleolus to nuclear membrane, shrinkage of axon, and increase in mitochondria and lysosomes. (Composite drawing after Bowsher, D., and Kreutzberg, G. In Minckler, J., editor: Pathology of the nervous system, vols. I and III, New York, 1968 and 1971, McGraw-Hill Book Co.)

to neurons, indicating a transfer sequence.[11] Such techniques also may be used to determine rates of flow through the axon.[3,9]

CYTOCHEMISTRY

The techniques of cytochemistry have been particularly useful in the study of neuronal regeneration and development. It was through the use of quantitative methods for examining RNA and protein levels that it became possible to establish the pattern of metabolic events in nerve regeneration. Ultramicrochemical techniques have also had important applications. It has been found that a reciprocal relationship exists between a neuron and its surrounding glia. If a neuron's supply of RNA and succinic dehydrogenase is depleted through function, high concentrations are found in the surrounding glia. The material in glia then presumably moves into the neuron. Ultrastructural studies indicate that the glia send processes that penetrate deeply the nerve cell bodies, presumably furnishing an avenue for exchange.[11]

PRIMITIVE AND SIMPLIFIED NEURAL SYSTEMS

The vertebrate nervous system is much too complicated for straightforward analysis of cell-to-cell interactions. This is very important, since the receptor cell translates its perception into electrical activity and passes it on to another cell. In this cell it is probably modified and passed on to the next. This process is called *integrative activity.* In the CNS of certain invertebrates, particularly in the stomach of certain crabs and the optic tract of certain marine snails (nudibranchs), there are small collections of nerve cells (ganglia) that have a single nerve tract leading in and out. Because there is a finite number of neurons, both the output and input can be monitored or stimulated, and recording electrodes can be placed in each of the cells to see how electrical activity in one cell affects the others.[7] In favorable cases a number of microelectrodes can be placed in individual cells and the outputs connected with a computer so that the neurons are seen to converse with one another. Some of the most important data concerning cell-to-cell interaction is being gathered in this manner.

BEHAVIORAL EXPERIMENTATION

Important data of another sort has been gathered from a combination of classic experimental behavioral studies and neurophysiology. After carefully conditioning cats to salivate by ringing a bell when being fed, the conditioning was extinguished by ringing the bell for some time without a reward. When the cat was anesthetized, its response to the bell indicated *suppression* rather than extinction of the condition response. The information was suppressed, but it was still present. Electrophysiologic and transectional studies have established two important facts: (1) storage of information occurrs in the receptor cell (prior to the first synapse); and (2) each tract possesses a parallel tract moving in the opposite direction and has the role of determining if the incoming stimuli are significant. Insignificant stimuli are filtered out, offering a highly developed example of integrative activity in a feedback control system.[5]

NEUROPHARMACOLOGY

A good deal has been learned in the field of neuropharmacology by physiologic and biochemical studies of the effects of drugs on nervous system function or metabolism. Some of the most interesting and useful work today is being done with certain orb-weaving spiders. Certain spiders build very regular webs, and when these are destroyed, the spiders immediately begin reconstruction. In a typical experiment the spider is either injected with or fed a given drug. In the feeding experiments an eviscerated fly is often filled with the drug. After drug administration, the web is destroyed. The drug affects the way in which the spider rebuilds the web. Amphetamines cause the spider to build haphazard, irregular webs, while barbiturates put it to sleep before web-building is completed. D-lysergic acid (LSD) leads to the building of a more elaborate web, with more lines more narrowly spaced than would naturally be the case. Serum from some mentally disturbed patients has also led to the building of abnormal webs, suggesting that chemistry rather than behavioral background was responsible for the observed aberrations in both donor and recipient behavior.

Attempts have been made to modify intelligence in humans by the use of drugs. In an average medical class, a significant increase in retention of information was obtained by use of the drug tricyano-2-amino-propene. There is also reason to believe that memorized data is stored in one of the fractions of RNA. Some of the early work was done with planarian flatworms.[1] The specific experiments are as yet inconclusive, but there is a substantial and growing body of evidence that indicates that RNA taken from the nervous tissue of one individual will influence the behavior of another. However, the implications of these experiments are significant enough to emphasize their status as new ideas rather than firmly established experimental procedures.

REFERENCES

1. Corning, W. C., and Ricco, D.: The planarian controversy. In Byrne, W. L., editor: Molecular approaches to learning and memory, New York, 1970, Academic Press, Inc.
2. David, G. B., Brown, A. W. and Mallion, K. B.: On the distribution of synaptic end-feet (boutons terminaux) in the central nervous system of the cat, J. Physiol. **147**:55, 1959.
3. Droz, B., and Leblond, C. P.: Axonal migration of proteins in the central nervous system as shown by autoradiography, J. Comp. Neurol. **121**:325, 1963.
4. Gray, E. G., and Guillery, R. W.: Synaptic morphology in the normal and degenerating nervous system, Int. Rev. Cytol. **19**:111, 1966.
5. Hernandez-Teon, R.: Modification of electric activity in trochlear nucleus during attention in unanesthetized cats, Science **123**:331, 1965.
6. Hydén, H.: The neuron, New York, 1967, American Elsevier Publishing Co., Inc.
7. Kennedy, D., Selverston, A. I. and Rember, M. P.: Analysis of restricted neural networks, Science **164**:1488, 1969.
8. Levi-Montalcini, R.: Chemical stimulation of nerve growth. In McElvey, W. D., and Glass, H. B., editors: Chemical basis of development, Baltimore, 1958, The Johns Hopkins Press.
9. Lubinska, L.: Outflow from cut ends of nerve fibers, Exp. Cell Res. **10**:40, 1956.
10. McMasters, R. E.: Regeneration of the spinal cord in the rat: effects of piromen and ACTH upon the regenerative capacity, J. Comp. Neurol. **119**:113, 1962.
11. Palay, S. L.: The role of neuroglia in the organization of the central nervous system. In Rodahl, K., and Issekutg, B., editor: Nerve as a tissue, New York, 1966, Harper & Row, Publishers.
12. Ramon y Cajal, S.: Degeneration and regeneration of the nervous system, translated by May, R. M., Oxford, 1928, Oxford University Press.
13. Vizoso, A. D.: The relationship between internodal length and growth in human nerves. J. Anat. London **84**:342, 1950.
14. Weiss, P.: Genetic neurology. In Problems of the development, growth and regeneration of the nervous system and its functions, Chicago, 1950, University of Chicago Press.
15. Windle, W. F., editor: Regeneration in the central nervous system, Springfield, Illinois, 1955, Charles C Thomas, Publisher.

CHAPTER 15

FUNCTIONAL ORGANIZATION AND MAINTENANCE

JEFF MINCKLER

ACTIVATING AND INHIBITING SYSTEMS

The individual synapses in a nervous system probably cannot operate physiologically on a simple direct cell-to-cell basis as usually illustrated (Fig. 15-1). They most likely are dependent for effective impulse transfer upon accessory neurons in a related pool (Fig. 15-2). Provision is made in the CNS for almost numberless sources and routes for accessory neural activity. These contribute to a final neural act as demonstrated in a final-common-path discharge (Fig. 15-3). While a functional system (such as touch) may deliver the main signals to a group of neurons as the *primary source,* the effectiveness of the ensuing signals is dependent upon correlated activity of synaptic terminals from other *accessory sources* (Fig. 15-4). The input in any synaptic area thus arises from many sources, and output can either concentrate in one route or diverge to many succeeding synaptic areas. In this way signals in neural groups can be concentrated or dispersed. This type of process occurs in myriads of patterns, which are thus modified or conditioned by the interaction of accessory neurons apart from the main chains. This concept of required accessory neuronal support has given rise to the notion that special neuronal systems must operate constantly as an alerting or suppressing mechanism for effective overall neural function. This activator (and inhibitor) system has its most elaborate representation in the reticular formation, but it probably operates almost universally in the human CNS during waking periods. The system is an expression of the function of myriads of short *internuncial neurons* and related convergent, divergent, and feedback fiber systems. Their structural patterns are presumptive neural models of considerable complexity (Figs. 15-2 and 15-3).[18]

Internuncial chain complexes are well represented in the short *spinospinalis* pathways of the spinal cord (Fig. 15-5). These are nonmyelinated or finely myelinated fibers that make up a strikingly neuron-dense neuropil. Somewhat similar in makeup are the short *arcuate fibers,* which pass from gyrus to gyrus in the cerebral cortex (see Chapter 21). *Convergent* patterns have many representations in the CNS and are generally regarded as a means of concentrating impulses, with a net result of increased sensitivity (Fig. 15-6). An example in an afferent complex is the olfactory convergence, by which a single olfactory mitral cell is brought into relationship with about 18,000 chemoreceptors. It is estimated that some cells of the brainstem reticular formation are subject to synaptic influence from as many as 4,000 sources; this is an example of an interlinking complex. A somewhat similar convergence in an output pattern occurs to final-common-path cells, whereby enormous numbers of circuit units are reduced to a few hundreds or thousands of contact points at the final cell that delivers the impulse to the effector (Fig. 15-3). *Divergent* patterns also are widespread and account for the fact that a pain stimulus, for example, can take alternate routes to reflex and conscious centers. The routes can be descending, transverse to the opposite side, and ascending. The patterns are commonly represented as in Fig. 15-7. In the reticular formation of the brainstem, for example, it is estimated that a single cell-

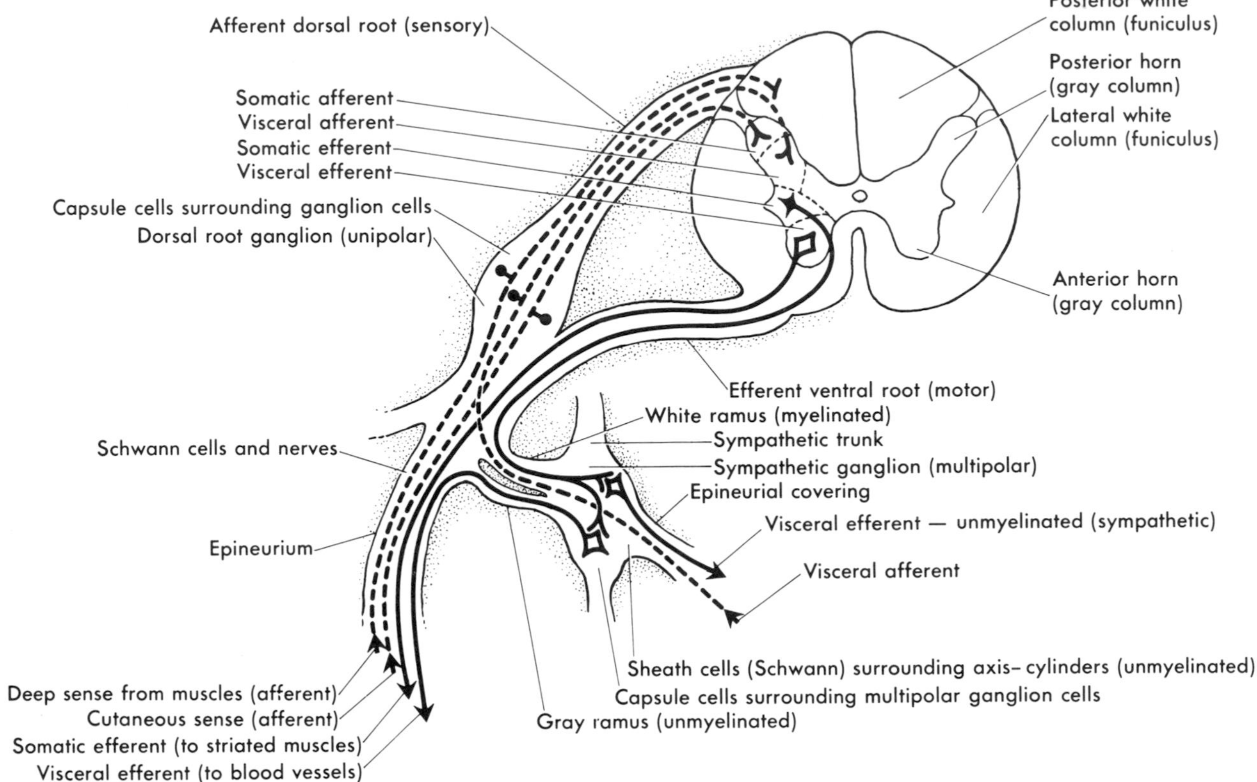

Fig. 15-1. Segmental receptor-effector system of CNS in diagrammatic transverse view.

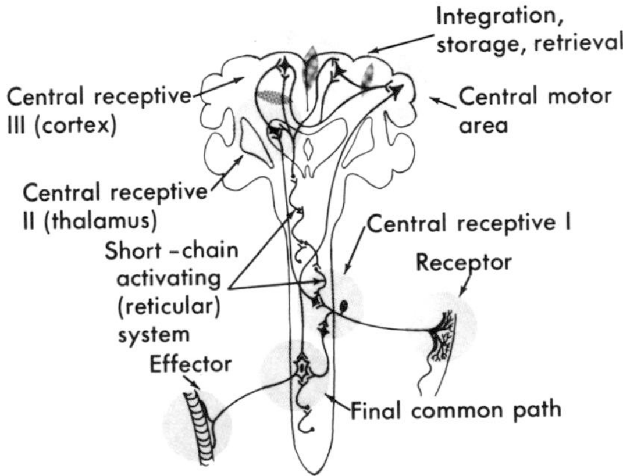

Fig. 15-2. Composite neural function diagram. Receptor complex is delivered to a primary central receptor field (*I*), which is regulated in part by the short-chain reticular system. Second receptive field (*II*) (thalamus) is reached by both lemniscal fibers and short chains. Central receptive cortex (*III*) has diverse delivery patterns through integrative fields to central motor area. Information reaches final-common-path area, which is also subject to short-chain activation in order to reach effector.

firing can be distributed to as many as 25,000 synaptic fields. *Feedback* patterns in neuronal pools are well-known modifiers of input in defined areas. Such a system is presumed to operate within the cerebral cortex as well as other areas (Fig. 15-8). Inhibiting complexes are often considered feedback fiber systems on physiologic grounds. Many feedback systems involve combinations of neurocircuitry, hormones, and extraneural blood chemical levels (such as renal-hypothalamic-posterior pituitary-antidiuretic hormone). Others involve both neurocircuitry and neuromuscular complexes (see Chapter 22).[7,14]

Reticular system (formation)

Reviews of the functional organization of the human nervous system have classically presented this system as *afferent* and *efferent* components linked by a complex *integrative* system. Recognition has gradually come about that special sets of neurons function in activation, inhibition, and synchronization of neural effort.[10] These neurons

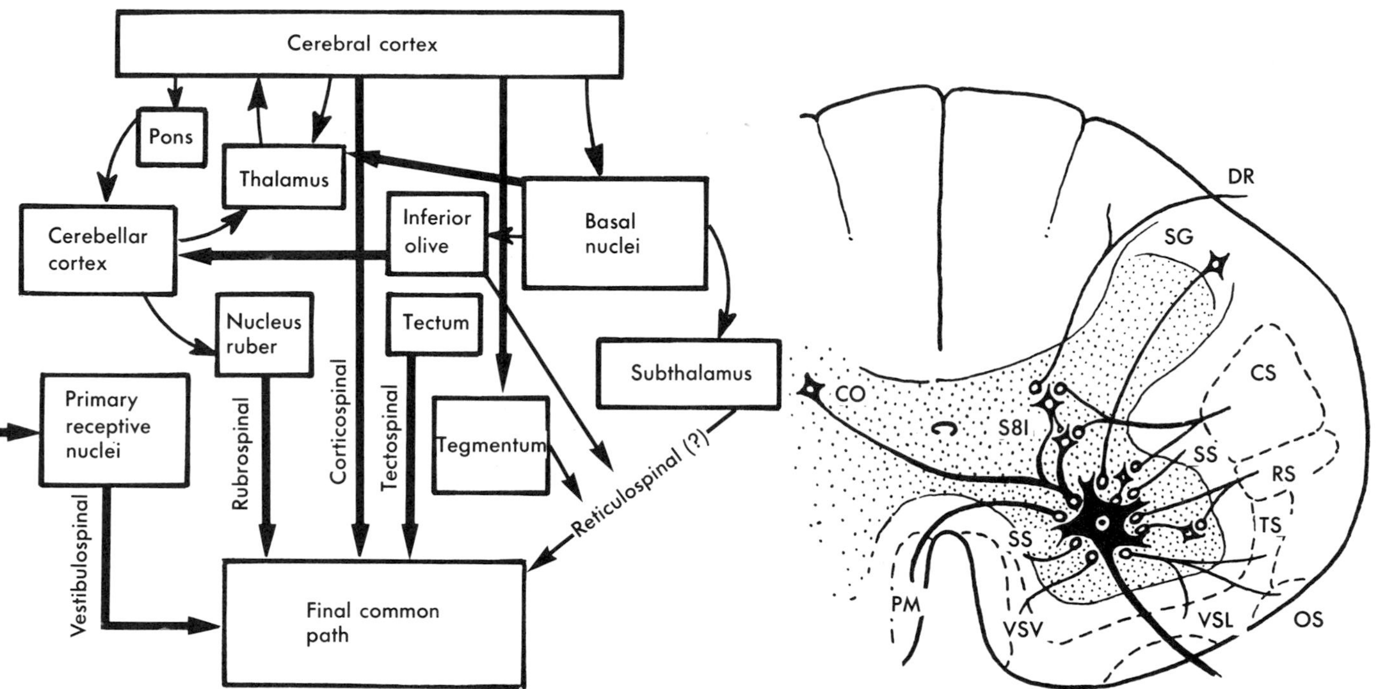

Fig. 15-3. Final-common-path complex is represented as arising in numerous diverse sources and delivered by many alternate routes. On right is diagram of the complex relating to a single cell. *DR* = dorsal root; *SG* = substantia gelatinosa Rolandi; *S* and *I* = sensory and internuncial; *CO* = commissural; *CS* = corticospinal; *RS* = rubrospinal; *TS* = tectospinal; *OS* = olivospinal?; *VSL* = lateral vestibulospinal; *VSV* = ventral vestibulospinal; *PM* = ventral corticospinal, including premotor; *SS* = spinospinalis.

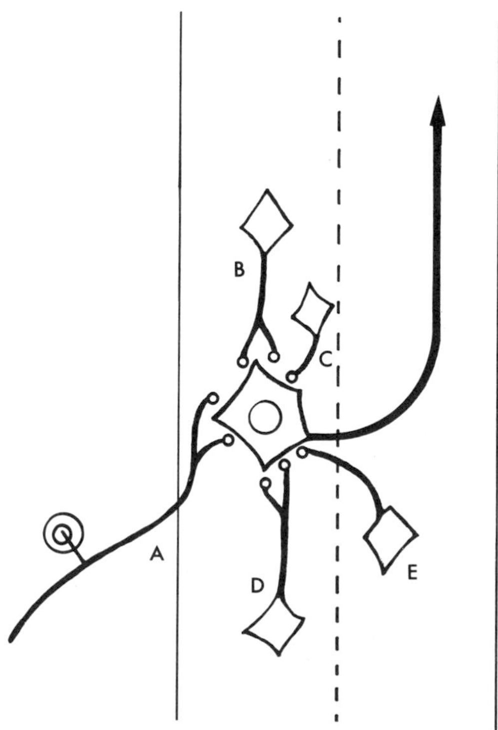

Fig. 15-4. Primary receptive system (*A*) to primary receptive area. Accessory systems include descending (*B*), internuncia (*C*), ascending (*D*), and commissural (*E*) sources, which activate or inhibit the continuum of a single sensory modality.

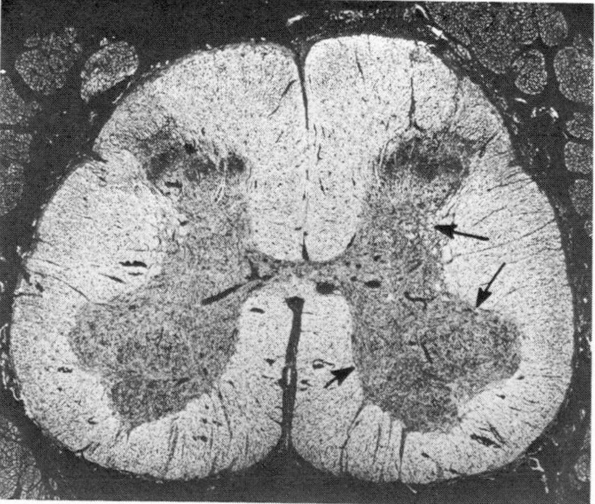

Fig. 15-5. Spinospinalis pathway in the lumbar spinal cord occupying the marginal gray-white junctional area *(arrows)*.

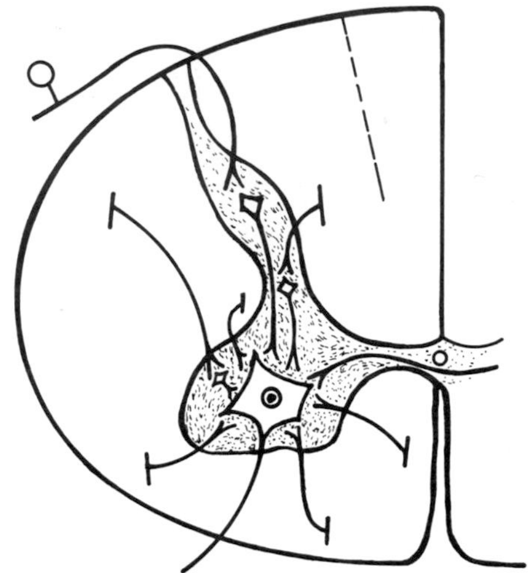

Fig. 15-6. Diagrammatic representation of *convergent* neuro-circuitry (see Fig. 15-3).

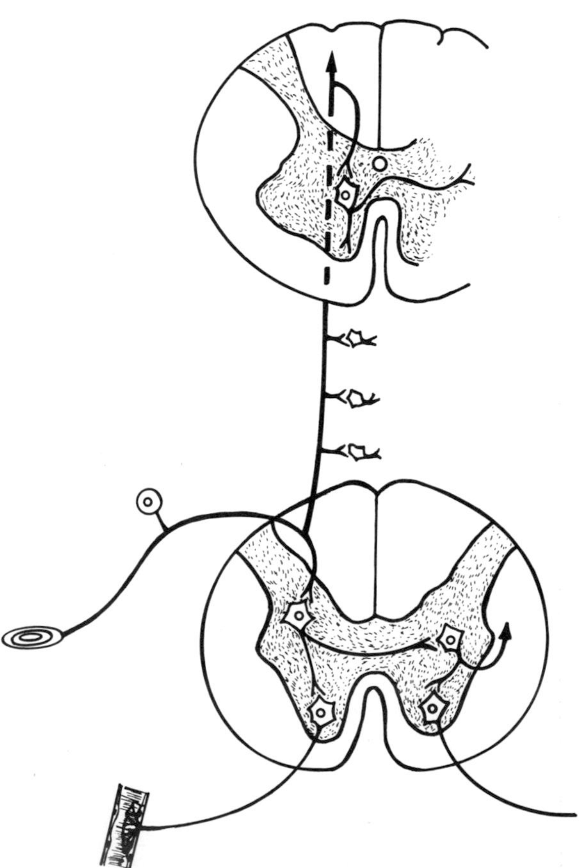

Fig. 15-7. Diagrammatic representation of *divergent* neuro-circuitry.

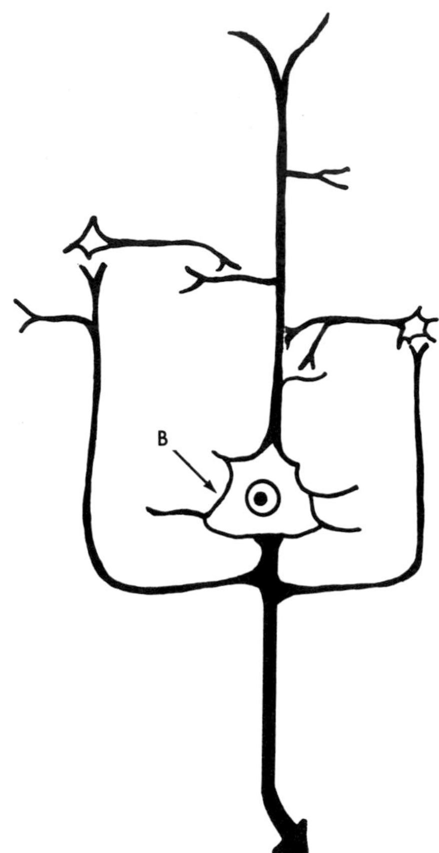

Fig. 15-8. Diagrammatic representation of feedback neuro-circuitry. (Betz cell (*B*) model.)

are essential to the operation of the principal modality pathways, but they are not part of these afferent and efferent chains themselves. Similarly, while they are not specific segments of integrating systems, such as commissures, they must be operative to effect integrative activity. The reticular system represents the nonspecific multisynaptic ascending and descending neuronal chain systems of lower animals. In animals that are phylogenetically lower than mammals, long-chain systems with few synapses *(the lemniscal systems)* are far less conspicuous. The specific modality pathways are phylogenetically late neural aquisitions. These pathways (such as cutaneous and deep sense) reach the peak of competence and specificity in man. It is not surprising, therefore, that the ancient reticular system of nonspecific, multisynaptic character has been overshadowed in man by the more easily demonstrated principal nervous pathways.

The anatomy of the reticular formation almost defies structural definition because of its ubiquity

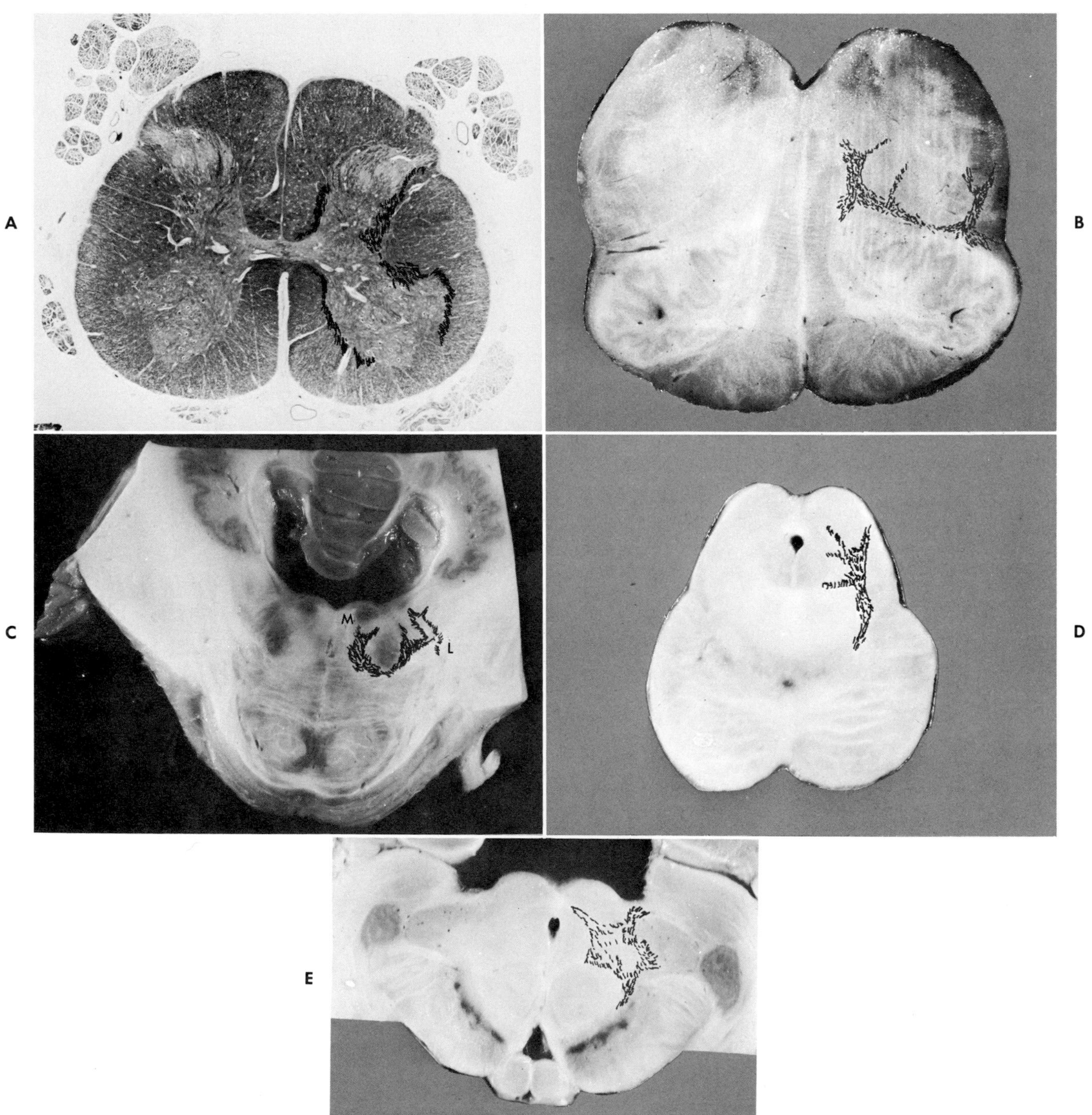

Fig. 15-9. Reticular formation (stippled). **A,** In spinal cord; **B,** in medulla; **C,** in pons (*M* = medial tegmental path, *L* = lateral tegmental tract); **D,** in lower midbrain; **E,** in upper midbrain.

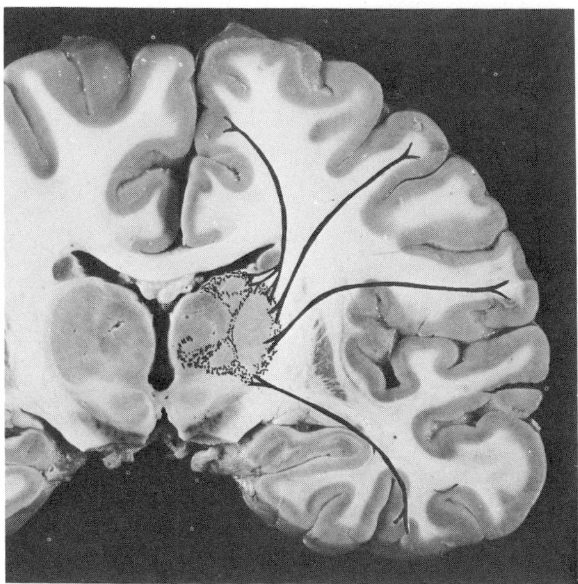

Fig. 15-10. Reticular thalamic nuclei (stippled on right) with projections and radiations to and from "silent" cortical areas.

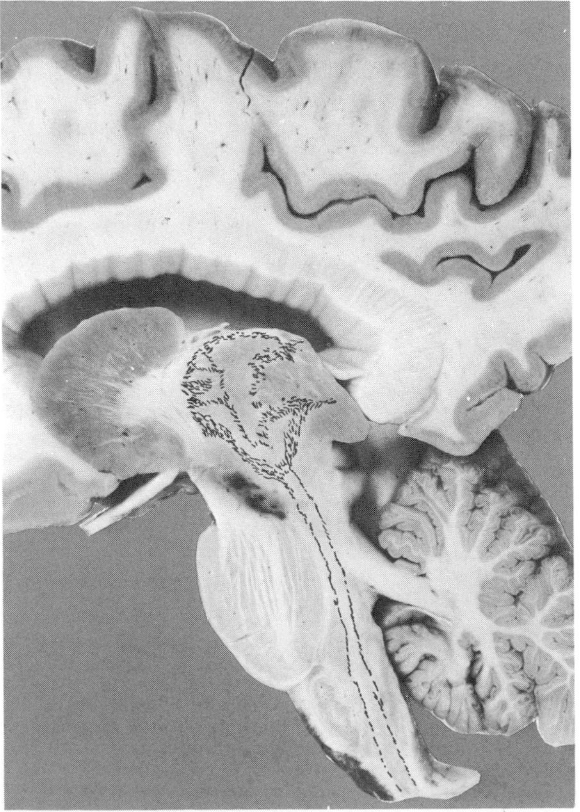

Fig. 15-11. Parasagittal brainstem with reticular formation stippled in.

and scattering. Short relay systems that qualify to be included exist everywhere. In the spinal cord the reticular units probably comprise more than half of the neurons in the gray matter, particularly in the dorsal horns. The principal fiber masses are represented in the spinospinalis (propriospinal) tracts. These lie circumferentially in a marginal position relative to the spinal gray matter (Fig. 15-9, *A*).

The fibers and cells of the spinal reticular system interlink with the reticular formation of the medulla via spinoreticular and reticulospinal tracts. The medullary part of the system is termed *reticuloreticular* (Fig. 15-9, *B*). The nuclei of this component of the medulla are diffuse, and the cells and fibers organize to some degree into medial parts (central tegmental tract) and lateral parts. The two parts are presumed to relate mainly to descending and ascending pathways, respectively. The reticuloreticular pathways continue throughout the tegmentum of the pons and midbrain (Fig. 15-9, *C* to *E*). The pretectal region also possesses short connecting fibers and scattered nuclear clusters, which qualify as part of this system. In the diencephalon the reticular formation is represented by the so-called *nonspecific nuclei* and their related connecting fibers (Figs. 15-10 and 15-11). These nuclei include those of the midline (paratenial, paraventricular, reuniens, and rhomboid), the intralaminar group (central, centromedial, parafascicular, centrolateral, and paracentral), part of the *lateral nuclear group* (ventral anterior), and the *reticular thalamic nucleus* (see Chapter 21). Connections of the reticular nuclei are elaborate and complex. The neural input into the reticular formation includes multisynaptic and collateral chains from the spinal cord, the cerebellum, the hypothalamus, the spinal and cranial nerves, and the cerebral cortex, limbic system, and basal nuclei. The output is directed in both ascending and descending directions to the cerebral cortex, basal nuclei, and cranial and spinal nerve nuclei, particularly those that are autonomic. Special note should be taken of the massive, diffuse projections from the nonspecific thalamic nuclei to the cerebral cortex in unassigned or nonspecific functional areas (Fig. 15-10). The core of reticular substance throughout the spinal cord and brainstem and up through the diencephalon has been called the *centrencephalic system*.

Functions of the reticular system. All known major pathways pour collaterals into the reticular formation. The system therefore represents an alternate means of conveying signals arising in the specific modalities from the principal paths to many relay stations and reflex systems. In general this system is regarded as a route by which a stimulus pattern can influence other neural activity rather than as an alternate pathway for conveying sensation to conscious centers. Most of this influence is directed to reflex and nonvolitional activity. By being fed into the reticular formation, the modality seems to lose its specificity. In some instances, however, (light touch, for example) the reticular route appears to be used as an alternate conducting system with preservation of the specific sensation. Another function is that of alerting or preparatory activation (sometimes inhibition) of neuronal pools, so that normal major pathway or integrative sequences can be carried out. Some degree of localization is apparent in the facilitory-inhibitory function. Experimental stimulation of the rostral part of the brainstem reticular formation (midbrain and thalamus) produces facilitation, while inhibition results from stimulation of the caudal part (medullary). It appears that the reticulospinal tract represents an important extrapyramidal motor pathway from basal nuclei to the final-common-path cells. The system is regarded phylogenetically as the most ancient component of the extrapyramidal units. In nonphysiologic situations (direct stimulation, experimental injury, disease processes, anesthesia) the reticular formation seems particularly related to respiratory, cardiovascular, autonomic, and postural phenomena. These activities are largely reflex and are certainly vital functions. The reticular system thus enters into numerous emotional and behavioral responses in either suppressing or facilitating them. As a component of the alerting and arousal mechanism, the converse might be expected, and the system does play a role in sleep and coma.*

NEURON-GLIAL RELATIONSHIPS

As mentioned previously, the wrapping patterns of oligodendroglial membranes are related to the myelin sheaths of central axons (see Chapter 10), and astroglia contribute prominently to the neuropil fiber complex. There are, in addition, recently demonstrated functional and spatial ties between glia and neurons. Astrocytic processes cover a substantial part of the surface membrane of central perikarya (see Chapter 10). A small segment of surface is also related to capillaries and occasionally to microglia, and the remainder (up to fifty percent) relates to boutons as the receptive part of the synaptic complex. The relationship of the astrocytic process to the cell body has been found to serve two additional functions. First, the astrocytic cytoplasm is capable of undergoing rapid changes in volume, principally by imbibing water. As a consequence, the surface relationship at the synapse can be greatly altered by increase or decrease of the relative area covered by astrocytic processes versus boutons.[15] The second major functional relationship lies in the prospect of metabolic exchanges between astrocytes and nerve cells.[8,13] It is possible that glia cells represent a reservoir of energy-rich components for neuronal use as well as a major storage compartment for fluids and some metabolites. From combined chemical, structural, and physiologic information Giacobini has related biologic properties of glia to suggested functions, as illustrated in Fig. 15-12.[9]

FLUID EXCHANGES AND THE BARRIER SYSTEM

As in other tissues, a great deal of responsibility for maintenance of the functionally organized brain relates to fluid exchanges and transport of metabolites (see Chapter 12). In the exchanges of fluids and metabolites the CNS presents the following two features that are somewhat unique among tissues: (1) the *interstitial compartment* is small or virtually absent; and (2) the blood-to-brain

Biologic properties	*Probable functions*
Slow electrical activity	Electrolyte and fluid exchanges (transport of Na^+ and Cl^-, plasma → glia)
Pulsatile activity	Regulation of CO_2 and NH_3 (glia ⇌ neuron)
High oxidative metabolism	Control of blood flow to neurons
	Supply of energy to neurons
Specific localization of a CO_2 hydration mechanism	Storage of glycogen
	Proteolytic activity
	Myelination

Fig. 15-12. Biologic properties, *left,* and probable functions, *right,* of neuroglia. (After Giocabini.)

*For an extended review of reticular anatomy and function see reference 14.

interface exhibits a highly complex restrictive transfer of some substances, thus establishing a *barrier system*.[4,6,21] Electron microscopy has established the paucity of interstitial space (see Chapter 8).[12,16] This finding has focused attention on transcellular rather than intercellular routes for metabolic exchanges. It has also stressed inclusion of glial elements in considerations regarding transcellular transport. This idea arises from the combined perivascular and perineuronal relationships of the glia through the sucker feet to vessels and from the broad contact of glial processes on nerve cells (Fig. 15-13.)[13] In the barrier system it is necessary to acknowledge the differences in site for transfer. The sites of special interest include at least the following four interfaces: (1) *blood-brain,* which refers to the interface between the capillary wall and the brain substance directly; (2) *blood-CSF,* which is *represented* in the choroid plexus; (3) *CSF-brain,* which handles transfer from CSF into brain through the ventricular lining or pia-glial membrane; and (4) *CSF-blood,* which deals with exchanges from CSF directly into the blood vessels of the subarachnoid space or via the special organs for this process in the pacchionian granulations or their equivalents in the meningeal spaces of the spinal cord (Fig. 15-14).

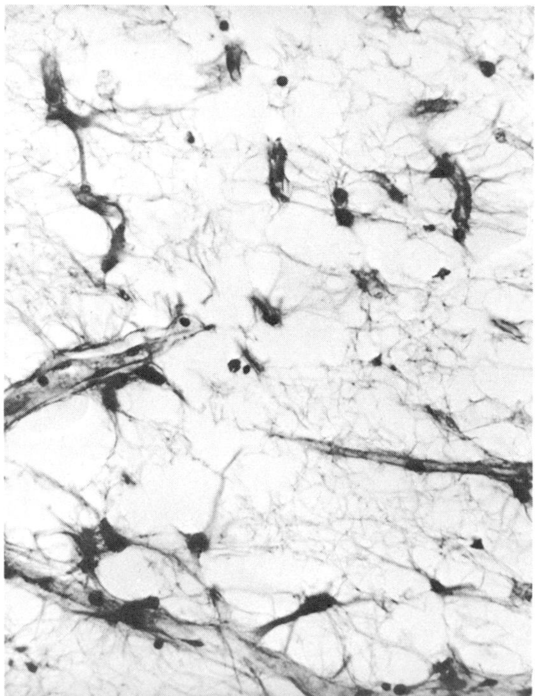

Fig. 15-13. Glial relationships to vessels and cells.

Despite the immense amount of inquiry into the nature of the barrier system, the anatomic sites remain undefined. Attention has been focused upon vascular endothelium, the basement membrane, the membranes of glial cells, pia-glial membrane, intercellular gap substance, and even upon the intercellular junctions in the case of intervening epithelial-type cells. None of the sites qualifies as singly accountable, and the notion of a single barrier factor has largely been abandoned.[4] Instead, a great many factors appear to operate to restrict fluid or metabolite exchanges in nervous tissue. These factors include the following: anatomic substrate (such as double membranes and basement membrane added to cell membrane); passive filter effect of some membranes; size and charge of particles being transported; tissue affinity of the transport substance; lipid solubility; ionization; metabolic needs of the interrelating substance and tissue; metabolic rate of the transport material; metabolite capability and lability of the holding compartment.[6] The behavior of the major physiologic substances related to the barrier system is reviewed in the following paragraph.*

Water is practically unrestricted in transport in nervous tissue and does not appear to be subject to barrier effect. *Inorganic monovalent ions* (Na^+, K^+, Cl^-, HCO_3) figure prominently in the investigation of the barrier systems because of their importance in fluid formation and retention, os-

*For review of clinical features, experimental procedures, and pathologic implications see references 3, 4, and 20.

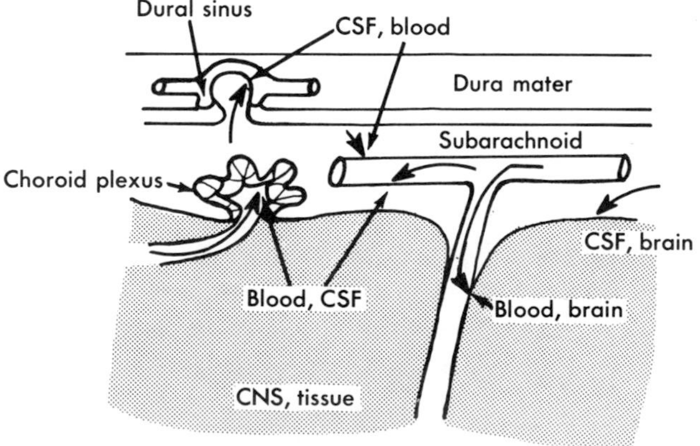

Fig. 15-14. Barrier systems *(large arrows)*.

motic effects, pH, and electric gradients in membranes.[3,6] These ions enter the brain substance from the blood, but with delays implying a barrier effect. The mechanism is unsettled, but may be enzyme-dependent (carbonic anhydrase). This idea arises from equivalent behavioral features to the transport activity in kidney tubules and from the fact that the enzyme concentrates in choroid and glial cells.[9] *Phosphate* ions are restricted in uptake through the blood-brain barrier, but less so through the CSF-brain interface. These ions may require a specific carrier mechanism or may adjust to metabolic needs. *Nutrients* are particularly important exchange items. Amino acids display barrier-like effects, but this may be more related to uptake variation than to transport restriction. This activity may be a reflection of metabolic need. The transport models for amino acids probably vary greatly with the protein makeup and metabolic requirements. *Glucose* is subject to a distinct barrier effect, but the mechanism remains in doubt. Simple diffusion is insignificant, and a special transport mechanism permitting rapid glucose transfer must be operative. Part of the regulation is apparently related to metabolic need, although a *carrier-facilitated* diffusion has been postulated. *Ethyl alcohol* and other lipid-soluble substances pass readily into the brain and are delayed in their concentration in CSF. The method of passage is presumed to be direct capillary diffusion.[6] *Nonphysiologic exchanges* and influences related to the barrier system are important indicator and therapeutic items, with applications in experimental pathology and clinical medicine. These exchanges and influences include acid dyes (trypan blue), heavy metals, blocking agents, metabolic inhibitors, barrier inhibitors, inert extracellular substances (such as india ink, sucrose, manitol) isotopes, anesthetics, drugs, and various barrier-damage indicators in the form of tracers.[4]

METABOLIC ACTIVITY

The metabolic rate of the brain exceeds by about twenty times the average for the rest of the body. This rate is enhanced by neural firing, which places a significant segment of the overall CNS metabolic load in neuronal activity. The accessory metabolic importance of the glial elements has already been noted. The source of the required energy is mainly in carbohydrate metabolism; reserve energy stores are exceedingly meager. The lack of reserve energy shows the absolute necessity for uninterrupted delivery of nutrients and oxygen to the CNS and explains the dramatically adverse effects of deprivation. The metabolic activities of the nervous system display special topographic features (such as the cell membrane, mitochondria, and the synapse), as well as specific chemical features (such as synthesis of proteins, carbohydrate management, lipid metabolism, water and electrolyte balance).*

SECONDARY SYSTEMIC INFLUENCES ON THE NERVOUS SYSTEM

It is obvious that the nervous system cannot operate physiologically as an isolate. It is, in fact, more dependent on intersystem cooperation than most tissues. Consequently, it is impossible to discuss the organization and maintenance of the nervous system without constant reference to the supportive activities of most of the other systems—cardiovascular, respiratory, muscular, gastrointestinal, renal, reticuloendothelial, endocrine, skeletal, and integumentary.

The *cardiac output* is a vital factor in CNS maintenance. Perfusion of the brain with adequate blood is only one of many major physiologic features dependent on cardiac action. Exchanges at the capillary level are a function of *arterial and venous flow*. They are dependent upon the arterial wall capability and upon *muscular* and *respiratory action* for venous return. In the pulmonary system *ventilation* must be assured to maintain the appropriate alveolar carbon dioxide tension related to the required metabolic activity. The ventilatory activity in the pulmonary system must function with diffuse physiologic *perfusion* to accomplish proper oxygen saturation in the pulmonary circulation. *Diffusion* of the gases in the interchanges between alveolus and capillary blood is a complex pulmonary function upon which cerebral internal respiration is dependent. *Transport* of oxygen is dependent not only upon the vascular system, but also upon the hematopoietic system, which provides red cells. Time and amount of delivery of oxygen to the CNS are both critical.

The gastrointestinal tract also is closely tied to the maintenance of nervous tissues. This tie operates through provision of *nutrients* and *vitamins* (particularly B_1) and through relationships of the liver and pancreas that are not fully understood but are evidenced by the frequent correlation of pathologic lesions in the two systems. Renal effects on the nervous system have diverse influences, including electrolyte and fluid balance, control of

*For a review of the neurochemical and metabolic phenomena associated with the function and maintenance of the nervous system see Chapter 12 and references 1, 5, 17, 19, and 22.

pH, elimination of toxic substances, control of blood pressure and flow, and control of various enzyme systems and consequent cellular metabolism.

The muscular system cannot be separated from the nervous system in terms of physiologic function. Consequently, there is reciprocal interdependence. The integument is important to the nervous system, as it houses the neural units that are in environmental contact. It thus becomes an integral part of the normal nervous system.

The skeletal system provides the unique closed-box protection of the CNS and figures prominently in excursions and maintenance of intracranial pressures and the attendant effects on blood flow and CSF.

REFERENCES

1. Barron, K. D.: Enzyme histochemistry of the central nervous system. In Minckler, J., editor: Pathology of the nervous system, vol. I, New York, 1968, McGraw-Hill Book Co.
2. Bodian, D.: Neurons, circuits and neuroglia. In Quarton, G. C., Malnechuk, T., and Schmitt, F. O., editors: The neurosciences, New York, 1967, The Rockefeller University Press.
3. Bowsher, D.: Cerebrospinal fluid dynamics in health and disease, Springfield, Illinois, 1960, Charles C Thomas, Publisher.
4. Broman, T., and Steinwall, O.: Blood-brain barrier. In Minckler, J., editor: Pathology of the nervous system, vol. I, New York, 1968, McGraw-Hill Book Co.
5. Cohen, M. M., and Snider, R. S.: Morphological and biochemical correlates of neural activity, New York, 1964, Harper & Row, Publishers.
6. Davson, H.: Physiology of ocular and cerebrospinal fluids, London, 1956, J. & A. Churchill.
7. Eccles, J. C.: The physiology of synapses, Berlin, 1964, Springer Verlag.
8. Galambos, R.: A glia-neural theory of brain function, Proc. Nat. Acad. Sci. U.S.A. **47**:129, 1961.
9. Giacobini, E: Metabolic relations between glia and neurons. In Cohen, M. M., and Snider, R. S., editors: Morphological and biochemical correlates of neural activity, New York, 1964, Harper & Row, Publishers.
10. Glees, P.: Neuroglia: morphology and function, Philadelphia, 1955, F. A. Davis Co.
11. Grundfest, H.: Pathophysiologic mechanisms in plural transmission. In Minckler, J., editor: Pathology of the nervous system, vol. I, New York, 1968, McGraw-Hill Book Co.
12. Hager, H.: Electron microscopy. In Minckler, J., editor: Pathology of the nervous system, vol. I, New York, 1968, McGraw-Hill Book Co.
13. Hydén, H.: The neuron, New York, 1967, American Elsevier Publishing Co., Inc.
14. Jasper, H. H., editor: Reticular formation of the brain, Boston, 1958, Little, Brown and Co.
15. Kreutzberg, G.: Degeneration and regeneration of peripheral nerves. In Minckler, J., editor: Pathology of the nervous system, vol. II, New York, 1971, McGraw-Hill Book Co.
16. Luse, S.: The neuron. In Minckler, J., editor: Pathology of the nervous system, vol. I, New York, 1968, McGraw-Hill Book Co.
17. Nachmansohn, D.: Chemical and molecular basis of nerve activity, New York, 1959, Academic Press, Inc.
18. Penfield, W., and Roberts, L.: Speech and brain mechanisms, Princeton, New Jersey, 1959, Princeton University Press.
19. Quarton, G. C., Melnechuk, T., and Schmitt, F. O.: The neurosciences, New York, 1967, The Rockefeller University Press.
20. Tourtellotte, W. W.: Cerebrospinal fluid and its reactions in disease. In Minckler, J., editor: Pathology of the nervous system, vol. I, New York, 1968, McGraw-Hill Book Co.
21. Tower, D. B.: In American Neurological Association: Properties of membranes and diseases of the nervous system, New York, 1962, Springer Publishing Co., Inc.
22. Young, I. J.: Neuroenzymology. In Minckler, J., editor: Pathology of the nervous system, vol. I, New York, 1968, McGraw-Hill Book Co.

PART IV Neural pathways

CHAPTER 16

GENERAL SENSORY SYSTEMS

JEFF MINCKLER

The neural parts mediating general sense, both somatic and visceral, lend themselves structurally to discussion in three categories: (1) *cutaneous sense;* (2) *deep sensibility;* and (3) *general visceral afferent* systems. The first two reach conscious levels in the usual physiologic circumstance. Cutaneous sensations register as *pain, temperature,* and *light* (*nondiscriminative*) *touch.* It is perfectly clear that many such afferent impulses operate at reflex levels only and consciousness occurs only in special circumstances (such as appreciation of an item of wearing apparel). Similarly, deep sensibility registers consciousness of sensations arising in noncutaneous tissues, such as *pressure, stretch, vibration, position, movement, intensity,* and *placement.* In many circumstances these are consciously registered, but such sensations enter into reflex connections even more prominently than cutaneous (postural maintenance, for example). The *discriminative* features of touch (*two-point, size, texture, form, stereognosis*) follow pathways that are common to those of deep sensibility to conscious centers and are discussed with them. The prominent *reflex* and *cerebellar routes* for deep sense provide a separate section of immense importance because of magnitude of reflex-control systems related to muscle and tendon activity. The general visceral afferent system characteristically is relatively insensitive to the usual stimuli that are effective in the somatic systems. *Pain* is certainly prominent in some visceral diseases, and visceral referral to cutaneous areas is the commonest manifestation of *referred pain* (see p. 277). *Temperature* (heat) is appreciated in the esophagus and lower rectum, but not elsewhere. Thermal stimulation elsewhere (such as in the pleura) elicits reflex responses but no consciousness other than that related to the reflex. *Complex sensations* (hunger, thirst, fullness, satiety, nausea, sexual sensations, and anal and bladder sensations) arise in the general visceral afferent system in ways that are often obscure. All the general sensations mentioned arise in *receptors,* which vary greatly in structure and function but which have some features in common.

Receptors are the end-organs that are in environmental contact either externally or viscerally. They operate as transducers in converting energy of diverse sources (heat, light, chemical, mechanical) into the electrical energy associated with depolarization and the nervous impulse. The structures are therefore *thermoreceptors, photoreceptors, chemoreceptors,* or *mechanoreceptors.* In some instances the same receptor is responsive to more than one type of stimulus. Pain appears to be elicited by intense stimulation of most receptors, particularly when tissue damage occurs (*nociceptors*). This may be a matter of stimulus intensity but also may be related to the release of irritating chemicals (histamine or kinins?) from destroyed tissue. Also, in some circumstances, a wide degree of latitude in the spectrum of the stimulus is displayed by receptors; for example, radiation beyond the wave length of visible light is sometimes appreciated either by photoreceptors in the eye or by direct stimulation of the CNS.[5] The basic mechanism of stimulation undoubtedly varies with the type of receptor, but in general an effective stimulus operates by nonselectively increasing the permeability of the receptive membrane to ions. This disrupts the resting potential by depolarizing the surface membrane (see Chapter 13).

CUTANEOUS SENSE

The special nerve endings in general body skin, mucous membranes of nose and mouth, teeth, orbital contents, and meninges that mediate *pain,*

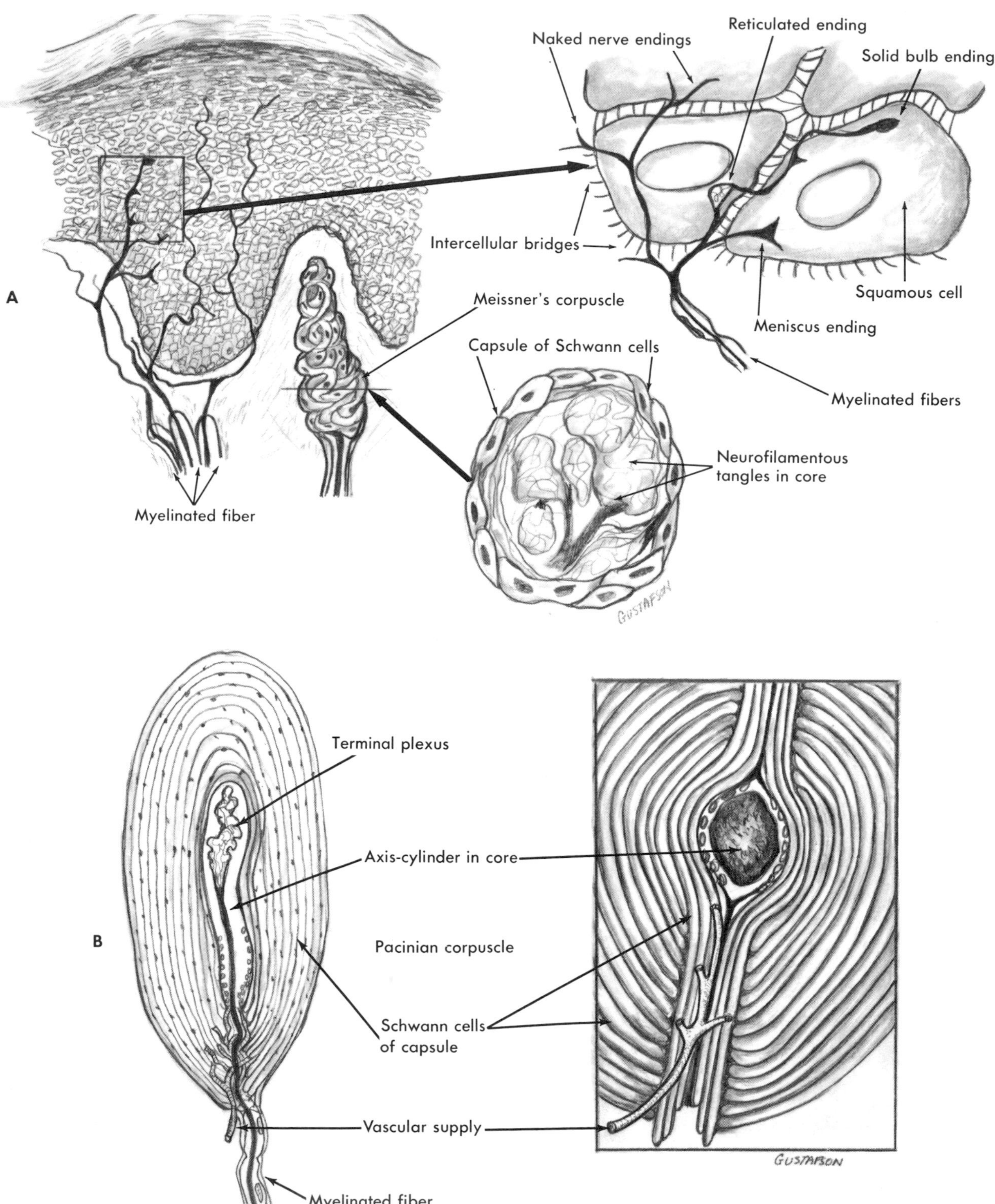

Fig. 16-1. Diagrams of receptors. **A,** Naked nerve endings and Meissner's corpuscle in skin; **B,** Pacinian corpuscle showing Schwann cell membrane organization of laminated body (right); **C,** plexus of Bonnet around hair follicle; **D,** Golgi-Massoni body, longitudinal and cross section; **E,** Krause bulb; **F,** Ruffini corpuscle.

temperature, and *light touch* are of several types. There is segmental overlapping in all cutaneous areas. This differs in extent in different parts of the body, but the usual representation is distribution to a full segment plus a half-segment on either side. This means that each area has at least two segmental supplies, but many areas probably have more (see Chapter 7).

Free, or *naked, nerve endings* are believed to be sensitive to *pain* (as well as to touch), but in general pain appears to be elicited whenever tissue in the areas listed above (and in periosteum, joints, and arterial walls) is damaged. The implication is that naked nerve endings pick up stimuli that give rise to the sensation of pain probably both from mechanical disruption of the ending membranes and from liberation of chemical irritants in damaged tissue. The prototype of this free ending is a fine fibril that is part of a ramifying axis-cylinder within epithelium and adjacent connective tissue. In general the naked nerve endings are thought to be incarcerated within cells and probably carry a unit membrane wrapping, as most so-called interstitial elements do. These fibrils appear to be devoid of independent structural covering, having lost any semblance of sheath before they penetrate the epithelium. These terminals branch dichotomously and form frequent *nets* (Fig. 16-1). A structural variation is the *meniscus,* or flattened disk, occuring either as a terminal or a widened structure along the filament (ending of Merkel-Ranvier) (Fig. 16-1). The meniscus is believed to relate to pain and itching and to touch.

Temperature, or thermal reception, probably is also picked up by naked nerve endings, but this sense is generally assigned to the complex *bulbs of Krause* and *corpuscles of Ruffini.* Through these structures the sensations of *cool* and *warm* and particularly *change* or difference in temperature are appreciated. It is claimed, for example, that a difference of one degree Fahrenheit can be appreciated by the backs of the hands. *Freezing* and *burning* sensations, as they intensify, become confused with pain. The end-bulbs of Krause are located in the dermis of the skin, the glans of the penis and clitoris, the nipples, the conjunctiva, and the mucous membrane of the tongue. They measure in most areas from 20 by 40 to 30 by 100 μ and are largest and most numerous as *genital end-bulbs.* Under the light microscope the Krause bulbs ap-

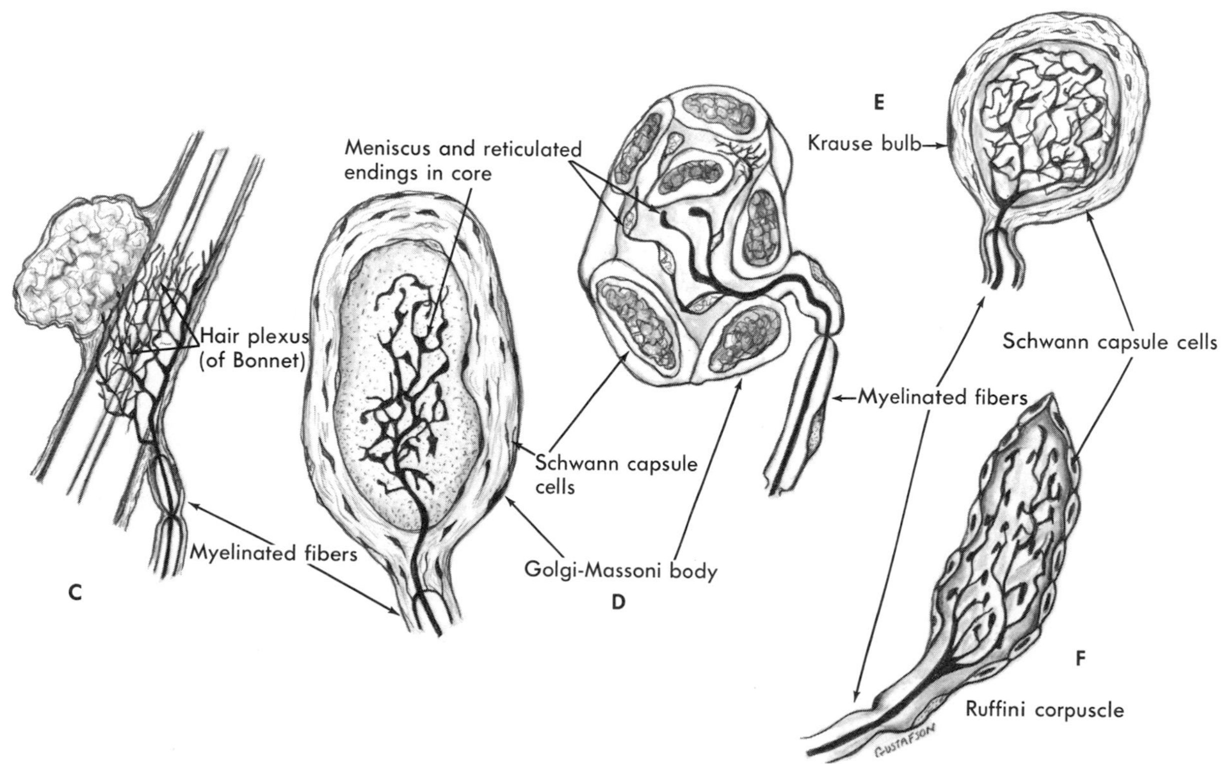

Fig. 16-1, contd. For legend see opposite page.

pear to be a complex tangle of neurofibrils covered by a capsule of connective tissue (probably Schwann cells) (Fig. 16-1). The neural fibers may form tiny nets within the tangle, simulating the internal structure of Golgi-Mazzoni bodies (Fig. 16-1). The corpuscles of Ruffini are elongate, complex terminals (60 by 300 μ), which are distributed throughout subcutaneous tissues but are most numerous in the deep dermis of the fingers. They appear under the light microscope to be made up of a tangle of multibranched axis-cylinders in a core and capsular mixture of Schwann cells.

Touch sensations in the skin and other tissues seem to be related to the most complex of the nerve endings and to the greatest variety. *Menisci* (tactile disks) are thought to respond to touch stimuli as well as to pain. *Plexuses of Bonnet* represent multibranched axis-cylinders lying between the bases of hair follicles and their surrounding connective tissue. Movement of the hairs elicits the sensation of touch through these endings. *Meissner's corpuscles* are the best known tactile endings and concentrate in density in the dermal papillae of the hand and foot, where they number about twenty per square millimeter. They also occur in the tip of the tongue, the lip, the nipple, the conjunctiva, and the anterior surface of the forearm. They vary greatly in size, with an average maximum dimension of 100 μ (Fig. 16-1). It appears clear that the endings are a combination of nerve filaments and Schwann cells.[1] *Corpuscles of Golgi-Mazzoni* represent fine tangles and nets of neurofibrils in a capsule of Schwann cells (Fig. 16-1). They occur in the subcutaneous tissue of the fingertips, the external genitalia, the conjunctiva, and periosteum. They measure 75 by 150 μ and present a granular center and laminated capsule under the light microscope.

Touch also is sensed by *Pacinian corpuscles* (of Vater-Pacini), which, however, appear to be primarily related to pressure sense. These are the most complex and well known receptors. They are from 1 to 4 mm. in length and are ubiquitously distributed in subcutaneous and other tissues. Because of their size they possess their own blood supply in a vascular plexus entering with the axonic stem. A Schwann myelin sheath continues up to the end-organ and becomes continuous with the lamellated covering. Electron microscopy has established that the central neural core occupies a cleft that is capped bilaterally and concentrically by individual lamellae arising in separate cytoplasmic processes of Schwann cells. The interlamellar spaces contain collagen; this is consistent with the Schwann cell origin.[2,3] The axis-cylinder in the central core ramifies extensively in the distal part of the organ. Under the light microscope the core appears to be largely fluid, and the margin of the core contains numerous Schwann cell nuclei (Fig. 16-1).

Cutaneous sensory neurons (first-order)

First-order neurons in this system are *receptor neurons,* in contrast to *synaptic neurons,* which receive their impulses from other neurons. This means that their pickup signals arise in their own nerve-ending receptors, as previously outlined. This configuration places these neurons in environmental contact through the skin. The fibers mediating cutaneous sense vary in speed of conduction from 0.5 to 15 meters per second, with the larger fibers being the more rapid conductors. The cutaneous sources of these impulses are represented in the diagrams of segmentation, p. 134. The cell bodies of these cutaneous afferent neurons (relatively small cells in accordance with their fiber size) lie in dorsal root and cranial nerve ganglia, which may be summarized as follows: (1) from general trunk and extremity surfaces—in the *dorsal root ganglia* of the spinal nerves; (2) from the skin of the face, from the orbit, mouth, nasal cavity, and paranasal sinuses, and from the meninges of the anterior and middle cranial fossae—in the *semilunar ganglion* of cranial nerve V (trigeminal); (3) from the postauricular region and part of the external auditory meatus—in the *geniculate ganglion* of cranial nerve VII (facial); (4) from the posterior third of the tongue—in the *superior ganglion* of cranial nerve IX (glossopharyngeal); and (5) from behind the ear, part of the external auditory meatus, and from meninges around the transverse sinus in the posterior fossa—in the *jugular ganglion* of cranial nerve X (vagus).

These cutaneous first-order fibers enter the CNS to end synaptically in relationship to the *primary receptive nuclei* for pain, temperature, and light touch (see Chapter 6). These nuclei include *nuclei cuneatus and gracilis, chief sensory nucleus* of cranial nerve V, *nucleus of the descending root* of the trigeminal nerve, and the *substantia gelatinosa Rolandi* (Figs. 16-2 and 16-3). It should be remembered that the last three nuclei are continuous from the spinal cord up to the middle of the brainstem.

Of the cutaneous fibers those mediating *touch* are the coarsest and enter the spinal cord in the most medial position among the fibers in the root. This position brings them directly into the pos-

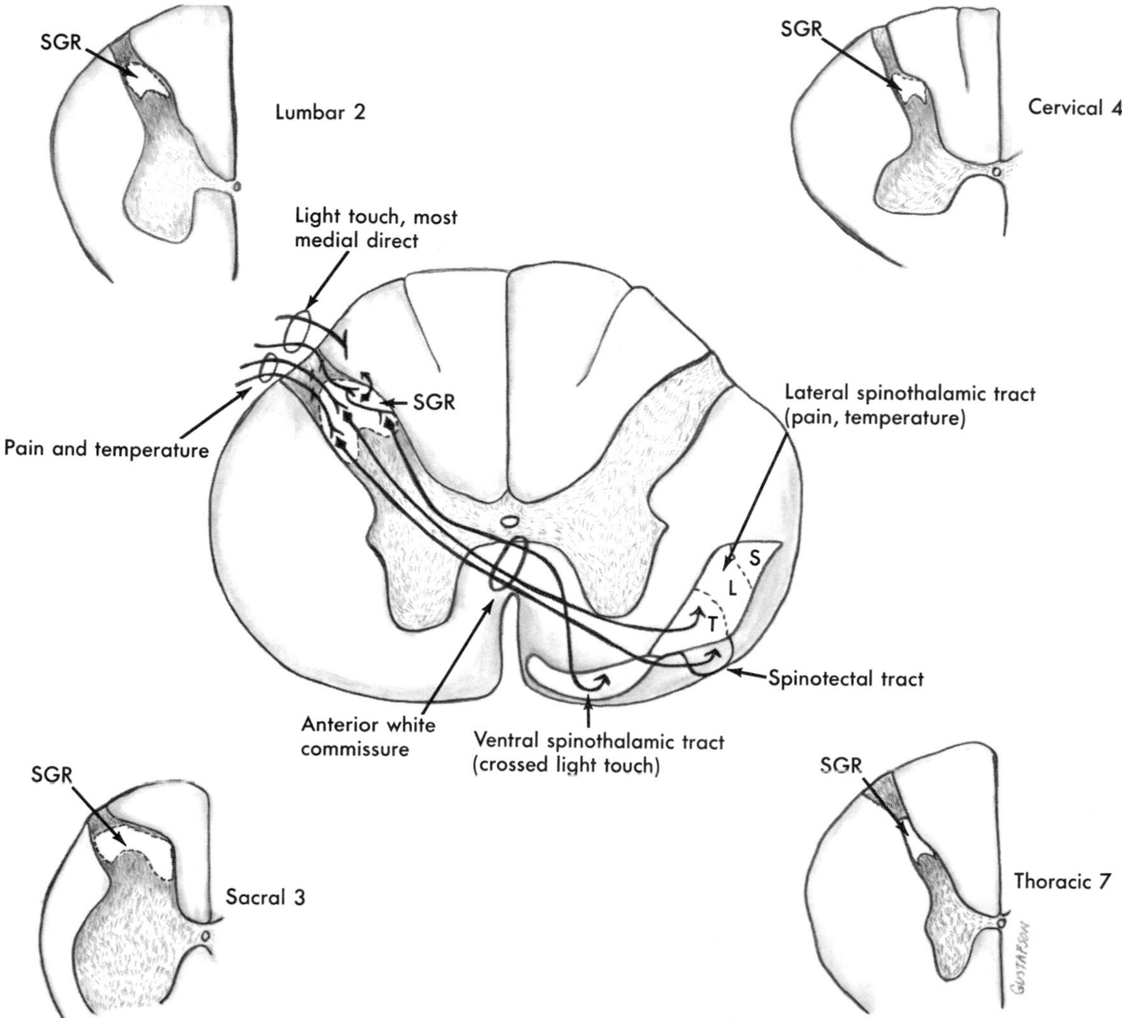

Fig. 16-2. Primary cutaneous receptor nuclei in cord. Substantia gelatinosa Rolandi (*SGR*) variations at indicated levels. Lamination of secondary ascending spinothalamic fibers is shown in central figure.

terior funiculus. The exact course of these fibers is uncertain. Light touch however is definitely separated from pain and temperature, as well as from discriminative touch at this level centrally. It is presumed that some of the fibers ascend in the posterior funiculus. In this case those arising in the lower extremity would ascend in the fasciculus gracilis to the nucleus gracilis, and those from body areas above mid-thoracic would ascend to the nucleus cuneatus through the fasciculus cuneatus (Fig. 16-4). While most touch sensation from the body is transmitted upward in the spinal cord on the homolateral side, some touch sensation moves to the opposite side. However, this is no doubt accomplished by neurons of the second order, with cell bodies located in the nucleus proprius. Touch fibers from the face region pass in the ascending tract of the trigeminal nerve to terminate in the chief sensory nucleus. In the face region light touch is less readily dissociated from tactile discrimination. In summary: while primary receptive nuclei for light touch remain uncertain, it is probable that at least three nuclear groups are involved; (1) nuclei of the posterior funiculus (*cuneatus and gracilis*); (2) *nucleus proprius* of the dorsal horn of the spinal cord; and (3) *chief sensory nucleus* of the trigeminal nerve (Fig. 16-3). These represent the probable origin for second-order neurons in the cutaneous pathway for touch.

Pain and *temperature* are mediated by fine fi-

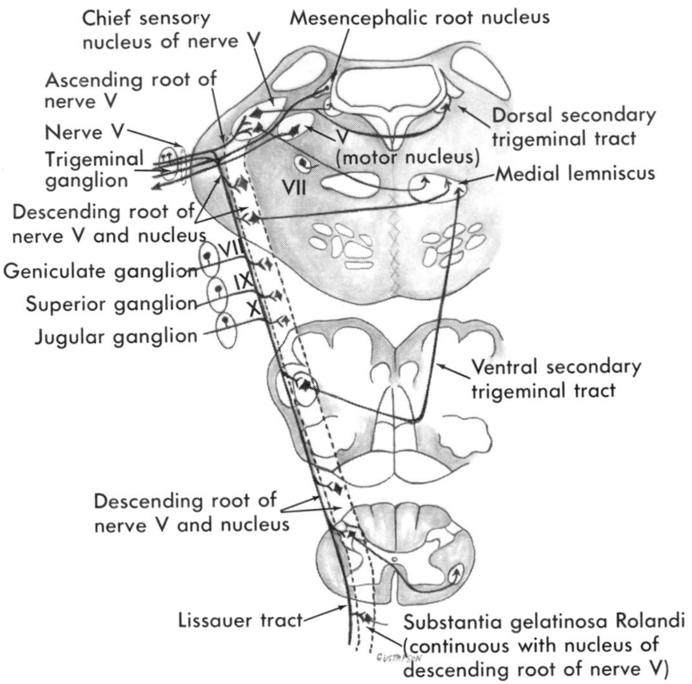

Fig. 16-3. Primary cutaneous receptor nuclei in brainstem. Note that the descending root nucleus is continuous below with the substantia gelatinosa Rolandi. The two secondary trigeminal tracts fuse into the trigeminal lemniscus at the midbrain level.

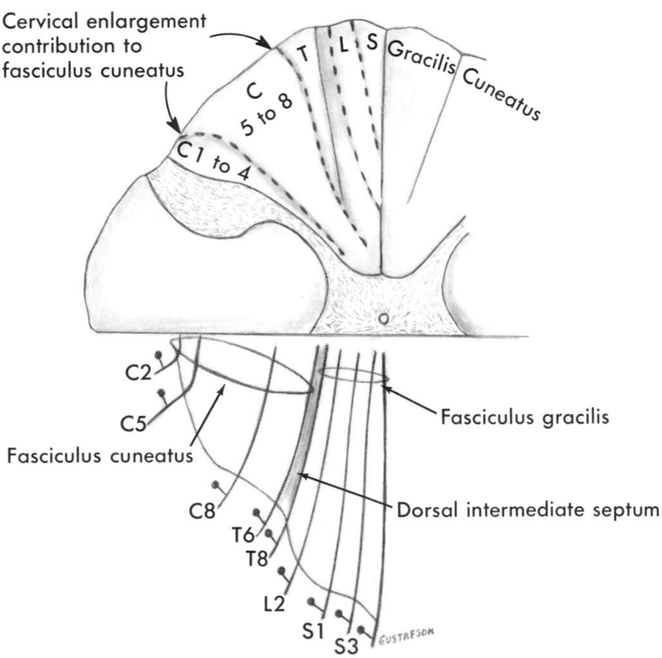

Fig. 16-4. Formation of fasciculus gracilis from below midthoracic level and of the fasciculus cuneatus from incoming fibers above that level. Note size of the contribution from upper extremity.

bers that occupy the lateral part of the dorsal root as it enters the cord (Fig. 16-2). They enter the *dorsolateral fasciculus of Lissauer* and quickly terminate within one or two segments in the nucleus *substantia gelatinosa Rolandi*. From the head region pain and temperature enter mainly through the trigeminal nerve, but also through nerves VII, IX, and X. All these turn downward into the descending root of the trigeminal nerve and terminate in the nucleus of that root (*nucleus of the descending root*). This root nucleus is continuous below with the substantia gelatinosa Rolandi. Of the branches of cranial nerve V, the ophthalmic pain and temperature fibers descend farthest in the descending root (to cervical segments); the maxillary fibers descend an intermediate distance, and the descending mandibular fibers extend the shortest distance (to the lower third of the medulla). In summary, pain and temperature neurons terminate primarily in the *substantia gelatinosa Rolandi* and in the *nucleus of the descending root* of cranial nerve V. These nuclei are the locations of nerve cell bodies of second order in the pain and temperature pathways.

Accessory connections

The traditional representation of the incoming fibers is placing of the terminals in specific primary receptive nuclei. It is recognized however that this is an oversimplification. The incoming fibers divide dichotomously with production of both ascending and descending limbs (Fig. 16-2). Usually the ascending limb is represented as the route to the primary receptive nucleus. It is presumed that the descending limb terminates in relationship to cells that form short reflex paths; hence, this limb avoids the ascending pathway of cutaneous "information" to conscious centers. The reflex connections may in some instances pass to final-path cells on the same side. For the most part they probably pass to internuncial cells of the dorsal horn (nucleus proprius), where they enter into reflex patterns with cells affecting either side. In general, such connections are divergent in character (see Chapter 15) and contribute to either activating or inhibiting complex responses. Another accessory linkage is the diverse input to the primary receptive nuclear field, which must be regarded as capable of operating either as activator or inhibitor to the function of the direct cutaneous pathway. Neurons of many sources undoubtedly bear on the receiving cells within these nuclei and contribute to the responses that arise from the total complex. The impulses that arise in second-order neurons and ascend to the thalamus are therefore a composite expression of many neural actions that probably extensively involve the short locally interconnecting neurons (*spinospinalis*).

Ascending neurons to the thalamus (second-order neurons)

Neurons of second order in the cutaneous system carry pain, temperature, and light-touch sensations from the primary receptive nuclei to the thalamus. Touch (direct touch) travels from the cuneate and gracile nuclei through fibers that cross at midline as *internal arcuate fibers* to join the *medial lemniscus* in its dorsal part (Fig. 16-5). Some direct touch probably travels by stages up the same side, using substantia gelatinosa relays or the spinospinalis reticular formation, and eventually crosses gradually to the medial lemniscus. Crossed light touch is even less certainly identified and passes from the nucleus proprius to the *ventral spinothalamic* tract of the opposite side (Fig. 16-6). As the ventral spinothalamic tract ascends, it gradually moves laterally to join the lateral spinothalamic tract and spinotectal tract, which as a group form the *spinal lemniscus*. Touch fibers in both the medial and spinal lemnisci ascend to the ventral nucleus of the thalamus and end in relationship to third-order thalamic cells. Touch from the face travels from the chief sensory nucleus of cranial nerve V via *dorsal* and *ventral secondary trigeminal tracts* (both crossed and uncrossed) to the ventral nucleus of the thalamus. The two secondary trigeminal tracts fuse as they ascend to form the *trigeminal lemniscus* before the fibers enter the thalamus.

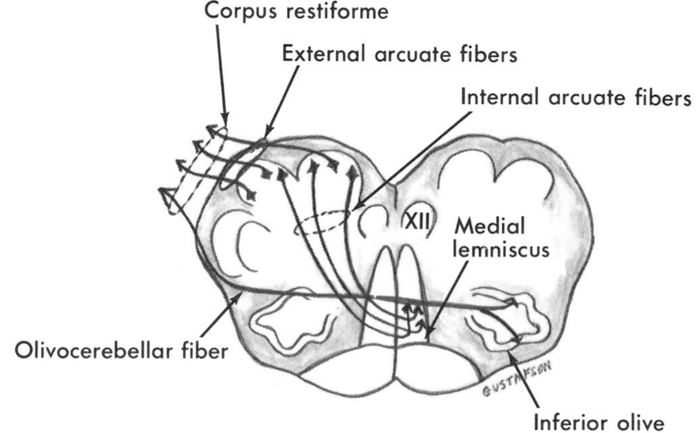

Fig. 16-5. Connections of cuneate and gracile nuclei in contributing the external arcuate fibers to the corpus restiforme and the internal arcuate fibers to the medial lemniscus for ascent to the thalamus.

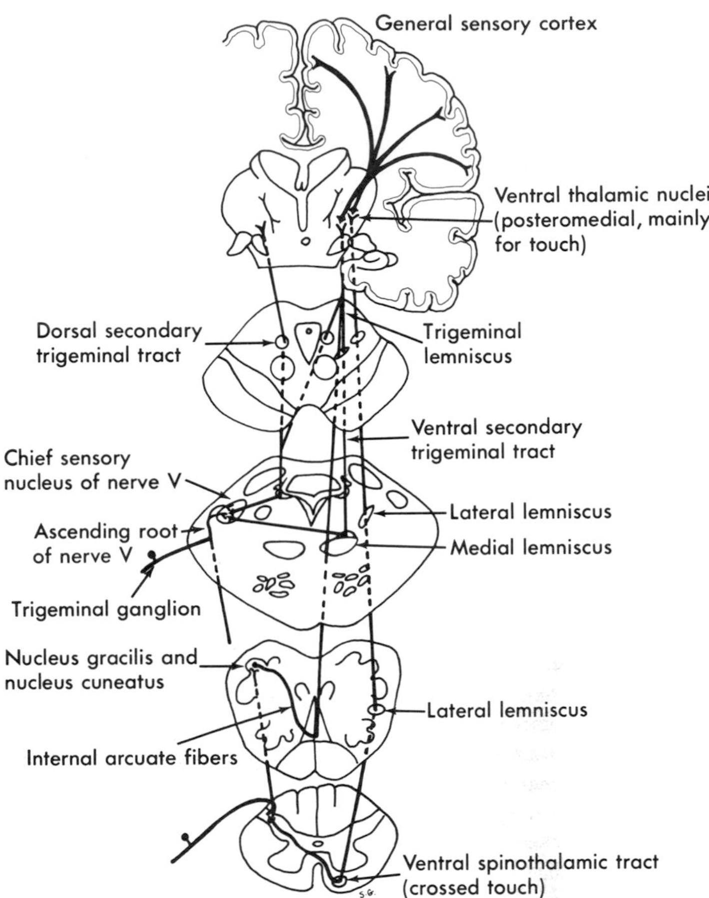

Fig. 16-6. Ascending touch pathways to the thalamus and cortex.

Pain and temperature secondary tracts from the general body arise in the nucleus substantia gelatinosa and pass in fibers that cross in the spinal *anterior white commissure* to ascend as the lateral *spinothalamic tract* of the opposite side (Figs. 16-7 and 16-16). As the fibers cross in midline and ascend, they are joined by incoming fibers from higher crossings on their medial side. This moves the lowermost accessions laterally so that a laminar pattern occurs in the spinothalamic fasciculus, with sacral fibers most superficial and more deeply placed lumbar, thoracic, and cervical fibers in that order (Fig. 16-2). The tract joins the spinotectal and ventral spinothalamic tracts to form the *spinal lemniscus,* by which the pain and temperature impulses reach the ventral nucleus of the thalamus. From the face region pain and temperature secondary neurons arise in the *nucleus of the descending root* of cranial nerve V. The fibers pass upward via the *ventral secondary trigeminal tract* to join the trigeminal lemniscus; they then continue to the ventral nucleus of the thalamus. Most fibers are crossed. The positions of the lemnisci are illustrated topographically in representative sections in Fig. 16-7.

Thalamic radiations (third-order neurons)

Thalamic radiations are projections from the thalamic nuclei to the postcentral gyrus, the somesthetic area of the cerebral cortex. As stated previously, the medial, spinal, and trigeminal lemnisci convey cutaneous sensations as axon bundles of secondary neurons to the ventral nucleus of the thalamus. The cell bodies of this nucleus are the third-order neurons of the lemniscal system. They convey these cutaneous sensations through the *posterior limb* of the internal capsule (general sensory portion) via the *corona radiata* to the cortex

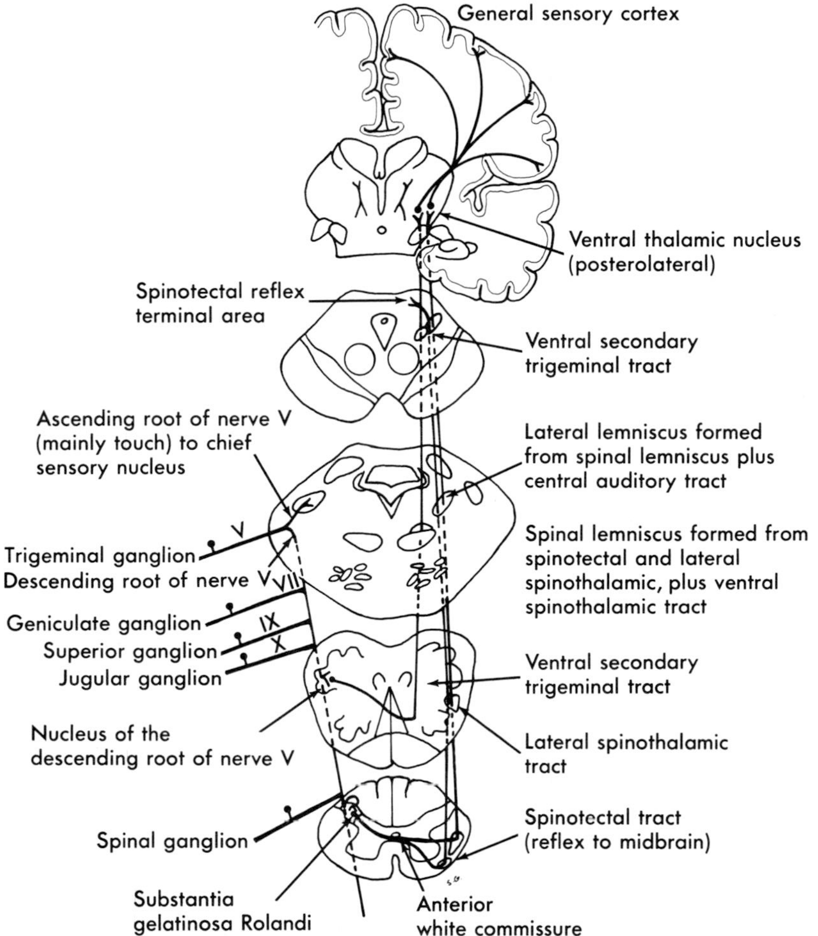

Fig. 16-7. Ascending pathways for pain and temperature to thalamus and cortex.

of the *postcentral gyrus* and adjacent gyri. This is the *general somesthetic area.* The representation correlating the body regions with the cortical receiving area is outlined in Fig. 16-8. Note that the body image is inverted, with face inferior and lower extremity superior in the cortical representation.

Reflex connections

It should be recalled that reflex connections are available in profusion at all nuclear stops. Some such connections aggregate in bundles as specific tracts, such as the *spinotectal tract,* a long reflex bundle terminating in the roof of the midbrain (Fig. 16-2). This bundle enters into the makeup of the spinal lemniscus and brings cutaneuos sensation into almost direct relationship with eye muscle responses in the midbrain. Many such long reflex relationships are present.

Referred pain is the sensation of pain received from an area that is considerably removed from the point of stimulation. This is usually considered to be cerebral misinterpretation of localization. For example, the usual location of pain associated with stimulation in the fourth cervical segment is the skin of the shoulder. In the event of irritation of the diaphragm (supplied by the phrenic, fourth cervical segment) this stimulation may be misinterpreted as coming from the shoulder, or *referred* to the shoulder. Many similar examples occur with the primary stimuli in the viscera (such as ureter, heart).[4]

The cutaneous system is summarized in Figs. 16-6 and 16-7.

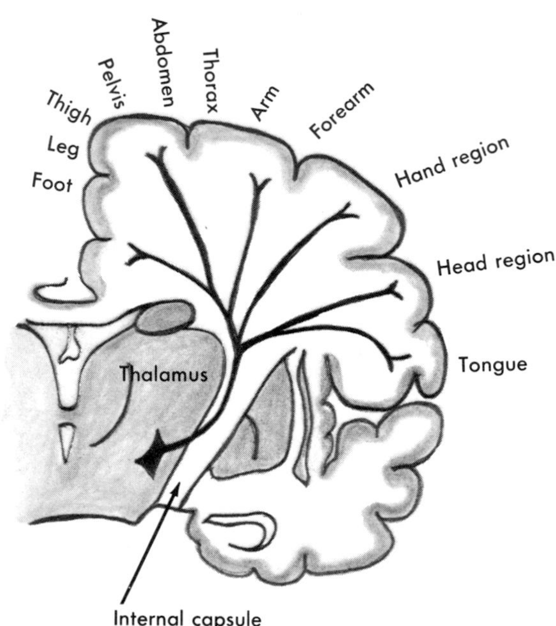

Fig. 16-8. Vertical regional distribution of somesthetic systems to sensory cortex.

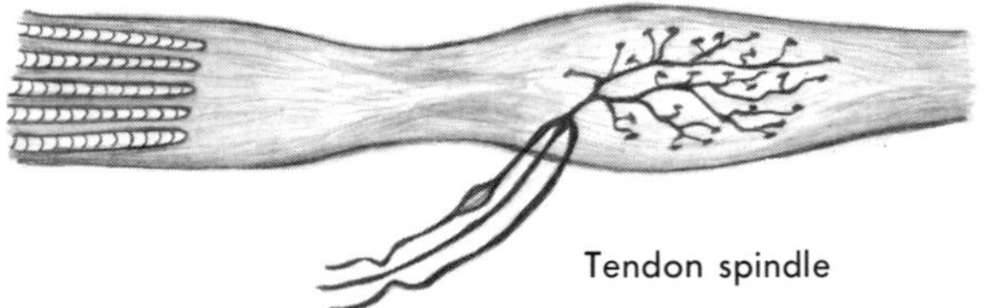

Fig. 16-9. Diagram of tendon spindle.

DEEP SENSIBILITY AND TACTILE DISCRIMINATION

Receptors

Special endings that are adapted to responding to pressure in deep tissues, stretch effects, vibrations, position sense, recognition of movement or change, differences in intensity, and placement are *deep sensibility* receptors. While they are essentially mechanoreceptors mediating somewhat the same sensations as cutaneous receptors, they differ in several important ways. They are picked up by deeply placed receptors. They travel more rapidly over bigger fibers, and they are, for the most part, routed differently in the CNS. The types of receptors that are susceptible to deep-sense stimulations probably include the Krause end-bulb in tendons, the Golgi-Mazzoni bodies in periosteum (also for pressure in skin of fingers and genitalia), free nerve endings that terminate in deep tissues, and Pacinian corpuscles, which are widely distributed in deep tissues (see p. 270). Of major importance in this system are the receptors in muscles and tendons (*spindles*). It is estimated that as many as half of all nerve fibers entering muscle are afferent fibers and arise in sensory receptors in those structures. Some of these nerves enter into pathways that reach conscious levels, but most undoubtedly operate in complex reflexes that regulate integrated muscle activities.

Tendon spindles (Golgi organs) are situated in tendons adjacent to the termination of muscle (Fig. 16-9). They measure 0.2 by 1.3 mm. and give rise to myelinated nerve fibers. Tendon spindles represent a complex nerve plexus ensheathed in cytoplasmic membrane of unknown origin (Schwann cell ?) and include collagen fibers. They are excited by stretch and contribute to muscle sense.

Muscle spindles are large endings (0.04 to 0.4 mm. in diameter and up to 13 mm. in length), which play a major role in muscle coordination and in the servomechanisms regulating muscle activity. The spindles concentrate in the center of the muscle and appear in density in relation to the refinement of muscle movements (most numerous in distal limb muscles). The organ is made up of two to ten specialized muscle fibers (*intrafusal fibers*) running parallel within an isolated capsular field. The capsule attaches at either end to the connective covering of regular muscle fibers (*extrafusal fibers*). This arrangement (Fig. 16-10) makes the spindle susceptible to mechanical stretch and contraction of the adjacent muscle, but in a different manner from that associated with tendon spindles (see Chapter 22). The afferent components associated with spindles include small naked nerve endings, which may be pain terminals, and the two special endings that characterize the Golgi organ, *annulospiral endings* and *flower spray endings.* The annulospiral endings are helical in pattern and encircle the central cluster of intrafusal fibers. They give rise to the large myelinated fibers (8 to 12 μ) leaving the spindle. The flower spray endings are multibranched in small rings and coils and appear within the spindle at one or both pole positions of the annulospiral endings. Motor fibers also are in the complex, but these will be reviewed later (see Chapter 22). The flower spray endings give rise to small myelinated fibers of 3 to 7 μ in diameter. The two afferent endings are sensitive to stretch and contraction in ways that are somewhat uncertain, but they regulate through rapid reflex paths the controlled muscle activity that is so important in posture and sustained contraction.

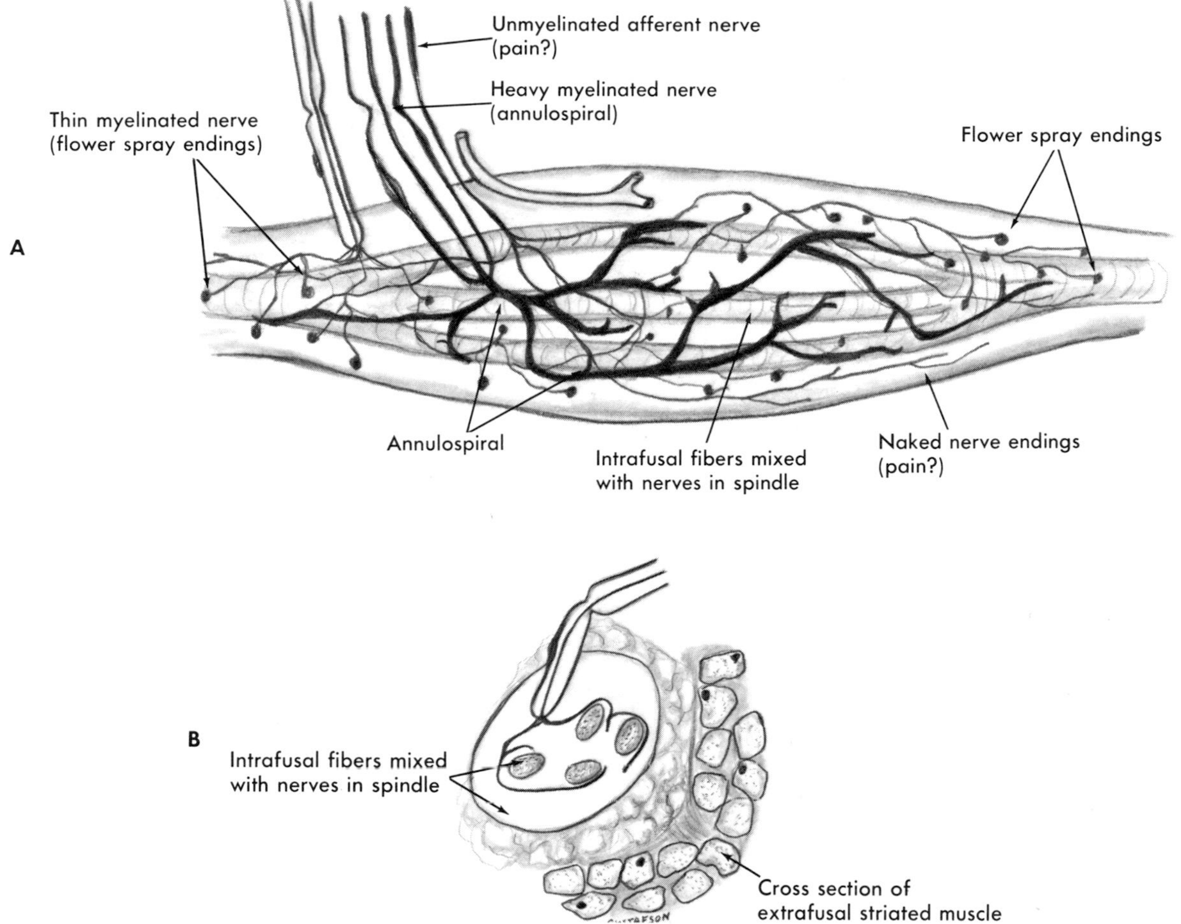

Fig. 16-10. Diagram of muscle spindle. **A,** Note three types of contributing fibers (unmyelinated, heavy myelinated, and thin myelinated), each relating to a different function of the spindle; **B,** cross section.

Sensory neurons (first-order)

Impulses of the discriminative cutaneous senses (two-point, size, texture, form, stereognosis or three-dimensional appreciation) are transmitted centrally with the sensations from deeper body parts, such as muscles, tendons, joints and bones (deep pressure, kinesthetic, position sense or proprioception, and vibratory sense). They are mediated through large fibers (4.0 to 22.0 μ in diameter), which conduct the impulses at a rapid rate (15 to 120 meters per second). The cell bodies (large cells) are located in the dorsal root ganglia for general body deep sense and discrimination, and in the ganglion of cranial nerve V for the head region. A special *central* unipolar ganglion (the *mesencephalic nucleus* of nerve V) probably mediates muscle sense from the muscles of mastication and possibly others. The location of the cells and the course of the deep-sense fibers from the muscles supplied by cranial nerves III, IV, VI, VII, and XII are unknown (see Chapter 6). The muscles supplied by cranial nerve XI probably send their afferent fibers through spinal segments. It is assumed that deep sense from muscles supplied by cranial nerves IX and X enters the CNS through the same nerves. In general, the deep-sensibility neurons direct their impulses in one of two major routes: (1) to *conscious centers,* and (2) to *cerebellar and reflex centers.* The latter center is especially important in this system, as compared to the cutaneous system.

The circuit to conscious centers for first-order neurons mediating discrimination and deep sense from the general body is via the dorsal funiculus. The large incoming fibers divide into short descending and long ascending filaments in the pos-

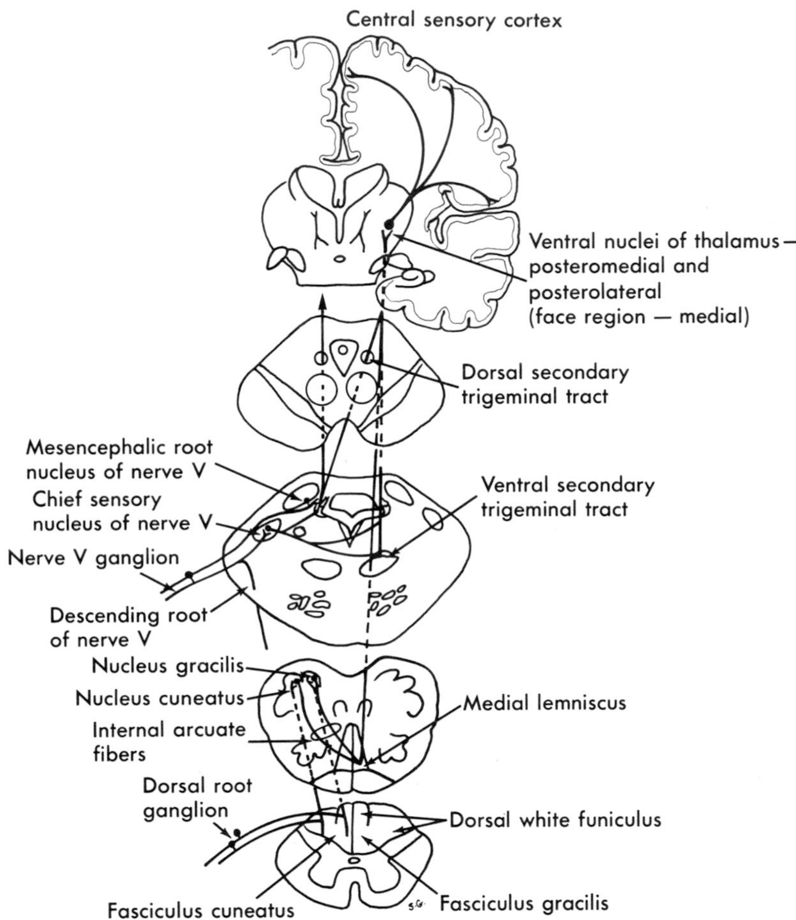

Fig. 16-11. Direct pathways for deep sensibility and discriminative sense to thalamus and cortex.

terior funiculus. Descending fibers are short (two or three segments) and aggregate in the *interfascicular,* or comma, *tract of Schultze* (Fig. 16-11) to terminate in the dorsal horn. Those ascending fibers enter low in the spinal cord and are carried more medially as additional fibers are added by the successive nerve roots in upward progression. Thus, deep-sense fibers from the lower extremity form the *fasciculus gracilis,* and those entering higher in the cord form the *fasciculus cuneatus* (Fig. 16-4). These tracts terminate in the two nuclei of the same names, adjacent to the cell bodies of second-order neurons. The course of fibers of the deep-sense system entering through nerve V (also nerves III, IV, VI, VII, and XII) remains unknown. It seems generally accepted that the mesencephalic nucleus of nerve V represents the cell bodies of deep-sense fibers from muscles of mastication. Just how much of this nucleus is similarly employed for other head-region muscles is unknown (see Chapter 6). All the nerves mediating deep sense from the head region, particularly nerves V and VII, seem to make fairly direct reflex connections with efferent fibers to the muscles through the motor nuclei of nerves V and VII.

Second- and third-order neurons

The *second-order* pathways mediating tactile discrimination and deep sensibilities from the head region are unknown. It is presumed that they move to the thalamus with the secondary trigeminal tracts, although they may ascend by relays. Deep sense from the general body have their second-order neurons arising in the nucleus gracilis and nucleus cuneatus. The fibers cross as *internal arcuate* fibers and enter the *medial lemniscus,* by which they ascend to the ventral nucleus of the thalamus (Fig. 16-11).

Third-order neurons pass from the thalamus into the posterior limb of the internal capsule, by which they are routed to the postcentral gyrus or general somesthetic area. As in cutaneous sensation, deep sense is represented for the *lower extremity and trunk* in the *upper third* of the postcentral gyrus, for the *upper* extremity in the *middle third,* and for the *head* and *neck* in the *lower third* (Fig. 16-8).

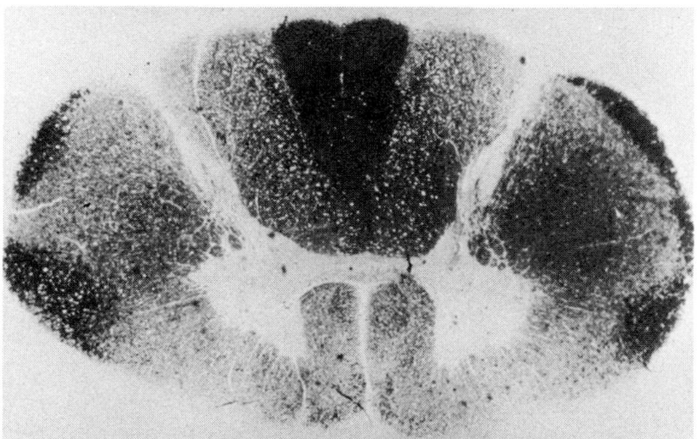

Fig. 16-12. Degeneration in tracts of cervical cord after transection at lower thoracic level. Note definition of fasciculus gracilis and of lateral dorsal and ventral spinocerebellar tracts. (Marchi stain.)

Circuits to the cerebellum and reflex connections

A few afferent fibers in the deep-sense system project through their ascending branches directly to the cerebellum via the posterior funiculus and inferior peduncle (corpus restiforme). The vast majority however reach the cerebellum in relays. *Reflex* and *cerebellar connections* for deep sensibility are particularly abundant and deviate from the direct pathway in the followng prominent ways. The first-order neurons from the general body terminate by short collaterals adjacent to the cells of the *dorsal nucleus of Clarke* (or bordering cells) (Fig. 16-11). This is presumed to represent termination of deep-sense primary neurons from the lower extremity and has an equivalent reflex termination for the upper extremity in the *cuneate nucleus.* Second-order neurons from both these sources enter the inferior cerebellar peduncle (corpus restiforme) and terminate adjacent to Purkinje cells of the cerebellar cortex (primarily of the

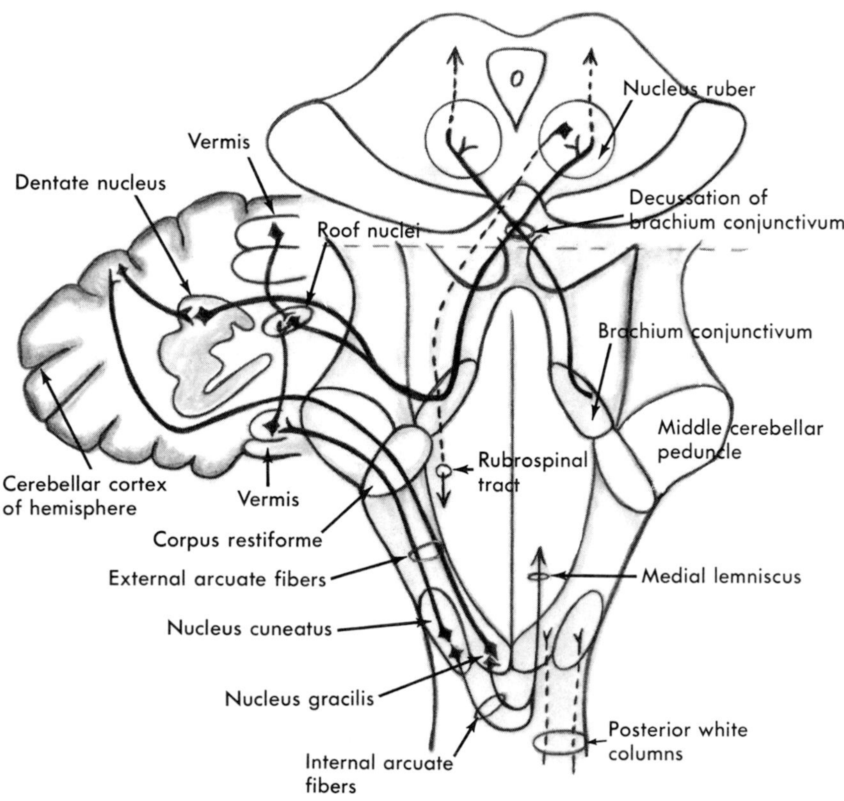

Fig. 16-13. Ascending deep sensibility pathways with cerebellar connections.

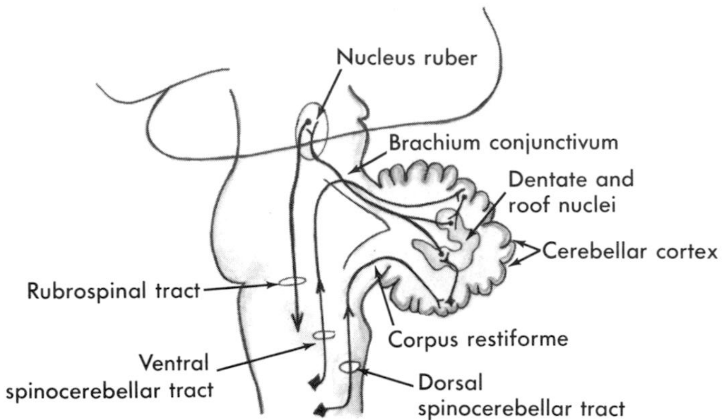

Fig. 16-14. Dorsal and ventral spinocerebellar pathways to cerebellum in longitudinal diagram. (Compare Fig. 16-12.)

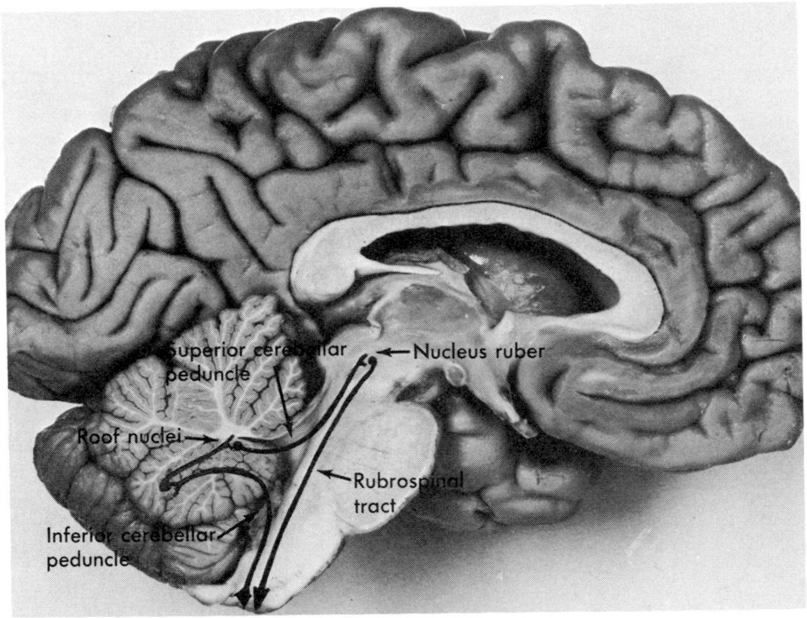

Fig. 16-15. Cerebellar connections superimposed on midsagittal section.

vermis). Fibers from the cuneate nucleus (fewer from the nucleus gracilis) pass directly to the cerebellum via the external arcuate tract and corpus restiforme (Fig. 16-5). The routing from Clarke's column and border cells is directed through both a *dorsal* and a *ventral spinocerebellar tract* (Fig. 16-12) of the same side, with the dorsal tract entering the cerebellum via the *corpus restiforme* and the ventral tract via the *brachium conjunctivum* (Figs. 16-13 and 16-14). (For details of cerebellar connections [Fig. 16-15] see Chapter 22.)

The first-order neurons from the head region probably have cell bodies in both the semilunar ganglion and in the mesencephalic root nucleus, although the location is far from certain. It is established however that deep-sense neurons terminate near the motor nuclei of the cranial nerves for reflex connections. Other first-order neurons in the reflex pathway terminate adjacent to dorsal horn second-order neurons, which cross to the opposite side or remain homolateral for immediate reflex connections with final-common-path cells. All ascending deep-sense fibers constantly give off collaterals for reflex connections in the dorsal gray

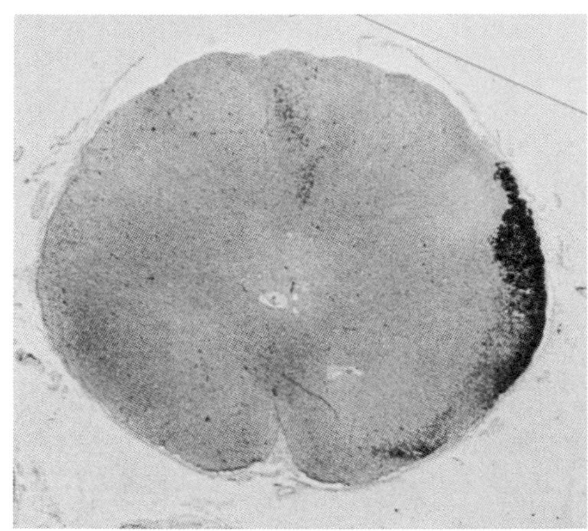

Fig. 16-16. Lower medulla after thoracic spinothalamic tractotomy; note "spread" to spinocerebellar tracts. (Marchi stain.)

matter and in the ventral horns. Still other second-order neurons cross to ascend in the *spino-olivary tract* to the *inferior olivary nucleus.* Here the impulses are relayed to the cerebellar cortex of the opposite side via the *olivocerebellar tracts* in the corpus restiforme (Fig. 16-13). From the cerebellar cortex these impulses are relayed to the dentate nucleus, and thence either to the red nucleus or the thalamus via the brachium conjunctivum, which decussates in the midbrain. The impulses thus can be returned to the spinal nuclei via the crossing *rubrospinal* tract or continue from the thalamus to the somesthetic area of the postcentral gyrus.

The pathways for deep sensibility and discriminative sense are summarized in Figs. 16-11 and 16-13.

GENERAL VISCERAL AFFERENT SYSTEM

The general visceral afferent system operates continuously with little conscious recognition. Almost the whole activity is carried out by reflex, with the autonomic system providing the motor limb of the reflexes. As mentioned previously, pain and temperature are appreciated slightly, and referred pain can be an important sensation generated in this system. The topography therefore has more than usual significance, and the recognized segmental relationships of viscera are summarized in Fig. 16-17.

Receptors

Free nerve endings occur in viscera primarily related to epithelium. Since no sensation arises there, these nerve endings are presumed to respond to contact-induced stimuli as the afferent component of reflex mechanisms. Pacinian corpuscles occur in viscera and in the peritoneal membranes. These corpuscles are thought to be responsive to pressure as elsewhere. Golgi-Mazzoni corpuscles occur in pericardium, and menisci appear in heart muscle. They are presumed to be stimulated by distention. Afferent receptor systems in smooth muscle fibers that simulate spindles are described by Larsell. Dense nerve nets occur in the carotid sinus adventitia, where they function as pressoreceptors. Nerve nets that are presumed to be chemoreceptors, dependent upon the CO_2 or O_2 concentration in the blood, also appear in the carotid sinus.

Sensory neurons (first-order)

The visceral afferent neurons arise in vessel walls and viscera. They have their cell bodies in dorsal root ganglia for the general body and in the ganglia of cranial nerves VII (geniculate), IX (petrosal), and X (nodose). The diameters of the fibers transmitting visceral impulses vary greatly (from 0.8 to 8.0 μ), and the rate of transmission varies accordingly. A special topographic relationship exists in the spinal cord. Visceral afferent fibers (except from blood vessels) enter only in cervical segment 4, thoracic segments 1 through 12, lumbar segments 1 through 3, and sacral segments 2 through 4. The relationship is a topographic one only and ties these fibers to the only neural channels available to the viscera. Fibers from blood vessels enter all segments through dorsal roots. In cervical segment 4 and in sacral segments 2 through 4, the first-order fibers end in relationship to cells of Stilling's cervical and sacral nuclei (see Chapter 6). In thoracic segment 1 through lumbar segment 3, the first-order neurons end in relationship to cells lying near the base of the dorsal gray horn (Fig. 16-17). In the visceral afferent cranial nerves VII, IX, and X the distribution of central fibers arising from soft palate, adjacent pharynx, auditory tube, and middle ear is through the *facial nerve.* The middle ear, auditory tube, pharynx, anterior epiglottis, border of soft palate and uvula, palatine tonsils, and carotid sinus deliver their impulses via the *glossopharyngeal nerve.* Afferent fibers from the epiglottis to the transverse colon are transported by the *vagus nerve.* All are directed centrally to the *solitary fasciculus,* with termination of these first-order neurons in the nucleus of that bundle (Fig. 16-17).

The central pathways for transmission of visceral afferent sensations to conscious levels are not

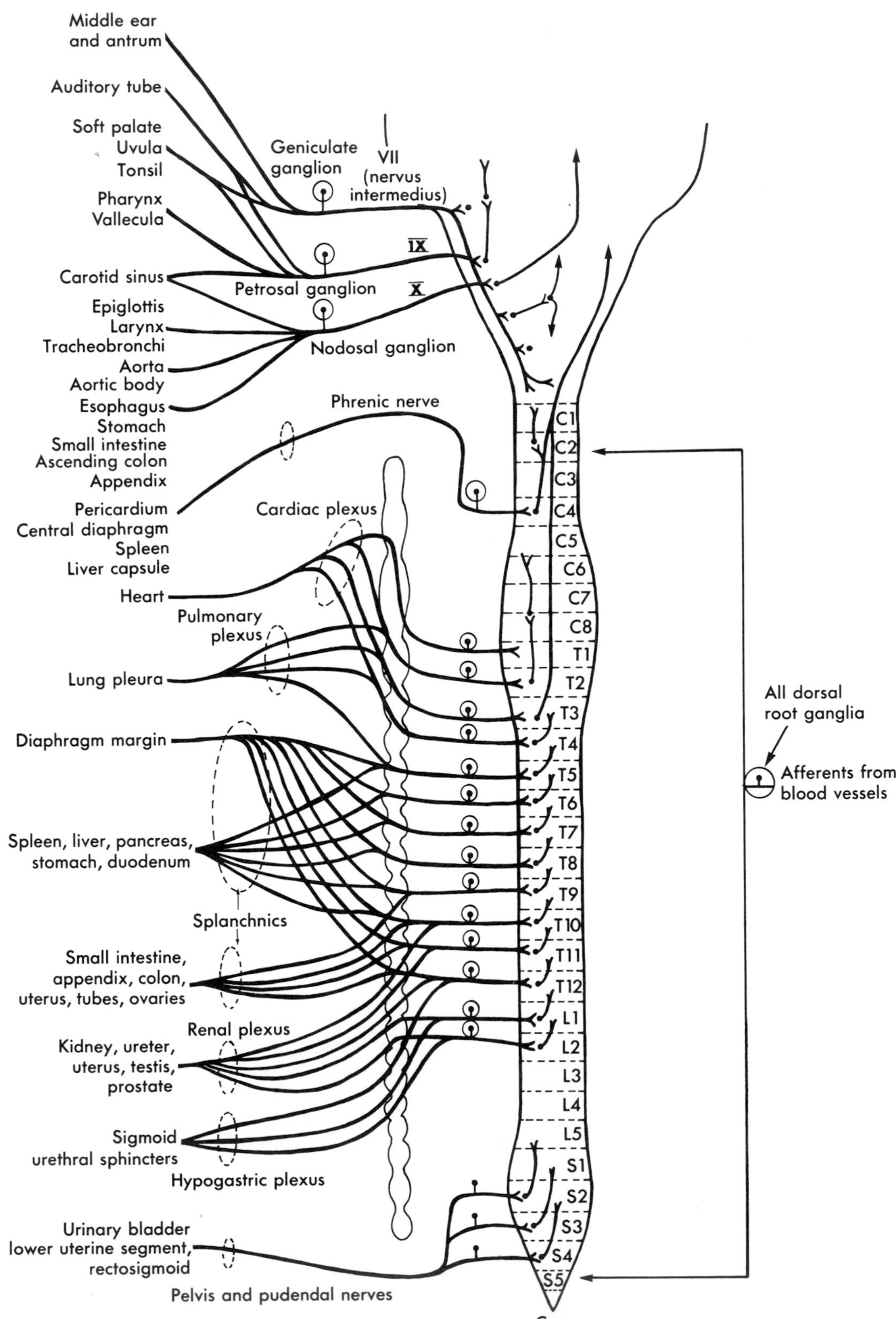

Fig. 16-17. General visceral afferent system. Afferent vessel nerves from cranial sources are via the afferents shown (upper left).

known. It is assumed they travel by short paths of the *reticular formation,* eventually reaching the thalamus, and then to the cortex for appreciation. Most important are the reflex connections to the secretory, respiratory, cardiac, vasomotor, and general visceromotor centers, which in turn regulate autonomic responses in reflex patterns below conscious levels (see Chapters 20 and 21). These are recognized components of the reflex control of vital centers, and their importance is self-evident. Despite this, it remains presently impossible to trace the central pathways of these critical afferent systems.

The general visceral afferent system is summarized in Fig. 16-17.

REFERENCES

1. Cauna, N., and Ross, L. L.: The fine structure of Meissner's touch corpuscles of human fingers, J. Biophys. Biochem. Cytol. **8**:467, 1960.
2. Luse, S.: The Schwann cell. In Minckler, J., editor: Pathology of the nervous system, vol. I, New York, 1968, McGraw-Hill Book Co.
3. Pease, D. C., and Quilliam, T. A.: Electron microscopy of the pacinian corpuscle, J. Biophys. Biochem. Cytol. **3**:331, 1957.
4. Ruch, T. C., and others: Neurophysiology, ed. 2, Philadelphia, 1965, W. B. Saunders Co.
5. Zeman, W.: The effects of atomic radiation. In Minckler, J., editor: Pathology of the nervous system, vol. I, New York, 1968, McGraw-Hill Book Co.

CHAPTER 17

GUSTATORY AND OLFACTORY SYSTEMS

JEFF MINCKLER

GUSTATORY SYSTEM

The *receptors* of this special visceral afferent system mediate the sensation of *taste.* These are chemoreceptors and the pickup of stimuli is through *taste buds,* which are distributed over the tongue, on the palatine arch, soft palate, posterior wall of the oropharynx, the posterior surface of the epiglottis, and, in rare cases, elsewhere in the oropharynx and larynx. The taste bud is a laminated onion-like end-organ to which the end filaments of cranial nerves VII, IX, and X are applied (Fig. 17-1). The buds are oriented perpendicular to the mucosal surface and are most numerous in vallate troughs, but they occur on surface epithelium as well. Each bud is made up of *neuroepithelial cells,* which are narrow and elongate and concentrate in the center of the organ. At the surface extremity these cells possess short hairs that are the specific chemoreceptors. The neuroepithelial cells are intermingled with elongate *sustentacular cells,* which are shaped like orange wedges, with narrowing at either extremity. These focus at the mucosal surface into the margins of a pit, forming the inner taste pore (Fig. 17-1). The hairs of the neuroepithelium extend into the pore. Some sustenacular cells are distinguished by greater width at the base of the bud where they provide the basal cells. The supplying nerve fibers enter the taste bud at this basal position and ramify throughout the organ to terminate about the surfaces of neuroepithelial elements.

Dissolved substances to be tasted stimulate the hairs and are applied within the surface pit via the pore. The nerve filaments of cranial nerves VII, IX, and X apply to the neuroepithelial elements in the distribution shown in Fig. 17-2. Note that nerve VII supplies the anterior two-thirds of the tongue. Nerve IX supplies the posterior third, and nerve X part of the posterior third and the "extra" buds, such as those on the posterior aspect of the epiglottis. The physiology of perception of taste is closely tied to olfaction. Taste itself appears to be limited to salty, bitter, sweet, sour, alkaline, and metallic. These are essentially those specific tastes that are appreciated even if olfaction is erased by holding the nose.[5]

First-order neurons from the anterior two-thirds of the tongue travel via the chorda tympani of the facial nerve (sometimes via the petrosal nerves) and have their cell bodies in the *geniculate ganglion.* The fibers mediating taste over the glossopharyngeal nerve have their cell bodies in the *petrosal ganglion,* and those over the vagus nerve in the *nodose ganglion.* All these first-order neurons for taste have their primary receptive centers in the *nucleus of the solitary fasciculus,* which they reach by descending in the *fasciculus solitarius* (Fig. 17-3). Note that the solitray tract and nucleus cross midline in the lower medulla as the *commissure infima* and its nucleus. The *second-order neurons* for taste arise in the nucleus of the solitary fasciculus and probably ascend to the thalamus via the *medial lemniscus* of the opposite side. A more laterally placed secondary gustatory tract has also been hypothsized, but the course this tract takes in man remains in doubt. There are a great many reflex connections from the nucleus of the solitary fasciculus to motor and secretory centers in the medullary area (especially the nucleus ambiguus, the salivatory nuclei, and the reticulospinal tracts).

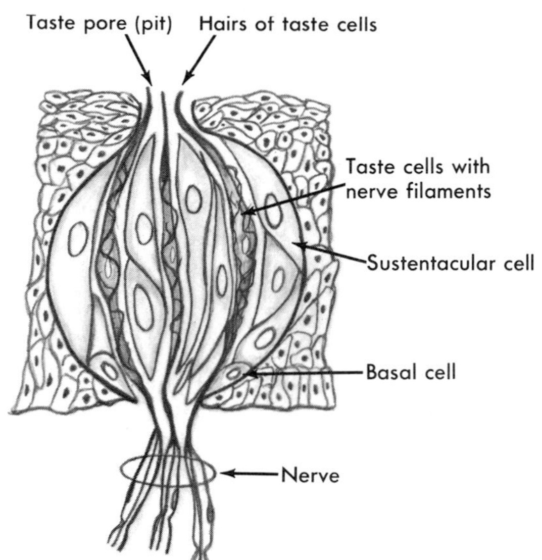

Fig. 17-1. Diagram of components in taste bud.

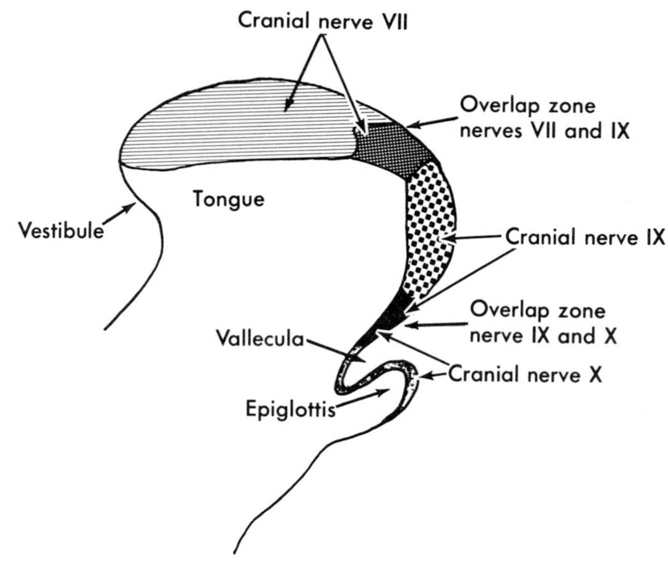

Fig. 17-2. Distribution of cranial nerves VII, IX, and X to taste bud areas of tongue. Some overlap also occurs across midline.

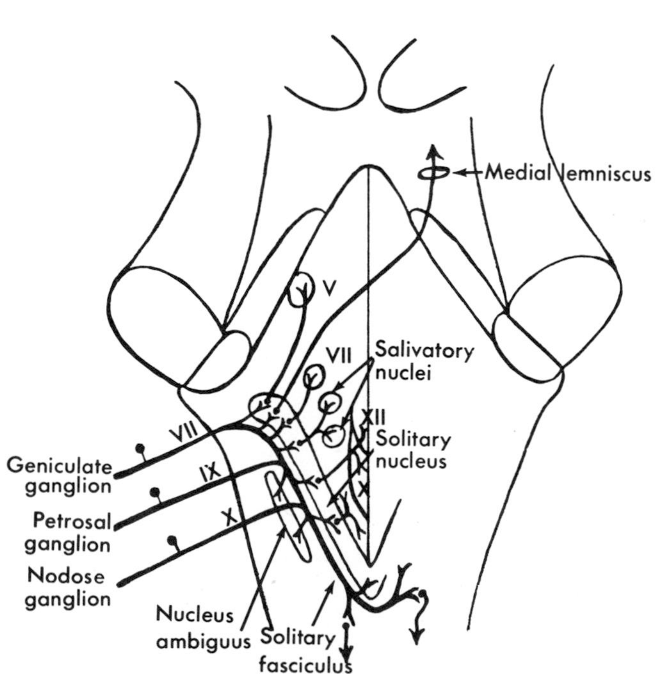

Fig. 17-3. The solitary fasciculus and its nucleus. Relationship to medial lemniscus as directly as shown is uncertain.

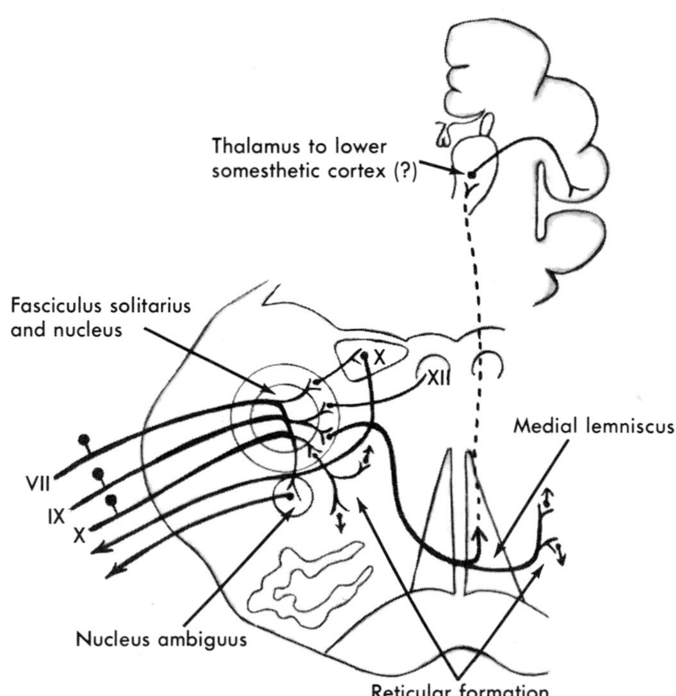

Fig. 17-4. Presumed gustatory route to cortex. Position of primary sensory cortical area is uncertain.

The ascending fibers en route to conscious centers terminate in the posteromedial part of the ventral nucleus of the thalamus. The *third-order neurons* in the thalamic relay carry fibers to the gustatory cortical center, which is presumably located in the inferior part of the postcentral gyrus.[1] The gustatory system is summarized in Fig. 17-4.

OLFACTORY SYSTEM

The *olfactory filaments,* or nerves, and the *olfactory brain,* or *rhinencephalon,* mediate the sense of smell. The gross parts involved are here arbitrarily restricted to include: cranial nerve I, represented by the olfactory filaments, the olfactory bulb and tract, and the olfactory areas (lateral, intermediate, and medial). The cortical representation lies in the amygdaloid nucleus and the pyriform area (lateral), the anterior perforated substance (intermediate), and in the subcallosal and parolfactory areas (medial). Like other parts of the telencephalon, these are closely related to the thalamus, parts of which appear to be almost wholly olfactory or related closely to allied visceral functions. It is traditional in descriptive neuroanatomy to include septal parts, the hippocampus, dentate gyrus, and fornix with the olfactory system. While the olfactory system undoubtedly relates to these parts (as to other cortical fields), they are probably more appropriately discussed with the limbic system, which in human neurology relates more closely to memory, emotion, and visceral experiences than to olfaction (see Chapter 22).[4]

Nerves

The olfactory nerves themselves provide the chemoreceptors for the sense of smell. These are bipolar neurons, with the cell bodies located within the olfactory mucous membrane (Fig. 17-5). The receptor mechanism is effected through a short dendritic stalk, which projects to the mucosal surface (for peripheral distribution see Chapter 6). The olfactory epithelium possesses *sustentacular* supporting cells, which relate to nerve endings of cranial nerves V for general sensibility of the area (such as pain, touch). Some sustentacular elements are short and broad and occupy a position along the epithelial basement membrane as *basal cells.* The *olfactory cells* are scattered among the sustentacular cells as the special-sense receptors. Each olfactory cell possesses a tuft from six to eight cilia, or short hairs (2 μ in length), which project from the nasal surface of the dendrite. The *olfactory cilia* project from a vesicular swelling of the dendrite, the *olfactory vesicle.* The cell body is inserted into the path of the axon in typical bipolar fashion (Fig. 17-5).[2] About 200 million filaments from the

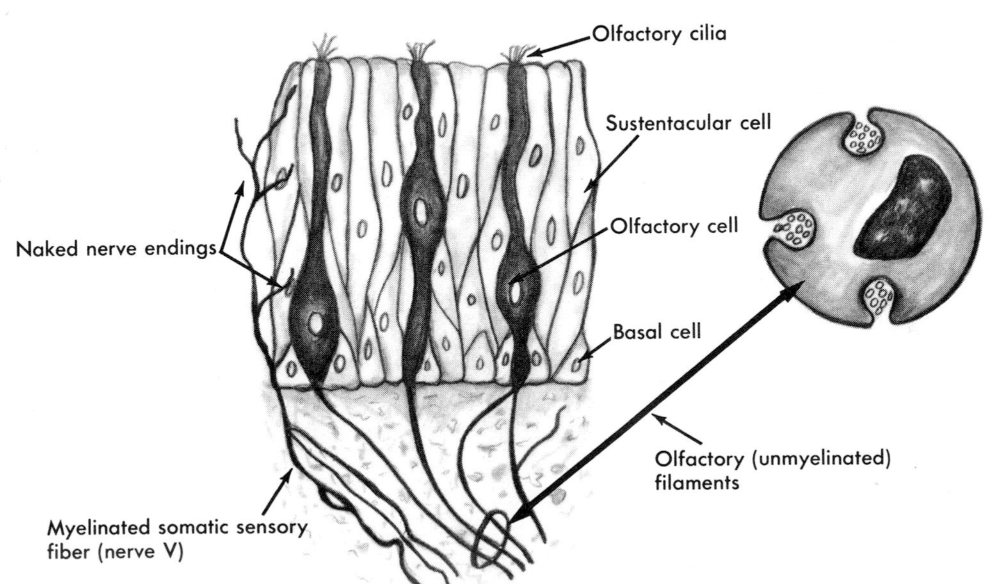

Fig. 17-5. Diagram of olfactory neuron and olfactory filament. On right is cross-sectional diagram of probable manner of Schwann membrane wrapping of multiple filaments.

same number of receptors aggregate as nonmyelinated nerves (eighteen to twenty per side) to enter the olfactory bulbs. The minute, slow-conducting filaments are bound in fascicles within Schwann cell membranes, with many filaments to one mesaxon (Figs. 10-13, 10-14, 10-31, and 17-5).[3]

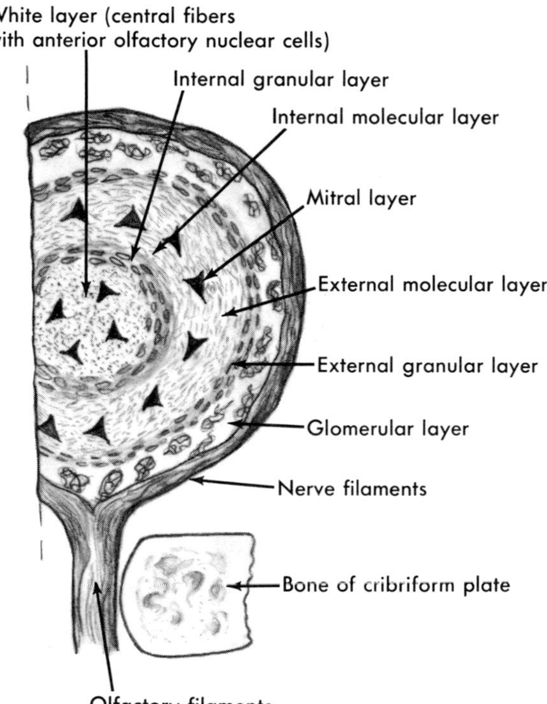

Fig. 17-6. Diagrammatic composite of lamination in olfactory bulb and relation to olfactory filament.

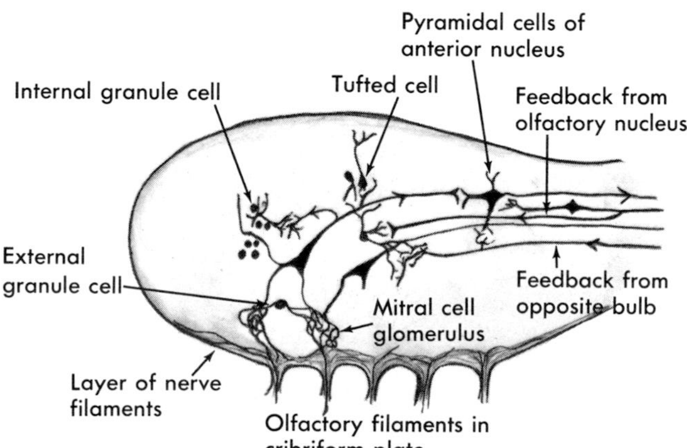

Fig. 17-7. Diagram of mitral connections and feedback systems in bulb and tract.

Bulb

The *olfactory bulb* houses the primary receptive cells for the incoming olfactory impulses. The bulb is an expansion of a central tract and consequently sometimes possesses remnants of an ependyma-lined cavity. The structural details of the adult human olfactory bulb bears little histologic resemblance to the idealized composite developed from animal tissue (Fig. 17-6). It is presumed that the minimized importance of the human olfactory system corresponds to its relatively poorly developed state. The outer rim of the bulb is made up of a *layer of nerve filaments.* These centrally adjoin a *glomerular lamina,* made up of tuft-like synaptic junctions between the incoming filaments and mitral cells (Figs. 17-6 and 17-7). Adjacent to the glomerular lamina is the *external granular* layer, made up of small granular cells and tufted cells. Internal to the granular layer is an *external molecular* layer, made up of the processes of the mitral cells. Next is the *mitral cell* layer, which is in a single row of large multibranched cells whose dendritic processes extend outward to form the glomerular junctions with the incoming olfactory filaments. An *internal molecular* layer lies next to the mitral cells, and inwardly adjacent to this layer is an *internal granular* layer. At the center of the bulb are the aggregated axons of the mitral cells, which form the *stratum album* (white layer). These distribute through the olfactory tract to the olfactory areas. *Anterior olfactory nuclear* cells are scattered irregularly throughout the white layer. The olfactory tract is represented by the white stratum, with a few scattered cells of the anterior nucleus.

The connections within the bulb are presumed to be: (1) *olfactory filaments to mitral cells;* (2) *granular cells* and *tufted cells interconnecting* among themselves and between *granular and mitral cells;* (3) *mitral cells to central nuclei* and *anterior olfactory nuclei* as second-order neurons; and (4) *mitral* and *anterior nuclear cell feedback to granular cells* (Fig. 17-7). This complex interconnecting undoubtedly accounts for the remarkable sensitivity of olfaction. Less well understood is the precise discriminative ability displayed by this special visceral sense. This ability is presumed to be based on combinations of stimuli rather than on special adaptation of individual receptors.[2,5]

Olfactory areas

Three olfactory subsystems arise as the tract carries inwardly to divide into the medial, intermediate, and lateral olfactory striae (Figs. 17-8 to 17-10). The *medial olfactory stria* turns medially at

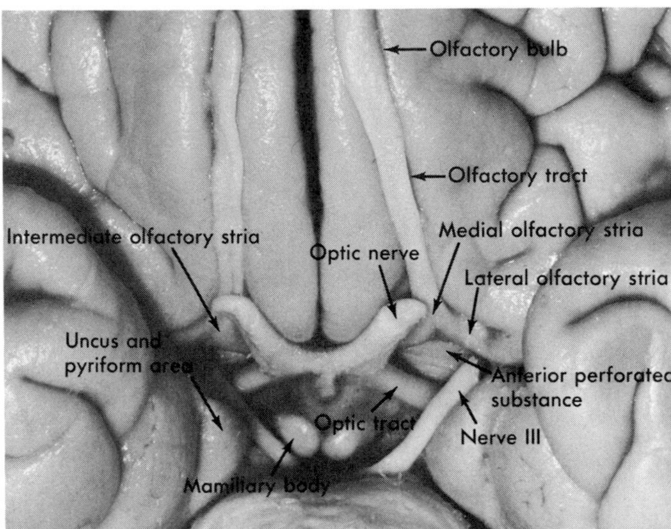

Fig. 17-8. Olfactory tracts and striae relating to hypothalamic and medial temporal lobe structures (uncus).

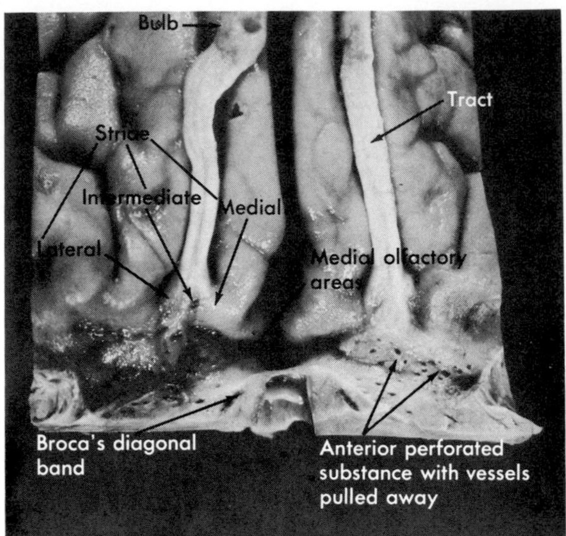

Fig. 17-9. Olfactory striae and anterior perforated substance.

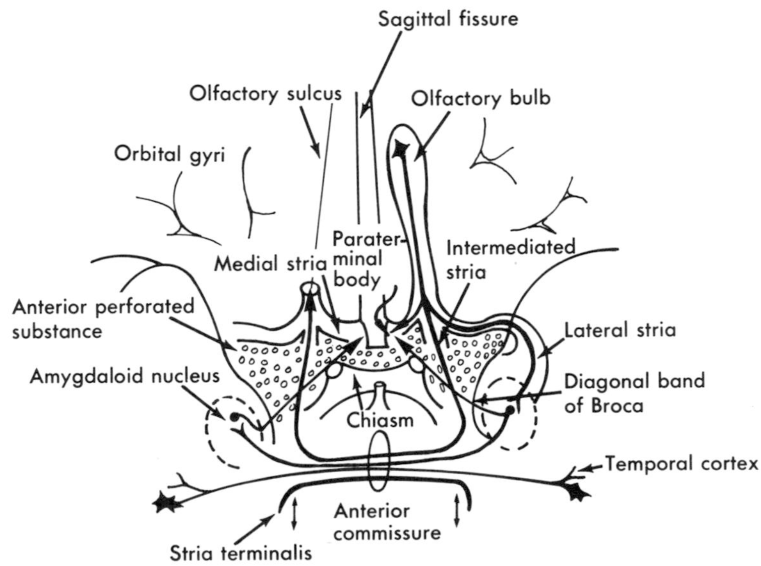

Fig. 17-10. Diagram of connections through olfactory striae and Broca's band.

the olfactory trigone and terminates in the medial olfactory areas identifiable as the parolfactory area (of Broca) and the subcallosal gyrus (Fig. 17-11). Third-order neurons continue from these nuclei to the habenular nucleus via the stria medullaris thalami, to lower centers via the olfactotegmental tract, and to the amygdala via the stria terminalis (Fig. 17-10). Other reflex connections can be extended through the habenular commissure, the habenulopeduncular fasciculus, the interpeduncular nucleus, the dorsal tegmental nucleus, and the dorsal longitudinal fasciculus to lower centers and the hypothalamus (Fig. 17-14). The medial olfactory area is associated with the lateral olfactory area by the *diagonal band of Broca* (Fig. 17-10).

The *intermediate olfactory area* (anterior perforated substance) (Fig. 17-9) is reached by the intermediate stria. Third-order neurons from this area pass to the caudate nucleus, which lies immediately above (Fig. 17-14). Other tertiary fibers pass to lower centers and to the habenular nucleus by routes that are the same as those from the medial area. There are also connections to the opposite amygdala via the anterior commissure. This commissure may also be used in interconnecting the bilateral olfactory tracts via the intermediate area.

The *lateral olfactory area* is made up of the pyriform area (limen of the insula and cortex of the uncus) and the amygdaloid nucleus (Fig. 17-12). The lateral stria mostly contains the axons of the mitral cells and supplies this lateral area. Third-order neurons from the lateral area join the olfactotegmental tract to lower nuclei and give off collaterals to the hypothalamus. Reflex connections also pass to the habenular complex via the stria medullaris thalami (Fig. 17-13). The opposite lateral olfactory area is related via the anterior commissure and probably less directly through the stria terminalis. The medial olfactory area (subcallosal gyrus) is connected to the lateral area through the diagonal band of Broca. This passes between the anterior perforated substance and the hippocampus, which are traditionally linked to olfaction. These nuclei are probably better viewed as cortical segments of the limbic lobe, which relates to olfac-

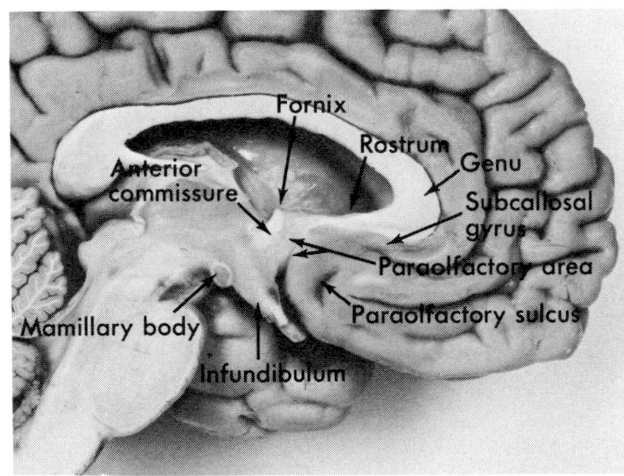

Fig. 17-11. Parolfactory area.

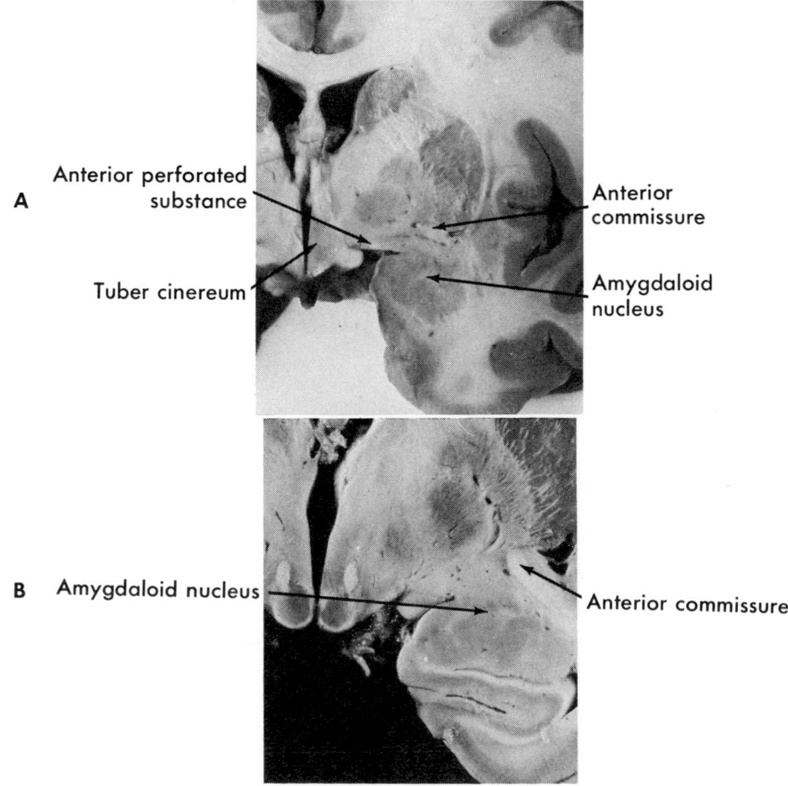

Fig. 17-12. A, Amygdaloid nucleus at level of tuber cinereum; **B,** amygdaloid nucleus at level of mamillary bodies.

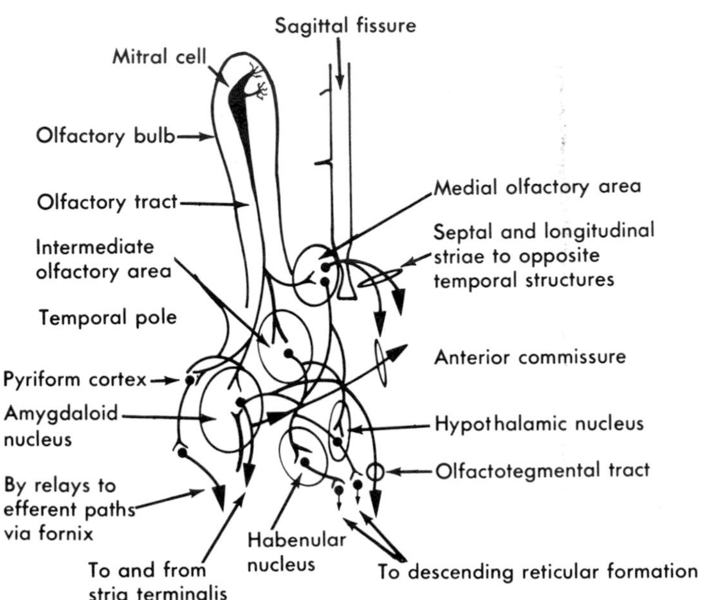

Fig. 17-13. Olfactory area connections.

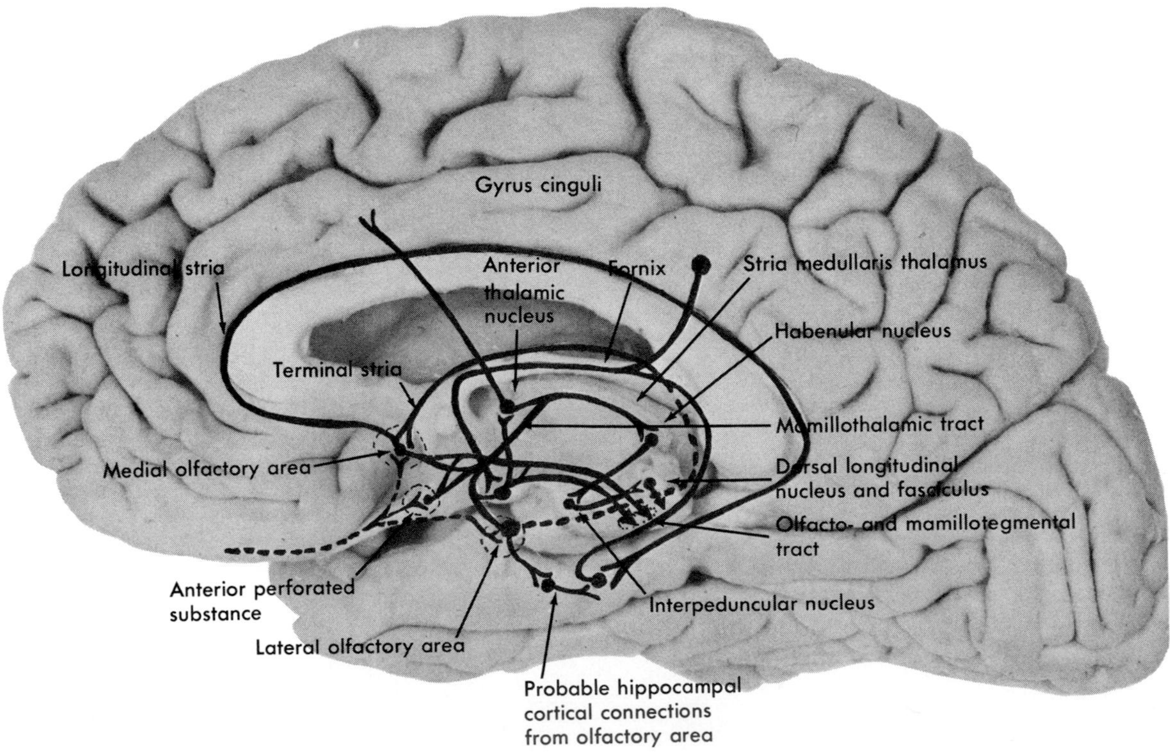

Fig. 17-14. Diagrammatic summary of olfactory pathways superimposed on medial view of brain.

tion only in the overall visceral tie to autonomic functions. It should be noted that the olfactory system does not utilize the thalamus as a way station to the cortex.

All olfactory areas relate to descending reflex connections, which are closely interconnected with the hypothalamus (Fig. 17-13). The olfactory system is summarized in Fig. 17-14.

REFERENCES

1. Bornstein, W. S.: Cortical representation of taste in man and monkey, Yale J. Biol. Med. **12**:719, 1940.
2. de Lorenzo, A. J.: Electron microscpoic observations of the olfactory mucosa and olfactory nerve, J. Biophys. Biochem. Cytol. **3**:839, 1957.
3. Gasser, H. S.: Olfactory nerve fibers, J. Gen. Physiol. **39**:473, 1956.
4. Livingston, K. E., and Escobar, A.: Anatomical basis of the limbic system concept, Neurology **24**:17, 1971.
5. Patton, H. A.: Physiology of smell and taste, Ann. Rev. Physiol. **12**:469, 1950.

CHAPTER 18

VESTIBULAR SYSTEM

JEFF MINCKLER

The human vestibular system essentially constitutes a reflex mechanism for the maintenance of equilibrium. The system operates in conjunction with muscle and tendon sensory systems, from which impulses that mediate awareness of motion, posture, change in position, turning, preservation of visual fields, and acceleration arise. The cerebellum is the main central organ related to these functions. It seems doubtful that direct cerebral cortical representation exists in this system. Appreciation is therefore presumed to be secondary in nature, with origin in the related muscle afferents. The peripheral organ involved in the receptor mechanism for equilibration is part of the internal ear. This structure is made up of a membranous, labyrinthine complex occupying a series of fixed canals in the petrous bone (Fig. 18-1).

The *bony labyrinth* is made up of a vestibule, three semicircular canals, and a cochlea (see p. 295).[1] The bony vestibule is an ovoid compartment (5 by 5 by 3 mm.), which is partially divided by a vestibular crest into an anteroinferior recess (spherical) and a posterosuperior recess (elliptical). The spherical recess contains the membranous *saccule,* and the elliptical recess contains the membranous *utricle* (Fig. 18-2). The vestibular, or oval, *window* is an aperture on the medial aspect of the spherical recess of the vestibule related to the saccule and to the vestibular periotic space of the cochlea (Fig. 18-2). Cribriform areas provide the apertures into the vestibule for nerves to both saccule and utricle. The cochlear round window (Fig. 18-2) relates to the tympanic periotic space of the cochlea. Both the oval window and the round window are bridged by mebranous coverings. The foot-plate of the stapes overlies the oval window membrane on the middle ear aspect. The basal turn of the cochlea extends to the region of the saccule, and the bony canals of the cochlear cecum and spherical recess communicate by a tiny canal. This contains the *ductus reuniens,* which links the saccule with the cochlear duct. A very small bony canal near the round window (*cochlear aqueduct*) connects the periotic scala tympani with the subarachnoid spaces. This opens on the inferior surface of the petrous bone just medial to a position between the carotid canal and the jugular fossa and is related to a tubular prolongation of the meninges (Fig. 18-3, *A*). A bony canal (*vestibular aqueduct*) extends from the medial wall of the vestibule to the posterior petrous surface just behind the internal acoustic meatus. This conveys the endolymphatic duct, which arises from two small ducts of the membranous labyrinth (one each from the utricle and saccule) and passes to the dural layers (Fig. 18-3, *B*). The vestibule also has an elliptical aperture connecting it with the scala vestibuli of the cochlea. The remaining openings of the vestibule are those related to the semicircular canals.

There are three semicircular canals (1 to 1.5 mm. in diameter and 12 to 33 mm. long), designated as superior, posterior, and anterior. Their planes are in the relationship of the corners of a cube. The lateral canal is horizontal, the posterior takes the vertical plane of the petrous ridge, and the anterior is at right angles to both. The posterial canal is thus almost at right angles to the ridge and vertically oriented (Fig. 18-1).* While the positions change somewhat, the anterior and posterior canals make an approximate 45-degree angle with the sagittal plane. Each canal represents about

*For details of growth and orientation see reference 4.

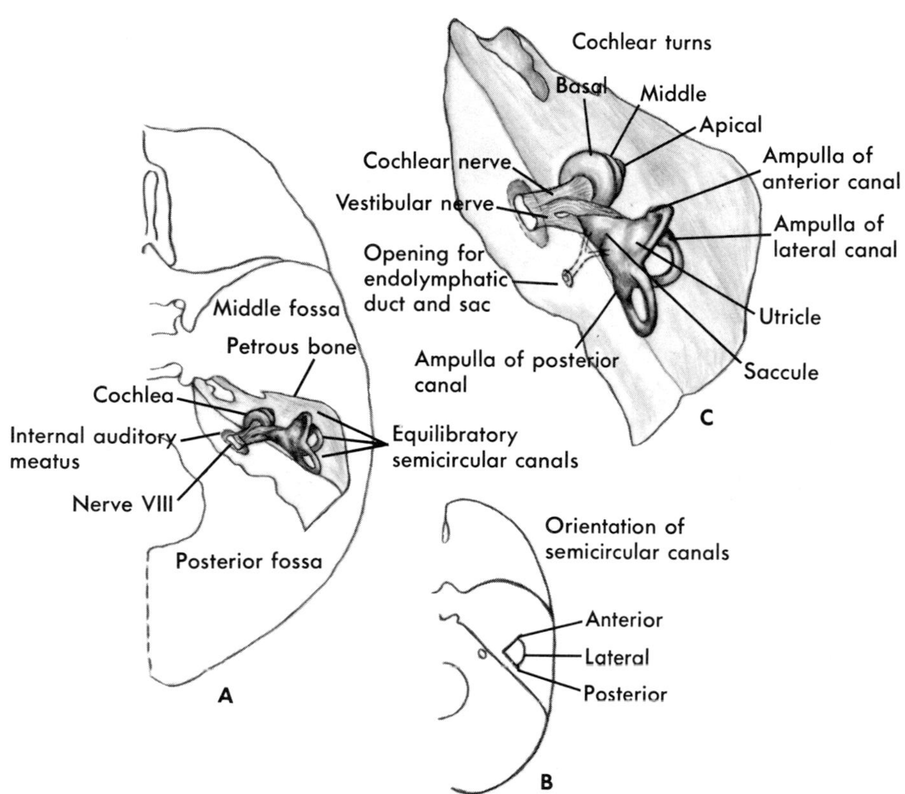

Fig. 18-1. Semicircular canals. **A,** Topography with base of skull; **B,** orientation of planes from above; **C,** details of topography in view from above and slightly medially.

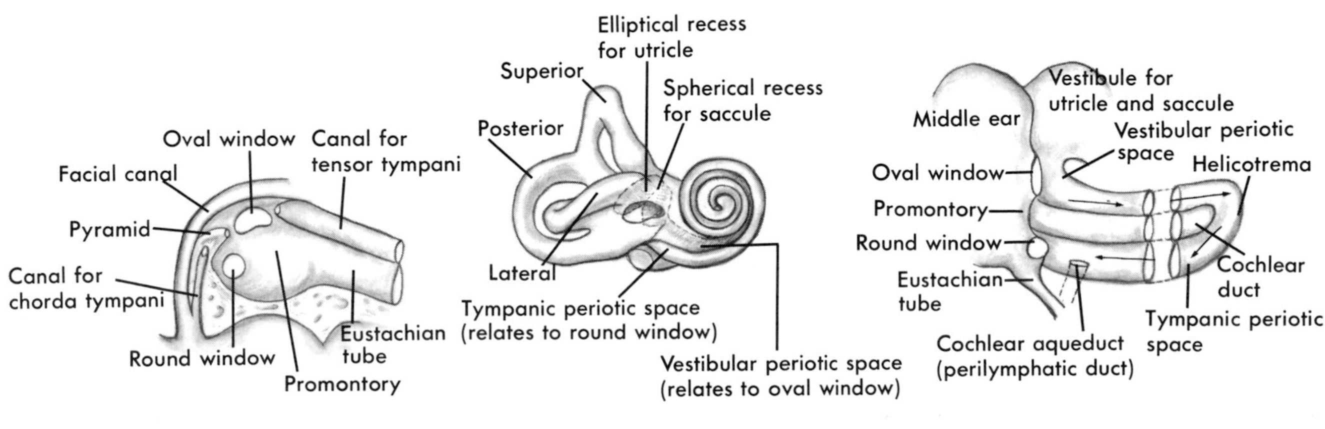

Fig. 18-2. Windows in medial wall of right middle ear. **A,** View of medial wall; **B,** relationship of windows to internal ear structures; **C,** coronal diagram relating windows to vestibule and periotic spaces.

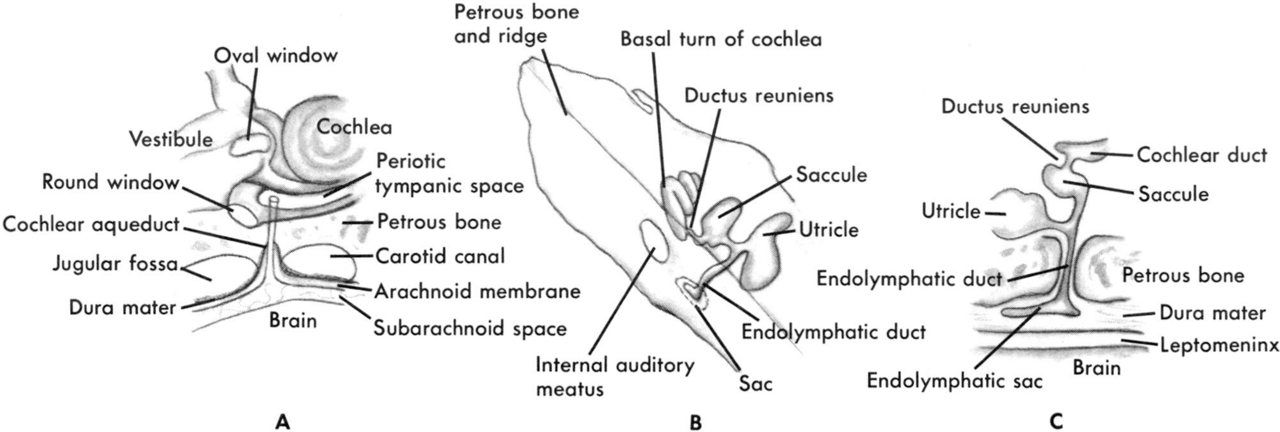

Fig. 18-3. A, Cochlear aqueduct connecting periotic tympanic space (periotic fluid) with leptomeningeal space (CSF); **B,** vestibular aqueduct connecting membranous labyrinth (endolymph) with dural layer just posterior to internal auditory meatus; **C,** diagram showing endolymphatic continuity from cochlear duct, saccule, and utricle to dural layer.

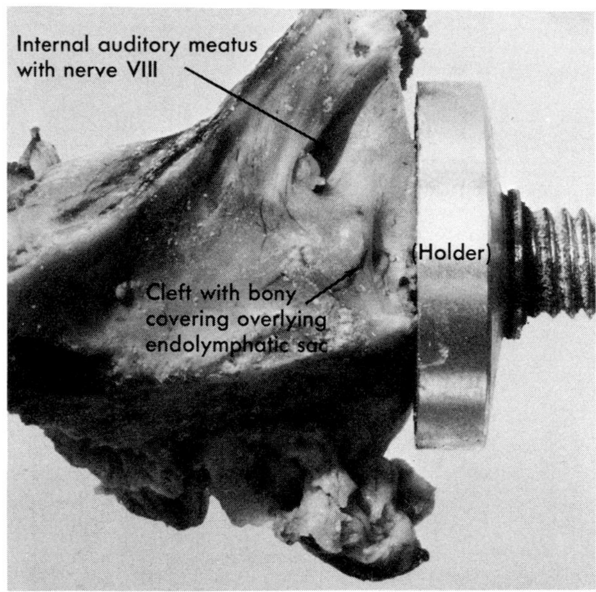

Fig. 18-4. Medial view of left petrous bone showing cleft for endolymphatic sac.

two-thirds of a circle, with the extremities arising in the vestibule. However, the anterior and posterior canals fuse in a single crus, so five rather than six openings relate them to the vestibule. At one extremity of each canal near the point of attachment to the utricular bony recess, the semicircular canals expand as *ampullae* (anterior, posterior, and lateral) (Fig. 18-5).

The *membranous labyrinth* of the inner ear related to equilibration is a fibromembranous, tubular channel that lies within the bony labyrinth. The sac attaches by fibrous strands to the periosteum of the bony canal and is otherwise separated from it by *perilymph* fluid. The membranous tube is filled with a separate fluid, the *endolymph.* This fluid is continuous throughout the membranous system, including the cochlear duct within the cochlea, the saccule and the utricle within the vestibule, and the semicircular ducts within the canals. The cochlear duct connects with the saccule via the ductus reuniens. The saccule connects indirectly with the utricle through the ducts leading into the ductus endolymphaticus. This carries into the endolymphatic sac on the posteromedial petrous surface (Fig. 18-4). All the semicircular ducts connect with the utricle near their ampullary extremities (Fig. 18-5). In general, the membranous ducts occupy one-third or less of the cross-sectional area of the bony canal. The membranous labyrinth is typically made up of three layers. The outer is loose fibrous tissue that blends with the trabeculate supporting structures in the perilymphatic spaces. The middle layer is a tunica propria, or basement membrane, related to a denser fibrous stratum. The lining is an ectodermal epithelium that shows many adaptations in forming the specific receptors of the inner ear.

The endolymph of the membranous canal is viscid, contains 1.6 percent solids and a trace of albumin, and is probably nutritive for the bloodless, specialized epithelium it bathes. It is replenished constantly and displays customary turnover of its chemical components. The fluid is known to have its origin in the area vascularis of the cochlear duct (see p. 310). A specialized secreting epithelium probably also exists near the ductus reuniens. Presumably there is an outflow pathway via the ductus reuniens to the saccule, although this is controversial. The flow pattern and exchanges of this segment of endolymph are poorly understood. The endolymph of the semicircular canals and utricle has the same chemical characteristics as that of the cochlear duct. Its origin may well be partially in the cochlea. A probable additional source is the secreting cells of the crescentic cellular planes at the borders of the cristae in the ampullae of the semicircular canals. It is presumed that the outflow is via the endolymphatic duct and sac, and that absorption takes place there. Some fluid is undoubtedly absorbed locally within the membranous labyrinths.

The periotic fluid, or perilymph, is similar to CSF. It is less viscid and contains more protein than endolymph. It also has a lower potassium and a higher sodium content. Since perilymph communicates with CSF through the cochlear aqueduct, the fluid is presumed to arise in CSF. Its circulation and metabolic features remain uncertain.

RECEPTORS

The special sensory receptors in the vestibular part of the inner ear occur in five areas: in the ampullae of each of the three semicircular canals, in the utricle, and in the saccule (Fig. 18-5). Specially adapted *hair cells* represent the mechanoreceptors subject to stimulation by turning the head, change of movement, acceleration and deceleration, or by any of the various test devices employed. The exact role of the labyrinthine components in equilibration remains controversial. It seems quite certain that the semicircular canals are involved only in rotational responses. On the other hand, the utricle probably responds to linear acceleration and tilting. The function of the human saccule remains uncertain. It may function as a receptor for slow vibrations rather than contributing to the vestibular complex.

In longitudinal section the ampullae display a partially dividing, transverse septum, or *crest* (crista), occupying approximately one-third of the lumen width. The crest bridges crescent-shaped plates of differentiated cells on each extremity of the septum. These form the *semilunar planes,* whose cells are probably secretory glands and may contribute endolymph to the pool in the vestibular part of the endotic duct system (see p. 310). The crest is covered by a gelatinous ridge, the *cupula,* which incorporates the projecting cilia of the underlying hair cells. The hair cells occupy the surface and upper sides of the crest and blend there with intermediate cells, which blend with the general epithelium of the duct. Movements of the cupula occur with rotation. This movement bends the cilia of the hair cells, starting the neural impulse (Fig. 18-7).

Hair cells occupy the outer two-thirds of the layer of neuroepithelium (Fig. 18-6). The intervening cells are supportive, and these nuclei tend

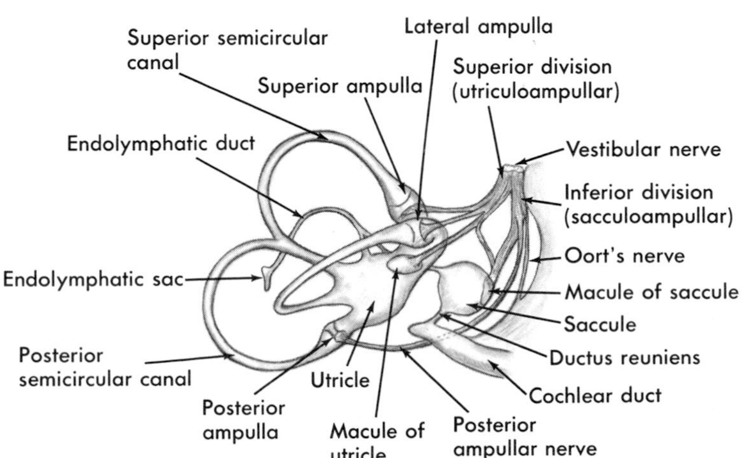

Fig. 18-5. Topography and relationship of semicircular canals and their ampullae; utricle, saccule, and their maculae; cecum of cochlear duct with duct reuniens; and vestibular nerves with Oort's bundle.

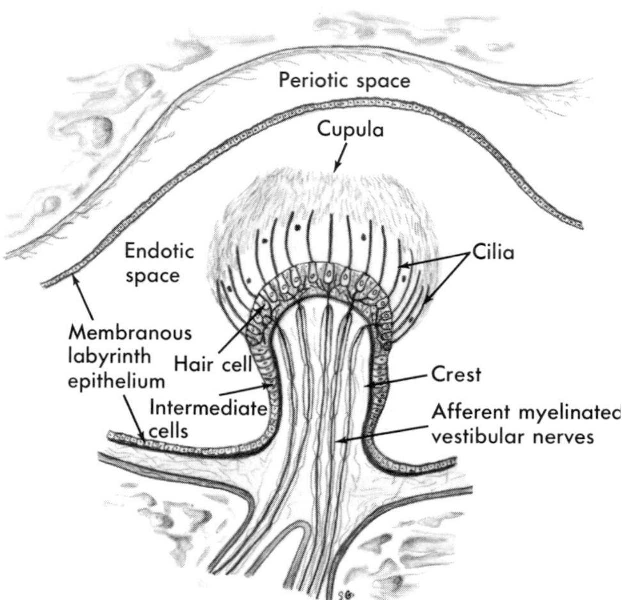

Fig. 18-6. Crest in ampulla of semicircular canal.

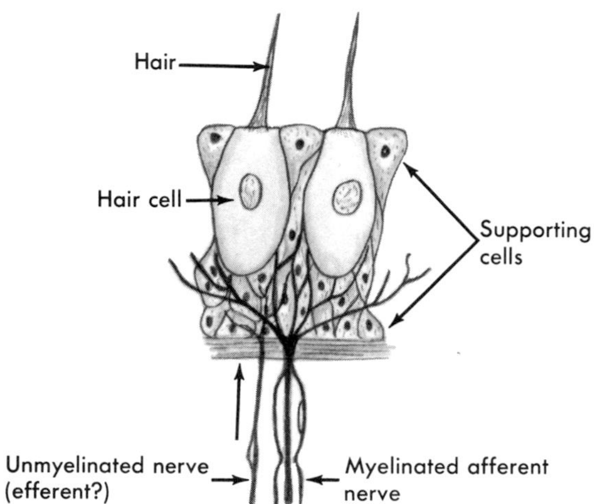

Fig. 18-7. Details of hair cells of crista in neuroepithelium.

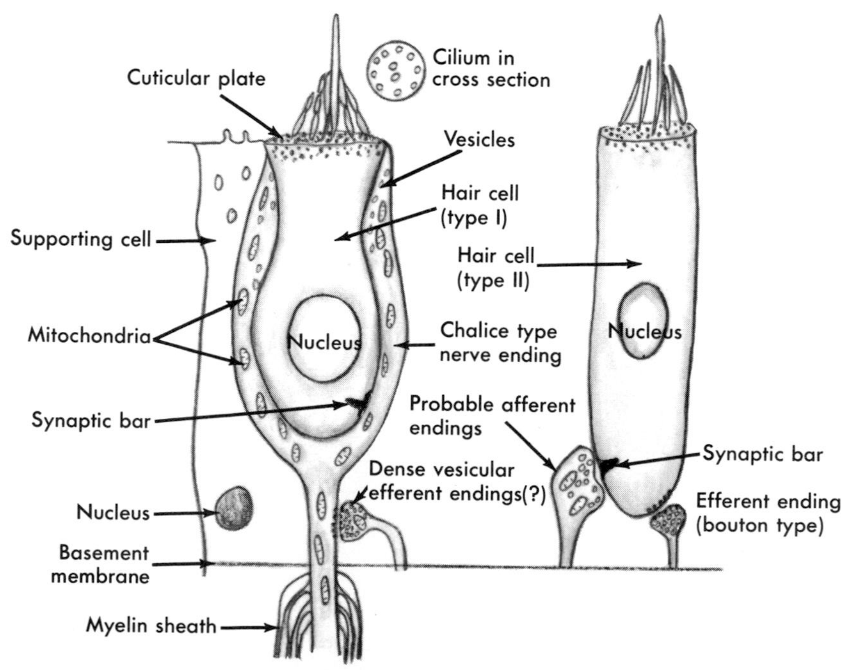

Fig. 18-8. Idealized composite from light and electron microscopy showing chalice ending on hair cell (type I) and two types of bouton endings, one relating to synaptic bars and presumed to be afferent and the other (more vesiculated and electron-dense) presumed to be efferent. Both types relate to both type I (bottle-shaped) and type II (cylindrical) hair cells (see Chapters 8 and 19).

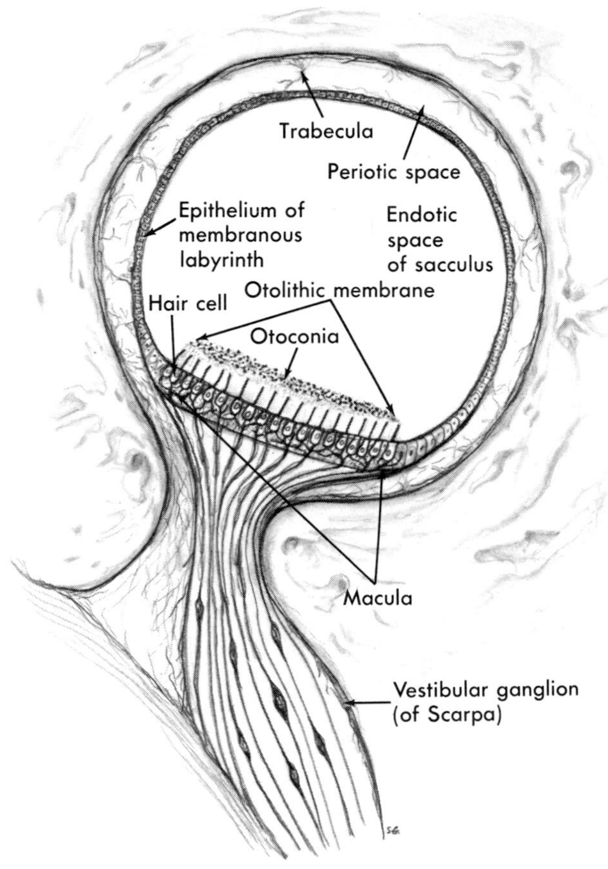

Fig. 18-9. Macula—diagram of histology.

to aggregate along the base of the epithelial layers. The long, cylindrical *supporting cells* form the semilunar plane, where they are apparently specialized. The specific sensory cells are of two types: (1) short-necked bottle shape (type I) with a deep cup-shaped (chalice) nerve ending related to it, and (2) a more elongate cell with a pointed infranuclear region (type II). Cells of the latter type have associated nerve terminals in the form of knobs, which may be either granular or nongranular. Similar endings also occur on the cells related to the chalice endings (Fig. 18-8). The round granular endings with prominent vesicles and great electron density suggest synaptic knobs because of their structure, implying that incoming neural influence is brought to bear on the neuroepithelium of the crista.[2,6] The less dense, afferent knobs relate to a synaptic bar on the receptor. A cuticle is formed on the free surfaces of the cells, and from this the hairs protrude. Ultrastructural details are illustrated in Figs. 18-7 to 18-8.*

The ampullary receptor organs have something of a structural counterpart in both the utricle and the saccule. These possess hair cells as the main receptor cells but are disposed in flat, rounded aggregates called *maculae* (Fig. 18-9). The mechanism of action is somewhat different from that in the ampullae, and the function is thought to vary. As mentioned, the ampullar sensory organs are stimulated by rotatory movements, while the macula of the utricle is related to gravity effects. The function of the macula of the human saccule is not definitely established, but it may be more related to vibratory appreciation than to equilibration. Structurally however the macula sacculi (1.5 mm. in diameter) and macula utriculi (2 by 3 mm.) are similar. The saccular organ is oriented perpendicularly in the parasagittal plane, with hairs directed laterally. The utricular macula is horizontally placed, with hairs directed upward. The cilia are somewhat shorter than those of the cristae, and they project into a thin (22 μ), jelly-like membrane *(otolithic membrane)* filled with crystals of calcium carbonate and protein (Fig. 18-9).[3] These *otoconia* measure 3 to 5 μ and appear to function in response to gravitational effects. The relationship of the macular sensory cells to nerve fibers is the same as in the cristae. It is presumed that efferent impulses also reach these receptors.[7]

VESTIBULAR NERVE

The nerve of equilibration is part of the nerve VIII complex and arises in two divisions, a superior and an inferior. The superior division (utriculo-ampullar) originates in the macula of the utricle and in the ampullae of the anterior and lateral semicircular canals. The inferior division (sacculo-ampullar) is derived from the macula of the saccule and from the ampulla of the posterior semicircular canal. *Oort's bundle* (vestibulocochlear anastomosis is a branch of this latter division. This may be a bundle of efferent nerves entering the cochlear division of nerve VIII after passing with vestibular fibers from the brainstem (Fig. 18-5). Cross sections reveal an aggregated bundle of unusually small myelinated fibers in the distal part that probably represent Oort's bundle (p. 325). The *vestibular ganglion* (of Scarpa) lies along the roots within the internal auditory meatus (Figs. 18-9 and 19-7). The cells are bipolar and are partially

*For review of ultrastructural details see reference 3.

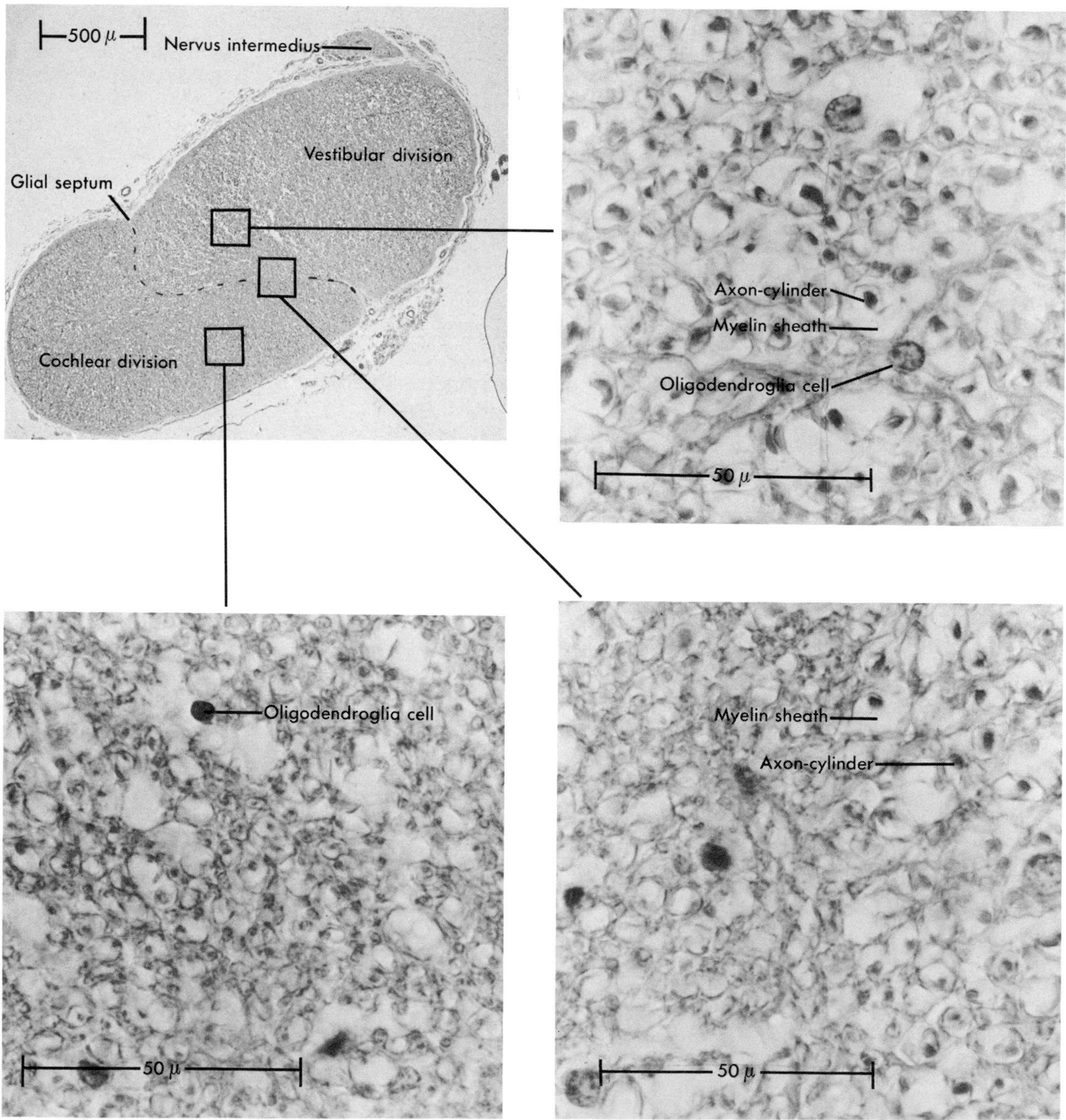

Fig. 18-10. Nerve VIII in cross section showing comparative size of fibers in cochlear and vestibular divisions. (Courtesy Dr. Max Powers.)

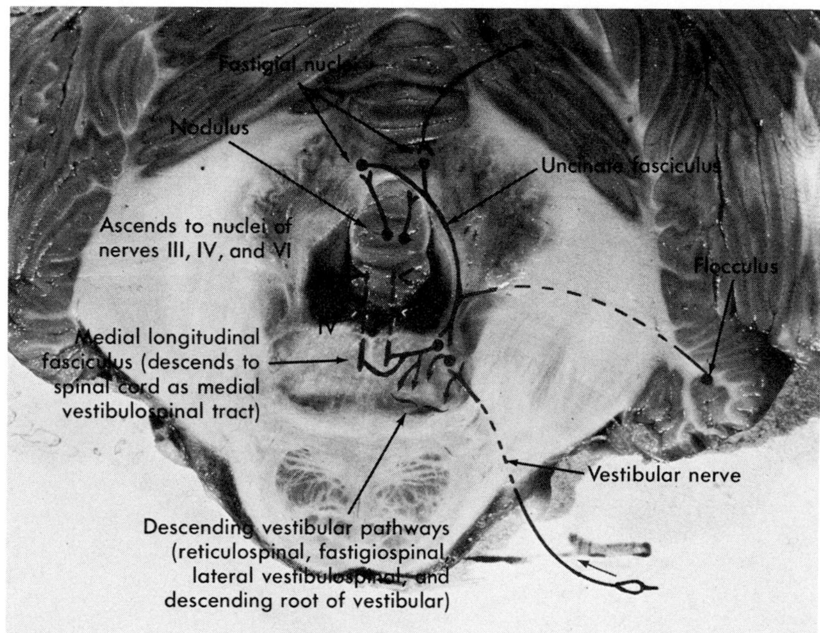

Fig. 18-11. Vestibular connections to cerebellum drawn as an overlay on cross section near the entrance of the vestibular nerve.

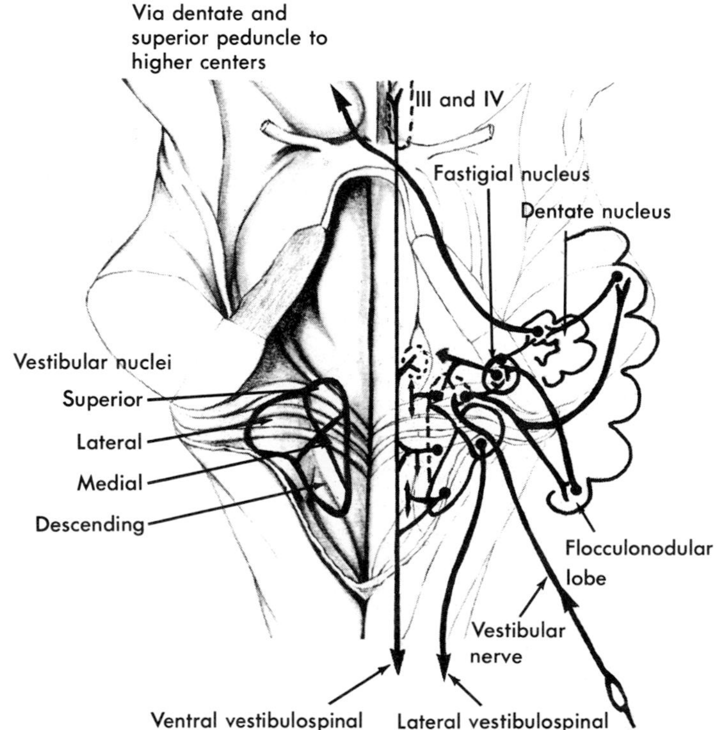

Fig. 18-12. Diagram of dorsal view of brainstem with placement of vestibular complex as an overlay.

myelinated, as are both the proximal and distal axons. The last myelin carries to the dendritic zones distal to the cell bodies. Unmyelinated fibers are abundant in the nerve and probably represent autonomic filaments.[7] The fibers of the vestibular nerve number from 14,000 to 24,000, with an average of 19,000. They are larger than the fibers of the auditory division, with which they blend slightly as the nerves course together (Fig. 18-10). The glio-Schwannian junction (Obersteiner-Redlich zone) is irregular, with glial cells extending outward from the brainstem one or more centimeters (Fig. 10-20). The nerve joins the brainstem immediately lateral to the take-off of cranial nerve

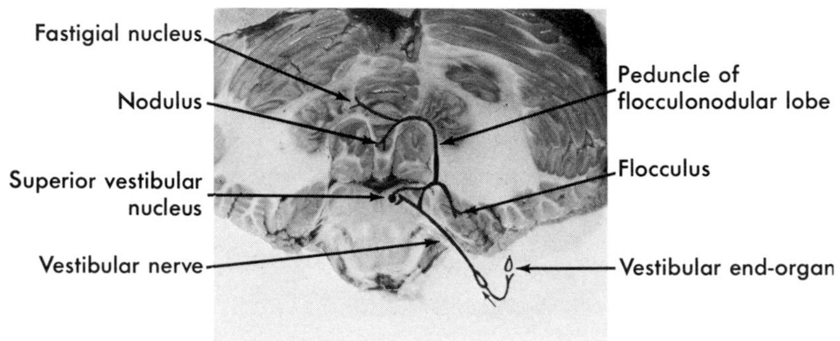

Fig. 18-13. Relationships of the flocculonodular lobe projected on a cross section of the stem and cerebellum.

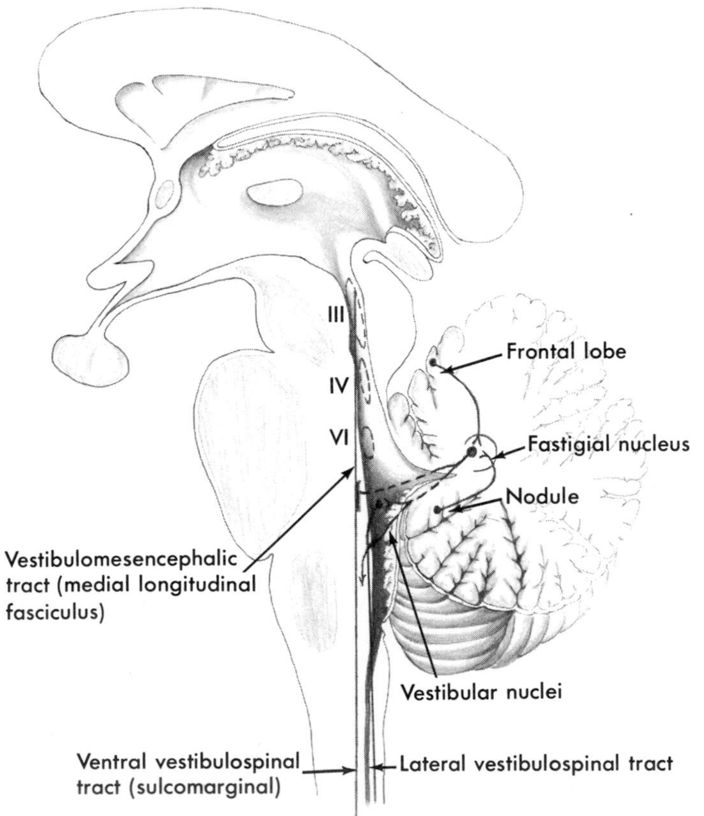

Fig. 18-14. Vestibular pathways in side-view diagram.

VII. Here the vestibular division separates from the auditory nerve, which passes over the corpus restiforme. The vestibular division penetrates the brainstem and passes ventral and medial to the corpus restiforme and lateral and posterior to the descending root of the trigeminal nerve (Figs. 18-11 to 18-12).

NUCLEI

Some of the fibers of the vestibular nerve terminate around cells that are interspersed among the entering fibers (*intraradicular nucleus*). The remaining parts of the nerve divide into an *ascending* and a *descending* root. The ascending root is directed to the cerebellar cortex of the same side, to the fastigial nucleus of the same side, and to the superior vestibular nucleus (of Bechterew) (Fig. 18-11). The cerebellar cortical parts involved include the flocculus and its peduncle, the nodulus (flocculonodular lobe), and the uvula (Fig. 18-13). Other anterior cerebellar regions relate in an efferent manner to the fastigial nucleus but do not seem to receive fibers directly from the vestibular complex. The fibers directed to the cerebellum terminate in the cortex and effect synapses, with cerebellar cortical outflow principally to the fastigial nucleus of the opposite side. Others pass to the brainstem to end in relationship to the vestibular nuclei. Here they probably feed into the descending reticular system (reticulospinal). The incoming vestibular fibers, which pass to the fastigial nuclei, terminate on both sides. The returning fibers comprise the *uncinate fasciculus* (of Russell) and, arising principally in the opposite fastigial

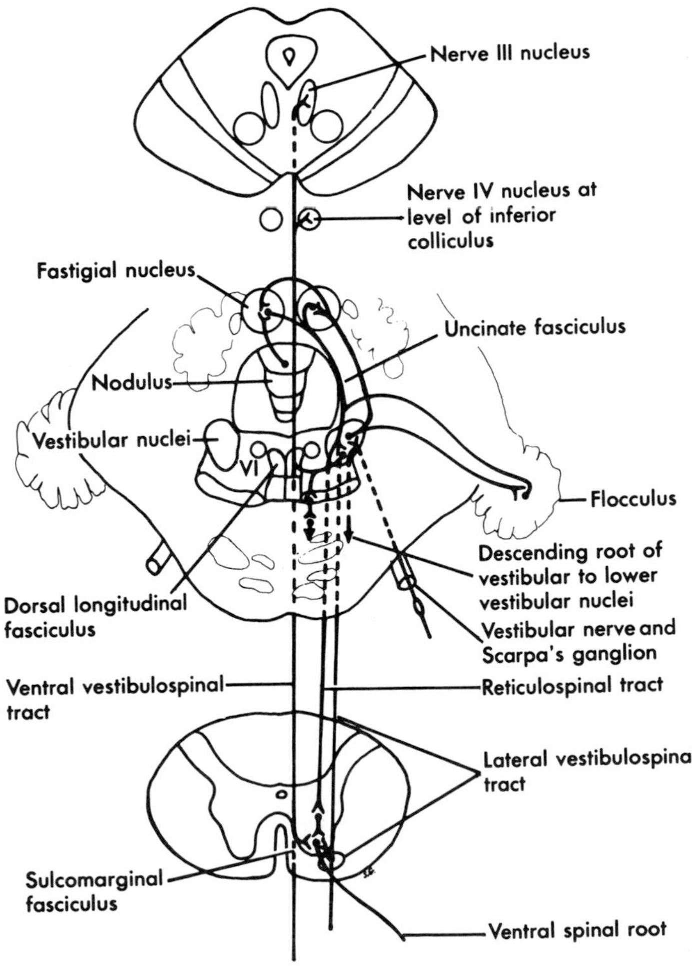

Fig. 18-15. Summary diagram of vestibular reflex connections.

nucleus, pass in an arch ventrally and downward into the vestibular nuclei and into the reticulospinal pool. Those ascending vestibular nerve fibers that terminate in the superior vestibular nucleus bear on connections that relate not only to the cerebellum as previously outlined, but to the medial longitudinal fasciculus as well.

The descending root of the vestibular nerve terminates in three vestibular nuclei, lateral (of Deiters), medial (of Schwalbe), and inferior (spinal). These are distributed as shown in Fig. 18-11 and link to the superior vestibular nucleus in the following connections. The lateral vestibulospinal tract arises from the lateral nucleus and descends to the final paths of the lower stem and spinal cord (Fig. 18-14). Downward-directed fibers from both the medial and spinal nuclei descend in the medial longitudinal fasciculus (ventral vestibulospinal fasciculus) and end around final-path cells of the spinal cord. The terminal spinal group of fibers of this tract makes up the *sulcomarginal fasciculus* (Fig. 18-15). Nuclei (of the medial longitudinal fasciculus) are interjected along this multisynaptic pathway. The ascending fibers that arise in the vestibular nuclei have their origins in the medial and superior nuclei. The ascending route is via the medial longitudinal fasciculus (vestibulomesencephalic), which is directed principally to the nuclei of cranial nerves VI, IV, and III (Figs. 18-14 and 18-15). It is probable that equilibration related to the upper extremity is located in the acoustic area near nucleus VI, and that equilibration related to the lower extremity is located in the lower part of the vestibular nuclear cluster.

REFLEXES

While sensations related to equilibration are well recognized, it is impossible to relate a specific cortical area to this sensation. The tracts from the vestibular complex do not possess a known direct ascending route to the thalamus and cortex. It appears probable that equilibration as perception arises secondarily from the many reflex relationships. The principal reflex connections are summarized in Table 18-1. The vestibular nuclei appear to relate mainly to ocular movements, to auditory responses, and to posture. Cerebellar influence obviously affects vestibular responses. Thalamocortical ties in the vestibular complex relate principally through audition, vision, and complex

Table 18-1. Principal reflex connections of the vestibular nuclei

Nucleus	Via tract	Termination
Superior vestibular nucleus	Nucleocerebellar	Fastigial nuclei Cerebellar cortex (flocculus, nodule, uvula)
	Ascending medial longitudinal fasciculus	Ocular nuclei
Medial vestibular nucleus	Ascending medial longitudinal fasciculus	Ocular nuclei
	Descending medial longitudinal fasciculus	Spinal motor nuclei
Lateral vestibular nucleus	Lateral vestibulospinal fasciculus	Spinal motor cells
Inferior vestibular nucleus	Descending medial longitudinal fasciculus	Spinal motor cells
Fastigial nucleus	Uncinate fasciculus	Vestibular nuclei and reticular formation
Cerebellar cortex	Projections	Fastigial nucleus possibly via dentate to higher centers

sensations, such as nausea, deep sense, and pressure. Disturbances in equilibration are manifested principally in dizziness, nystagmus, nausea, and vomiting. These are elicited by lesions in the peripheral pathways and in the vestibular nuclei. Dizziness can be evoked by electrical stimulation of the temporal lobe anterior to the auditory area.[5] There is also experimental evidence that the region of the medial geniculate body relates to equilibration. Nausea and vomiting are certainly related to hypothalamic activity. In a similar manner many thalamocortical regions relate to equilibration. At present however these pathways remain clouded, and the circuitry to these centers is obscure.

The vestibular system is summarized in Fig. 18-15.

REFERENCES

1. Anson, B. J., and Donaldson, J. A.: The surgical anatomy of the temporal bone and ear, Philadelphia, 1967, W. B. Saunders Co.
2. Engström, H., and Wersäll, J.: The ultrastructural organization of the organ of Corti and of the vestibular sensory epithelia, Exp. Cell Res. Supp. 5:460, 1958.
3. Iurato, S.: Submicroscopic structure of the inner ear, Elmsford, New York, 1967, Pergamon Press, Inc.
4. Minckler, T.: Physical growth. In Minckler, J., editor: Pathology of the nervous system, vol. I, New York, 1968, McGraw-Hill Book Co.
5. Penfield, W., and Roberts, L.: Speech and brain mechanisms, Princeton, New Jersey, 1959, Princeton University Press.
6. Rasmussen, G. L., and Windle, W. F.: Neural mechanisms of the auditory and vestibular systems, Springfield, Illinois, 1960, Charles C Thomas, Publisher.
7. Wersäll, J.: Electron microscopic studies of vestibular hair cell innervation. In Rasmussen, G. L., and Windle, W. F., editors: Neural mechanisms of the auditory and vestibular systems, Springfield, Illinois, 1960, Charles C Thomas, Publisher.

CHAPTER 19

AUDITORY SYSTEM

JEFF MINCKLER

The neural system that is adapted to detection of sound waves in the air constitutes the hearing mechanism. A complex system of transducing devices converts the air movements to neural signals. The neural signals arise in the internal ear through receptors (hair cells) in the organ of Corti. The transducers in this conversion occupy the external, internal, and middle ear compartments.

EXTERNAL EAR

The external ear includes the auricle and the external auditory canal. The canal is lined by squamous equithelium and possesses ceruminal glands and hairs. It is supported by discontinuous cartilage bars and adjacent bone.

TYMPANIC MEMBRANE

The canal terminates at a *tympanic membrane* (drum), which separates the external from the middle ear compartment. The membrane is 0.1 mm. thick at its center and is suspended from a cartilaginous ring by fibrous ligaments attached to the margin. It displays a quadrant pattern and a flaccid membrane oriented about a central tent-like inward projection, the *umbo* (Fig. 19-1). The anterior inferior quadrant is characterized by a reflecting cone of light. The anterior superior quadrant joins the flaccid membrane superiorly and is bounded behind by the ridge manubrium of the malleus. The posterior superior quadrant overlies a segment of chorda tympani nerve, which lies deep to it. The anterior boundary of this quadrant is limited by the manubrium and superiorly meets the flaccid membrane. This quadrant conveys major vessels and sensory nerves (nerve V) of the membrane along the manubrial contour. The posterior inferior quadrant possesses marginal vasculature, as do the other quadrants, but is otherwise less complex. The flaccid membrane (of Shrapnell) is a somewhat triangular membrane superior and slightly anterior to the prominence (lateral process) of the malleolus (Fig. 19-1). It is bounded in front and back by malleolar folds.

The histologic features of the membrane include a thin squamous membrane on the external surface that is continuous with the skin of the external auditory canal. The main body of the membrane is a fibrous substantia propria made up of a radial lamina that is external to circular fibers of connective tissue. The lining on the deep surface is cuboidal mucous membrane, which is continuous with the ciliated respiratory membrane of the middle ear cavity (Fig. 19-2).

MIDDLE EAR

The cavity of the *middle ear* is continuous with mastoid air cells and with the eustachian tube, which connects to the nasopharynx (Fig. 19-3). The *ossicular chain* is made up of the linked auditory ossicles (malleus, incus, and stapes). The handle (manubrium) of the malleus attaches throughout to the tympanic membrane. This bone is subject to the inward pull of the tensor tympani, whose tendon attaches to the medial side of the root of the manubrium. The muscle draws the bone medially, and therefore tenses the attached membrane. The head articulates with the incus, whose long process inserts into the head of the stapes. The foot of the stapes is inserted into the oval window. Thus, the transmission of forces through the ossicular chain begins with movement of the tympanic membrane and terminates with movement of the membrane covering the oval window. Action of the stapedius muscle, which inserts on the posterior aspect of the stapedial neck, rocks the stapes vertically so that the posterior part of the base depresses the

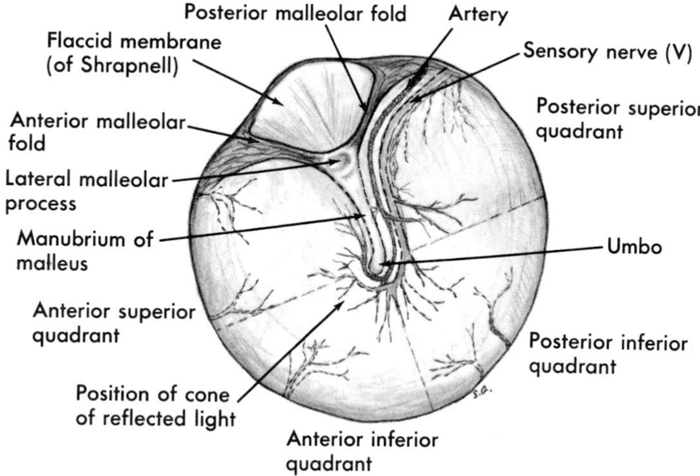

Fig. 19-1. Tympanic membrane of left ear as viewed through otoscope.

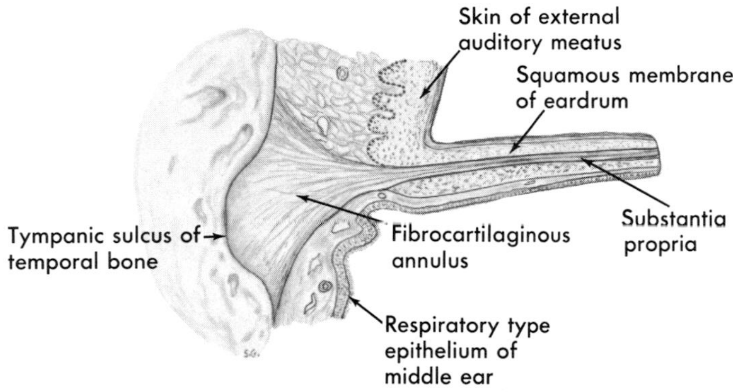

Fig. 19-2. Tympanic membrane—histology.

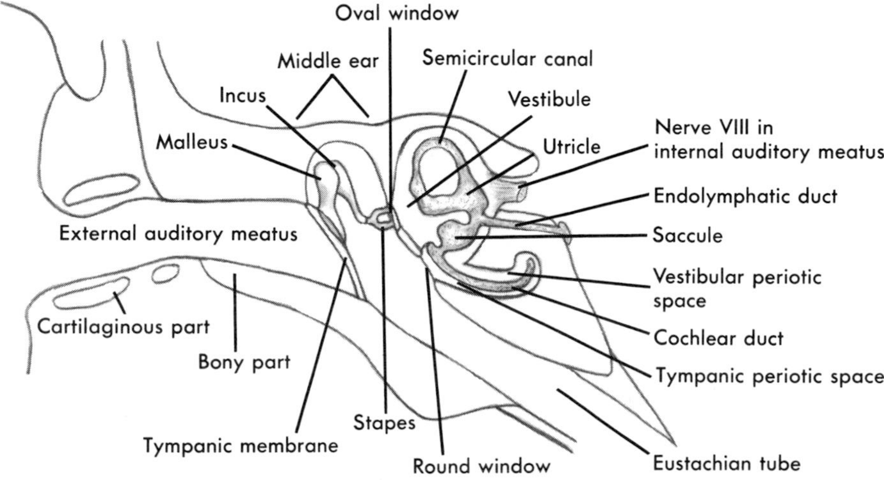

Fig. 19-3. Diagram showing compartmentation of ear into external, middle, and internal parts.

oval window membrane (Fig. 19-4). The action through the ossicular chain is such that the amplitude of membrane excursion from tympanic to oval window is reduced by about one-third. The movement of the stapes foot-plate is about 0.04 mm. in response to pressure from the ossicular chain. At the same time, the increase in pressure at the stapes is ten times the pressure imparted at the tympanic membrane.[22,23]

Below and slightly behind the oval window is a second membrane-covered bony opening, the round window (Fig. 18-2). This membrane moves in a counter direction to the membrane underlying the stapedial foot-plate. It operates therefore in response to ossicular chain movement and is part of the transducing mechanism, by which fluid movements within the internal ear are imparted to hair cell neural receptors (Fig. 19-4).

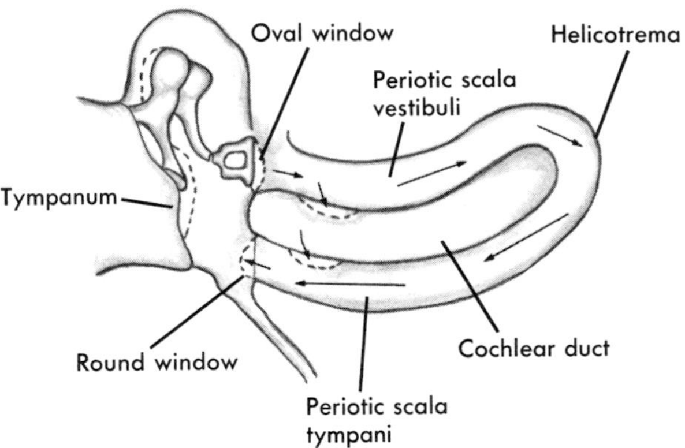

Fig. 19-4. Coronal diagram relating oval window to vestibule and vestibular periotic space, and round window to tympanic periotic space. Dotted lines show effects of movement of tympanum and ossicular chain on membranes of oval and round windows. Represented is effect of high frequency vibration on basal turn area.

INTERNAL EAR

The *internal ear* is made up of a series of labyrinthine bony canals containing the membranous canals (membranous or otic labyrinths) of both the vestibular and auditory apparatuses. The equilibratory system has been reviewed (see p. 294), and the present discussion is directed to the cochlea and structures related to hearing. The topographic relationships of the internal ear are illustrated in Figs. 18-1 to 18-5.

Bony labyrinth

The framework supporting the otic labyrinth is essentially a bony canal lined with periosteum. It forms a coiled cylinder that completes two and three-fourths turns, forming basal, middle, and apical (the three-quarter turn) segments in a gross cone-shaped structure. Castings of the bony labyrinth usually measure 9 mm. across the base and 5 mm. in the vertical axis to the apex. The cone-shaped central bony axis is the *modiolus* (Fig. 19-5). Projecting from the modiolus about half the diameter of the bony canal and wound in a spiral pattern around it is a bony ridge, the *spiral lamina.* This ridge partially subdivides the bony canal into a space on the basal side of the ridge and one on the apical side of the ridge. This division is completed by a fibrous membrane, the *basilar mem-*

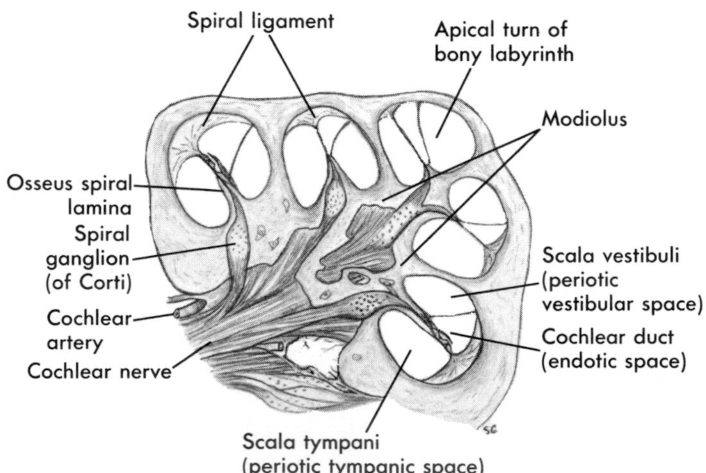

Fig. 19-5. Modiolus in diagram showing separation of two periotic spaces by cochlear duct.

brane, stretching between the spiral lamina and the outer wall periosteum. It attaches to the outer wall by the spiral ligament. The two canals thus formed (30 mm. long) connect at the apex via the *helicotrema.* The spaces form the *scala tympani* (basal side) and *scala vestibuli* (apical side) as *periotic spaces* bordering the *otic* or *membranous* labyrinth (Fig. 19-6). These spaces are filled with periotic fluid, or *perilymph,* which is thus continuous from scala vestibuli through the helicotrema to the scala tympani. The scala vestibuli relates via the vestibule to the *vestibular* (*oval*) *window,* which is covered by a membrane to which the foot-plate of the stapes is attached. The scala tympani relates in its basal turn to the round window, which is closed by a membrane (secondary tympanic membrane) (Fig. 19-4). Waves transmitted to the periotic fluid in the vestibule and scala vestibuli are in turn transmitted via the helicotrema and the scala tympani to the secondary tympanic membrane, covering the round window. This is a significant feature in theories pertaining to the mechanisms of stimulation of the neural receptors in the cochlea.

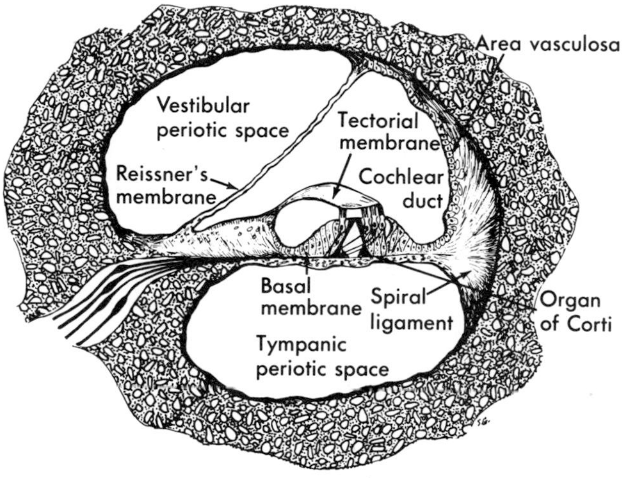

Fig. 19-6. Diagram of details of periotic spaces and cochlear duct.

The bony central cone of the modiolus is penetrated by channels that house the cochlear nerve. The bundles of fibers reaching the cochlear apex form the central cone of the aggregated nerve at the base of the modiolus. The remaining fibers twist around this cone, so that the fibers from the basal turn are applied most superficially (Fig. 19-7). Near the base of the bony spiral lamina the spiral canal accommodates the spiral ganglion (bipolar cells), from which the cochlear fibers project into the organ of Corti.

Membranous labyrinth

The membranous canal related to the cochlear bony canal is the *cochlear duct* (scala media). This duct relates to the bony labyrinth in much the same way that the semicircular membranes relate to the bony canals in the vestibular system. The duct is essentially a blind, fibrous, thin-walled.

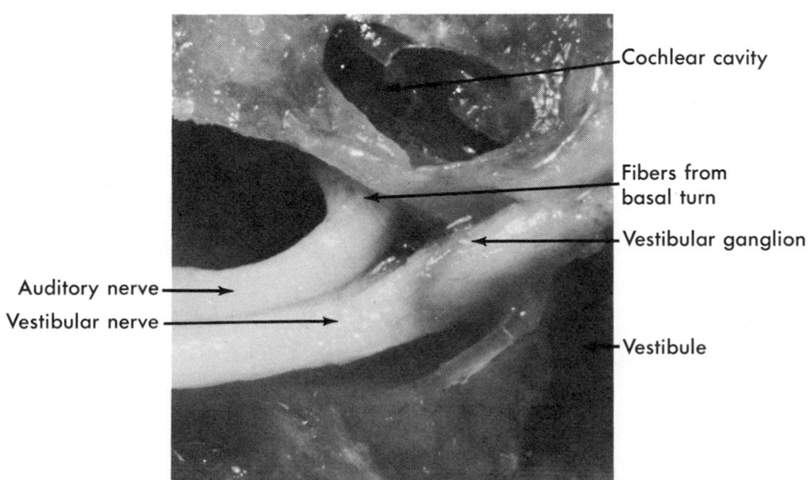

Fig. 19-7. Gross dissection of cochlear and vestibular nerves deep in the meatus. Note spiral wrapping pattern of cochlear nerve, which places fibers from the basal turn superficial to the middle and apical turns. (Apical are central in nerve.)

epithelium-lined pouch that has several complex adaptations. The duct follows the course of the bony labyrinth of the cochlea and is open only near the basal extremity, from which the *ductus reuniens* extends to join the saccule (Fig. 18-3). The cochlear duct adds to the septum, dividing the bony canal into the two periotic spaces. The duct is triangular in cross section and is definable as a three-sided figure with apex oriented centrally and base laterally (Fig. 19-6). One side lies adjacent to the basilar membrane, limiting the scala tympani. This side carries the organ of Corti, or spiral organ. The base of the triangle overlies the spiral ligament, which is attached to the outer wall along the periphery of the bony canal. Secreting epithelium is applied to this surface, and prominent vascularity forms the area vascularis. This complex produces the endotic fluid, which fills the scala media. The third side forms the vestibular, or Reissner's, membrane, which borders the scala vestibuli (Fig. 19-6).

Organ of Corti

This complex structure supports the prime receptor mechanism for hearing. As previously stated, the organ is fixed to the *basilar membrane,* which bridges from the *spiral bony lamina* to the *basilar crest* of the *spiral ligament.* The spiral bony lamina is perforated by canals that transmit the branches of the cochlear nerve into the organ complex at this point. On the endotic side of the bony lamina the connective tissues are piled into the *spiral limbus,* which is concave on the outer side, forming the *internal spiral sulcus.* The limbus and sulcus are lined by cuboidal to columnar epithelium, which become *border cells* near the hair cell–bearing area (Fig. 19-8). Extending from the peak (vestibular lip) of the limbus is the *tectorial membrane,* which overlies the hair cells. The hairs project into the substance of the membrane, although this relationship distorts beyond recognition in the usual histologic preparation (Fig. 19-8).

The supporting cells and structures of the organ of Corti play an important role in the complex manner of stimulation of the receptor (hair) cells (Fig. 19-8). On the external aspect of the inner spiral sulcus are *border cells,* which apply to the inner hair cells. Immediately external to the inner hair cells and limited to the lower half of the width of the organ are the bodies of the *inner phalangeal* cells. These cells give rise to extending rigid processes (phalanges), which project to the surface of the organ and then expand into broad plates. These plates of the phalanges join adjacent plates to contribute to the formation of the limiting *reticular* membrane. Two similar heavy phalanges arise in *basal* cells immediately external to internal phalangeal cells. These are the *rods* or *pillars of Corti* and define the triangular *inner tunnel* by fusion at the apex. The expansions at

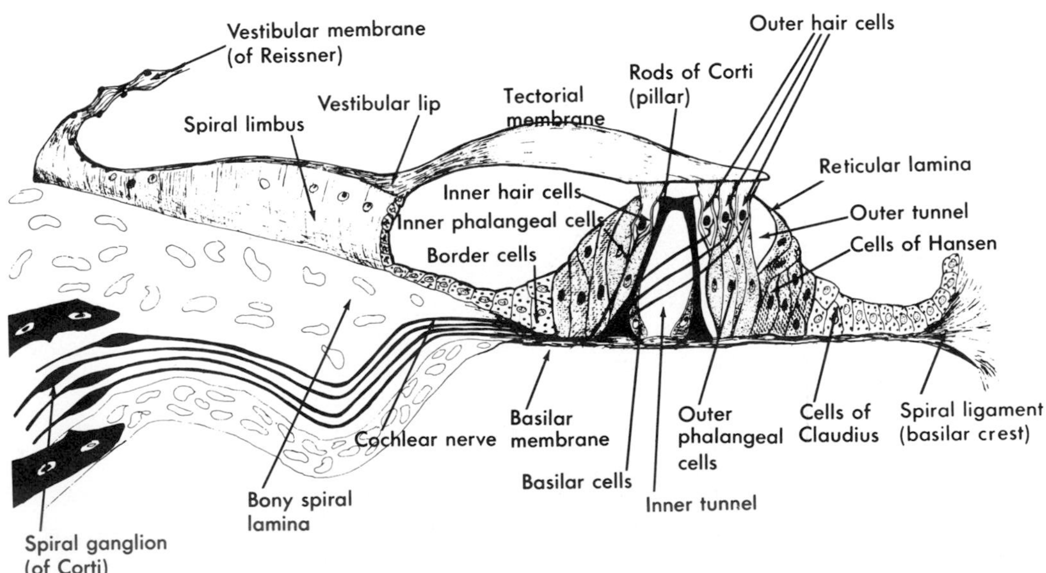

Fig. 19-8. Diagramof organ of Corti.

the apex join the head-plates of phalanges and contribute the reticular membrane, into which the free borders of the hair cells insert. External to the outer rod is the *space of Nuel,* which separates the rod from the outer rows of phalangeal cells (Deiter's cells). The processes of these cells also contribute broadened head-plates to the reticular membrane. These immediately surround the outer rows of hair cells. Lateral to the head-plates is the *outer tunnel,* supported laterally by the *cells of Hensen.* These cells blend with the *cells of Claudius,* which continue into the specially adapted secretory cells of the area vascularis. The secreted endotic fluid of the scala media appears to serve a nutritive transport function as well as its role in hearing.

Because the basilar membrane is closely related to pitch, careful measurements have been most instructive. The membrane is wider at the apex (0.5 mm.) than at the basal turn (0.08 mm.) and displays an uneven change in width throughout its 32 mm. length.[22] The average width in the basal turn is 0.21 mm., in the middle turn 0.34 mm., and in the apical turn 0.36 mm. At the base the membrane is responsive to 20,000 vibrations per second. Comparative values along its length include: at 5 mm. from the base, it responds to 8,195 vibrations per second; at 7.33 to 9.5 mm. from base, 4,096 vibrations per second; at 9.5 to 12 mm., 2,048 vibrations per second; at 15 mm., 1,024 vibrations per second; and at the apical extremity (32 mm. from base), 16 vibrations per second. The maximum human range of audible vibrations per second thus varies from 16 to 20,000 (compared to 30 to 35,000 vibrations per second in dog and up to 98,000 per second in bat).[17] It is evident that appreciation of low frequencies is initiated by stimulation of the apical turn, and that of high frequencies is related to basal-turn stimulation. Despite the appearance of the basement membrane and the designation of its basal fibers as auditory strings, the organ probably does not function in any way as a vibratory membrane.

Receptors. The special mechanoreceptors in the organ of Corti that are sensitive to impulses generated by sound waves are the *hair cells* (Fig. 19-8). According to Bredberg,[4] these number about 16,800 in each ear. They are arranged in an inner row, averaging 3,400 cells (range from 2,800 to 4,000) on the basement membrane near the bony spiral

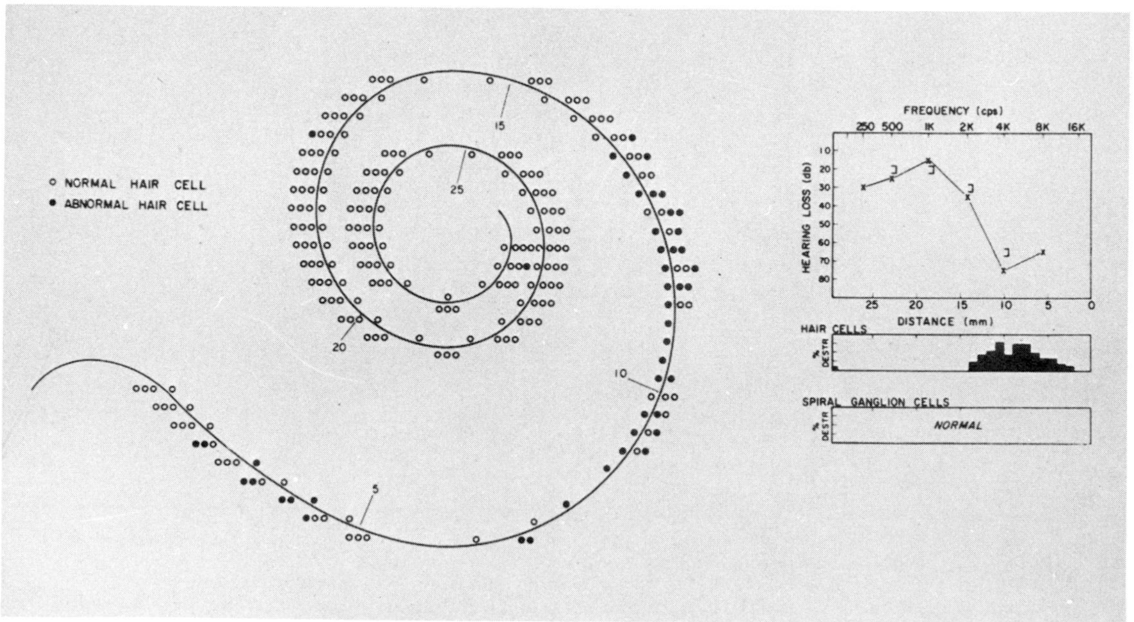

Fig. 19-9. Graphic representation of hair cells with correlated audiometric reading and percent destruction of hair cells and spiral ganglion cells. (From Igarashi. In Minckler, J., editor: Pathology of the nervous system, vol. III, New York, 1972, McGraw-Hill Book Co.)

lamina of the *modiolus*. Approximately 13,400 hair cells (range from 11,200 to 16,000) are disposed more distally in an outer group. These hair cells occur in three rows in the basal cochlear turn, in four rows in the middle turn, and in five rows in the incomplete apical turn. Their distribution can be graphically displayed as in Fig. 19-9, which is an illustration of sample counts of hair cells in a projected pattern as though viewing the cochlea from above (cochleogram).[4,11] Hair cells degenerate and disappear with age (the inner layer primarily at the base, the outer layers overall). Hearing seems to be more disturbed with hair cell loss in the basal turn.[4,11]

Mechanisms of stimulation. The cilia of the hair cells project to touch or embed in the *tectorial membrane,* while the upper surface edge of the body of each hair cell is firmly fixed in the rigid *reticular lamina* (Fig. 19-8). This lamina is rigidly fixed by the triangular *rods* of Corti to the base of each basilar fiber and by the phalanges of the phalangeal cells. The basilar fibers, the rods, and the reticular lamina move as a unit as the basilar membrane responds to fluid waves. As the membrane moves upward, the whole complex moves upward and inward, hinging at the narrow membranous base of the spiral sulcus. Similarly, the entire complex moves downward and outward as the basal membrane moves downward. Thus, with vibrating motions imparted to the basilar membrane, the processes of the hair cells, through fixation to the tectorial membrane, are subject to bending or sheering. This movement excites the receptor potential. The manner of transfer of this potential to the related filaments of the cochlear nerve is not clear. Whether chemical or physical, this excitation is transmitted to the nerve endings that form basket-like receptacles at the bases of the hair cells (Fig. 19-10). A good deal of attention is merited by the synaptic relationship of the hair cells and by the structural details that account for their remarkable behavior.

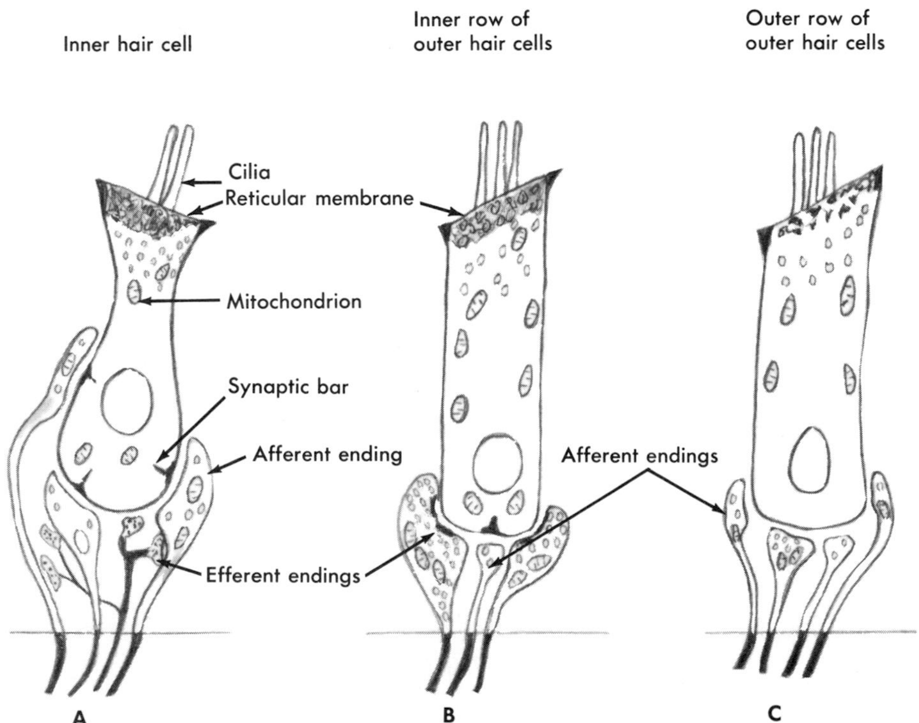

Fig. 19-10. Nerve ending relationships of cochlear hair cells diagrammed as composite information from experimental animals (notably guinea pig). A, Inner hair cell with pale afferent endings predominating. A few "efferent" terminals, which have greater electron density, end against the afferent terminals, as well as the receptor; B, first outer hair cell row. The electron-dense terminals are large and numerous and presumably represent efferents to this row principally in the basal area; C, second and third outer hair cell rows, which possess smaller cochlear afferents and fewer electron-dense efferents.

The inner and outer hair cells probably subserve different functions, although the exact nature remains obscure. The inner cells project through the reticular membrane and produce a continuous double row of cilia (ten to sixty per cell) through the length of the cochlea. The outer cells are located more deeply in the reticular membrane and present their cilia (forty to 120 per cell) in an irregular pattern of three or four rows in a w configuration on the surface of each cell. The sheering forces applied would thus affect the inner and outer hair cells differently.[1,8,10] The inner hair cells closely resemble those of the vestibular membranes. They possess ultrastructural features that distinguish them from the outer hair cells (Fig. 19-10). The related nerve endings are particularly noteworthy and fall into two main groups: (1) heavily granulated endings with prominent electron density, and (2) pale-staining terminals. The latter suggest by structure a regular pickup terminal (type I) and are regarded as cochlear nerve endings. They usually relate to synaptic bars in the hair receptors (Fig. 19-10). The dense endings, by contrast, are filled with synaptic vesicles and large mitochondria (as viewed with the electron microscope) and may represent efferent terminals (see p. 298). The two types of endings are mixed around inner hair cells, with a predominance of cochlear afferents. The dense terminals designated type II are conspicuous among the outer hair cells and concentrate in the basal extremity of the cochlea, with fewer near the apex. They also are more numerous on the proximal, or first, of the three rows of outer hair cells (Fig. 19-10). As in the semicircular canals, the structural features of the dense endings suggest incoming neural connections and probably represent the terminals of the olivocochlear bundle of Rasmussen. However, their exact origin remains controversial.

The many concepts of receptor pickup in the organ of Corti must take into account the structure and behavior of the basal and tectorial membranes, the physical and chemical features of the fluids related to the receptors, and the structural and behavioral characteristics of the receptors themselves. Added to this are the synaptic connections of the hair cells and the quantitative features related to the afferent volleys arising from hair cell stimulation. At present no single theory seems to fit all the requirements to explain auditory pickup. The theories advanced are mutually supportive.[3,22,23]

In connection with the sensitivity of the generation of receptor potential in hair cells, the ionic peculiarities of the endolymph of the scala media becomes significant. This endolymph (in contrast to perilymph, which is similar to CSF and has a relatively high sodium concentration and twice the protein of CSF) is secreted by the *area vascularis* of the outer wall of the cochlear duct and possesses a high concentration of potassium, simulating intracellular ionic content. Its protein content is relatively low. This establishes a relatively high positivity in the fluid of scala media compared to the periotic fluid and establishes an endocochlear potential. The outer surfaces of the hair cells adjacent to the tectorial membrane are bathed in endolymph. An endocochlear potential is thus added to the natural membrane potential of the hair cell, nearly doubling the latter potential. It is thought that this unusually high membrane potential in the hair cells accounts for their striking sensitivity to movements of the hairs. It is probable that the fluid bathing the bases of the hair cells and their related filaments in the tunnel is specially adapted in terms of ionic properties and also differs from perilymph (cortilymph).

Nerve fibers (*first-order afferent*) of the cochlear nerve on the cochlear side of the spiral ganglion arise as aggregates of finer, more distal filaments. These peripheral nerve filaments (dendritic zones ?) arise from a position of contiguity with several or many hair cells, and each hair cell is contacted by several separate filaments. At least two types of contact points exist between hair cells and nerve fibrils, a small, finely granulated bulb and a larger, richly granulated terminal (Fig. 19-10). The physiologic meaning of the different terminals is not known. It is possible that one type is part of an efferent feedback system that functions in inhibition of auditory input. The peripheral distribution from Corti's (spiral) ganglion is in the following two distinct patterns: (1) *radial fibers,* which radiate from the foramina of the bony spiral lamina outward to one or more inner hair cells or between the rods of Corti to deviate basally half a turn and innervate many outer hair cells in a row; and (2) *spiral fibers,* which form intraganglionic and internal and external spiral bundles that follow the multirow spiral pattern of hair cells and bring several in touch with the same filament (Fig. 19-11). The filaments aggregate into fine fiber bundles entering the modiolus adjacent to the *spiral ganglion.* These aggregated fibers add Schwann cells and some myelin sheaths, which are continuous with the sheaths over the ganglion cells. It is presumed that these filaments are parts of the dendritic zones of the bipolar cells of Corti's ganglion. Some of the filaments undoubtedly represent efferent

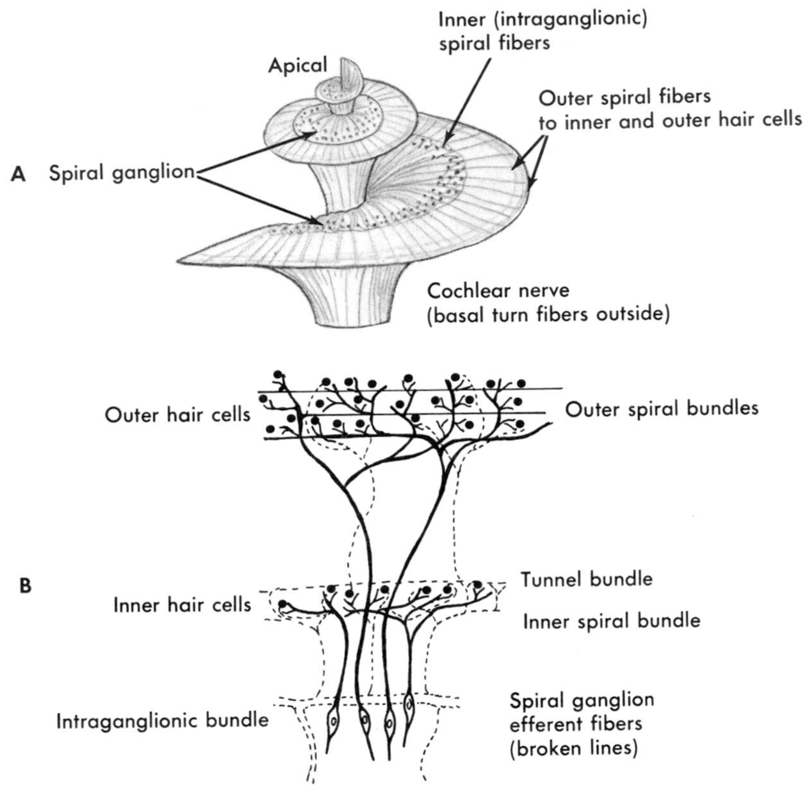

Fig. 19-11. A, The distribution of nerves in the spiral organ; **B,** the probable relationships of efferent nerves are shown in broken lines. These probably make up the bulk of the intraganglionic bundle, the inner spiral bundle, and the tunnel bundle.

fibers leading into the cochlea. Loss of nerve filaments in the modiolus relates better to loss of inner hair cells, but those relationships are not fully established.[4]

Spiral ganglion (Corti). The ganglion of Corti occupies the spiral canal of the modiolus (Fig. 19-5) and exhibits varying cellular density in the various turns. The cells number roughly 1,200 per mm. in the basal turn of the cochlea, 1,100 per mm. in the middle turn, and progressively diminish to 600 per mm. in the apex. They outnumber the hair cells by approximately 2 to 1. The 30,000 cell bodies of the *spiral ganglion* measure 13 to 16 μ and are in general somewhat smaller than those in the vestibular ganglion (of Scarpa), which measure from 19 to 27 μ in diameter. The cells are bipolar (Fig. 19-11) and are frequently myelinated. The capsule cells in this location (as well as others) contribute a myelin sheath to the ganglion cells that is equivalent in all respects to, and continuous with, the sheath contributed by the Schwann cells of the more centrally located axis-cylinders. The exact relationship of the number of fibers in the human cochlear division of nerve VIII to the number of spiral ganglion cells has not been established with certainty, but the ratio is probably 1 to 1.[16,17] The efferent fibers in the nerve are proportionately few and probably aggregate in their own bundle (of Oort?), which grossly connects to the basal cochlear turn (Fig. 18-5).

ACOUSTIC NERVE

Cranial nerve VIII measures 17 to 19 mm. in the adult. The nerve represents a combination of *cochlear* and *vestibular* components and also includes fibers of facial nerve (VII) origin, part of the nervus intermedius of Wrisberg. Efferent fibers probably also contribute to the nerve, although the number and nature of such fibers in man are not established. This complex structure would account for discrepancies in comparative counts of fibers and ganglion cells, but these data are not presently

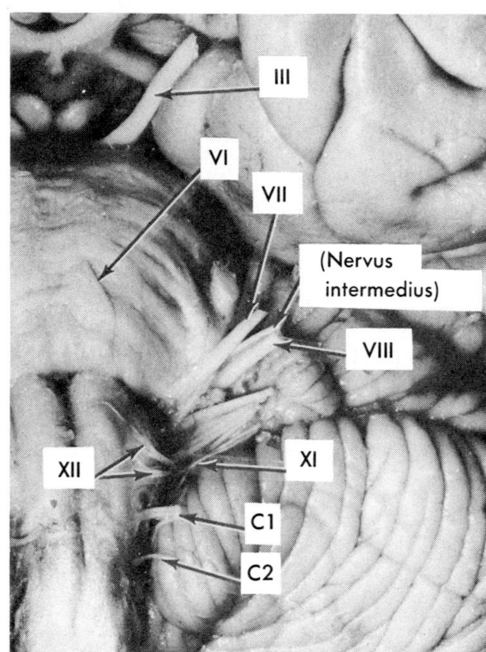

Fig. 19-12. Relationships of nerve VIII at brainstem.

available. The human cochlear nerve has been estimated to contain an average of 31,000 fibers.[16,17] This figure is in close agreement with Guild's estimate of 30,00 spiral ganglion cells. The other fibers of the human nerve remain quantitatively obscure.

The centrally directed axons that arise from spiral ganglion cells and serve the apex of the cochlea take a central course in the cochlear nerve (Fig. 19-7). Fibers arising lower in the cochlea are added to the nerve in a more peripheral position. The fibers from the right ear twist clockwise and those from the left counterclockwise, and each side displays as many turns as the coil of the cochlea from which it arises. The basal fibers thus are straight or are twisted only slightly compared to those of the apex. The fibers arrive at the cochlear nuclei presumably arrayed in the orderly pattern of the uncoiled cochlea. The cochlear division of the acoustic nerve is closely related to the vestibular division in the internal auditory meatus and lies lateral to this latter division as it reaches the inferior cerebellar peduncle. At this point the cochlear division passes dorsal to the inferior peduncle, while the vestibular division penetrates the medulla between the inferior peduncle and the spinal tract of the trigeminal nerve (Fig. 19-12). The first-order neurons principally terminate adjacent to cells of the *dorsal* and *ventral* cochlear nuclei (Fig. 19-13),

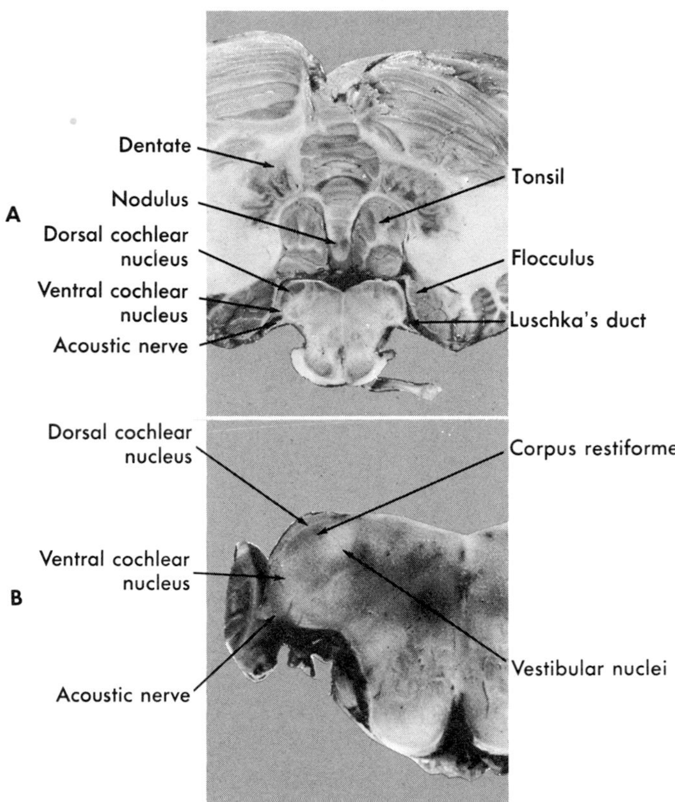

Fig. 19-13. A, Cochlear nuclei and relationship of Luschka's duct; **B,** enlargement showing relationship of nuclei to corpus restiforme.

with a few fibers reaching the cells of the *superior olivary complex*.

The cochlear fibers range from 3 to 10 μ in diameter, with the vast majority exhibiting diameters between 5 and 7 μ (Fig. 18-10). Like the fibers of other nerves attached directly to the CNS, the acoustic nerve fibers possess a Schwann cell covering in the distal part (usually within the internal auditory canal) and glial (oligodendroglial) covering in the proximal part (Fig. 18-11). This *glio-Schwannian junction* (Obersteiner-Redlich zone) occurs at the opening of the canal and is 10 to 13 mm. from the brainstem in men and 7 to 10 mm. from the brainstem in women. Near the same junction, perineurium (of fibroblastic tissue) on the peripheral part joins an extension of pia mater proximally along the nerve. Similarly, the fibrous tissue of the neural wrappings in the internal auditory canal are replaced by gliogenous cells and fibers in the intracranial part of the nerve. These relationships are thought to be important in the development of Schwannian and neurofibromatous tumors of nerve VIII that arise within the canal and project inwardly to occupy the cerebellopontine angle. A further distinguishing structural feature of the Obersteiner-Redlich zone is the concentration of corpora amylacea on the glial or proximal side of the junction (Fig. 18-11). This feature is somewhat related to aging and is basically a manifestation of an error in carbohydrate turnover. Corpora amylacea become prominent only after the middle years.

COCHLEAR NUCLEI

These nuclei are clustered around the entry pathway of the cochlear division of cranial nerve VIII at the junction of the pons and medulla. The total nuclear mass measures from 3 to 5 mm. in a longitudinal axis and as much as 7.5 mm. in maximum dimension in a line from the most medial part of the medial nucleus around the corpus restiforme to the dorsomedial aspect of the dorsal nucleus. The combined volume of the dorsal and ventral nuclei is from 17 to 19 cu. mm. in the adult. By relationship to the corpus restiforme a *ventral* nucleus and a *dorsal* nucleus (*acoustic tubercle*) can be defined. The ventral nucleus is divided by the cochlear nerve into a ventromedial part, which lies medial to the nerve, and a ventrolateral part, which extends along the floor of the lateral recess (of Luschka). This subdivision has a common extension around the recess and therefore appears in what is ostensibly cerebellar white tissue. A direct relationship of cochlear fibers to cerebellum has been postulated, but it is not established for man. The ventrolateral components account for about two-thirds of the total volume of the ventral nucleus. Carried dorsally around the inferior cerebellar peduncle, the cochlear nuclei are compressed into a waist (intermediate part) and expand again more dorsally into the dorsal cochlear nucleus (Fig. 19-13, *B*).[5] All the extensions of the nuclear groups are continuous, but there are some differences in cellular conformation in terms of dominance. It is assumed that the human cochlear fibers deliver impulses to all cell types within the nucleus.[13] The possibility of a tonal differential (tonotopic pattern) at the cochlear level has been hypothesized for man based on the pattern in the cat. This pattern suggests a serial representation of the spiral organ, with fibers from the basal turn (high frequencies) terminating in relationship to ventromedial cells, and the fibers from the apical turn (low frequencies) terminating along the dorsolateral edge.

The nerve cells of the entire cochlear complex number from 100,000 to 200,000 on each side, with approximately two-thirds of these occupying the ventral segment.[7] This is in contrast to an estimated 88,000 total cells on one side in the Rhesus monkey[6] The cellular density however appears to be greater in the dorsal part of the human nucleus. The densities vary from 10,000 cells per cu. mm. in the ventral nucleus to more than 15,000 cells per cu. mm. in the dorsal nucleus. The numerical ratio of receiving cells to delivering afferent cochlear fibers is approximately 7 to 1 in man.[7] It is generally conceded that each cochlear nerve fiber makes contact with approximately one hundred cells in the cochlear nuclei and that all cell types participate.[1] This is not established in man, and it is impossible at present to decipher the function of each of the cell types. It is presumed that the small stellate cells are internuncial and that the large cells give rise to longer ascending or connecting fibers.

The roles of glia in neural activity, in metabolic responsibilities, and in compartmentalization and storage of electrolytes and fluids have prompted estimates of glial densities in the nuclei at 126,000 to 265,000 per cu. mm. Of these thirty-three percent are astrocytes, fifty-two percent oligodendroglia, and the remainder are indeterminable in routine sections.[7] The labile nature of these cells is reflected in the extreme variability in their numbers.

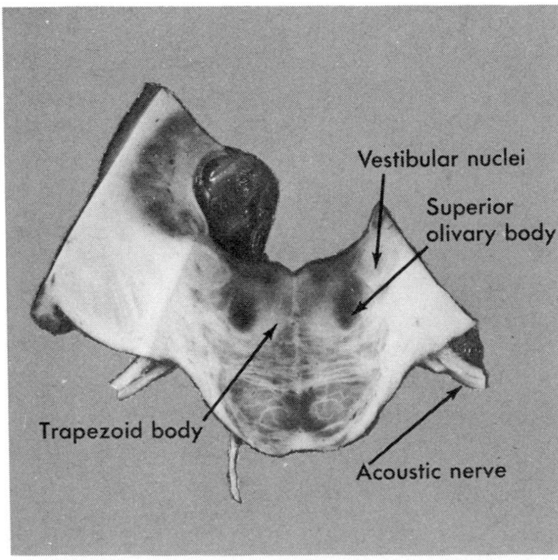

Fig. 19-14. Superior olivary complex and trapezoid body viewed from above. Plane a few millimeters above that of Fig. 19-13, *B*.

Connections of the cochlear nuclei

Theories of the distribution patterns of second-order fibers arising in the human cochlear nuclei are based on those patterns in animals, which are in themselves somewhat uncertain. At least two ascending patterns seem generally accepted. (1) Fibers arise in the ventral cochlear nucleus and pass transversely through the medial lemniscus. They then join the trapezoid bodies to cross and turn superiorly as part of the lateral lemniscus of the opposite side. The cells of origin are presumed to be the larger, rounded elements that dominate this nucleus. Contrary to findings in other animals, no structurally distinctive lamination of these cells exists in man. (2) Fibers from the cells of the dorsal cochlear nucleus pass medially, deep to (not in) the stria medullaris, cross their opposites in a midline decussation, and join the lateral lemniscus above the superior olive to ascend to the midbrain and thalamus (Fig. 19-14). While most of these fibers cross, some turn to join the lateral lemniscus of the same side. The cells of origin of these fibers are presumed to be the large, spindle-shaped cells that are so distinctive in this nuclear group. The remaining efferent connections of the nuclei are shorter internuncial units that are impossible to establish with certainty in man. Based on experimental forms, these connections probably include: (1) fibers from the ventral cochlear nucleus to the superior olive of the same side and (less certainly) the opposite side via the trapezoid body; (2) fibers from both nuclei via the trapezoid body to the trapezoid nucleus of the opposite side; (3) a crossing bundle above the trapezoid body (commissure of Held) that passes from both the dorsal and ventral nucleus to the opposite side; (4) fibers from the dorsal cochlear nucleus directly into the lateral lemniscus of the same side; and (5) a short-chain relay system ascending via the reticular formation (Fig. 19-14). The origin of fibers feeding into the cochlear nuclei is even less certain than the distribution patterns. It is generally accepted however that a descending pathway, probably with multiple relays, bears on the cochlear nuclei and adds to the effective regulation of auditory input.

SUPERIOR OLIVARY AND TRAPEZOID COMPLEX

As the name implies, the superior olivary complex lies superior to the inferior olive in the lower part of the pons. The dimensions of the nucleus are roughly 7 mm. (longitudinal) by 5 mm. (side to

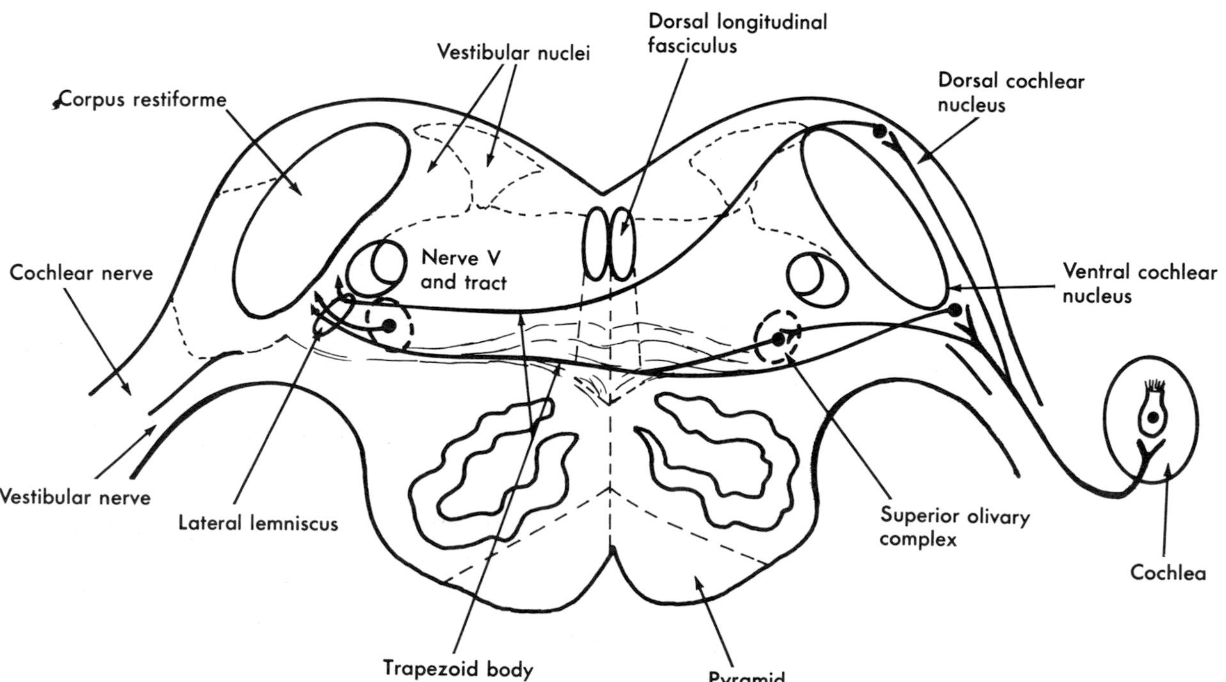

Fig. 19-15. Diagram of connections of cochlear nuclei and origin of lateral lemniscus.

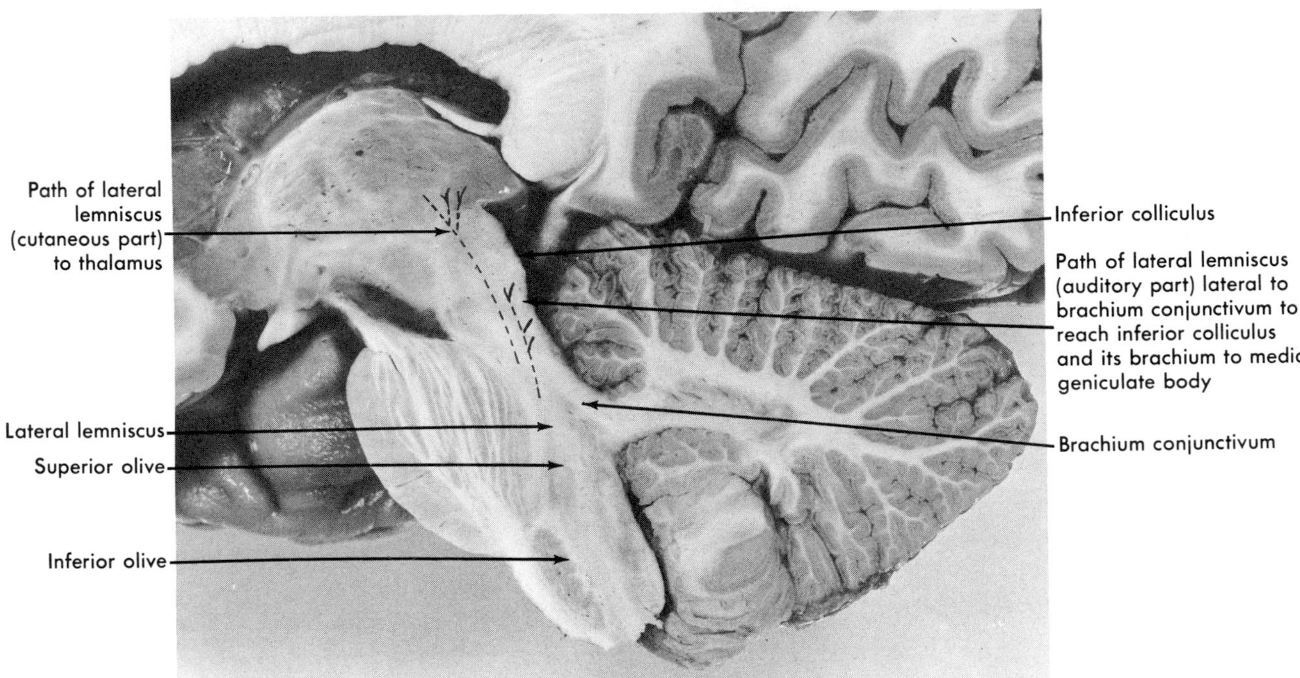

Fig. 19-16. Parasagittal section through superior olive showing longitudinal pattern of lateral lemniscus.

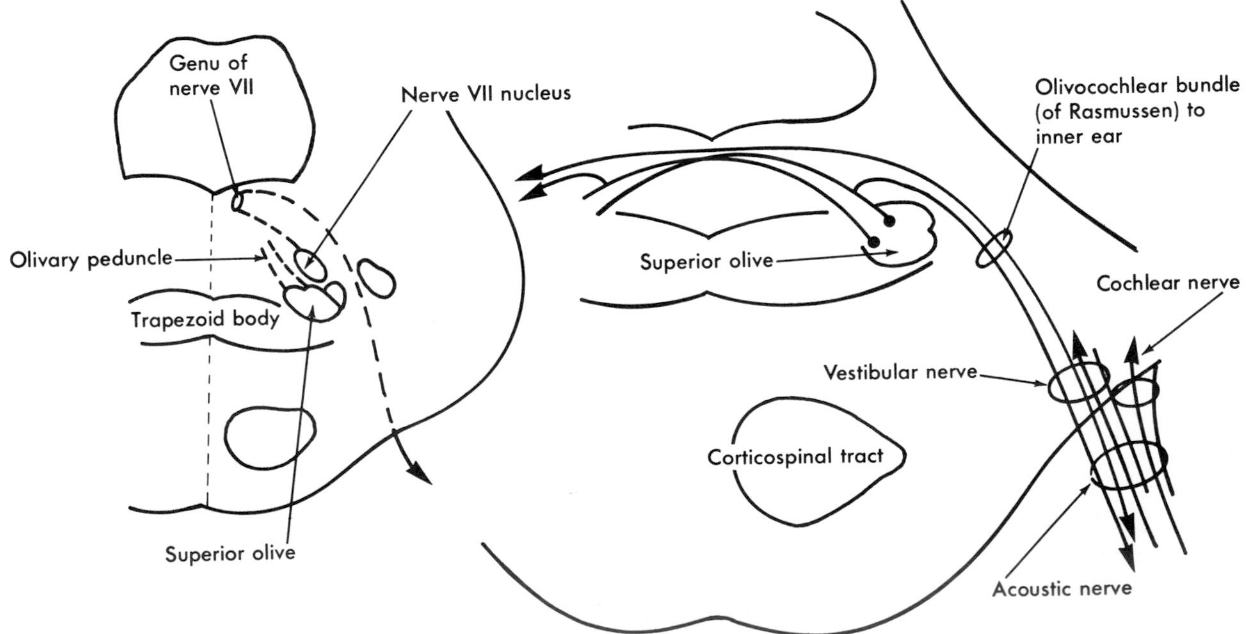

Fig. 19-17. Diagram of superior olivary complex and probable relationship of olivocochlear bundle.

side) by 4 mm. (dorsoventral) in maximum dimensions. It can be delineated in parasagittal brainstem section approximately 1 cm. lateral to midline, and in transverse section through the lower pons at the level of the cerebellar incisure, approximately midway between the origin of cranial nerve V and the lower border of the pons (Fig. 19-15). Its relationships to the tegmentum of the pons and to the lateral lemniscus stand out clearly in parasaggital section (Fig. 19-16). In transverse section the nuclear complex lies just medial to the terminal nucleus of cranial nerve V (trigeminal) and ventral to the nucleus of origin of cranial nerve VII (facial) (Fig. 19-17). Chow has estimated the number of cells in the superior olivary complex of the Rhesus monkey at 34,300.[6]

In finer detail, the human superior olivary complex is made up of at least three nuclear groups: (1) superior olive (lateral superior olive); (2) accessory superior olive (medial superior olive); and (3) nucleus of the trapezoid body. These nuclei vary greatly in their configurations, depending upon the level of sectioning (Fig. 19-17). The nuclear groups representing the superior olive proper in man probably are equivalent to the medial olivary group in animals, which display these nuclei more conspicuously. As sections are carried superiorly the nuclei come in close apposition to the ventral components of the ipsilateral nucleus of the lateral lemniscus. The nucleus of the trapezoid body lies ventral and on either side of the inferior half of the superior olive and is closely related by function. Among the cells comprising the superior olivary complex, at least two configurations stand out clearly: (1) those of the lateral superior nucleus and the trapezoid nucleus, which are characteristically round and plump and possess short processes; and (2) those of the medial superior olive, which are characteristically flattened and are spindle- to crescent-shaped. Malone regards the medial group, which is characterized by elongate flattened cells, as representing a visceral efferent-type nucleus (equivalent to autonomic final-common-path cells, such as in the spinal cord intermediolateral column).

Connections of the superior olivary complex

While the connections of the superior olive are based on anatomic studies in lower forms (particularly pigeon, cat, and primate), the following inferences are suggested for the nucleus in man. This complex may serve as a primary receptive center for incoming fibers from the cochlear nerve, and in this way joins the dorsal and ventral cochlear nuclei as a group. This pattern of cochlear nerve termination is represented in Rasmussen's auditory pathway[18] and probably must be considered to be a relationship to the nucleus of the trapezoid body (lateral part). Secondary receptive activity from cochlear sources certainly comes from both dorsal and ventral cochlear nuclei, with the ipsilateral fibers terminating in the lateral superior olive. The contralateral fibers, as well as those that are ipsilateral, terminate in the medial superior olivary nucleus.[21] It is probable that each nuclear group receives commissural fibers from the same nucleus of the opposite side, and there probably are intranuclear exchanges. Afferent fibers to the complex also arrive from more superior auditory pathway nuclei, and many of these connections probably arises in the auditory cortex (corticocifugal) and descend by many relays. It is common to assume that some of this transfer from higher centers is conveyed via the reticular formation to the superior olivary complex.[13,18] Some evidence, particularly electrophysiologic data, suggests that the route of transfer is extrareticular and probably close to, but separate from, the known ascending pathways. In addition, it probably has fewer synaptic relays.

Fibers that arise in the superior olivary complex are commonly represented as major contributors to the ascending auditory pathway. These relays travel via the trapezoid body to the opposite side and ascend directly up the lateral lemniscus of the same side. Relays are effected in the opposite superior olive, in the nuclei of the lateral lemnisci (dorsal and ventral) on both sides, and in the inferior colliculi. A few fibers appear to go directly to the geniculate bodies as the thalamic representatives of the pathway. Some fibers extend inferiorly from the complex to the upper spinal cord.[18] The efferent groups listed in the preceding paragraph appear to arise in the lateral superior olivary nucleus (at least in the cat) and probably in the bordering cells of the complex. The complex apparently contributes to the nucleus of nerve VI mainly through cells of origin in the nucleus of the trapezoid body. The relationship to the medial longitudinal fasciculus does not appear to be direct, but is assumed to exist through the reticular formation relays.

Olivary peduncle

Of particular importance is the efferent bundle arising from the superior olivary complex as the olivary peduncle (Fig. 19-17). In the human this bundle extends dorsally from the complex to the region of the floor of the fourth ventricle near the nerve VI nucleus and the genu of nerve VII. The fibers decussate to join the opposite vestibular nerve[18] and are believed to constitute the olivocochlear bundle of Rasmussen by joining the cochlear nerve via the vestibulocochlear anastomosis. Rasmussen has suggested that these fibers arise as visceral efferent carriers from the cells of the medial superior olivary nucleus and probably supply the cochlea itself, vasculature, or glands in this distribution area (Fig. 19-17). It has thus far been impossible to trace these fibers to their terminations by direct methods either experimentally or in man. Nonetheless, the possibility exists that these fibers do in fact extend to the inner ear, and Rasmussen[18] has adopted the notion that they might represent efferent innervation of hair cells. This is consistent with the fact that two types of fibers, coarse and fine, end in synaptic relationship with the hair cells. In addition, evidence in the cat points to the probable fact that the olivocochlear bundle terminates on the hair cells of the organ of Corti.[19] The idea is however not entirely supported by physiologic evidence.

With general agreement that an efferent bundle passes from the olivary complex to the cochlea via the cochlear nerve, there has been a concentrated effort to establish the function of such a bundle. The suggested functions include visceral efferent influence governing vascular or glandular action; influence directed to general or special metabolism of the cochlea; some neural process bearing on perception of sound; some process directly related to hearing; indirect effects related to responses through middle ear muscle activity; and an extension to the cochlea of gating influence on audi-

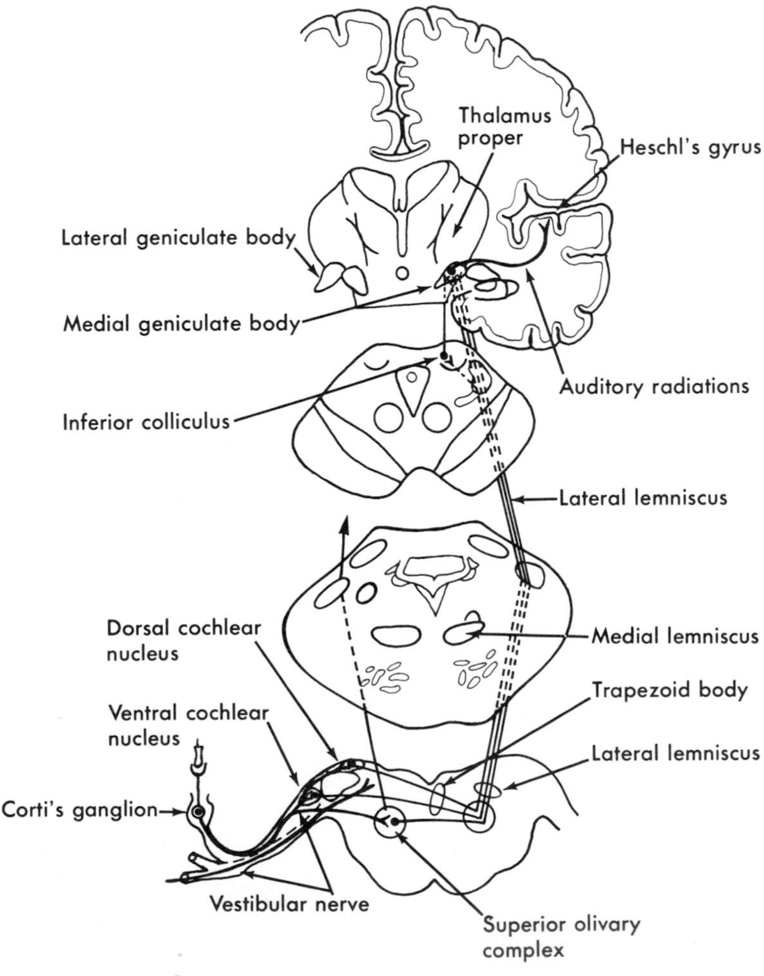

Fig. 19-18. Auditory pathway in diagram.

tory input as an effect arising in higher auditory centers. While both anatomic and electrophysiologic studies support the existence of Rasmussen's bundle and its profound effect on auditory input, its exact nature in man is not yet established. The central regulation of acustic input is undoubtedly remarkably complex and involves at least a corticocifugal feedback mechanism, which probably utilizes both the superior olivary complex and the cochlear nuclei in its relays.

LATERAL LEMNISCUS AND NUCLEI

The main ascending bundle in the auditory pathway is the lateral lemniscus (Fig. 19-18). To summarize, this tract probably receives contributions from the dorsal cochlear nuclei of both sides, from the ventral cochlear nucleus of the opposite side, and from the nuclei of the trapezoid bodies and the superior olives of both sides. The major source in bulk appears to be the trapezoid body, which abruptly turns superiorly on either side to continue as the lateral lemniscus. The nuclei of the lateral lemniscus serve as relay neurons in the ascending auditory pathway. It is possible that these nuclei relay impulses orginating in cochlear nuclei only. The nuclei of the lateral lemniscus occur in two major groups of cells, the *ventral,* which is the inferior group (two-thirds of the length of the nucleus), and the *dorsal,* which lies superiorly and dorsally and occupies the upper third of the cell mass. This latter nucleus lies close to the inferior colliculus (Fig. 19-18). In the Rhesus monkey there are 38,100 cells in the nuclei of the lateral lemniscus on one side.[6] The lateral lemniscus principally terminates in the homolateral inferior colliculus, but some fibers continue to the medial geiculate body without relay via the brachium of the inferior colliculus. There are probable interconnections side to side (between nuclei of the lateral lemniscus, particularly the dorsal), and some of the fibers cross in ascending to the inferior colliculus of the opposite side via the commissure of Probst. Corticocifugal relays of the descending auditory pathways probably course in the lateral lemniscus to terminate in the superior olive and possibly in the cochlear nuclei.[18]

INFERIOR COLLICULUS

The largest and most complex of the nuclei in the auditory system is the inferior colliculus. The cells of this nucleus in the Rhesus monkey are estimated to number 392,000.[6] The nucleus is bilaterally imposed in the ascending pathway as the major receptor of impulses transmitted through the lat-

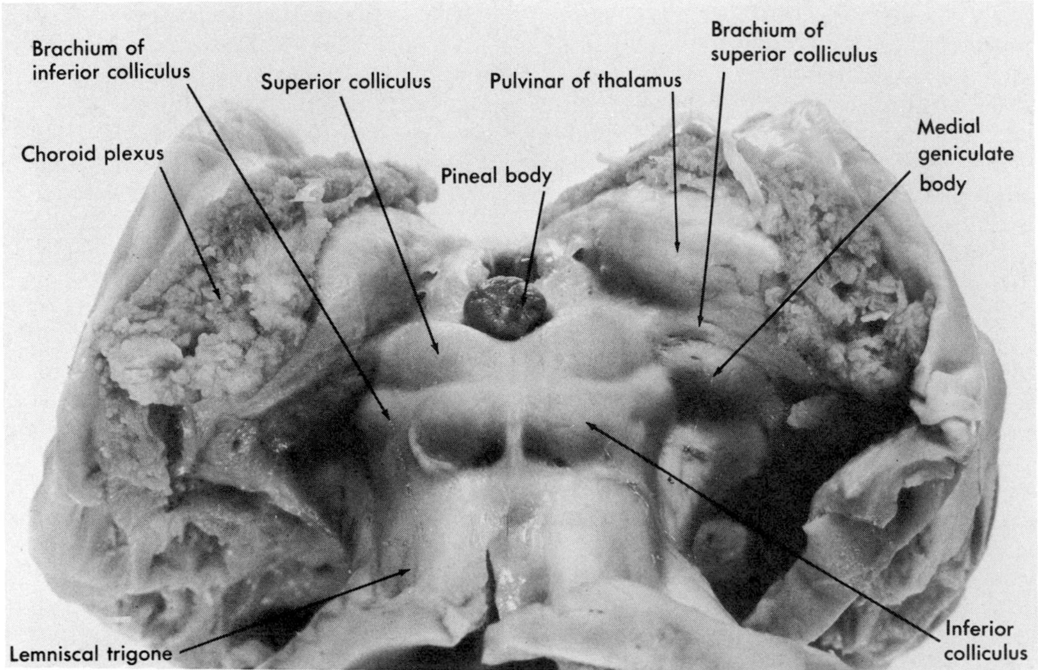

Fig. 19-19. Gross relationships of inferior colliculus, its brachium, and the medial geniculate body.

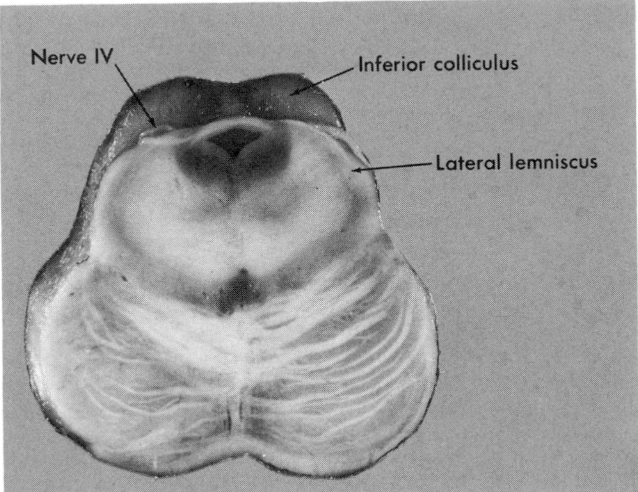

Fig. 19-20. Location of lateral lemniscus immediately below the inferior colliculus.

eral lemniscus. It projects to the medial geniculate body via the *brachium of the inferior colliculus* (Fig. 19-19). The inferior colliculus thus houses third-order (or higher) neurons of the major auditory pathway. The entering fibers from the lateral lemniscus spread over the nucleus in capsular form (especially ventrolateral) and enter at various levels. Some (probably few) of the lemniscal fibers pass the colliculus and go directly to the medial geniculate body via the brachium. An *intercollicular commissure* connects the two inferior colliculi, through which the ascending fibers from one side impinge on both nuclei (Fig. 19-20). This interrelationship of the two colliculi seems well established, but the volume of the bilateral transfer remains in doubt. A very few fibers from the lateral lemniscus may cross in the inferior intercollicular commissure and continue without relay via the branchium to the auditory cortex of the opposite side. Other possible efferent connections of the inferior colliculus include fibers to the superior colliculus, fibers to the nuclei of the pons, and contributions to the tectobular and tectospinal tracts, by which auditory influences are presumed to be imparted to eye, head, and trunk movements. The tectocerebellar tract imparts collicular influences to the cerebellum via the anterior medullary velum. There is probably also a returning cerebellotectal tract of uncertain cellular origin.

The inferior colliculus is characterized by dense cellularity, both neural and glial with prominent satelliting. The cell masses of the two sides fuse at midline dorsal to the central canal and in this area blend with the central gray matter. The human nuclei present no noticeable lamination or organization, and the cellular display in section seems quite haphazard. The cells are concentrated in a central area, the chief nucleus, in which two types can be distinguished, small spindle or pyramidal cells and medium-sized oval or triangular cells. Marginally the cells are less densely intermingled with the capsular strands of nerve fibers (Fig. 19-20).

It is evident that the inferior colliculi function in more than relay and reflex patterns. The nuclei not only start projections to the cortex via the thalamus, but probably also receive fibers from the cortex and play a role in the descending auditory pathway. Such descending paths from the inferior colliculus may be routed via the superior colliculus in man. From the distribution pattern of ascending fibers entering the colliculus, it has been assumed that the nucleus may display a spatial mechanism for tone reception. This finding would correspond to that in the cat. The complex interrelationships of the inferior colliculus and the superior colliculus serve to tie audiovisual relays, reflexes, and intergrative acts together at a subcortical level.

MEDIAL GENICULATE BODY

All ascending impulses from the lower auditory pathway probably relay through the medial geniculate body en route to the cortex (Fig. 19-21). A few exceptions in direct colliculocortical tracts have been claimed, but these are certainly quantitatively unimportant. This segment of the thalamus is thus generally accepted as the origin of the auditory radiations reaching the auditory cortex. These fibers course laterally from the geniculate body, pass through the sublenticular and retrolenticular portion of the internal capsule, and reach the auditory cortex by passing inferior to the insula (Fig. 19-22). The main supply of ascending fibers reaching the medial geniculate body is via the *brachium of the inferior colliculus.* These fibers arise for the most part in the cells of the inferior colliculus. Less certain is the origin of the relatively few fibers reaching the geniculate body via the brachium that do not arise in the inferior colliculus. Some of these may arise in the cochlear nuclei of both sides and possibly from the superior olivary complexes. These are undoubtedly numerically important, since the distal part of the brachium carries approximately a third more fibers than the proximal part.[9] Some direct connection exists between the lateral lemniscus and the medial geniculate body, and it is logical to include the

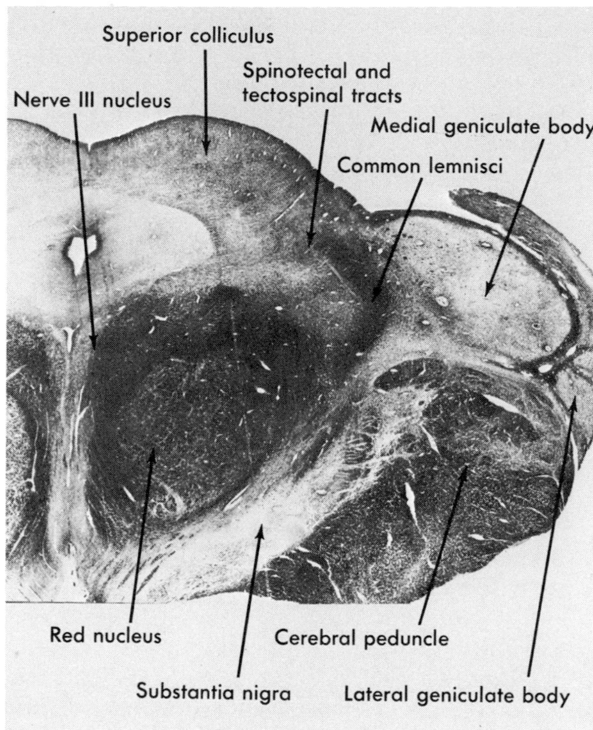

Fig. 19-21. Brainstem at level of medial geniculate body.

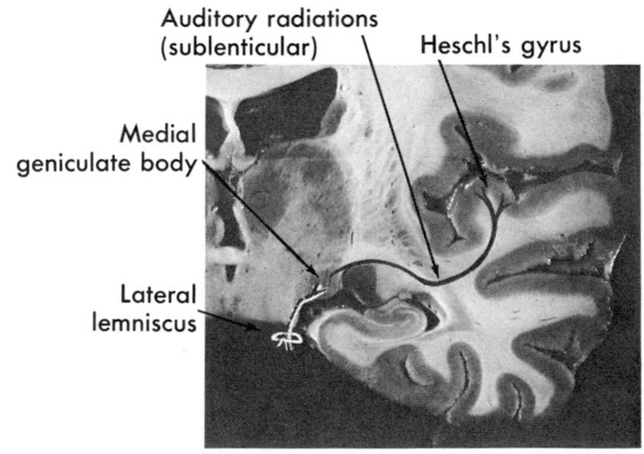

Fig. 19-22. Auditory radiations from medial geniculate body to Heschl's gyrus.

nuclei of the lateral lemniscus as possible sources of these fibers. In addition to the ascending bundles reaching the medial geniculate body, *descending fibers* from the auditory cortex terminate in the nucleus (corticogeniculate tract). The two nuclei interconnect through the *commissure of Gudden,* which courses with the optic tracts and optic chiasm from side to side. This commissure is incon-

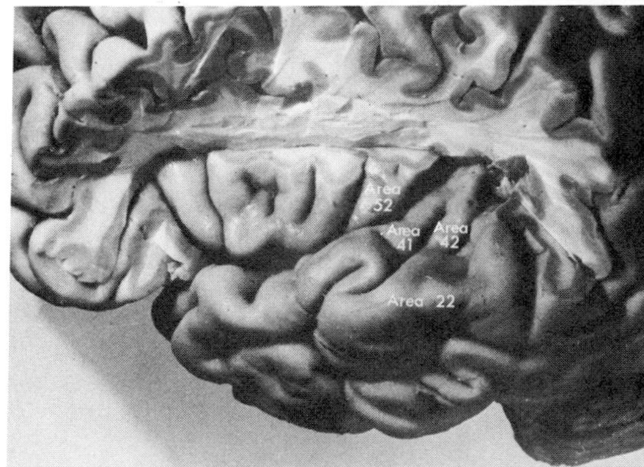

Fig. 19-23. Auditory cortex and related gyri. Overhanging frontoparietal tissue removed.

spicuous in man. The vestibular complex may be anatomically related to the geniculate body, but the paths remain obscure in man.

The histologic makeup of the medial geniculate body is divided in primates into the main small and medium-sized cellular concentration (*parvicellular nucleus*) in the dorsomedial part and a large-celled concentration (*magnocellular*) in the ventrolateral part. Small granular nerve cells are liberally sprinkled throughout the human geniculate body. The function of these cell types has not been determined for man, but experimental evidence in the cat suggests that they terminate in the homolateral gyrus of Heschl. The magnocellular component probably also projects to the primary auditory cortex as sustaining fibers and to secondary auditory cortical fields in the adjoining temporal and insural cortex (Fig. 19-23).

The structural details of the human medial geniculate body have been worked out by Jaeger and others.[12] The neurocellular complement numbers over 800,000 on each side, with slightly more on the right. The cellular density is 16,000 to 17,000 per cu. mm. Glial cells average 67,000 to 72,000 per cu. mm. The nuclei measure 9.5 by 5 mm. to 10 by 5.5 mm. and are slightly larger on the right. The volume varies from 36 to 68 cu. mm. No strong patterning or major cellular groupings appear in the human nucleus, although the larger cells tend to localize in the lateral and ventrolateral aspect (Fig. 19-21).

Thalamic level consciousness for pitch recognition probably exists in the medial geniculate body in man as well as cat. This is possibly established by cellular spatial representation within the main nucleus in a pattern reduplicating the pickup in the cochlea. Thus, low frequencies go to the inferior portion of the nucleus in cat, and the high frequencies travel to the dorsal region. Intermediate pitches are represented in an ascending spiral pattern between these extremes. This differential in pitch representation probably projects to the cortex (tonotopic pattern). It is important to recognize that hearing loss is slight or absent with unilateral destruction of the medial geniculate body. This fact illustrates the prominent bilateral representation in the auditory pathway at this level.

AUDITORY CORTEX

There is general agreement that the posterior, obliquely transverse gyri (of Heschl) on the superior surface of the temporal lobe are the primary auditory cortical centers (Fig. 19-23). Campain and others have shown remarkable variability in the gross configuration of the area.[5] It is therefore difficult to assign numbers to the various areas, but in general the numbering for topographic identity is that shown in Fig. 19-23. Presumably the thalamic radiations from the parvicellular portion of the medial geniculate body in the cat go to the equivalent of gyrus 41. Bordering zones, including adjacent insula and superior temporal gyri (both 52 and 22), are also auditory and probably correspond to the secondary auditory areas of lower mammals, which are supplied by the magnocellular part of the geniculate bodies. It has been noted that the geniculate architecture in the cat has no counterpart in man.[12] Massive lesions of the temporal lobe in man do correlate with retrograde effect in the geniculate body, but the individual cell distribution pattern is not known.[14] Efferent projections from the auditory cortex go to the medial geniculate body and the inferior colliculus of the same side *(corticogeniculate and corticotectal tracts).* There are numerous short association fibers between primary and secondary auditory cortical areas. Association fibers also go to the postcentral gyrus, the insula, and the inferior frontal gyri (Broca's area). The area also connects directly to frontal eye fields in primates. Commissural fibers connect one auditory area with its opposite through the corpus callosum. The secondary auditory areas (52, 42, and 22) also interconnect widely on both homolateral and contralateral sides.

The use of arbitrary reference numbers to identify cortical areas has been generally adopted for convenience and commonly follows the scheme of Brodmann (Fig. 21-7, p. 353). By this reference method the primary auditory area in the human brain is designated 41, which is the anterior gyrus of Heschl (Fig. 19-23). Area 42 is less certainly related and is sometimes called *para-auditory.* The secondary auditory areas (if some exist in man that match those of cats and primates) are designated area 52 (on the anterior insular border of area 41) and area 22 (on the temporal lobe side of the auditory area in the superior temporal gyrus) (Fig. 19-23).[5] If the primate parallel applies to man, the spatial pitch representation *(tonotopic pattern)* in area 41 (and 42?) would exhibit low tones localizing to the anterolateral portion and high tones to the posteromedial area. Similarly, if the parallel persists, the secondary areas (52?, 42?, and 22?) would exhibit a reversal in tonotopic pattern.

THE COMMISSURAL SYSTEM

Bilateral representation of auditory sensations is so striking that deafness does not occur on either side from unilateral lesions in the pathway above the cochlear nuclei. Slight diminution in acuity may occur on the side opposite the lesion, although even this is hard to demonstrate and difficult to interpret. This bilaterality is accomplished through the abundant crossings of the auditory pathways. In summary, these commissures include the following: (1) The *trapezoid body* conveys fibers from the olivary complex, trapezoid nucleus, and cochlear nuclei to the opposite lateral lemniscus. (2) The *commissure of Held* carries secondary fibers from the cochlear nuclei and superior olive to the opposite lateral lemniscus above the level of the trapezoid body. (3) The *commissure of Probst* crosses between the dorsal nuclei of the lateral lemnisci and carries fibers from these nuclei to the inferior colliculus and medial geniculate body of the opposite side. (4) The *inferior intercollicular commissure* interconnects the colliculi and probably carries crossing fibers from one colliculus to the opposite medial geniculate body. (5) The medial geniculate bodies interconnect through the *commissure of Gudden,* which passes with the optic tracts and chiasm. This is probably not important in man. (6) The *corpus callosum* interconnects the auditory fields on either side (probably areas 41, 42, and 22) by fibers that pass inferior to the insula and ascend to the commissure via the extreme capsule. Some fibers from area 22 pass via the tapetum to the posterior part of the callosal body. It is probable that the callosal fibers arise from infragranular cells and terminate in the supragranular layers of the opposite side (Fig. 19-19).

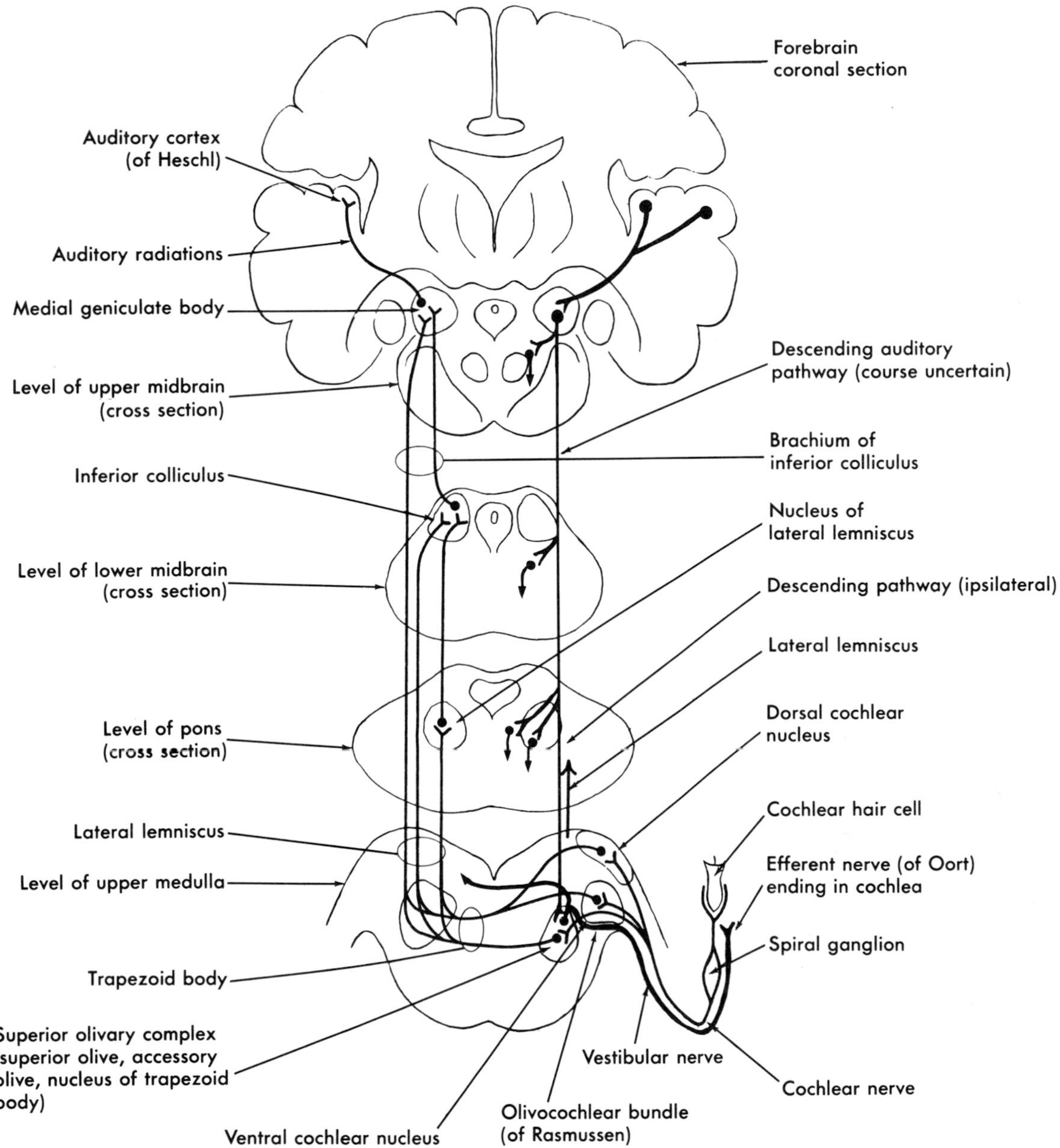

Fig. 19-24. Summary diagram of central auditory system with efferent system added on right.

THE DESCENDING AUDITORY CONDUCTION SYSTEM

The existence of a conduction chain from cortex to cochlea seems well established on experimental grounds. The anatomic features of this system and the function of each unit in man remain to be disclosed. Based on experimental studies of both anatomic and physiologic type it seems certain that projections from the primary auditory cortex (areas 41 and probably 42) and from secondary cortical area 22 pass to the medial geniculate body and inferior colliculus. The superior colliculus and pulvinar probably also receive fibers from the associational area 22, but these tracts are presumed to bear on audiovisual subcortical relays and integrative function rather than being directly concerned with the descending auditory pathway. Attention is focused on the inferior colliculus as a major corticocifugal way station in the descending auditory pathway. Relays presumably occur in the nuclei of the lateral lemniscus (particularly dorsal), and the main anatomic descending pathway is along the medial aspect of the lateral lemniscus (Monakow's bundle). Other short-chain descending paths with numerous relays are presumed to be available via the reticular formation and from both geniculate bodies and colliculi to the various brainstem nuclei. The short-chain systems eventually appear to terminate in the superior olive and cochlear nuclei. Unequivocal electrophysiologic demonstrations of these pathways remain to be disclosed, although reasonable certainty attends their structural existence (Fig. 19-24).

The terminations of the descending pathways, regardless of route, seem quite certainly to be in the nuclei of the trapezoid body, the superior olive, and (either directly or secondarily through these nuclei) to the cochlear nuclei. These patterns are known to exists in cats,[13,18] where they bring the upper auditory system in synaptic relation ship to the better-known olivocochlear system of fibers. This system (Rasmussen's bundle) arises in the cat in the superior olive and passing dorsally divides into a crossed component (eighty percent of the fibers) and a homolateral component (twenty percent of the fibers). The crossed bundle joins the vestibular fibers of the opposite nerve VIII, picking up the opposite homolateral component en route. These efferent fibers are probably joined by additional efferent fibers from the cochlear nuclei, and then they proceed to the cochlea along the acoustic nerve (Fig. 19-17). Along the nerve root the fibers remain a distinct bundle, which gradually adheres to the cochlear division (vestibulocochlear anastomosis) to enter the modiolus as the *bundle of Oort* (Fig. 18-5).

The intracochlear course of the efferent bundle is variously described as forming the spiral bundles of the cochlea, as winding around the spiral fibers, as carrying to the hair cells, and as being obscure. The existence of two types of nerve endings (heavily and lightly granulated) related to the hair cells has excited speculation and experimentation to determine if one of these might be an efferent synaptic contact. Special staining, degenerations, electrophysiologic, pharmacologic, and electron microscopic studies have thus far failed to establish the relationship with certainty.

REFERENCES

1. Ades, H. W.: Central auditory mechanisms. In The American Physiologic Society: Handbook of physiology, vol. I, Washington, D. C., 1959.
2. Austin, J. H., and Sakai, M.: Corpora amylacea. In Minckler, J., editor: Pathology of the nervous system, vol. III, New York, 1971, McGraw-Hill Book Co.
3. von Bekesy, G.: Experiments in hearing, New York, 1960, McGraw-Hill Book Co.
4. Boedberg, G.: Cellular pattern and nerve supply of the human organ of Corti, Acta Otolaryng. Suppl. **236**, 1968.
5. Campain, R., Jaeger, M., and Minckler, J.: The auditory cortex, Thesis. University of Denver, 1970.
6. Chow, K. L.: Numerical estimates of the auditory central nervous system of the Rhesus monkey, J. Comp. Neurol. **94**:159, 1951.
7. Crace, R., Jaeger, M., and Minckler, J.: The cochlear nuclei of man, Thesis, University of Denver, 1968.
8. Engstrom, H., Ades, H., and Hawkins, J.: Structure and functions of the sensory hairs of the inner ear, J. Acoust. Soc. Amer. **23**:1356, 1962.
9. Ferraro, J., Jaeger, M., and Minckler, J.: The brachium of the inferior colliculus, Thesis, University of Denver, 1969.
10. Hawkins, J. E.: Antibiotics and the cochlea, J. Acoust. Soc. Amer. **24**:448, 1952.
11. Igarashi, M.: Pathology of the inner ear end organs. In Minckler, J., editor: Pathology of the nervous system, vol. III, New York, 1971, McGraw-Hill Book Co.
12. Jaeger, M., Crace, R., and Minckler, J.: A quantitative study of the human medial geniculate body, Thesis University of Denver, 1967.
13. Lorente de Nó, R.: Anatomy of the eighth nerve, Laryngoscope **43**:1 and 327, 1933.
14. Minckler, J.: Communication disorders. In Minckler, J., editor: Pathology of the nervous system, vol. III, New York, 1971, McGraw-Hill Book Co.
15. Olszewski, J., and Baxter, D.: Cytoarchitecture of the human brain stem, Philadelphia, 1954, J. B. Lippincott Co.
16. Powers, M., and Minckler, J.: The eighth nerve of man, Thesis, University of Denver, 1968.
17. Rasmussen, A. T.: Studies on the VIIIth cranial nerve of man, Laryngoscope **50**:67, 1940.
18. Rasmussen, G.: Anatomical relationships of the ascending and descending auditory system. In Fields, W. S., and Alford, B., editors: Neurological aspects of auditory and vestibular disorders, Springfield, Illinois, 1964, Charles C Thomas, Publisher.
19. Schuknecht, H. F., and Woellner, R. C.: Hearing loss following partial section of the cochlear nerve, Laryngoscope **63**:441, 1953.
20. Spoendlin, H. H., and Gacek, R. R.: Electronmicroscopic study of the efferent and afferent innervation of the organ of Corti in the cat, Ann. Otol. **72**:660, 1963.
21. Stotler, W. A.: An experimental study of the cells and connections of the superior olivary complex, J. Comp. Neurol. **98**:401, 1953.
22. Wever, E. G.: Theory of hearing, New York, 1957, John Wiley & Sons, Inc.
23. Zemlin, W. R.: Speech and hearing science, Englewood Cliffs, New Jersey, 1968, Prentice-Hall Inc.

CHAPTER 20

VISUAL SYSTEM

JEFF MINCKLER

Commonly regarded as the most valued and important among the special senses, the visual system contributes enormously to all sensory input. Vision and audition relate particularly to language and writing, which are the specifically human associated motor acts of symbolic expression. The visual system (with the auditory system) therefore takes on special meaning in human neuroanatomy. Binocular vision is a product not only of light transfer through the refractive media of the eye and stimulation of a train of neural events, but also a product of remarkably coordinated neuromuscular acts that move the eyeballs and effect changes in focal depth. The basic neurology of vision therefore includes the innervation of the eyeball and its muscles and the modifiers of the refractive path, as well as the structure and function of the light-sensitive retina and the central neural pathways. Of lesser importance to vision, but of major neurologic importance, are the orbital and periorbital neuromuscular sets, including the eyelids.

ORBITAL REGION

The periorbital muscles and muscles of the lids impart significant facial expression and function in protection of the eye. Cranial nerve VII supplies the periorbital muscles. *Orbicularis oculi* is an eliptical muscle that surrounds the eye in palpebral, orbital, and lacrimal divisions. Contraction closes the eye, stretches the skin of the forehead, and probably compresses the lacrimal gland. The lateral margin of the orbital part aids in producing radiating wrinkles. While the muscle is principally attached to skin, it also applies to the orbital margin in part and to the tarsal plate of the upper lid. The *corrugator* muscle arises from bone near the frontonasal suture and inserts into the skin of the brow. Its contraction produces vertical wrinkles of the forehead (frowning). The *procerus* muscle arises from the nasal bone and associated cartilage and inserts in skin over the root of the nose. It draws the skin of the forehead down and wrinkles the skin across the root of the nose. The foregoing muscles are among the most expressive and operate in closing the lids, forcing tears by compressing the lacrimal gland, dilating the lacrimal sac and affecting the venous plexus of the lacrimal sac, stretching and furrowing the forehead (surprise, frowning), making transverse furrows at the base of the nose in expression of fierceness, and producing "crow's feet" at the orbital margins in expressing joviality.

Eyelids

The *levator palpebrae superioris* arises from the roof of the orbit and inserts in an aponeurosis that contributes three layers to the upper lid: (1) one layer to the deep surface of the skin of the lid, (2) one to the upper margin of the tarsal plate, and (3) a layer to the upper fornix of the conjunctiva. The second layer is smooth muscle and sustains the open lid involuntarily. The first and third layers elevate the lid voluntarily. The striated muscles of layers 1 and 3 are innervated by cranial nerve III (*oculomotor*). The middle smooth muscle layer (Mueller's tarsal muscle) is supplied by sympathetic nerves arising in the superior cervical ganglion (Fig. 20-1). The lower lid possesses no tarsal plate and operates primarily through the action of the orbicularis. Scattered smooth muscle fibers occur in the region of the infraorbital groove as the inferior orbital muscle of Mueller. The function is unknown. These smooth fibers, like the

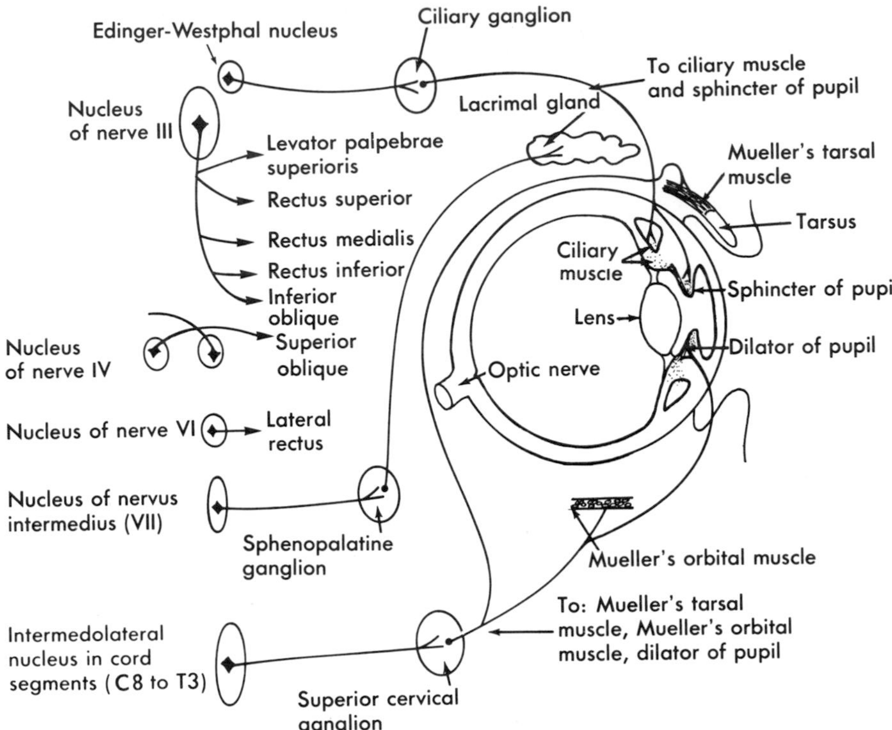

Fig. 20-1. Efferent innervation of eye.

tarsal muscle, are supplied by sympathetic fibers from cervical ganglia via carotid, cavernous, and ophthalmic periarterial nerve plexuses.

Muscles of the eyeball

The *superior, inferior, medial, and lateral rectus muscles* arise from a fibrous ring that surrounds the optic foramen at the back of the orbit. These muscles insert on upper, lower, medial, and lateral surfaces of the sclera and respectively turn the eyeball up, down, medially, and laterally. The superior and inferior recti also rotate and adduct the eye by virtue of their attachment slightly medial to the vertical midplane of the eye. The superior, medial, and inferior recti are supplied by cranial nerve III (*oculomotor*), and the lateral rectus by cranial nerve VI (*abducens*). The *superior oblique muscle* arises above the optic foramen medial to the superior rectus, passes through a fibrous pulley (trochlea) attached at the upper medial margin of the orbit, and passes backward and laterally to insert into the sclera between the superior and lateral recti behind the orbital equator. It rotates the eyeball medially and turns the eyeball to look downward and laterally. The superior oblique muscle is innervated by cranial nerve IV (*trochlear*). The *inferior oblique muscle* arises from the floor of the orbit lateral to the nasolacrimal canal. It passes below the eye laterally to insert on the sclera between the superior and lateral recti, posterior to the superior oblique. It rotates the eye laterally and cooperates with the superior rectus in turning the eye upward. The inferior oblique is innervated by cranial nerve III (*oculomotor*). Binocular vision is dependent upon cooperative multimuscular activity coordinated in both eyes (Fig. 20-1).

EYEBALL

The eye displays remarkable developmental precocity and attains approximately half of adult stature by birth (birth volume, 3.4 cc.; adult volume 7.7 cc.). Seventy-two percent of the average adult diameter of 24 mm. is attained by birth. However, the lens continue to grow throughout life.[6] The remaining parts exhibit some differences in growth patterns, but in general they have a steady increase to adult size after the rapid prenatal spurt. The general structural features are illustrated in Figs. 20-2 and 20-3.

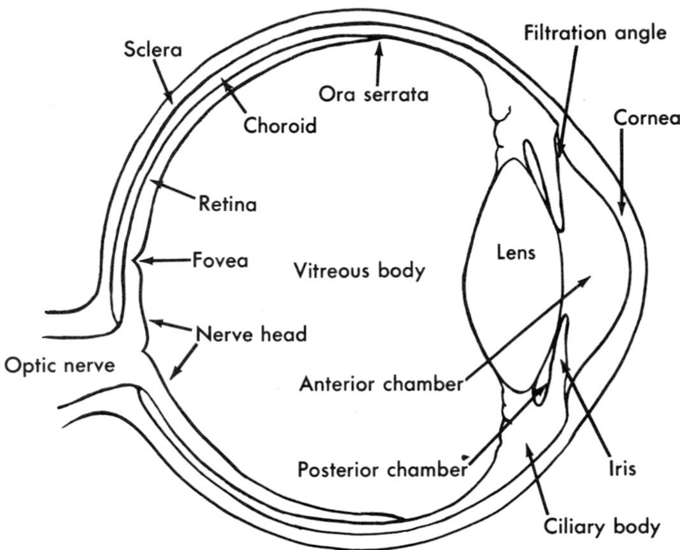

Fig. 20-2. Schematic of general anatomy of eye.

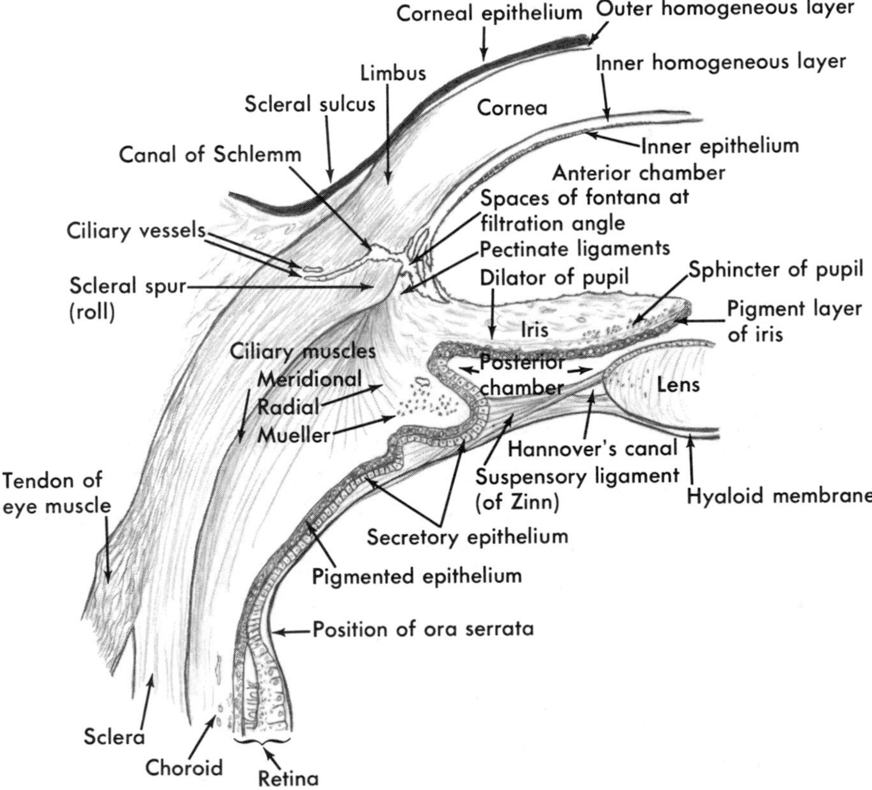

Fig. 20-3. Drawing of anterior part of eye.

Cornea

The transparent anterior sixth of the globe is the *cornea.* It measures 12 mm. horizontally by 11 mm. vertically on the average, and is 0.5 to 0.7 mm. in thickness. The cornea joins the sclera posteriorly at the *limbus,* which is a junctional zone about 1 mm. wide. The cornea is somewhat conical, with its greatest radius of curvature at the center. As a transparent light-transmitting component of the globe, the cornea is part of the refracting media (Figs. 20-2 and 20-3). The histologic make-up of the cornea is shown in Fig. 20-4. The outer epithelium is nonkeratinizing *stratified squamous* and is seated upon an *outer homogeneous lamina* (Bowman's membrane), which appears structureless under the light microscope. This membrane overlies the *substantia propria,* which makes up the main bulk (ninety percent) of the corneal thickness. The substantia propria contains corneal corpuscles, which are interspersed in approximately sixty parallel lamellae of fine collagenous fibrils in a matrix of hyaluronic acid sulfate. This substance serves to bind the collagen in this transparent part of the globe. The substance of the cornea is dry (compared to sclera, for example), and this feature may in part account for its transparency. On the deep surface the substantia propria is limited by an *inner homogeneous membrane* (of Descemet), which is covered on its inner surface by single-layered *inner epithelium* (Descemet's endothelium) of cuboidal cells. This inner layer is variously described as epithelium, mesothelium, and endothelium.

The cornea is avascular and possesses no lymphatics. It is therefore nourished by a transport mechanism involving the aqueous humor, which bathes the deep surface. The cornea possesses a rich nerve plexus that includes at least three types of nerves. Two types are coarse and are presumed to be sensory. They no doubt figure in the corneal protective reflexes (winking and lacrimal secretion) and are part of cranial nerve V distribution. These nerves are sometimes myelinated and show in a plexus pattern of considerable density. The third type of nerve is much finer and is presumed to be autonomic or trophic, although just what they innervate is not clearly understood. At the limbus extremity the corneal substance contains laminated corpuscles of the Kraus end-bulb type (see Chapter 16). Otherwise the endings are naked. They project into the outer epithelial layer from a subjacent plexus. The inner epithelium (Descemet's endothelium) does not appear to be supplied by nerves.

Of particular importance is the behavior of corneal tissue in homologous transplants. Because of the avascular character of the tissue and the restrictive barrier effect of the fluid supplying its metabolic needs, the cornea is unique in its transplantation and lack of rejection. Viable transplants lose both epithelial coverings very quickly, and these layers are replaced by host tissues in a matter of days. The stromal cells of the substantia propria apparently survive for long periods (years) and are only very slowly replaced by host tissue responses.

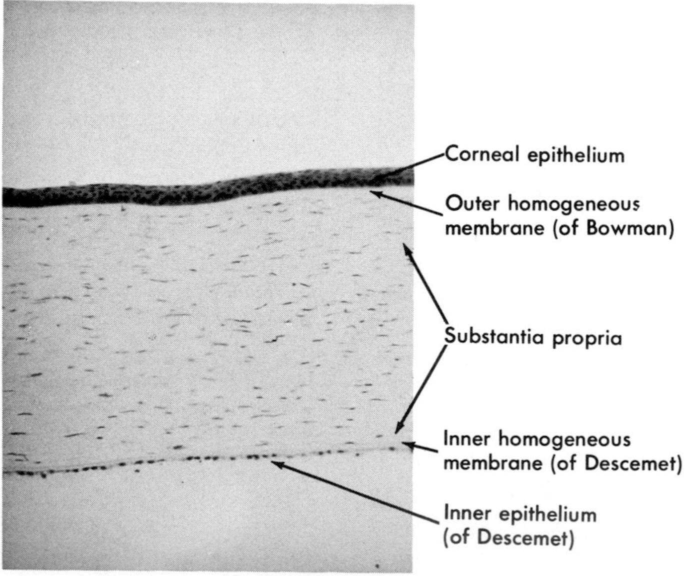

Fig. 20-4. Cornea.

Sclera

The dense, tough, opaque tissue (0.4 to 0.8 mm. thick) continuing posteriorly from the cornea is the sclera. This tissue is continuous with the dura mater, which wraps the optic nerve. Close to the limbus the sclera is thickened with a projection that is spur-like in section and extends inwardly as the scleral roll (or spur) (Figs. 20-3 and 20-5). Similar to dura mater, the sclera is made up of dense collagenous fibers containing flattened fibrocytes. At various places over its surface the sclera receives tendinous attachments from the ocular muscles. The deep surface relates to the choroid coat, where pigmented cells (lamina fusca) can be distinguished within scleral substance (Fig. 20-11). The sclera possesses a higher water content than the cornea, and dehydrating the sclera locally will produce transparency. Near the limbus the sclera possesses a circumferential depression where the cornea begins to project. This depression forms the *outer scleral sulcus.* Opposing this depression on the inner surface is a similar *inner scleral sulcus,* just on the corneal side of the scleral roll. At the posterior part of the globe at the optic nerve head the sclera forms a sieve-like disk (*lamina cribrosa*), which provides the holes for exit of the optic nerve fibers. At this point the nerves entering the disk make a 90 degree flexion turn. These nerves are supported at this site by a glial fiber (special spider glial cells from the optic disk) that overlies the disk with a wicker basket-like covering.

The sclera has few capillaries, but it is penetrated by fairly large arteries and veins. Arteries enter through the lamina cribrosa (central artery of retina) and through the posterior part of the globe (ciliary arteries). Venous return is via vortex veins, which leave the sclera anterior to the coronal equator of the globe. Nerves enter the sclera with the ciliary vessels. These fibers are trigeminal and protective.

Trabecula and filtration angle

A circumferential trabecular system bridges the angle of reflection between the corneoscleral junction and the base of the iris (Fig. 20-3). This *corneoscleral trabecula* occurs as a complex fine meshwork where the inner homogeneous membrane of Descemet terminates laterally (Schwalbe's line). The meshwork perforations (spaces of Fontana) relate to the scleral spur on its anterior aspect and eventually fuse peripherally in a circumferential venous sinus (canal of Schlemm). The filaments of the trabecula provide the *pectinate ligaments* at the *filtration angle* (Fig. 20-6). In this area the fluid of the anterior chamber (aqueous

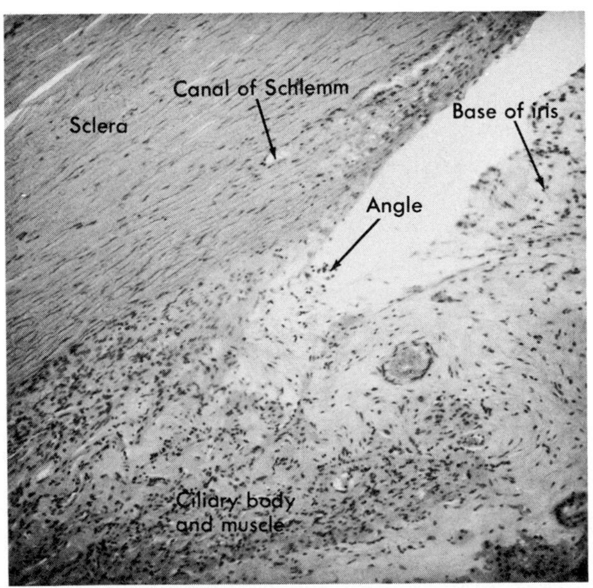

Fig. 20-5. Detail at filtration angle.

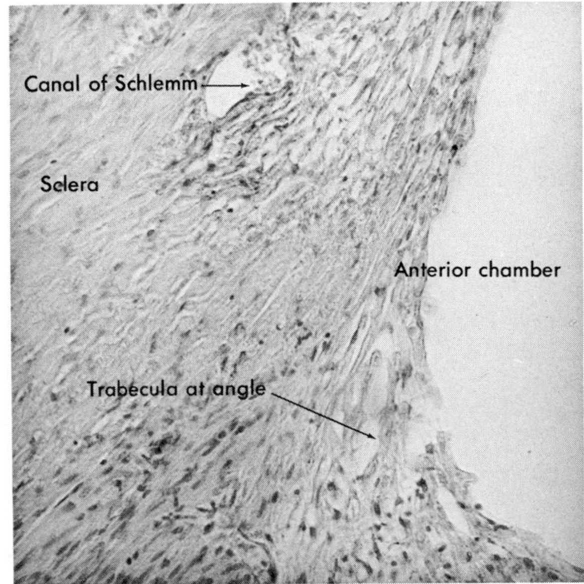

Fig. 20-6. Trabecula at angle.

humor) is reabsorbed into the venous system at the canal of Schlemm, which in turn connects to the anterior ciliary vessels. A parallel circulatory device exists for both CSF (see p. 207) and otic fluid (see p. 296). As the main mechanism of outflow for the fluid that arises in the posterior chamber of the globe, the filtration angle figures prominently in regulation of intraocular tension. Disturbances in tension (glaucoma) arise from muscular tension on the scleral spur by the meridional fibers of the ciliary muscle or from angle closure by tissue excursions in the area. The trabecula is richly innervated by fine nerve fibers from the ciliary plexus.

Iris

The iris relates to the ciliary body and the choroid as common parts of the *uvea* that are distinguished by pigmentation and vascularity. The iris is a complex circular diaphragm over the lens and possesses a central aperture (*pupil*), which is subject to variation in size. The iris separates the anterior chamber of the eye from the posterior chamber and baffles the course of ocular fluid as it moves from posterior to anterior chambers. The iris is made up of an anterior mesodermal stromal mass and a posterior pigmented epithelium. The stroma is covered on its anterior surface by a flattened mesodermal lining that continues laterally over the trabecula with the inner epithelium of the cornea. The stroma itself is continuous with that of the ciliary body. The iris contains two muscles with opposing action, a *constrictor* and a *dilator* (Fig. 20-7, *A* and *B*). The constrictor is smooth muscle of neuroepithelial origin and is innervated by parasympathetic fibers (nerve III via ciliary ganglion) (Fig. 20-1). The muscle is circular, and its fibers are placed on the distal posterior aspect of the iris. The dilator is atypical myoepithelium and stretches from the base of the iris to its distal part along the pigmented epithelium. It is activated by sympathetic stimulation (superior cervical ganglion from segments C8 and T1 to 3). The pigmented structure of the iris is in two layers, an anterior layer, which is intimately related to the dilator muscle, and a posterior or internal layer, which is continuous with the pigment layer of the ciliary body.

Ciliary body

This body forms a muscular ring around the inner surface of the globe at the level of the lens. It extends from the iris to the *ora serrata,* which is its saw-tooth posterior extremity at the junction of the ciliary body and retina (Fig. 20-3). It possesses a vascular stroma that is continuous with the iris and choroid. The external part is the bulky smooth ciliary muscle, which has three rather distinct parts: (1) meridional fibers, which connect the scleral role to the globe wall; (2) radial fibers, which radiate inward from the scleral role to the circular muscle; and (3) the circular ciliary mus-

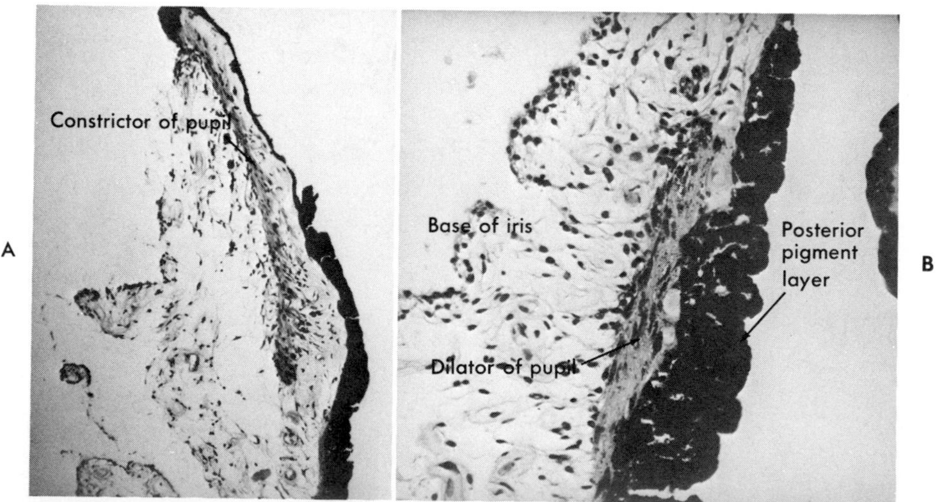

Fig. 20-7. Iris. **A,** Distal part with constrictor muscle along pigment layer; **B,** base of iris showing dilator fibers adjacent to pigment.

cle (of Mueller), which is circumferential at the base of the ciliary processes (Figs. 20-3 and 20-8). There are seventy ciliary processes, or folds, projecting toward the lens, to which they attach by ligaments. There is a complex nerve supply to the ciliary body arising in the ciliary plexus. The nerves are motor to the smooth muscles (pupil movements, accommodation, trabecular movements via the scleral spur, changes in iris-lens relationships), sensory to the area, vasomotor, and probably trophic in function. Occasional ganglion cells are displayed in the uveal tract, but these may represent degenerate bodies. The epithelial covering of the ciliary body is in two layers: (1) an outer pigmented layer, which is continuous with the pigmented uveal epithelium, and (2) a nonpigmented inner layer. The nonpigmented layer is the secretory epithelium, which produces the aqueous humor. This fluid is emptied into both the zonular chamber and the posterior chamber and has a flow pattern through the posterior chamber into the anterior chamber through the pupil. It is absorbed at the filtration angle. The secretory layer of cells is continuous posteriorly with the optic retina at the ora serrata.

Lens

The lens is an ectodermal derivative that continues to grow throughout life from cells persisting along its equator. In the adult the lens has average measurements of from 8 to 9 mm. transversely by 3.6 to 4 mm. anteroposteriorly. The radius of curvature on the anterior surface varies from 10 mm. to 6 mm. from a relaxed state to one in accommodation. The posterior radius of curvature similarly varys from 6 to 5 mm. The lens is transparent and elastic. It is held in place by a suspensory apparatus called the *zonula ciliaris* (of Zinn). This apparatus is made up of gelatinous extensions from the lens capsule, which is an elastic homogeneous protein membrane that keeps constant pressure on the lens to make it globular. The fibrillar character of the zonular substance in sections (Fig. 20-3) may be artifactitious. The zonula connects from the capsule of the lens to the surrounding ciliary body. The fibrillar precipitate within the zonula forms a canal (of Hannover) at the lens margin and additional chambers within its substance (of Minsky). Contraction of the ciliary muscle (of Mueller) relaxes the tension on the zonula and lens capsule, permitting the lens to assume a more globular shape. Accommodation for close vision is thus an active muscular effort. The lens includes the capsule (Fig. 20-10), an anterior single-layered epithelium, and a body of flat, hexagonal, ribbon-like fibers, which are nucleated and arranged radially in the cortex (Fig. 20-9). In the central part they are nonnucleated and smaller. They number about 1,400 at 3 years of age, compared to 2,200 in the adult. With age the lens becomes tougher, loses elasticity and transparency, and tends to become yellow. The lens is avascular, having lost the hyaloid arterial supply that existed during development. It has no nerve supply.

Vitreous body

The vitreous body is the gelatinous filling in the chamber between the lens and retinal internal limiting membrane (Fig. 20-2). Chemically it is a

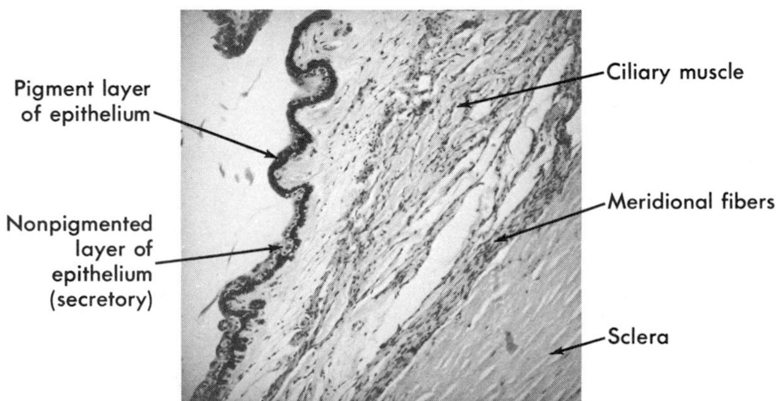

Fig. 20-8. Detail of ciliary body.

large-molecular, hydrated mucoprotein probably enmeshed in collagen filaments. It functions to hold the lens and retina in place and probably is nutritive to the retina. The vitreous body is fixed to the sides and posterior surface of the lens. The zonular structures are admixed with it and may in fact be derivatives of the vitreous body. The vitreous body functions as a hydrophilic colloid system. Its formation, transport mechanism, and turnover of metabolites are poorly understood. A remnant of the hyaloid canal system runs through this substance from the optic papilla to the posterior surface of the lens (canal of Cloquet). The vitreous body normally contains no vessels, no nerves, and only a few cells, most of which are migrating microglia (macrophages) of retinal origin.

Choroid

The choroid is continuous with the rest of the uveal tract (ciliary body and iris) and lies external to the retina, to which it provides nourishment. It varies from 0.2 to 0.3 mm. in thickness. The layers are described variously, usually to include four discernible laminae—outer epichoroid (suprachoroid), a vascular layer, choriocapillaris, and the basal or glassy membrane (of Bruch) (Fig. 20-11). The *epichoroid* joins the sclera by means of elastic fiber attachments and carries a dense nerve net associated with numerous pigment cells (chromatophores). The pigment appears to be melanin, although it differs from melanin pigment elsewhere in the body. This pigment accounts for color variation in the fundus. Ciliary vessels traverse this layer of choroid. Internal to the epichoroid is the *vascular layer,* which contains both large and medium blood vessels that are branches of ciliary vessels and vorticellar veins. The third layer, which is internally adjacent to the vascular layer, is the *choriocapillaris.* A supracapillary layer is sometimes defined as separating this layer from the overlying vascular zone. The choriocapillaris is a single layer of capillaries of very large diameter. These are rapid-shunting vessels

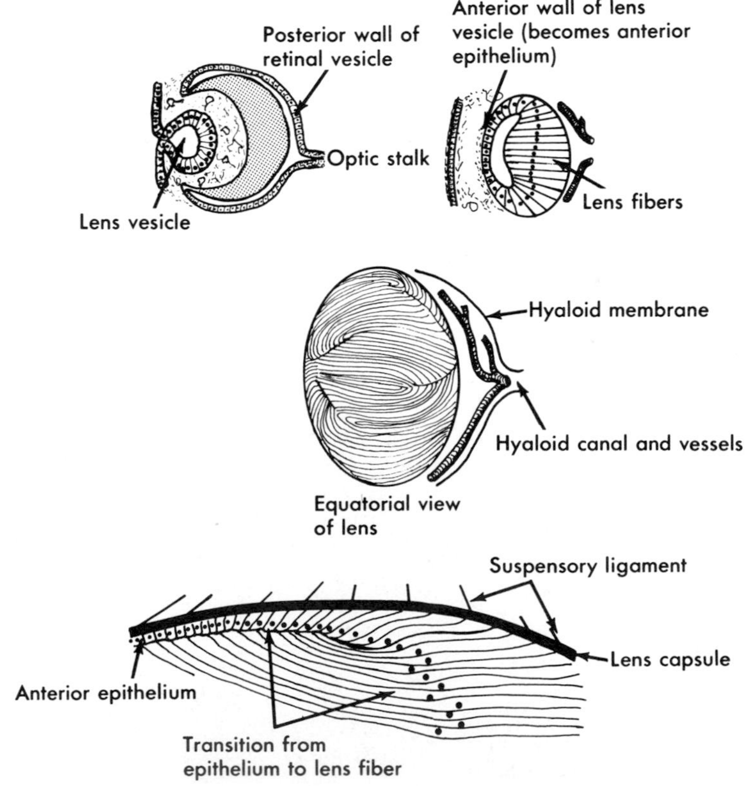

Fig. 20-9. Lens—schematic of development and structure.

from arteries to veins. The internal choroidal layer is *Bruch's membrane,* which includes an outer cuticle into which choroidal fibers are anchored and an inner basal (glassy) membrane applied to the pigmented epithelium of the retina. This last membrane is semipermeable and figures in transport of metabolites to the retinal photoreceptors.

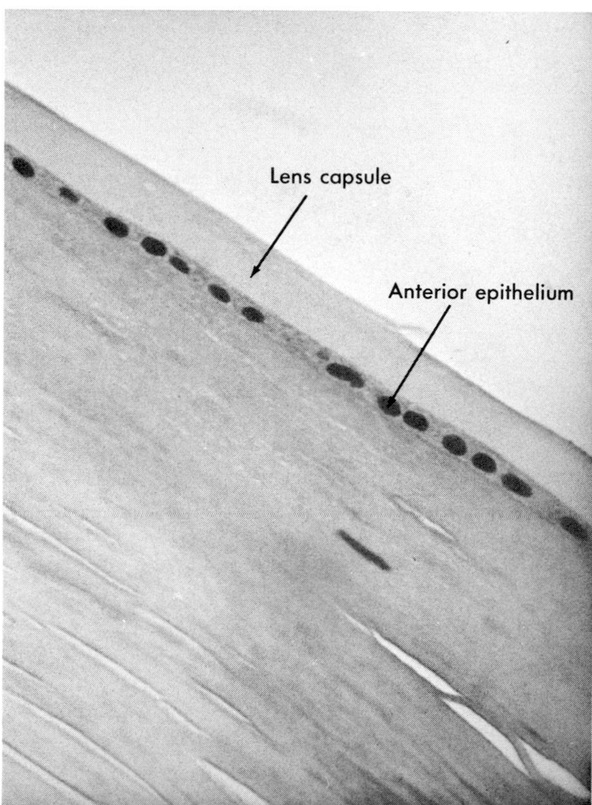

Fig. 20-10. Lens capsule. Clefts are artifacts.

Retina

As a derivative of the invaginated optic vesicle, the retina is wholly an extension of the CNS. The retina averages 0.5 mm. in thickness and covers the internal surface of the globe posterior to the ora serrata. The macula lutea (yellow spot) appears in the posterior retina in direct line with the pupil and slightly lateral to the nerve head. Its center (1.7 mm. in diameter) is a shallow depression, the fovea centralis. The retina attaches firmly to the choroid only at the ora serrata and at the optic papilla. It is absent over the papilla where the *blind spot* is formed. Elsewhere it separates easily from the pigment epithelium. The retina is made up of ten layers, which are reviewed from the external aspect to the internal in the following paragraphs (Fig. 20-12).

1. The layer of *pigment epithelium* develops from the outer layer of the optic cup, and hence is embryologically separated from the neural retina by a cleft. The layer binds tightly to Bruch's membrane by a hyalin cementing substance. The single-layered epithelial cells elaborate pigment, which migrates between the rods and cones in strong light and recedes (migrates outward) in dim light. It seems probable that the pigment epithelium produces and stores the photochemicals that are intermediaries in the stimulation of rods and cones as a response to light.

2. The layer of *rods and cones* includes the receptor extremities of the photoreceptors; these structures are designated by their shape in side view (Fig. 20-13). This layer is totally avascular and depends upon the choroid for nourishment. Rods possess an outer segment, which is made up of superimposed disks covered by a sheath that is open at the top. The outer segment has faint longitudinal striations, and the basal part incorporates

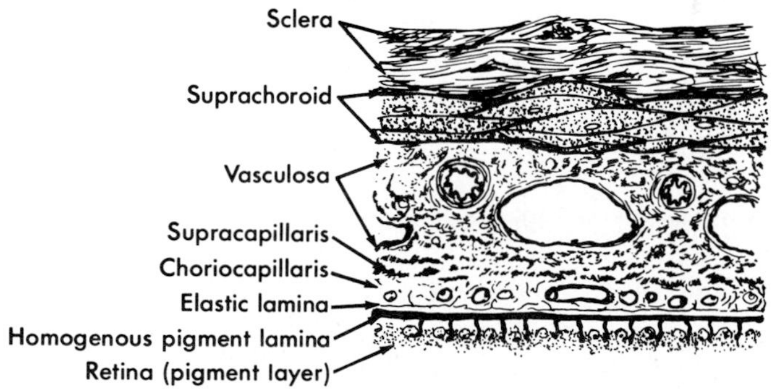

Fig. 20-11. Choroid layers.

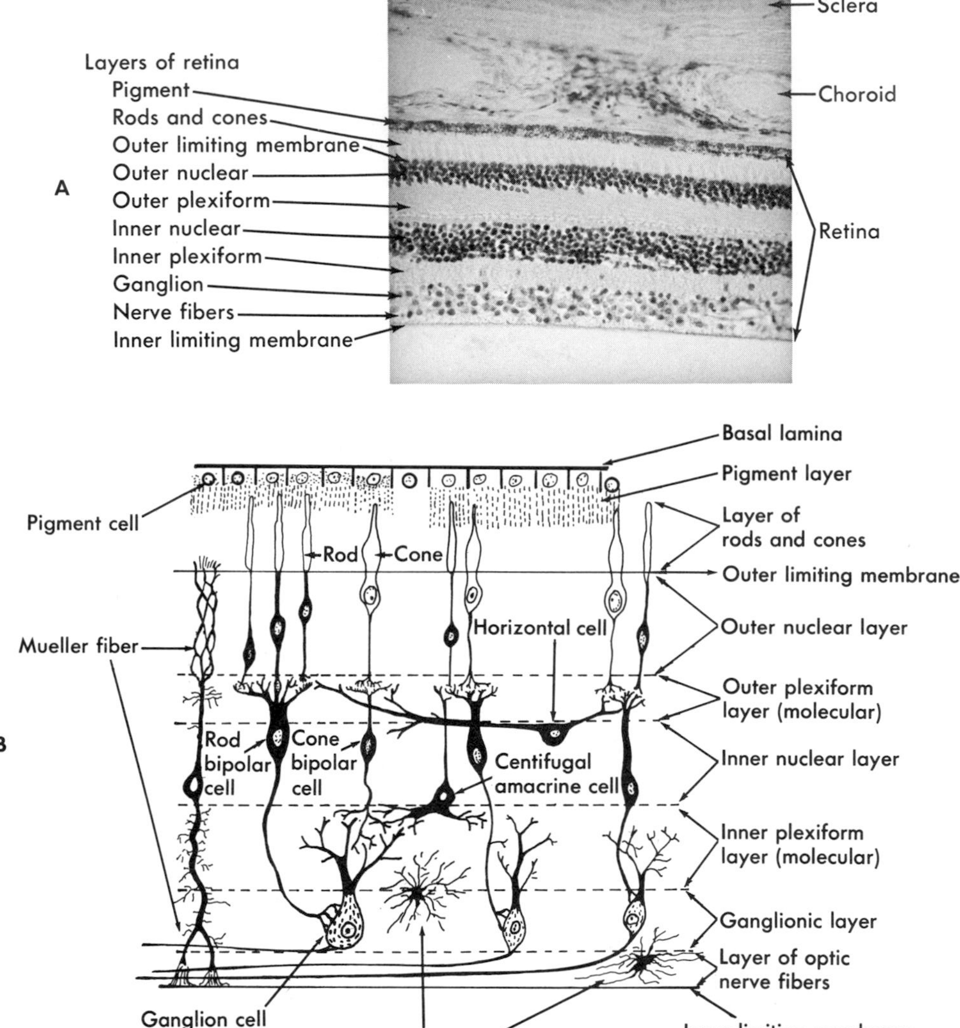

Fig. 20-12. A, Retinal layers. (H & E.) **B,** Schematic of retina and types of cells.

a fine fibril, the peripheral fiber, which arises from a diplosome at the junction of outer and inner segments. The external half of the inner segment contains highly refractile fibrils (lentiform body), while the internal half contains granular material (myoid). The nonfibrillated segment shortens in the dark.

The outer segment of rods contains rhodopsin (visual purple), which is bleached by light and probably represents the stimulating mechanism. This mechanism may be diagrammed as follows:

$$\text{Rhodopsin} \xrightarrow{\text{light}} \text{stimulating decomposition product} \longrightarrow \text{impulse initiated in rod}$$

The reaction is presumed to reverse in the dark and is capable of both a slow and a rapid reconversion. Rods are therefore presumed to facilitate vision in dim light and adaptation to dark. Vitamin A is part of the intermediate step in the slow reconstitution of rhodopsin.[11] Rods probably are also the main pickup endings for appreciation of movement. Rods vary in size from 1.5 to 3 μ by 40 to 60 μ in length and number about 120,000,000 in each eye. They do not occur in the fovea centralis but increase in density to the periphery.

Cones also possess an outer and inner segment. Both are shorter, and the inner segment is broader than in rods. The outer segment possesses no lon-

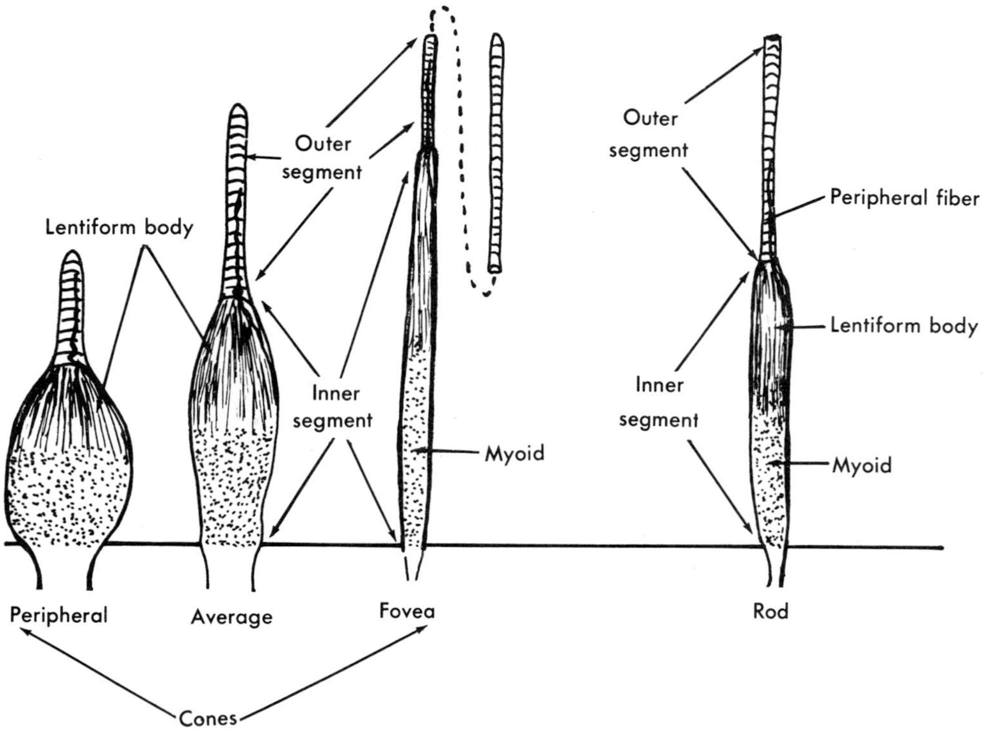

Fig. 20-13. Rods and cones.

gitudinal markings and is closed at its extremity. It has superimposed disks, but contains no rhodopsin. The fiber apparatus is the same as in rods, and both a lentiform fibrillated portion and a contractile myoid appear in the inner segment. Cones in the fovea centralis are elongate and narrow, and they become broad and stubby peripherally. Cones vary from 1.5 to 7 μ in width and from 22 to 85 μ in length. They number about 7,000,000 in each eye. The cones occupy the fovea centralis exclusively and are the pick-up endings for color vision and discriminative sight. Like the rods, cones penetrate the external limiting membrane by a narrowed "waist" and expand into a nucleated bulb within the external nuclear layer. The photochemical basis for cone activity is not established. Additional pigments probably function in cones much the way rhodopsin does in rods. A photochemical secretory mechanism has been hypothesized.

3. *Outer limiting membrane* is a sieve-like structure made up of flaring processes of elongate neuroglial fibers (of Mueller), which connect this layer to the inner limiting membrane adjacent to the vitreous body. The processes of the photoreceptors pass through this membrane and have their nuclei in the next layer (Fig. 20-12, *B*). The Mueller cells are not only supportive, but cover wide areas of rods with their cytoplasmic expansions. They probably function in metabolic exchanges similar to astrocytes in the general CNS.[1]

4. *Outer nuclear layer* is the laminated mass of nuclei belonging to the rods and cones (Fig. 20-12, *B*).

5. *Outer plexiform* (*molecular*) *layer* is the field of synaptic contact of the rods and cones with the dendritic and adendritic extremities of the bipolar cells (Fig. 20-12, *B*). Both rods and cones make contact with the bipolar cells via synaptic structures characterized by dendritic invagination from the bipolar elements. Electron microscopy reveals dendritic inroads within the rod terminals that vary somewhat with the animal studied (Fig. 20-14).[1,10] Both rod and cone terminals possess abundant synaptic vesicles, with concentration at the presynaptic membrane. The recessed dendritic receptors are more complicated in the cone synapses. An electron-dense elongate body (synaptic ribbon) appears as a distinctive component of retinal junctions. Dark adaptations accompanied by accumulations of vesicles occur at the presynaptic membrane.[1]

6. *Inner nuclear layer* is made up of the nuclei of the bipolar cells. These cells contain no Nissl

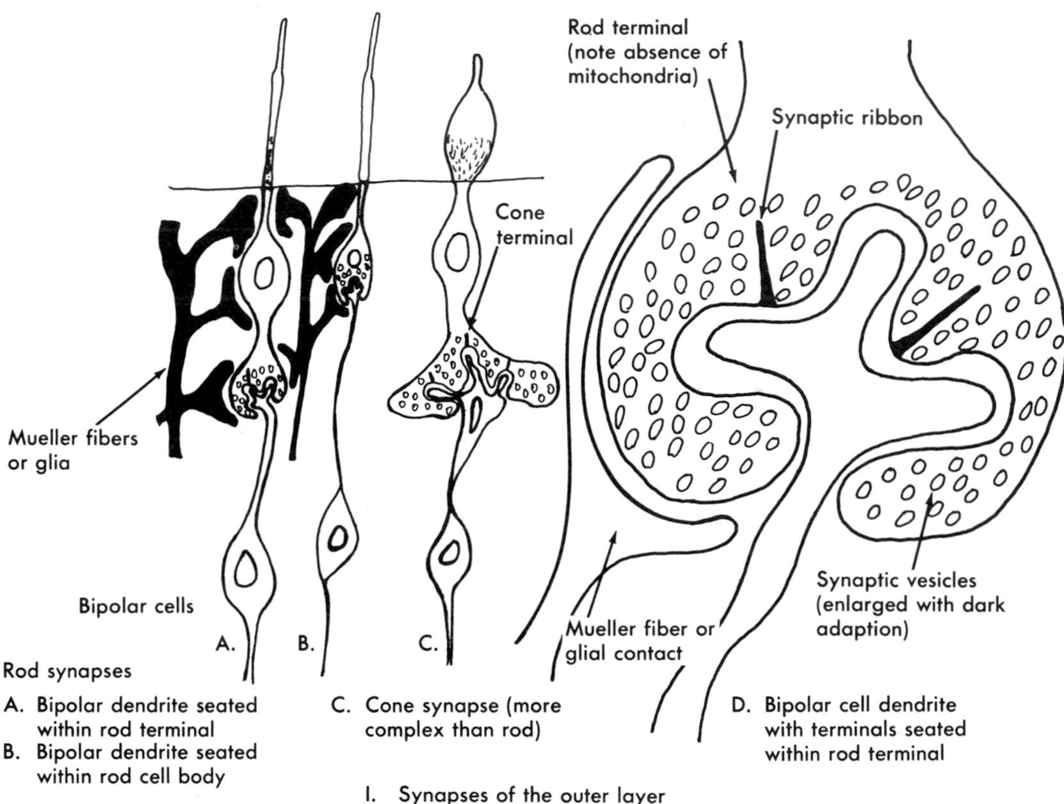

I. Synapses of the outer layer

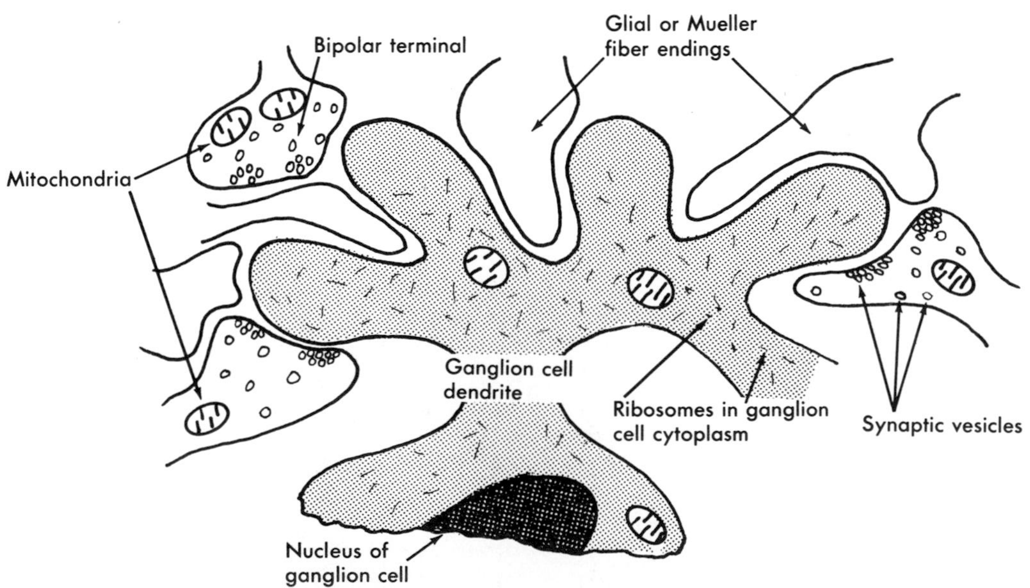

II. Synapses of inner layer to ganglion cell

Fig. 20-14. Composite electron micrographic character of retinal components.

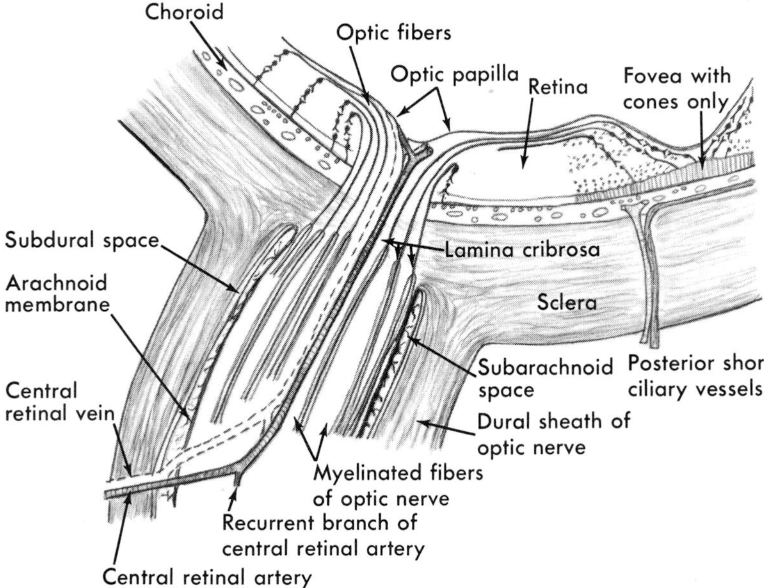

Fig. 20-15. Schematic of optic nerve head and vascular supply to eyeball.

granules and vary in shape from elongate, dendritic elements to cells that display no dendrites on their receptive extremity when viewed under the light microscope. Both those cells that link with rods (several) and those that link with cones (single or several) direct their impulses to ganglion cells (cetripetal). The nuclei of *Mueller's neuroglia* also occupy this layer. There are also *horizontal cells* (of Cajal), which interconnect with the synaptic junctions in the outer plexiform layer. The *amacrine* cells provide a feedback mechanism within the retina and pass from inner plexiform layer to outer plexiform layer, with their cell bodies located in this inner nuclear layer (Fig. 20-12, *B*). Blood vessels from the inner retina extend into this layer.

7. The *inner plexiform* (*molecular*) *layer* is made up of synaptic unions between bipolar cells and ganglion cells. The junctions are either axodendritic or axosomatic from both rod and cone bipolars. Some astrocytes are found in this layer (Fig. 20-12, *B*). The inner plexiform or synaptic layer is more complex in its interconnecting makeup than the outer layer. The Mueller cell expansions are fewer. Vesicles and mitochondria occur in some form at least, and the synaptic field is vast. The synaptic relationships however are not established for man in this zone. The functional physiology of this layer appear to be different from that of the outer layer. The inner layer of synapses appear to be cholinergic.[1]

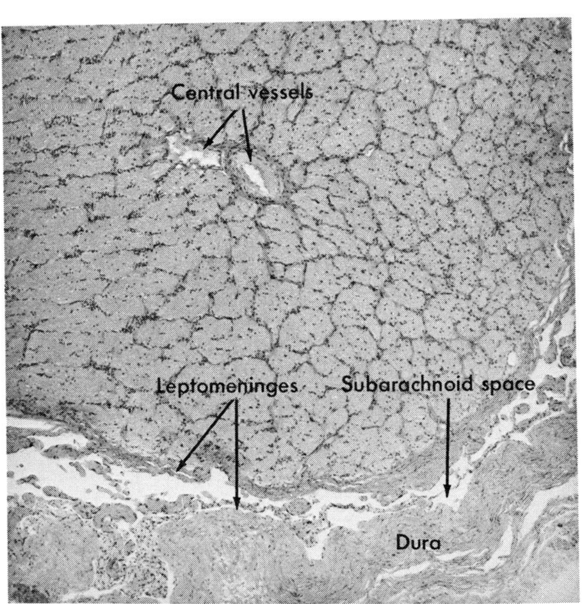

Fig. 20-16. Cross section of optic nerve with meninges and central vessels.

8. *The ganglion cell layer* houses the cell bodies whose axons project into the substance of the optic nerve. These vary from large to small cells and display mainly axosomatic synapses from rod bipolars. Astrocytes occur in this layer (Fig. 20-12, *B*).

9. *Layer of nerve fibers* are the axons of the ganglion cells. The layer is traversed by expanding Mueller fiber tufts. It contains astrocytes and microglia (Fig. 20-12, *B*).

10. *The inner limiting membrane* is made up of expanded terminal nets of the specialized neuroglial elements, Mueller fibers, which interconnect the two limiting membranes (Fig. 20-12, *B*).

Vessels and nerves of the eyeball

These are presented diagrammatically in summary form in Figs. 20-15 and 20-16.

VISUAL FIELDS AND BINOCULAR VISION

For an object to appear single the eyes respond so that the image simultaneously strikes specific positions on the nasal half of one eye and the temporal half of the other (Fig. 20-17). This synchronization requires coordinated muscle effort in convergence and proper accommodation. The projected visual pattern for the nasal half of the right eye, for example, will correspond to the projection from the temporal half of the left eye. These projections are the *visual fields* and arise by virtue of the crossing of the nasal retinal fibers in the optic chi-

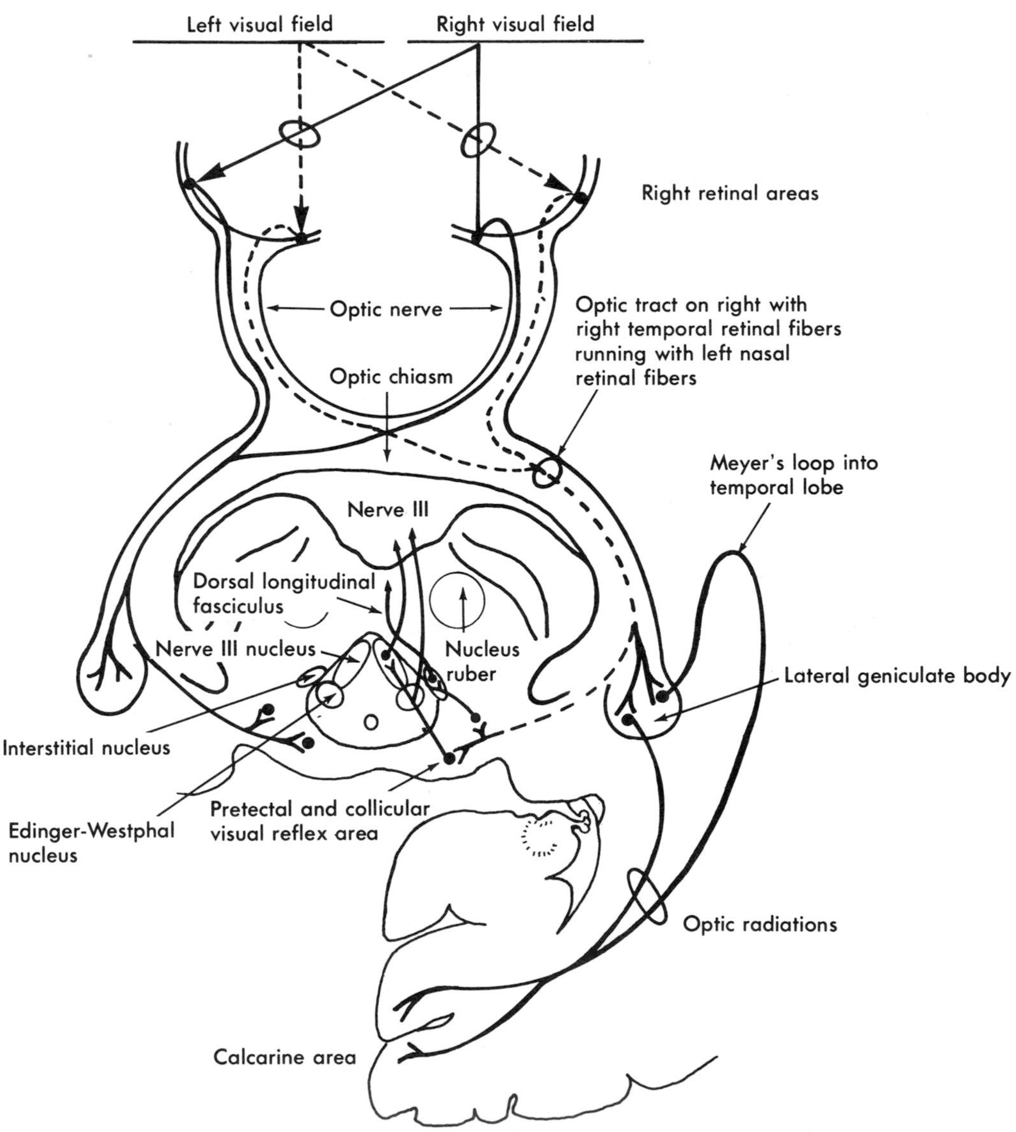

Fig. 20-17. Schematic of binocular retinal relationships to stimulation from visual fields.

asm to join the temporal fibers of the opposite eye in the visual pathways to the cortex. It has been convenient to map the retinal fields in quadrants (upper and lower external and medial) and to subdivide these as macular, paramacular, and peripheral retinal zones (Fig. 20-18). In each retinal field and on both the nasal and temporal sides of each eye there is a marginal zone that cannot be matched by the opposite eye in simultaneous stimulation. These therefore represent monocular fields.

OPTIC NERVE

The nerve fibers from the ganglion cells of the retina converge at the optic papilla to form the optic nerve head. This structure lies 3.5 mm. medial to and slightly above the macula lutea. The

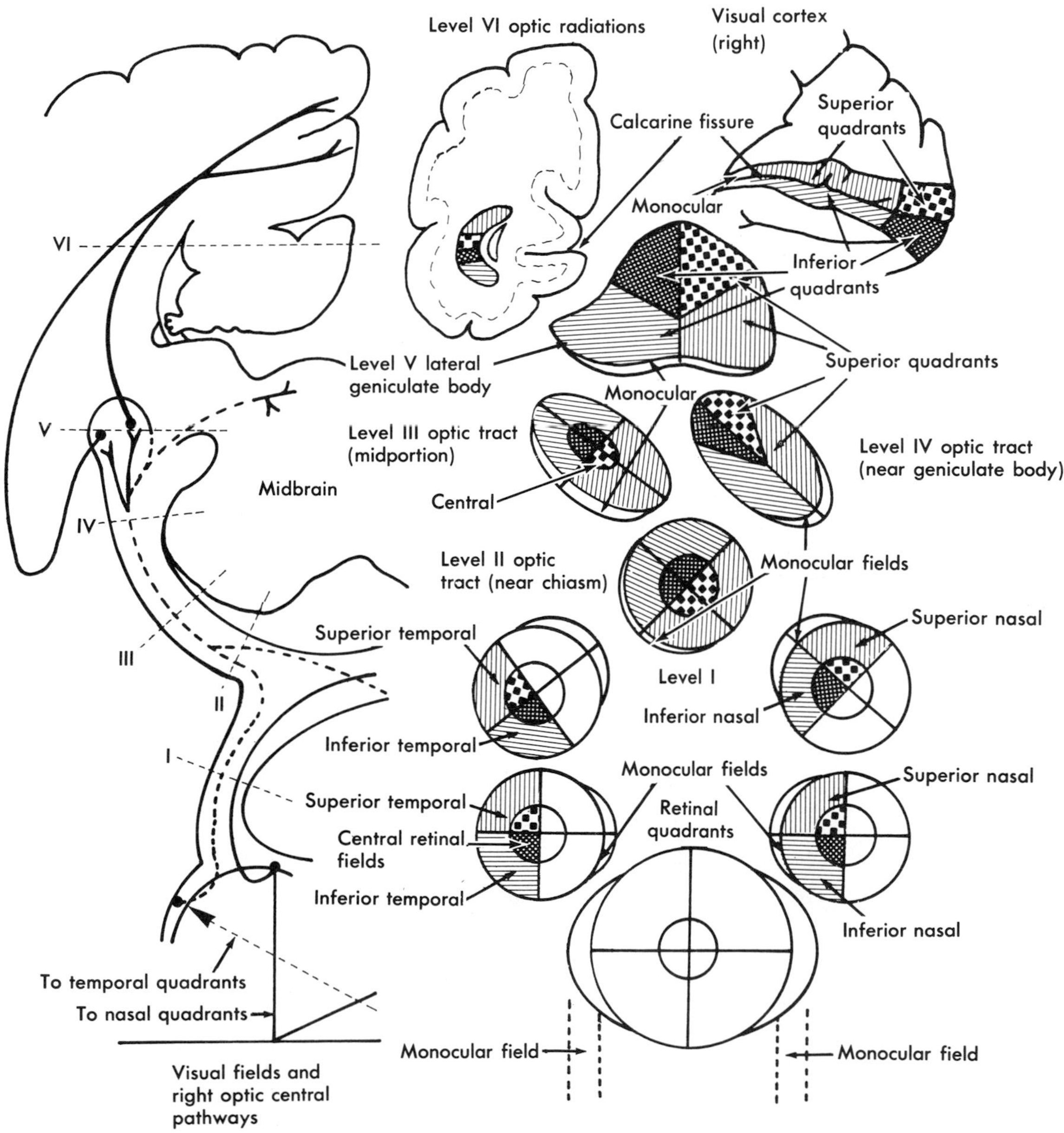

Fig. 20-18. Tract patterns through optic nerve, chiasm, tract, geniculate body, and radiations.

nerve head is 1.5 mm. across and is the site of edema, or swelling, as a response to intracranial hypertension. The fibers from the macula (papillomacular bundle) form the central core of the nerve. The fibers penetrate the glial basket of spider glial cells overlying the lamina cribrosa, which is the sieve-like perforated segment of the sclera (Fig. 20-15). Cross sections and distribution of the quadrants delivering fibers to the nerve are shown in Fig. 20-18. The nerve fibers number about 1.2 million on each side. The optic nerve is covered by a dural sheath, which continues into the sclera.

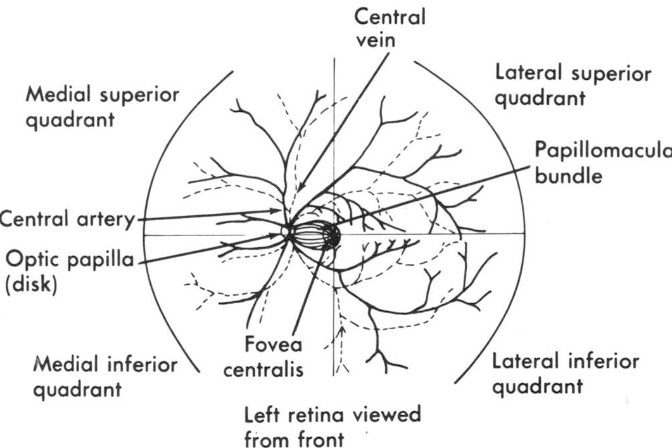

Fig. 20-19. Retinal areas and vessels diagrammed as viewed from front.

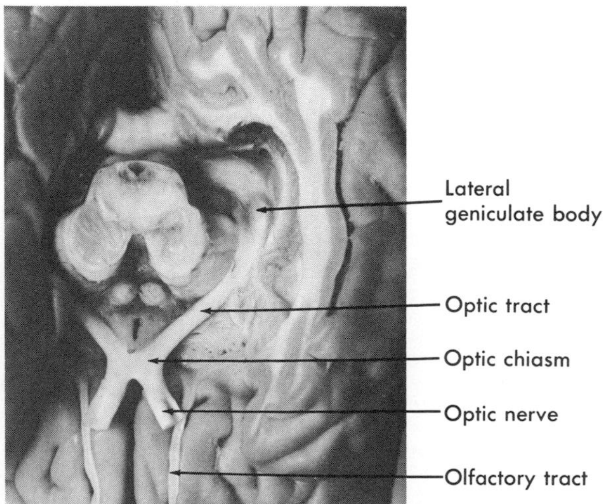

Fig. 20-20. Dissection of optic nerve, chiasm, tract, and lateral geniculate body showing relationships to midbrain and hypothalamus.

The leptomeninges and related spaces also continue to the junction of the nerve with the eyeball. The central vessels of the retina, both artery and vein, enter the optic nerve 1.5 to 2 cm. behind the eyeball (Figs. 20-16 and 20-19). These vessels bridge the subarachnoid space at the point of entry. The optic nerve is structurally the same as white matter within the brain. The fibers are myelinated by oligodendroglial wrapping, and the field contains astrocytes. Myelination usually ceases at the lamina cribrosa.

OPTIC CHIASMA

The fibers arising in the medial quadrants cross in the optic chiasma, while the lateral quadrants remain uncrossed to enter the optic tracts (Fig. 20-18). The same pattern of crossing is followed by macular fibers. The macular path remains centrally placed into the optic tract. The gross topography of the nerve, chiasm, and tract is shown in Fig. 20-20.

OPTIC TRACT

In its course from the chiasm the optic tract essentially wraps around the infundibulum and tuber cinereum. It then applies to the sides of the peduncle and terminates in the lateral geniculate body (Fig. 20-20). A few commissural fibers interconnect the two medial geniculate bodies via the optic tracts and chiasm (Gudden's commissure). This is probably unimportant in human physiology. The cross section of the tract (Fig. 20-18) displays the superior quadrants in a medial, slightly downward position, and the inferior quadrants lateral and slightly upward. The macular fields are central. Monocular fields wrap around the inferior aspect.

LATERAL GENICULATE BODY

This thalamic segment (metathalamus) represents the primary terminus of the fibers arising in the ganglion cells of the retina. The pattern of termination (Figs. 20-20 and 20-21) is as follows: superior quadrants to the medial aspect, inferior quadrants to the lateral aspect, and macular fibers to the superior and posterior part of the nucleus. Monocular fields are ventrally placed in a narrow rim. Coronal views of the lateral geniculate body provide a Napoleon-hat silhouette, which on close gross inspection is laminated in six strata (Figs. 20-22 to 20-24). The hollowed inferior portion is the hilus, and numbering this stratum as 1, the apex becomes 6. The first two layers have larger cells than the others (magnocellular). Experimen-

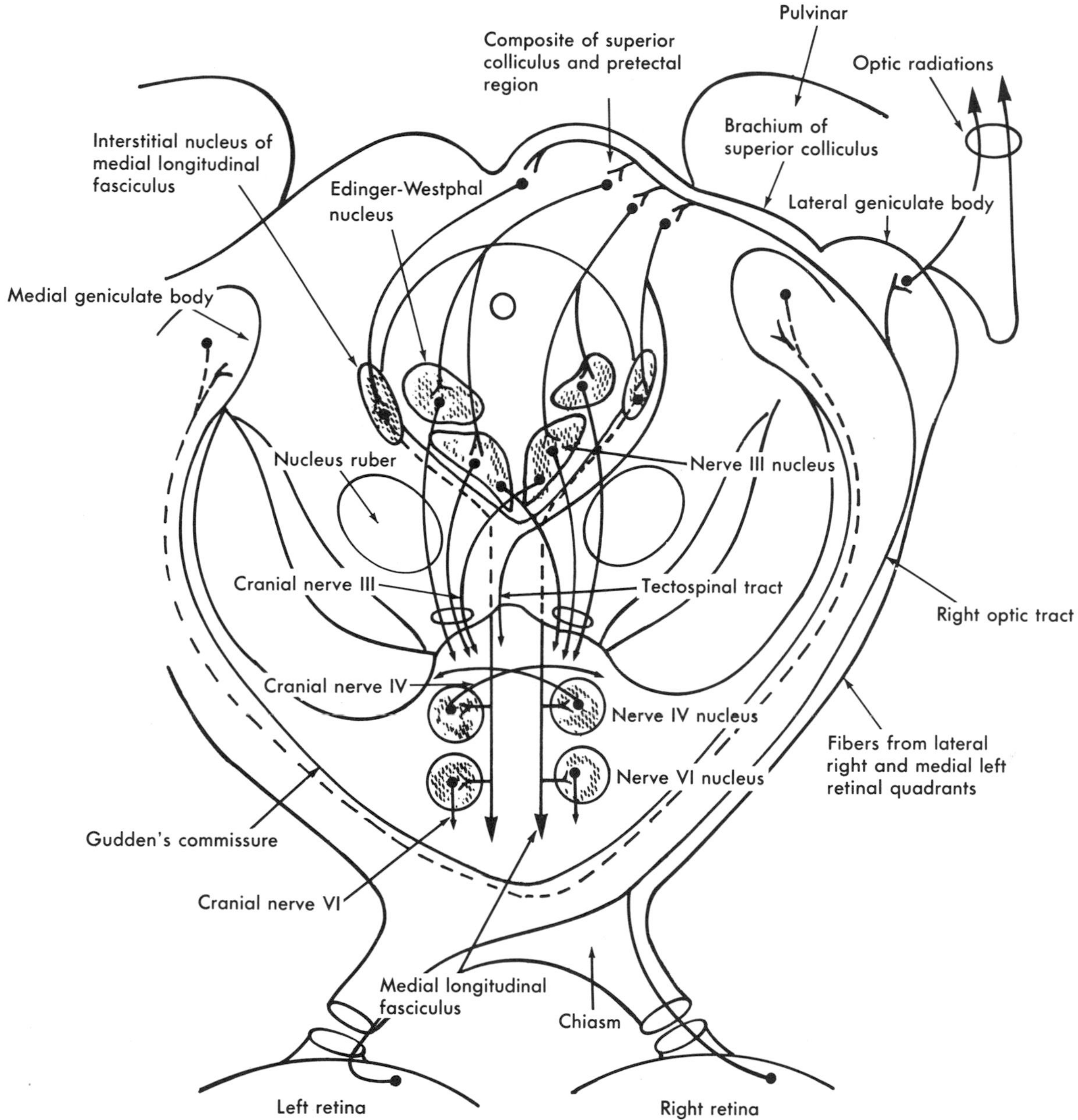

Fig. 20-21. Schematic of optic nerve terminations viewed from below, as in Fig. 20-20.

tal evidence indicates that the fibers from the contralateral eye (crossed) terminate in layers 1, 4, and 6, while the ipsilateral (temporal retina) fibers terminate in 2, 3, and 5.[2,4]

The terminals in the nucleus and the collaterals are not established for man. In general it is believed that successive collaterals are given off to cells between the main laminae, serving to intermix the representation of the two eyes. In addition, either collaterals or direct fibers from the retina are believed to extend to the superior colliculus (via the brachium of the superior colliculus) and probably the pretectal region for reflex connections. The lateral geniculate body may play a role in color vision, as demonstrated in the color sensitivity of its cells.[3,5]

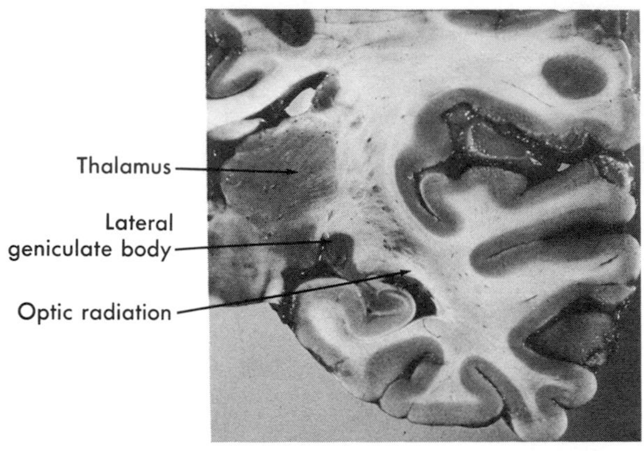

Fig. 20-22. Coronal section showing characteristic shape of lateral geniculate body.

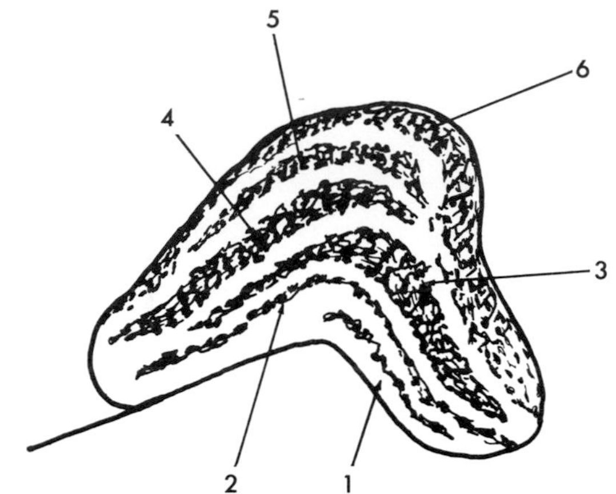

Fig. 20-23. Diagram of six laminae in lateral geniculate body.

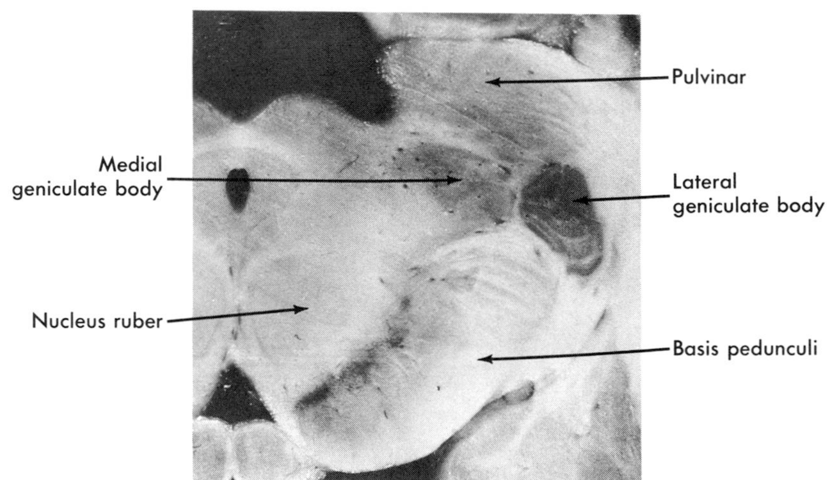

Fig. 20-24. Transverse section showing laminated lateral geniculate body and the bordering medial geniculate body at level of upper midbrain.

REFLEX CONNECTIONS IN THE VISUAL PATHWAY

The direct reflexes may be viewed in two sets—those relating to ocular and body movements and those relating to reactions within the eyeball itself. The ocular movements appear to be mediated through direct neuronal flow to nerve III nuclei from the superior colliculus and the pretectal region, the medial longitudinal fasciculus, and the periaqueductal nucleus (of Darkschewitsch). The reflex paths receive interrelating connections through the posterior commissure and contribute fibers to the medial longitudinal fasciculus (Fig. 20-21). This system relates to vertical reflex eye movements. Reflexes from the colliculus and pretectal region also relate to horizontal eye movements in a complex relationship with vestibular nuclei. These nuclei regulate conjugate deviation (simultaneous abducens and contralateral medial rectus stimulation) via the reticular formation and the medial longitudinal fasciculus. The tectal region is brought into relationship with trunk innervation via the tectospinal tract.

Reflexes for light and accommodation depend upon innervation of the constrictor of the pupil, the dilator of the pupil, and the ciliary muscle.

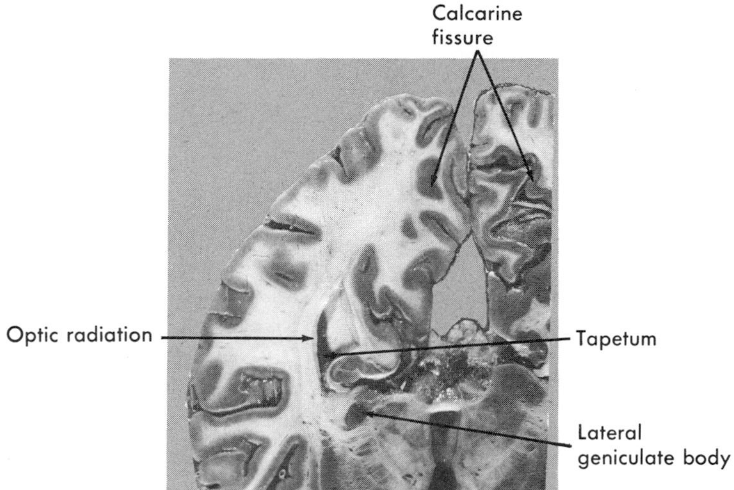

Fig. 20-25. Transverse section showing optic radiations.

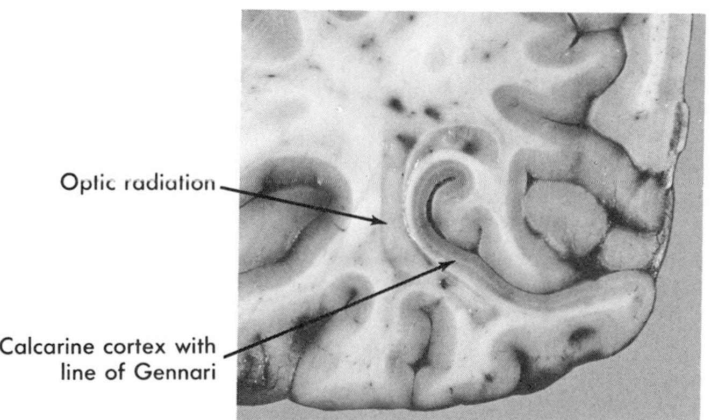

Fig. 20-26. Calcarine fissure showing line of Gennari.

Stimulation of the retina by light is carried to the pretectal region and then to the Edinger-Westphal nucleus. This area is presumably the source of preganglionic fibers to the ciliary ganglion. Parasympathetic postganglionic fibers innervate the constrictor of the pupil as a response to light (Fig. 20-1). The same pathway operates in stimulation of the ciliary muscle for accommodation. The response to light is sometimes absent, while accommodation persists (Argyll-Robertson pupil). The exact point of separation of these two circuits is unknown, but the idea is advanced that accommodation is placed more caudally in the pretectal Edinger-Westphal complex than responses to light. In contrast to that of light and accommodation, the dilator response is mediated from the pretectal region via the medial longitudinal fasciculus to sympathetic visceral efferent fibers in thoracic nerves 1 to 3. These initiate the preganglionic flow to the superior cervical ganglion, from which postganglionic fibers pass to the dilator muscle via the perivascular plexuses (Fig. 20-1). It should be noted that these reflex pathways divert from the pathways to the visual cortex. Thus, ocular movements and light and accommodation can persist as reflexes although cortical blindness exists.

CORTICAL CONNECTIONS OF THE VISUAL PATHWAY

The geniculocalcarine tract represents the optic radiations. These radiations leave the thalamic body through the posterior inferior portion of the

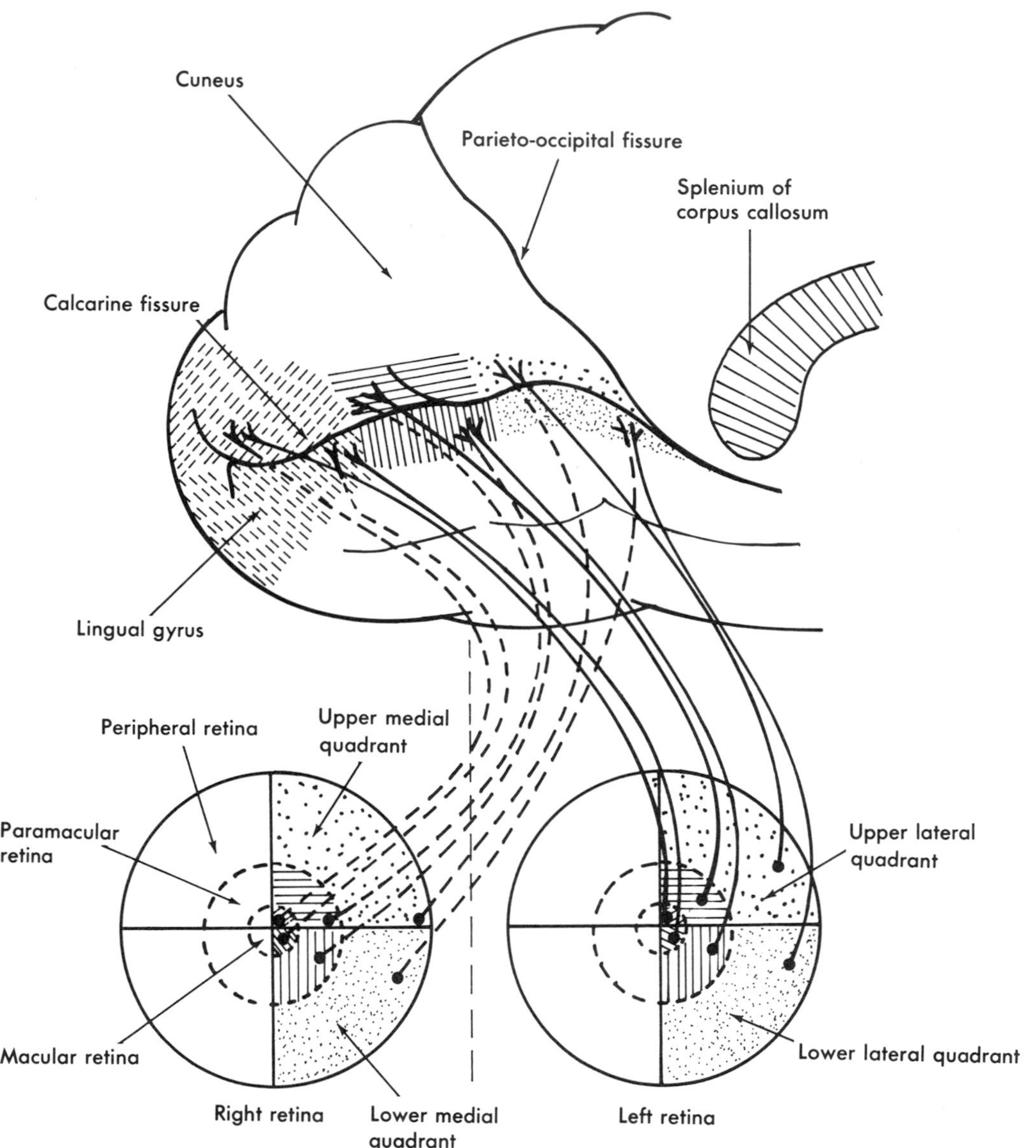

Fig. 20-27. Relationship of retinal area to visual cortex.

internal capsule (Fig. 20-25). The medial side of the lateral geniculate body gives rise to fibers that pass around the confluent part of the lateral ventricle to distribute in the cerebral cortex of the cuneus, which lies superior to the calcarine fissure (Fig. 20-26). This course brings the impulses arising in the superior quadrants of the retina to the superior aspect of the primary visual cortex. Opposing this activity, the fibers arising in the lateral part of the geniculate body pass laterally and anteriorly over the ventricle, with the anteriormost fibers directed into the temporal lobe as Meyer's loop. The fibers curve posteriorly to lie lateral and inferior to the posterior horn and progress to the lingual gyrus below the calcarine fissure (Fig. 20-27). Impulses derived from the inferior quadrants terminate in the inferior aspect of the visual cortex. Macular impulses from all quadrants are directed to the posterior third of the visual area, paramacular to the middle third, and peripheral to the anterior third. As seen in Fig. 20-25, most of the visual cortex is buried.

The *geniculocalcarine fibers, or optic radiations,* form a grossly distinct lamina in the lateral part of

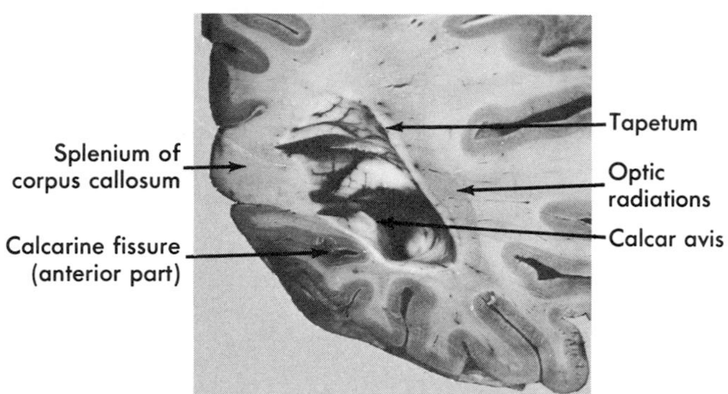

Fig. 20-28. Coronal section through sagittal strata of occipital lobe.

the *sagittal stratum* (Fig. 20-28). Medial to the tract are fibers projecting from the cortex to the thalamus and a narrow band of corpus callosum extensions (tapetum) that applies to the ventricular wall. Lateral to the optic radiations are association bundles, which interconnect parts of the cerebral cortex. Within the tract itself the upper quadrant is superior, the macular representation central, and the inferior quadrant inferior.

The parts of the thalamus other than the lateral geniculate body, such as the pulvinar, are controversial in their relation to the visual system. The pulvinar is probably more closely related to parietal functions. (For discussion of parietal functions and integrative features of the visual system see Chapter 21.)

REFERENCES

1. de Robertis, E.: Electron microscope observation on the submicroscopic organization of the retinal rods, J. Biophys. Biochem. Cytol. **2**:319, 1956.
2. Glees, P.: The termination of optic fibers in the lateral geniculate body of the cat, J. Anat. **75**:434, 1941.
3. Granit, R.: Receptors and sensory perception, New Haven, Connecticut, 1955, Yale University Press.
4. Le Gros Clark, W. E.: The laminar organization and cell content of the lateral geniculate body in the monkey, J. Anat. **75**:419, 1941.
5. Marks, W. B., Dobelle, W. H., and MacNichol, E. F.: Visual pigment of single primate cones, Science **143**: 1181, 1964.
6. Minckler, T., and Boyd, E.: Physical Growth. In Minckler, J., editor: Pathology of the nervous system, vol. I, New York, 1968, McGraw-Hill Book Co.
7. Polyak, S. L.: The retina, Chicago, 1941, The University of Chicago Press.
8. Polyak, S. L.: The vertebrate visual system, Chicago, 1957, The University of Chicago Press.
9. Scammon, R. E., and Wilmer, H. A.: Growth of the components of the human eyeball, Arch. Ophthal. **43**: 599, 1950.
10. Sjöstrand, F. S.: Ultrastructure of retinal rod synapses of the guinea pig eye, J. Ultrastruct. Res. **2**:122, 1958.
11. Wald, G.: Neurophysiology. In Field, R. A., McGoun, H. W., and Hall, V. E., editors: Handbook of physiology, Washington, 1959, American Physiologic Society.
12. Wolter, J. R.: Neuropathology of the eye and its adnexa. In Minckler, J., editor: Pathology of the nervous system, vol. I, New York, 1968, McGraw-Hill Book Co.

CHAPTER 21

THALAMUS AND CEREBRUM

JEFF MINCKLER

It is almost impossible to physiologically account for thalamic activity without including the cerebral cortex or to discuss the cerebral cortex apart from the thalamus. Consequently, they are treated together in this section. While the thalamus is seated primarily as a relay station between the systems subserving sensory pickup and the cerebral cortex, it also participates as an efferent way station in some motor systems. (For review of the thalamic parts related to the motor activity in the autonomic system, the neuroendocrine system, and the limbic system, see Chapter 22.)

THALAMUS

In an overview of the thalamus it is helpful to separate the anatomic segments into functional systems regardless of structural relationships. The three functional systems are: (1) specific relay nuclei, (2) associational nuclei, and (3) nonspecific nuclei. These divisions apply best to the thalamus proper, but include nuclei apart from this grouping. Definite specific relays are located in the metathalamic geniculate bodies. Hypothalamic structures are mainly concerned with limbic, autonomic, and neuroendocrine activities. The subthalamus also relates more to motor systems as does the epithalamus, which provides output pathways for limbic activities (see Chapter 22).

Specific relay nuclei

The major subdivisions of the diencephalon have been reviewed as thalamic nuclei (see Chapter 2). Some degree of localization of function in these several divisions has been implied in delivery of special afferent pathways to special areas of the thalamus (the specific primary relay nuclei). As third- or higher-order neurons, the thalamic cells in these relays act as mediators of the afferent impulses in transferring them to cerebral cortical areas.

The following specific relays have been noted. Cutaneous sense is received in both the posteromedial and posterolateral parts of the ventral nucleus and radiates from these nuclei via the posterior limb of the internal capsule to the general somesthetic area. Deep sensibility similarly goes via the posteromedial and posterolateral parts of the ventral nucleus and is transferred by radiations through the posterior limb of the internal capsule to the general somesthetic area. General visceral afferent impulses are principally reflex, but in some instances (such as pain, fullness, hunger) they reach conscious levels by multiple stages and eventually, through the medial lemniscus, terminate in the posterolateral part of the ventral thalamic nucleus (pain probably in the spinothalamic tract). From there the impulses go to the somesthetic area (often referred).

The gustatory system is probably also routed over the medial lemniscus to the posteromedial part of the ventral nucleus and then to the inferior part of the somesthetic area. The olfactory system, like all the visceral systems, relates to the hypothalamus in its integrative pathways. The cortical areas for olfaction include the subcallosal area, the anterior perforated substance, and the piriform field over the uncus. These cortical fields are reached directly by the olfactory tracts and represent rhinal area, or paleocortex. They possess no thalamic component that is intervening between the receptors in the nose and the cortex. These olfactory areas relate to the thalamus in their continuing efferent paths.

The visual system reaches the lateral geniculate bodies through the optic tracts and radiates from

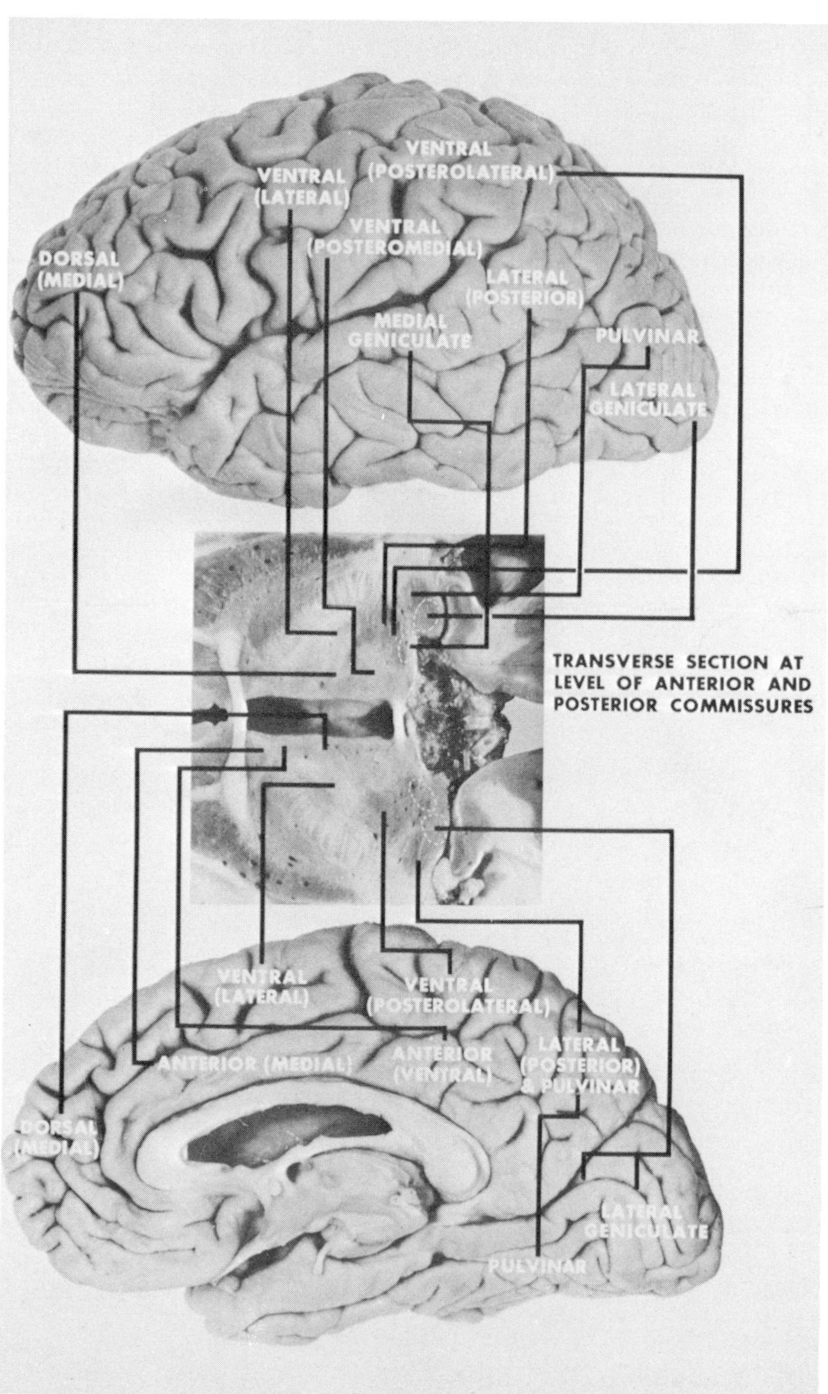

Fig. 21-1. Medial and lateral cerebral cortical views related to the thalamic nuclei and areas.

there to the calcarine area of the occipital lobe via the retrolenticular part of the internal capsule.

Little is known of thalamic connections of the vestibular system, except as it relates through vision, audition, deep sense, and pressure. A cortical center adjacent to the auditory fields is presumed to exist. The auditory system relays through the thalamic medial geniculate body to the auditory cortex in Heschl's gyri. These connections are considered well-established specific thalamic way stations to the cerebral cortex for the major afferent pathways.

There are undoubtedly similar thalamocortical radiations and projections for other thalamic fields that function in somewhat more obscure fashions. The anterior nuclear group relates specifically from the limbic pathway to the neocortex. In addition, it operates as a feedback to the cortex from the globus pallidus. These relationships have been established through identity of degenerative changes in thalamic nuclei as a consequence of destructive lesions of the cortex.[8] Elaborate integrative systems involve the entire central brain, including diencephalon, mesencephalon, and probably rhombencephalon. The known additional interrelationships of thalamic and cortical parts are summarized in Figs. 21-1 and 21-2.

It is well known that the entire thalamus operates in many functional capacities, not only as a way station in the major afferent systems.[4,7,11] In most parts of the thalamic nuclei, cerebral cortical representation is returned by projections from the same cortical areas that are supplied by the thalamic radiations. The returning fibers may not localize precisely in the source of radiations to the cortex, since the fibers to the cortex fan out more extensively than the reciprocal fibers, which tend to converge. Most thalamic parts are also interrelated by intranuclear connections. In addition to this varied and complex neural display of integrative character with some localization of function, the thalamus is also recognized as a center of appreciation (consciousness) of distinctive type. Animals, for example, can be shown to recognize changes in tone in the absence of auditory cortical tissue. The same tonal recognition may also reside in the medial geniculate body of man. At least some auditory consciousness is known to exist in the thalamus, although meaningful sounds require cortical representation. Similar thalamic con-

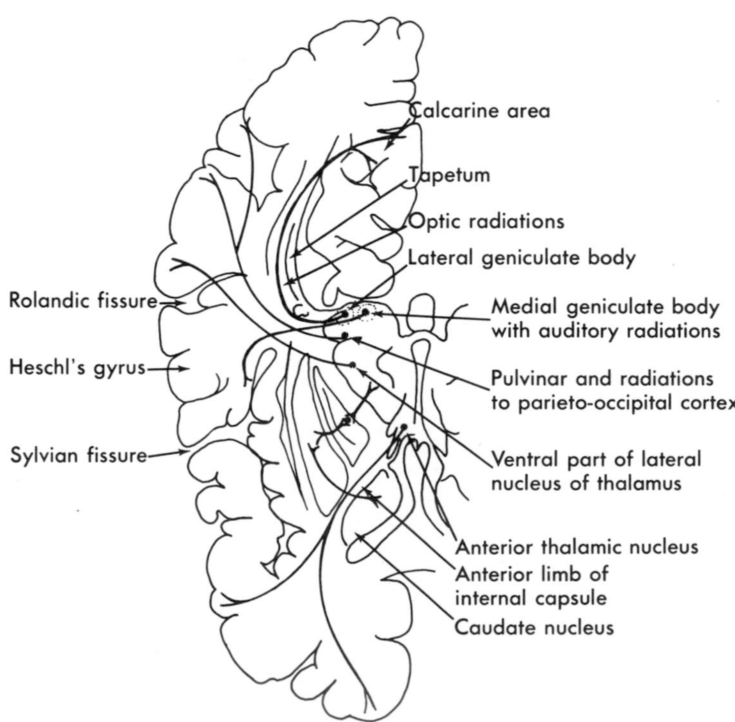

Fig. 21-2. Drawing of transverse section through thalamus showing radiations to cortex. Most have reciprocal returning fibers.

sciousness is demonstrable in other systems (pain, thermal, pressure, touch, for example).

Association nuclei

The specific association nuclei of the thalamus include the medial nuclear group and the dorsal part of the lateral nucleus (Fig. 21-3). The subdivisions of the latter are the lateral posterior nucleus, the lateral dorsal nucleus, and the pulvinar (Figs. 21-4 and 21-5). These nuclei receive no specific input from ascending pathways, but appear in many ways to operate as secondary relays to other diencephalic nuclei or to the cortex. They relate primarily to associational or integrative cortical fields, rather than to specific sensory or motor areas of the cortex. In this manner they also enter into feedback systems in the loop circuitry from cortex to basal ganglia to thalamic nuclei

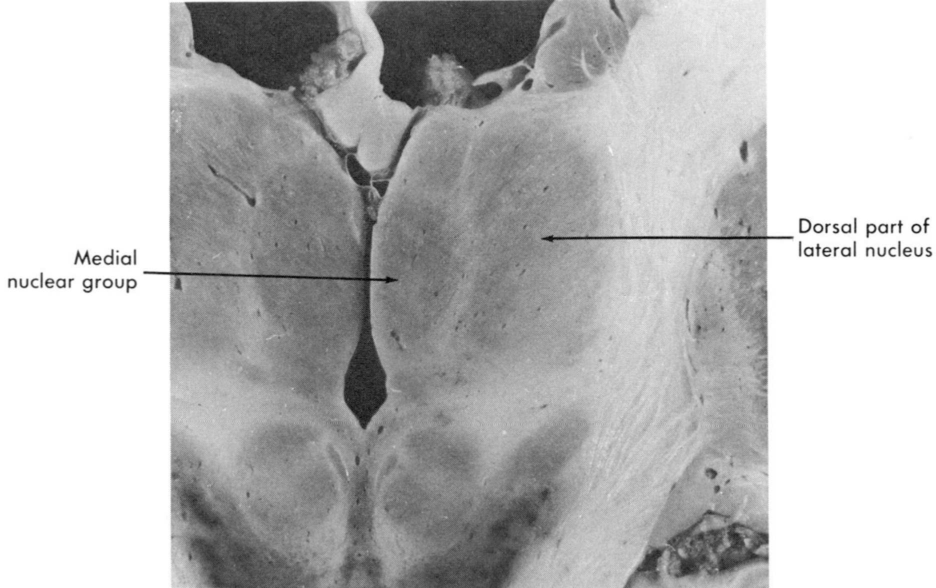

Fig. 21-3. Principal association nuclei of thalamus.

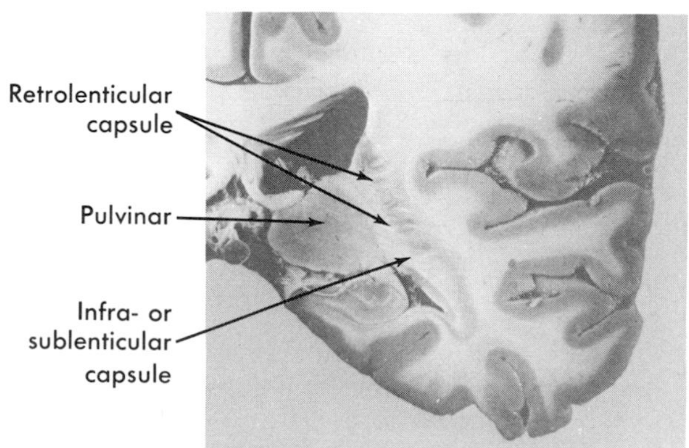

Fig. 21-4. Posterior pulvinar showing association radiations to and projections from cortex. Note fibers passing through, and posterior to, the lenticular remnants (retrolenticular internal capsule) and inferior to the lenticular remnants (infralenticular internal capsule).

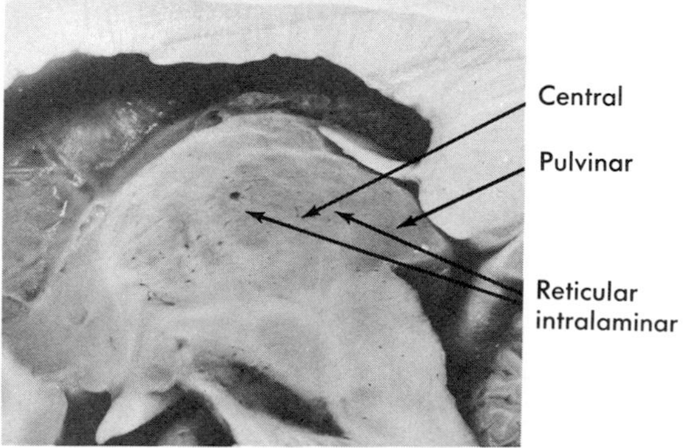

Fig. 21-5. Parasagittal section showing association and nonspecific thalamic nuclei.

back to cortex. Electrostimulation of these nuclei evoke widespread cortical responses. These associative cell groups display reciprocal cortical connections and in many ways suggest a function of combining integrative activity for different sensory systems.[7,12] For example, the input to the pulvinar, the largest of the association nuclei, is of diffuse origin (from the amygdala as well as other thalamic nuclei). No direct connection from either geniculate body seems to exist, nor are direct fibers from the somesthetic relays apparent. Nonetheless, the pulvinar has extensive reciprocal connections with parieto-temporo-occipital association areas, which undoubtedly process somesthetic, visual, and auditory interplay at the highest integrative level. The dorsal part of the lateral nucleus also connects prominently to association cortical fields and functions in ways that are still largely obscure.

Nonspecific nuclei (thalamic reticular substance)

These nuclear groups include the midline, lateral, reticular, and central cell masses that are abundant and generally classed as intralaminar (Figs. 21-3 and 21-6). They connect with the ascending reticular substance of the brainstem and interconnect widely among themselves and with other thalamic nuclei. Some also connect with basal ganglia. Their activity is consonant with short-chain reticular substance response elsewhere. While not specific in any definite functional set, these nuclei are essential in maintaining general thalamic activity. Their fibers do not reach the cortex, but they play a part in neuronal interactions that permit the direct and associational pathways to function.[4,11]

In summary, the thalamus functions as a relay for specific sensation and possesses some level of crude appreciation. Through these connections it also contributes to discrimination by relaying the pathways for the characteristics of quality and quantity. In addition, the thalamus contributes to affect through generating autonomic connections via collaterals and feedback systems to and from the cortex. The indirect integrative relays contribute enormously to the association phenomena that account for general integration of complex, mixed sensory information. The reticular components operate to reinforce, activate, inhibit, and synchronize thalamocortical exchanges.[7] All these functions are dependent in the physiologic state upon the integrity of cortical connections.

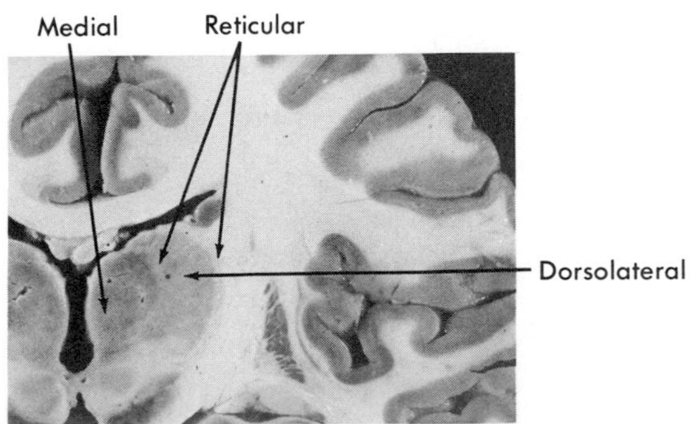

Fig. 21-6. Nonspecific and reticular nuclei of thalamus.

CEREBRAL CORTEX

The covering rind of the human brain (cortex) differentiates in the following three structural entities: (1) *paleocortex,* or paleopallium, which is olfactory and is a superficial nonlaminated cortical field related to olfaction; (2) *archicortex,* or archipallium, which is the hippocampal complex; and (3) *neocortex* (isocortex), or neopallium, which is the vast laminated cell mass overlying the bulk of the brain. The neopallium possesses a surface area of 200,000 to 250,000 sq. mm. and probably houses about 15 billion cells. The thickness varies from 1.5 to 3.5 mm., and the total weight is from 500 to 700 grams.[1,3,9] The convolutional patterns provide reasonably secure landmarks to specific areas. Topography is largely based on convolutional configuration. The present section relates the brain surfaces to function and interrelates the parts of the brain by fiber connections. As mentioned previously, the thalamus has a conspicuous reciprocal fiber exchange with the cortex. (For review of the volume and complexity of the major efferent paths from the cortex, see Chapter 22.) The present section deals with *sensory localization, structure of cortex, special cortical areas,* and the *organization of the white matter* interrelating the cortex with other parts of the CNS.

Cortical localization

Primary sensory localization. The general cortical landmarks have been reviewed (see Chapter 2) in terms of fissures, sulci, and lobes and by functional localization as *primary receptive areas.* It is convenient in detailing cortical characteristics to refer to an arbitrary spatial compartmentalization by a number system rather than by the longer descriptive terms (for example, area 8, instead of the posterior fourth of the intermediate frontal gyrus). The most widely accepted arbitrary number system is modified from Brodmann and is represented in Fig. 21-7. The centers discussed thus far represent primary receptive fields related to specific afferent pathways and include *general somesthetic* (areas 3, 1, 2, 5), *auditory* (area 41), *visual* (area 17), *gustatory* (areas 27?, 43?), *olfactory* (areas 25, 34), and *equilibratory* (anterior 22?) fields.

The *general somesthetic* (primary) area occupies the postcentral gyrus, with coronal specificity assigned from lower lateral to upper medial as follows: visceral abdominal at the buried opercular part of the gyrus; pharynx and tongue at lower fourth of lateral surface; teeth, gums, mouth, face, and eye through next fourth of lateral surface; hand and wrist over next fourth; arm, trunk, and leg through upper fourth of lateral surface; foot and genitalia on medial surface of hemisphere (see Chapter 16). In this pattern it is apparent that the segmental representation of the body is generally reversed. This does not hold for the cervical dermatomes, which are in the same vertical order in the sensory cortex as in the neck. In the representation of the hand the ulnar side lies above the radial. The general somatic sensations are not equally represented in either intensity or quality. For example, pain and simple sensations are only slightly related to the area in comparison to discriminative sensations. In this connection spatial relations appear to be best appreciated in the anterior part, weight and shape in the posterior part, and graduated intensity in the posterior inferior part. The limits of the somesthetic field seem quite constant in including a slight part of the precentral gyrus, all of the postcentral gyrus and the posterior half of the paracentral lobule, the anterior part of the superior parietal lobule, and often the anterior superior part of the supramarginal gyrus.

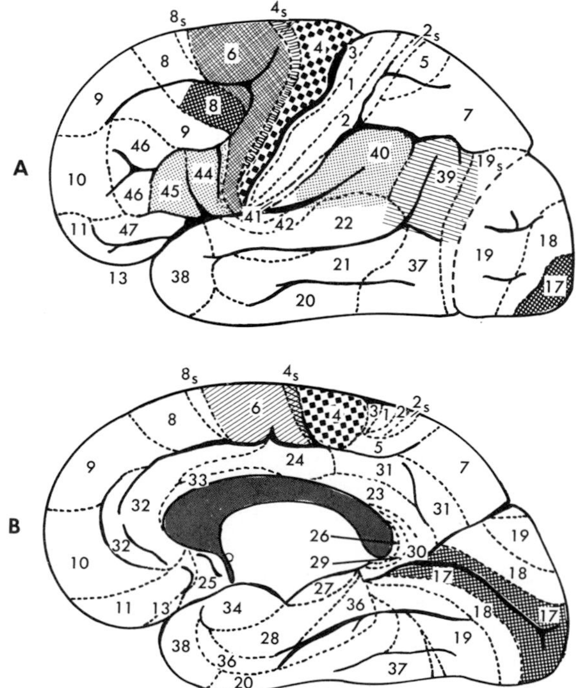

Fig. 21-7. Lateral, **A,** and medial, **B,** views showing cortical subdivisions. (After Brodmann.)

The *auditory area* is traditionally tied to Heschl's gyrus (area 41), with a somewhat confused inclusion of a second paralleling gyrus, area 42. In fact the gyral configurations vary enormously in the area. Only one in three brains possesses two bilaterally parallel transverse gyri of Heschl. The commonest configuration (forty-eight percent) is one transverse gyrus on the left and two on the right.[2] These features cause real difficulty in specific assignment of area numbers for refined cortical localization (see Chapter 19).

The *visual cortex* (area 17) is uniformly related to the calcarine fissure and has been previously reviewed (see Chapter 20). The visual cortex is also called the area striata because of the presence of the line of Gennari in the field.

The uncertainties surrounding the localization of primary fields for *gustatory, equilibratory,* and *olfactory* sensations have already been mentioned. While the human gustatory field remains controversial, the inferior part of the general somesthetic area (43) is usually credited. By tradition olfaction is assigned to the uncus and hippocampus in general, as well as to the parolfactory, anterior perforate area, and piriform cortex overlying the uncus (paleocortex). It is probable, at least in man, that the archicortex (hippocampal complex) is adapted to the more complex viscera-related activities of the limbic system (see Chapter 22). Equilibration is commonly assigned to the anterior part of area 22 and the external aspect of 41 and 42, because stimulation of the zone produces vertigo.[13]

Secondary sensory areas. Certain cortical fields are known to be functionally related to sensory complexes, commonly multiple, in a higher integrative level of activity. Assignment of cortical area is necessarily vague, and fiber pathways are impossible to follow because of the multitude of relays in the systems. In general the areas are physiologic extensions of the primary sensory complexes. It should be understood that these areas are focal concentrations of these associations and are richly interconnected. They are therefore dependent upon many anatomic systems for functional integrity, and they are not localizable in the same sense as primary receptive areas. Those generally represented as *secondary* sensory areas include: areas 5 and 7, which relate to general somesthetic sense; area 42 and possibly 51, which relate to audition; and areas 18 and 19, which relate to vision. The functions are not specifically known, but some interesting suggestions have been advanced. Area 42, for example, may possess an opposing tonotopic pattern to that existing in area 41. *Suppressive (S) zones,* which are quite specific for the somesthetic area (2 S) and for the visual association area (19 S), can be identified by electrical stimulation. The remaining secondary areas relate to the primary areas as extensions for qualitative change or in refinement of sensation.

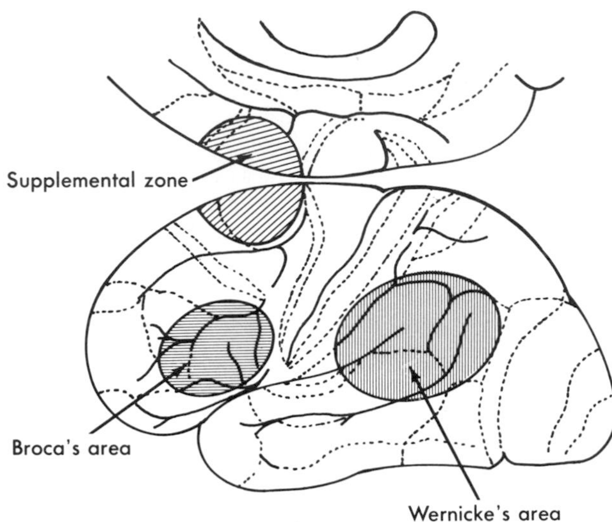

Fig. 21-8. Cortical areas relating to dysphasias. (After Penfield and Roberts.)

Association sensory zones. Of particular interest among sensory zones are the several classic cortical areas that are represented as localization fields for symbolic expression. Defects in the areas are presumed to relate to dysphasia, or impairment of speech, by interrupting the sensory side of the association pattern required in reading and hearing. The classic representations include: (1) auditory associations relating to the meaning of spoken words (*area 22*); (2) visual auditory associations, which combine visual and auditory symbols in understanding the spoken word and recognizing the printed word (combined posterior areas *22, 37,* and *39,* or *Wernicke's area*); (3) symbol association, by which words are recognized as symbols (*area 40,* supramarginal gyrus); and (4) symbol recognition association, by which printed words are recognized (*area 39,* angular gyrus).[10] This degree of specificity has been difficult to prove on the basis of physiologic and pathologic studies.[8,13] The most important sensory association area for speech and hearing has been identified as lying in the parietotemporal field, roughly corresponding to posterior areas 22, 40, and 39, and upper area 37 (Fig. 21-8).[13] The field is described as the posterior speech center and is localized to the left hemisphere, regardless of handedness. It may shift to the right during the period of development in the event of absence or early destruction of the left region.

Higher centers. Integrative action among primary, secondary, and associational zones has been postulated for frontal, parietal, and temporal cortical fields not otherwise assigned in either sensory or motor dominance. Association fibers are abundantly evident in all locations, but specific physiologic assignment is thus far impossible. Memory, emotion, intellectual activity, and all the complex cerebration having to do with volitional procedures are impossible to localize and probably must be be regarded as products of "total" cerebration, although (as determined from ablation experiments) only a fraction of cerebral substance seems to be activated in most experiences.

Intellectual functions, higher skills, memory storage, refined synergies, appreciation, and elaboration of thought are variously assigned to frontal, parietal, and temporal lobe areas not otherwise engaged. These represent cerebral functions of highest order and are not individually anatomically localized. Integrity of the cerebral fields listed is essential to the functions named.

Reticular formation and the cortex. The myriad of short-chain neuronal systems has been repeatedly referred to as providing pathways for almost every function. These systems provide interconnections from cortex to cord, with inclusion of thalamus, basal nuclei, and brainstem. Most important is the apparent continuous activity of this system of interneurons in activating synaptic transfer in most nuclei (see Chapter 15). Perhaps the most satisfactory cortical assignment of this multisynaptic system is in *arousal* or *inhibition,* either ascending or descending, in which the thalamus also plays an important part. As in other nuclear fields, the cerebral cortex undoubtedly requires continuing neuronal synaptic bombardment as a prelude to effective integrated discharges.

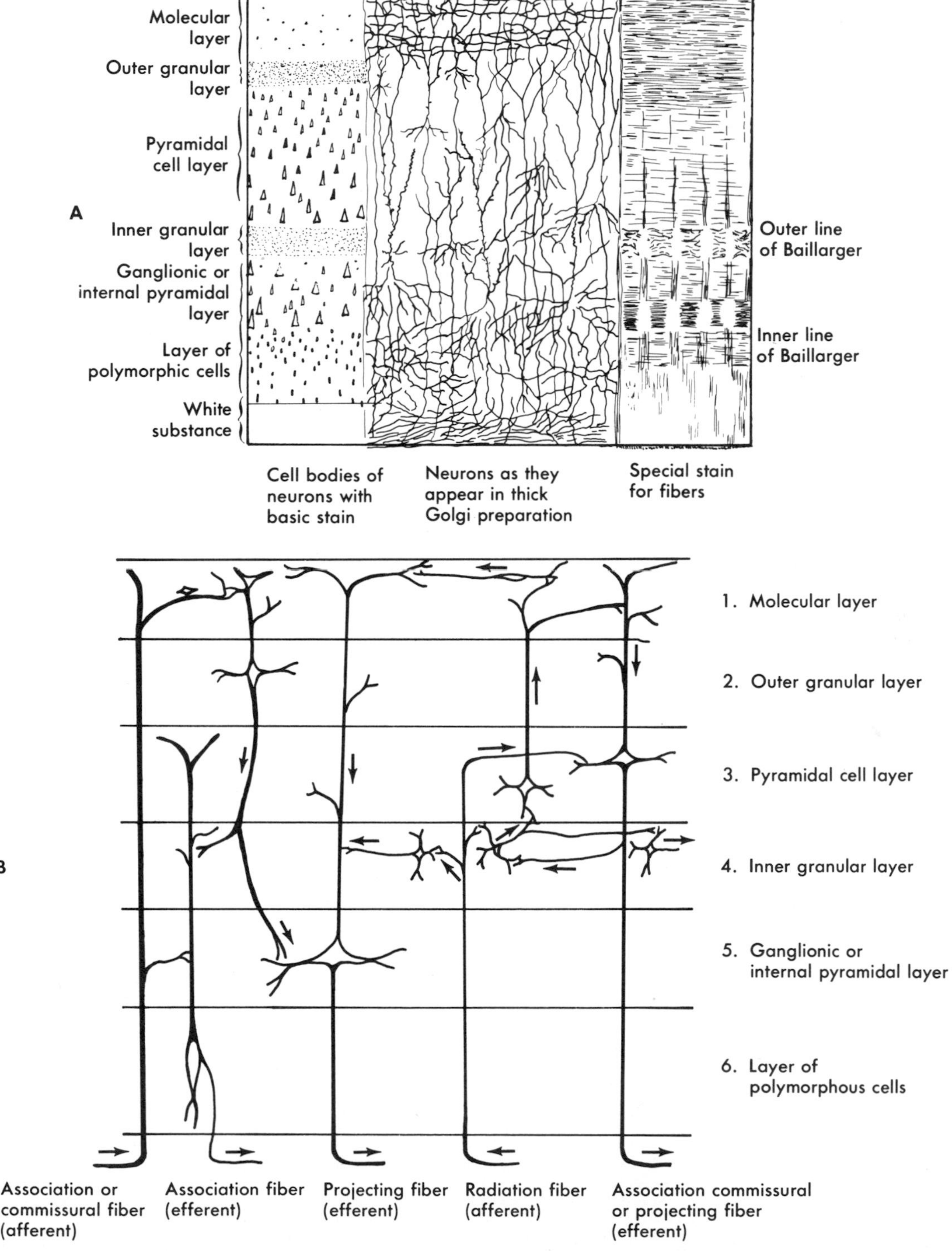

Fig. 21-9. A, Composite of cellular and fiber patterns of cerebral cortex comparing Nissl, Golgi, and silver methods; **B,** diagram of cortical interconnections. (After Lorenti de Nó.)

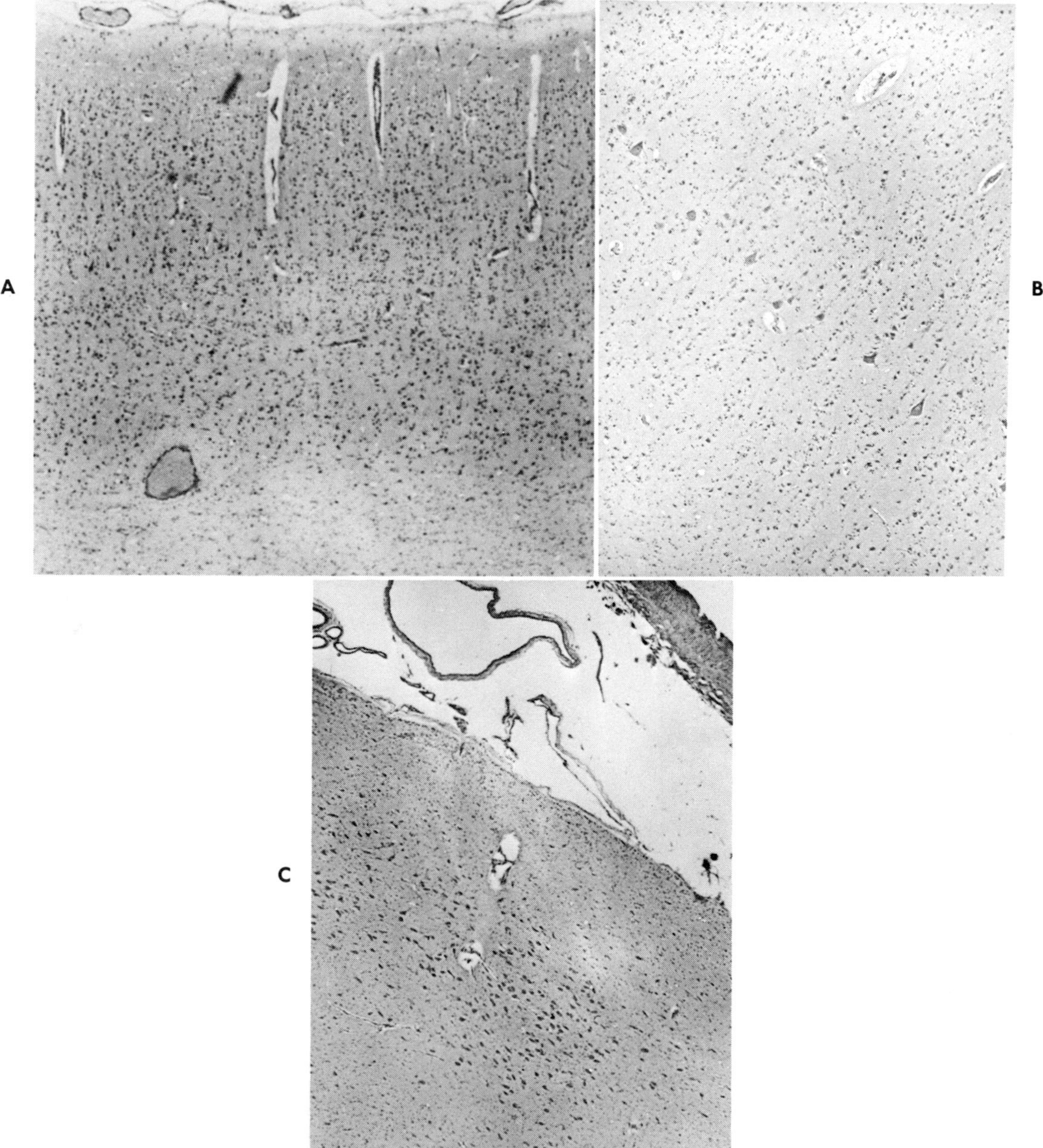

Fig. 21-10. A, Prototype of laminated "granular" cortex—somesthetic areas 1, 2, and 3; **B,** prototype of laminated "nongranular" cortex—motor area 4. (×45.) **C,** Prototype of nonlaminated cortex—anterior perforated substance, olfactory, or paleocortex.

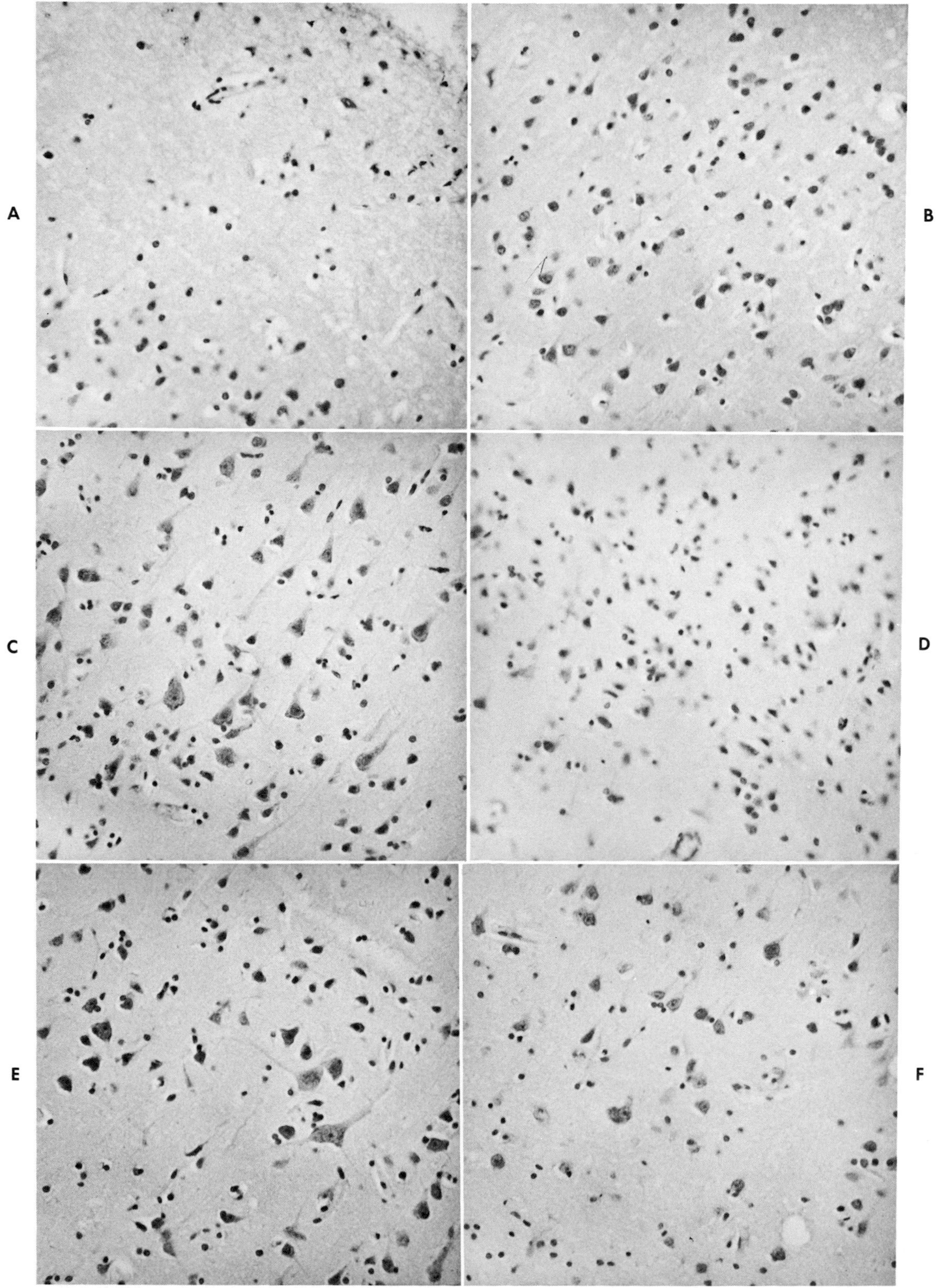

Fig. 21-11. Prototype cell patterns characterizing cortical layers from area 3. **A,** Molecular; **B,** external granular; **C,** external pyramidal; **D,** internal granular; **E,** internal pyramidal or ganglionic; **F,** polymorphous or multiform. (×312.)

Structure of cortex

Neocortex. The structural details relating to the human cerebral neocortex are represented best as a composite drafted from cell studies (*cytoarchitecture*) and from fiber studies (*myeloarchitecture*). The general relationships are diagrammed in Fig. 21-9, *A*, as a six-layered cell pattern with interconnections, as shown in Fig. 21-9, *B*.[6]

Cytoarchitecture. In general, the cortical layering can be characterized by lamination in granular or nongranular patterns (Fig. 21-10, *A* and *B*), or as nonlaminated (Fig. 21-10, *C*). The outer layer of a prototype area (such as area 3) as represented is layer I, *molecular*. It is relatively cell-free and represents a prominent synaptic field. The few cells (of Cajal) are oriented horizontally and seem to serve a correlative function. They are flattened or fusiform (Fig. 21-11, *A*). Layer II (*external granular*) is made up of small pyramidal and stellate cells of 10 to 12 μ in diameter. These cells interconnect within the cortex (Fig. 21-11, *B*). Layer III (*external pyramidal*) has large cells of from 30 to 35 μ and medium cells from 20 to 25 μ in maximum cell body dimension. These cells possess long dendrites arising in the molecular layer that attach to the external surfaces of the perikaryon, and shorter dendrites attaching to the base of the pyramid (Fig. 21-11, *C*). Layer IV (*internal granular*) is mainly granule cells, which are oriented perpendicularly. They possess short dendrites and axons. It is presumed that they are primarily receptive. A varying number of small pyramidal and stellate cells are admixed in this layer. One large elongate stellate type (of Martinotti) connects with the molecular layer. It is presumed that they are primarily receptive (Fig. 21-11, *D*). Layer V (*internal pyramidal*, or *ganglionic*) is dominated by large and medium-sized pyramidal cells. Their axons are directed to the white matter, but they give off collaterals that turn back into the cortex and pass toward the surface. This layer also includes fusiform and ovoid cells, whose axons are directed both deep and toward the surface (Fig. 21-11, *E*). Layer VI (*polymorphous*, or *multiform*) is characterized by a mixture of neuron types, including pyramidal, stellate, and fusiform shapes. (Fig. 21-11, *F*).

Embryologic and comparative anatomic studies suggest that the cortical layers external to the internal granular layer (*supragranular cortex*) are concerned principally with intracortical associations. These relate to higher associational or psychic functions. On the other hand, the layers deep to the internal granular layers (*infragranular cortex*) gives rise to projections that leave the cortex. These provide the projection fibers from the cortex and are in general related to organic and instinctive processes. While the intimate details of laminar connections in man remain obscure, the presumed interrelationships illustrated in Fig. 21-9, *B*, provide a working base derived from many sources. The principal receptive field is probably the internal granular layer. It follows then that the primary sensory cortical areas are relatively granular (Fig. 21-10, *A*). The auditory cortex is characterized by the unusual relative thickness of the granular layers and by the perpendicular orientation of these cells. The other primary receptive areas (somesthetic and visual, for example) are also basically granular in character, but they are less thick than the auditory cortex and are devoid of the fusiform cells of Cajal. The efferent fibers leaving the cortex make up the projections that pass to the thalamus, basal nuclei, brainstem, and cord. These arise in infragranular layers, and where efferent activity dominates (motor) the granular layers are relatively small, and the internal pyramidal layer is prominent (Fig. 21-10, *B*).

Myeloarchitecture. With special stains (Fig. 21-9, *A*) the fiber patterns within the neocortex produced a series of bands or stripes. These include *outer tangential bands* in the molecular layer; a *supragranular layer*, or outer line of Baillarger, in the external part of the internal granular zone; and an *infragranular layer*, or inner line of Baillarger, within the pyramidal area. The two lines of Baillarger fuse in the visual cortex to form the line of Gennari. These fiber tracts are made up of transverse axon collaterals from pyramidal cells, of basal dendrites from pyramidal cells, and of horizontal branches and terminals from fibers entering the cortex. The fibers that are oriented perpendicularly form masses of radiating filaments entering and leaving the cortex. Long association fibers traverse full thickness to terminate in the supragranular layers, particularly the molecular layer. These are oriented obliquely in the fiber mass in the cortex (Fig. 21-12). The radiations arising in the thalamus presumably terminate principally in the internal granular layer, where interneurons are abundant. The fibers projecting from the cortex include the bulky axons from the infragranular layers that are destined to leave the cortex, and the smaller filaments from supragranular layers that are directed to associations.

Allocortex. The paleocortex, or olfactory cortex, is topographically described in Chapter 17. The nonlaminated character of the anterior perforated substance (olfactory cortex) is shown in Fig. 21-10,

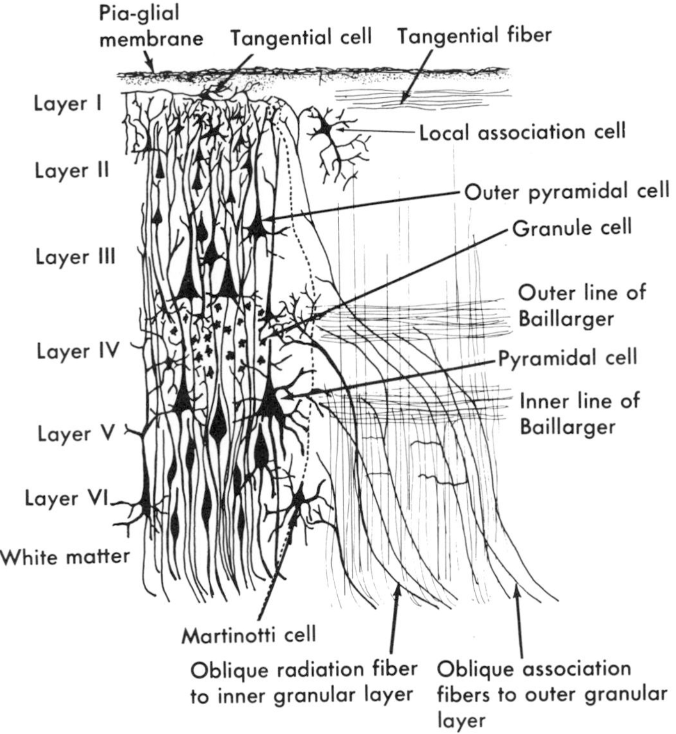

Fig. 21-12. Composite of Golgi and silver-stained cortex showing oblique cortical fibers. (After Rasmussen.)

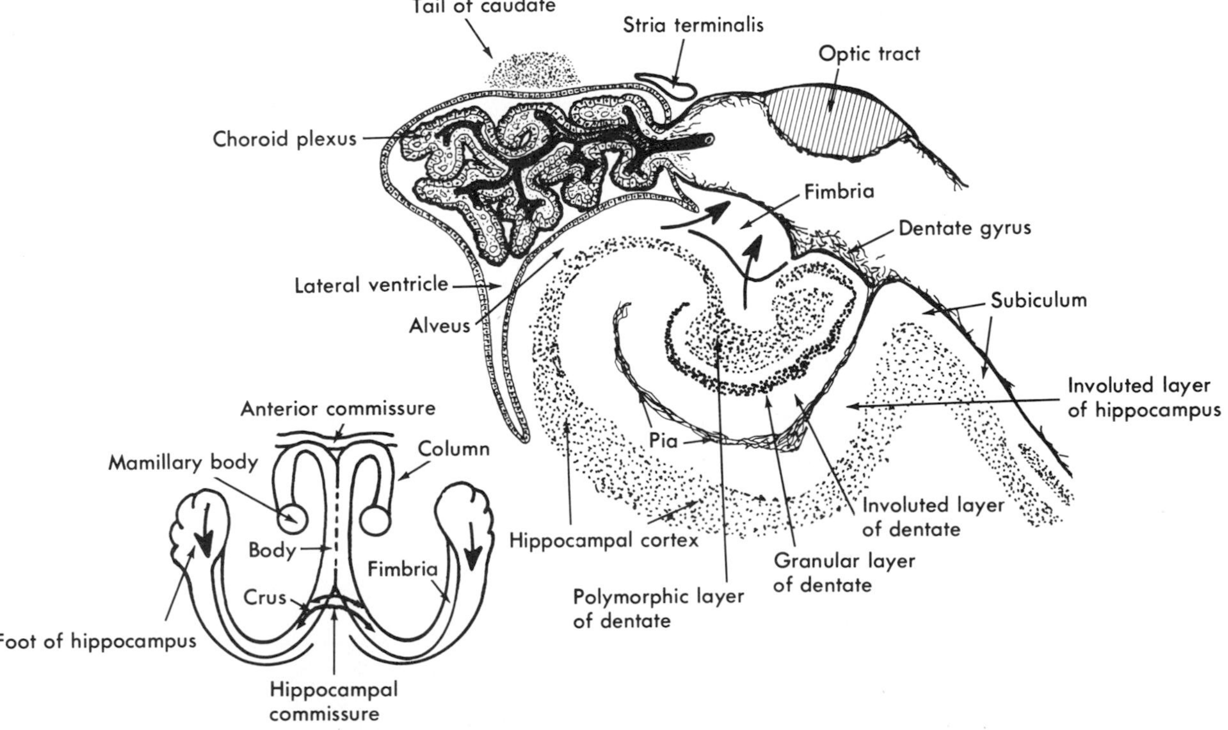

Fig. 21-13. Hippocampal cortex (archicortex) with insert showing efferent pathway through fornices and hippocampal commissures.

C. The archicortex displays the unique laminated configurations shown in Fig. 21-13, illustrating the hippocampus. This segment of the limbic brain has a markedly varied input from numerous afferent sources. The efferent path is via the fornices to the hypothalamus (see Chapter 22).

SPECIAL CORTICAL AREAS

Limbic system

A somewhat circular ring of cortical tissue including orbitofrontal, cingulate, hippocampal, and uncus portions are specially related to behavior and emotions (visceral brain) (Fig. 21-14). As a consequence, the function of these areas is closely tied to vegetative and metabolic activity of the hypothalamus and to other diencephalic nuclei, as well as to parts of the basal ganglia. This involves such complex sensations as pleasure, satiety, guilt, punishment, habituation, wakefullness, alertness, excitement, so-called psychic effects, and general autonomic activity, particularly as applied to endocrine responses. In general, the limbic cortical system seems to be associative in complex responses related to behavior. The limbic system is anatomically closely related to the olfactory cortical fields and to the amygdala, whose medial aspect derives extensive input from the olfactory complex (see Chapter 17). While olfactory input is dominant in some species, this sensory complex is less prominent in man, where visual, auditory, and general sensory influences play a greater role in complex behavioral responses. (For discussion of the limbic system and its autonomic features, and the motor complexes, see Chapter 22.)

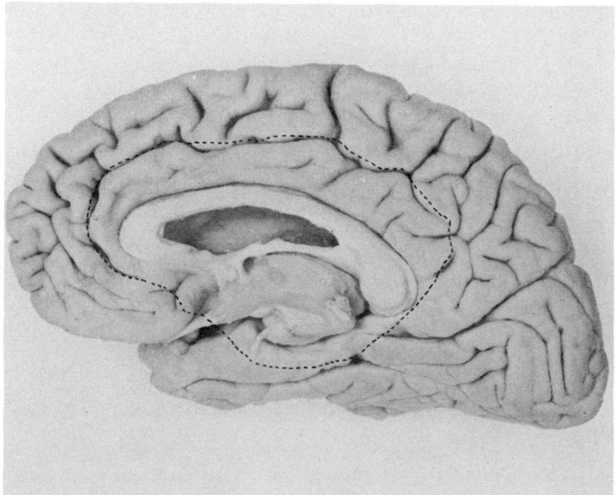

Fig. 21-14. Limbic lobe outlined on medial view of brain. The system includes the fornices (see Chapter 22).

Temporal lobe

As previously noted, auditory and vestibular localization in primary, secondary, and associational spheres can be directed to the temporal lobe. The neocortical part is closely related to the allocortical hippocampal complex of the limbic system. Visual ties are extensive and show up in the dysphasic features related to lesions of the temporal lobe. Part of the visual radiations pass into the temporal lobe via Meyer's loop and involve the area in visual phenomena (see Chapter 20). Because stimulation of the temporal pole gives rise to responses that relate to experiences (hallucinations and illusions), this region has been called the *psychic* cortex. Unilateral stimulation of the temporal cortex may elicit facial movements on either side. This ties the region to motor systems. In general, the temporal lobe has much unassigned cortical tissue that qualifies as integrative in function. A section from a "typical" association area (area 22) is shown in Fig. 21-15.

Insula

In general, the insular fields are poorly correlated with specific function in man. Area 52 may represent an associational or secondary auditory area (see Chapter 19). The island cortex may have some part in autonomic regulation or appreciation (such as nausea). Connections of the human insula remain uncertain.

Occipital lobe

Primary, secondary, and associative features of vision account for much of the occipital cortical function (see Chapter 20). In micro section the visual cortex is granular and is basically that of the prototype (area 3) shown in Fig. 21-10, *A*. Fibers entering the field largely terminate in the granular layer. The efferent fibers are short associational fibers to area 18.

Parietal lobe

The histologic character of the somesthetic area is shown in Fig. 21-10, *A*. This area relates by short associational fibers to the motor cortex and to the gyri behind it (both 5 and 7). The area also projects to basal nuclei and the thalamus, and sends and receives commissural fibers via the corpus callosum. Areas 40 and 39 relate to symbolic perception and display little specific cytoarchitectural detail. Area 19 relates to visual association and plays a

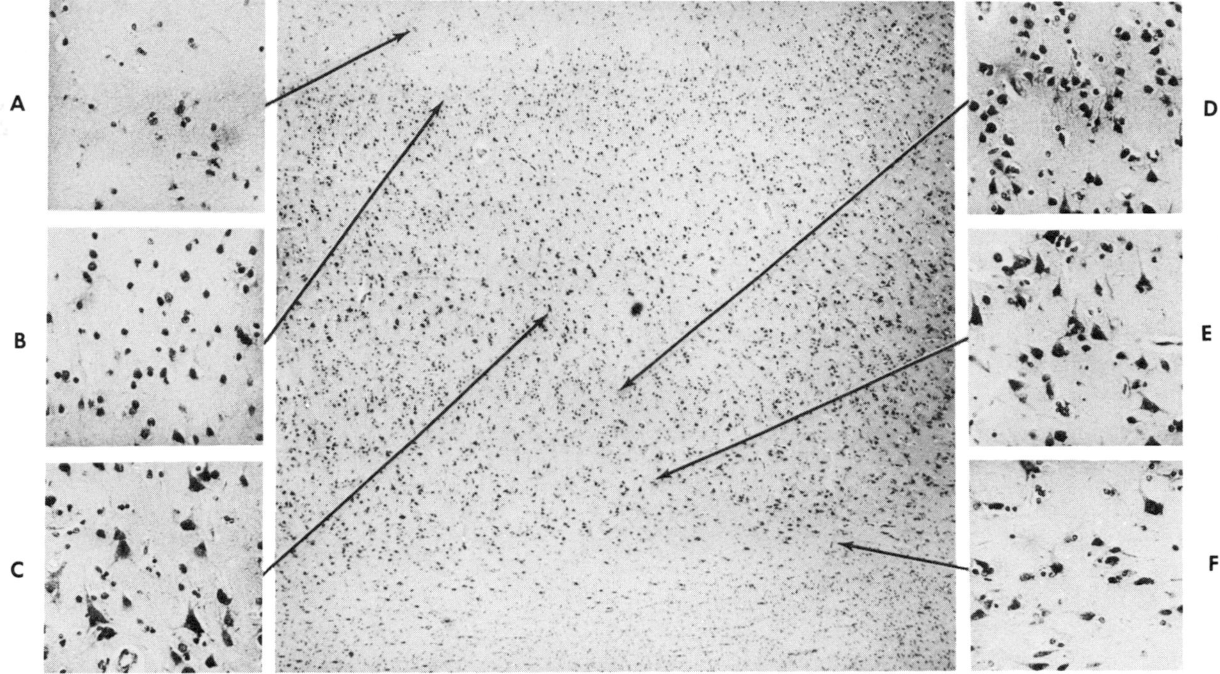

Fig. 21-15. Association area 22. Note supragranular prominence. **A, B, C, D, E,** and **F** are from layers I, II, III, IV, V, and VI, respectively.

role in following movements of the eye (opticokinetics). The superior parietal lobule above the angular and supramarginal gyri represents a field presumed to be integrative in its action.

Frontal lobe

The precentral gyrus is the motor cortex whose structural details are shown in Fig. 21-10, *B*. This area (4) is discussed in the following chapter in connection with the motor systems, as are areas 6 and 8 (premotor cortex), areas 44 to 47 (Broca's area of motor speech), and the supplemental motor field (6 and 8) on the medial side of the frontal lobe. The motor fields also have related suppressor (S) areas, 4 S and 8 S, which by stimulation will suppress output from the corresponding motor fields (Figs. 21-7 and 21-8). Areas 9 through 12 are prefrontal; this region has prominent reciprocal fiber connections with the dorsomedial nucleus of the thalamus (Fig. 21-1 and 21-2). It also projects directly to the hypothalamus. Its extensive ties to the limbic system suggest the prefrontal fields as the neocortex of that complex. Disturbances in the prefrontal area produce alterations in personality rather than intelligence. Ablation of the area or isolation (lobotomy) produces diminished *drive,* lessoned anxiety, released restraints, and profoundly altered state of mind, or *affect*. The area links to autonomic responses through the hypothalamus and enters into their display in emotional states.

ORGANIZATION OF WHITE MATTER

The parts of the cerebral cortex interrelate by fibers of two categories. Those that connect from cortex to cortex of the same side are *association fibers*. Those that connect from side to side are *commissural fibers*. A third type of fiber connection relates the cortex to nuclei outside the cortex, such as the thalamus, basal nuclei, brainstem nuclei, and the nuclei of the spinal cord. These form the *projections*. Fibers coming from outlying nuclei and entering the cortex are called *ascending projections*. When arising from the relatively small bulk of a nucleus such as the thalamic parts, these ascending projections are called *radiations* because of their fanning pattern.

Associations

Association fibers occur in two distinct patterns, *short* and *long*. The short association (arcuate) fibers pass from gyrus to gyrus, and in this route closely hug the cortical margin (Fig. 21-16). They possess distinct enough characteristics to persist in many conditions in which the long association bun-

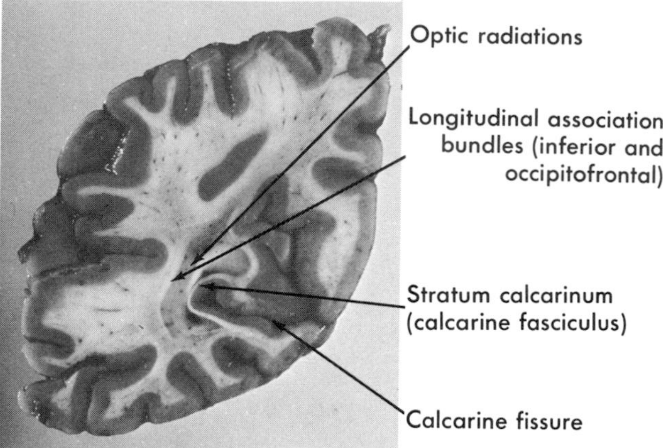

Fig. 21-16. Short association fibers exemplified in stratum calcarinum. Note vertical associations.

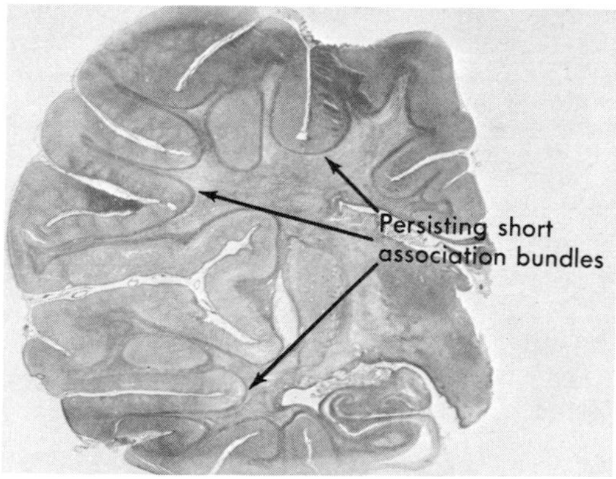

Fig. 21-17. Persistence of short association bundles in otherwise totally demyelinated brain.

dles degenerate (Fig. 21-17). Presumably they both arise and terminate in supragranular layers. A particularly prominent short association tract is the *stratum calcarinum,* which conveys fibers between upper and lower visual cortex.

The long association bundles interconnect more remote regions and organize into fairly distinct bundles in the following locations. The *uncinate fasciculus* passes from the frontal lobe in a hook-shaped configuration to the temporal pole (Fig. 21-18, *B*). The *inferior occipitofrontal fasciculus* passes from occipital to frontal areas in the white matter along the inferior border of the insula and claustrum. It fans out both occipitally and frontally (Fig. 21-18, *A* to *C*). The *superior occipitofrontal fasciculus* runs in a subcallosal position where the corpus callosum meets the internal capsule (Fig. 21-18, *C*). It probably feeds fibers into the caudate nucleus as well as interconnecting the cortical areas. The *inferior longitudinal fasciculus* passes from temporal to occipital cortex, running in the inferior temporal white matter (Fig. 21-18, *B* and *C*). The *superior longitudinal fasciculus* passes from frontal to parietal, occipital, and temporal lobes in a fanned-out pattern, as shown in Fig. 21-18, *B*. This fasciculus forms considerable bulk in the centrum semiovale and intermixes with fibers of the internal capsule and corpus callosum (Fig. 21-18, *C*). The *cingulum* occupies the main bulk of the gyrus cinguli and interrelates frontomedial cortex with parieto-occipital and temporal cortex on the medial sides (Fig. 21-18). A *vertical* association fasciculus passes from upper lateral to lower lateral occipital cortical areas (Fig. 21-18, *B*).

Commissures

The *corpus callosum* is the massive interhemispheric commissure that connects the right to the left cortex in almost all its parts. Area 21 on the lateral aspect of the temporal lobe, the suppressors zones (both motor and sensory, 4 S, 8 S, 2 S, 19 S), and area 17 of the visual cortex do not contribute fibers to the corpus callosum. Both the somesthetic and motor fields contribute relatively few fibers to the callosal exchange. Almost all others cortical areas interconnect by this means. Some do so on a symmetrical exchange pattern. Other areas are both symmetrical and asymmetrical, and in this relationship the corpus callosum receives collaterals from both long association and projection fibers (Fig. 21-19). The most abundant contributions arise from the cortical areas related to integrative activity. The function of the corpus callosum remains obscure insofar as specific neurologic deficits occur from lesions within it. The structure can be absent by agenesis, with the defect neurologically imperceptible, but so-called split-brain preparations have a profound effect on learning and retention.[14] The commissure undoubtedly relates during the periods of growth and learning to transferring of engrams, particularly of the higher integrative type, from one side to the other (see Chapter 23).

The *anterior commissure* interrelates areas 21 of the temporal lobes. It also relates the symmetrical olfactory fields (piriform area, amygdala, and anterior perforated substance) and connects the olfactory nuclei on one side with neocortex on the other (see Chapter 17).

The *hippocampal commissure* interrelates the

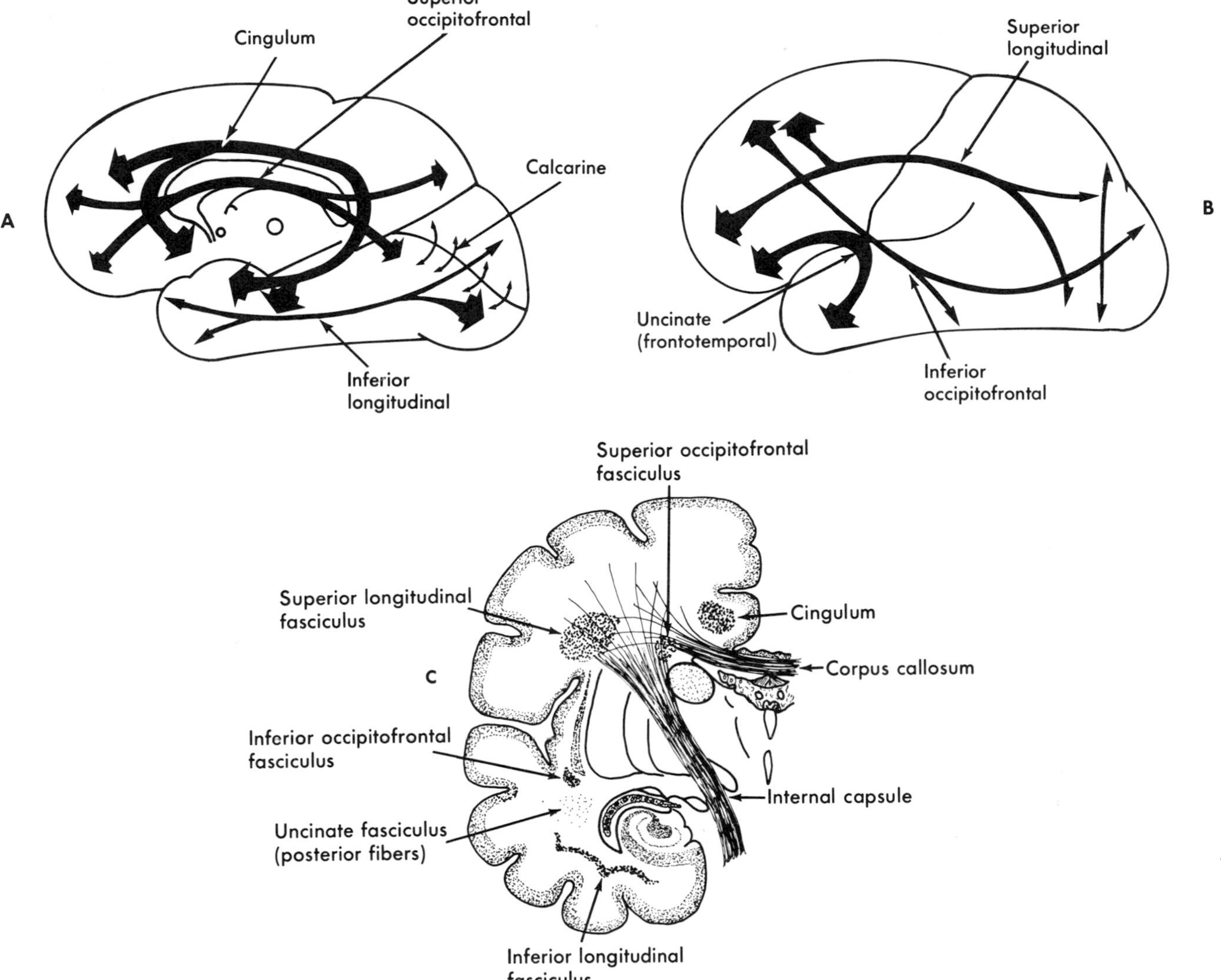

Fig. 21-18. A, Long association fibers projected on medial view of brain with stem removed; **B,** schematic of long association fibers projected in lateral view; **C,** placement of association bundles in coronal section.

hippocampal complexes of either side by passing from the crus of one fornix to that of the other (Fig. 21-17). Some temporal neocortex is undoubtedly involved in this interchange, as well as the hippocampal archicortex.

Numerous other commissures interrelate cerebral structures, but do so indirectly. These are the posterior, habenular, Gudden's, thalamic, and brainstem fiber crossings previously reviewed.

Projections

The masses of fibers arising in the cerebral cortex that leave the area for outlying nuclei are organized into the internal capsule. The radiations ascending in this fiber mass from thalamic nuclei have previously been mentioned. The makeup of the internal capsule relates parts of the structure to topographic markers that permit the following subdivisions (1) an *anterior limb,* which relates to the frontal cortex and passes in the cleft between the caudate head and the putamen (Fig. 21-20); (2) a *genu,* which is a knee-like bend in the capsule most evident in a transverse section (Fig. 21-20); (3) the *posterior limb,* which extends posteriorly from the genu between the lateral nucleus of the thalamus and the globus pallidus (Fig.

21-20); (4) a *retrolenticular* part, which is posterior to the lenticular nucleus (Fig. 21-4); and (5) a *sublenticular* part, which is inferior to the lenticular nuclei and best visualized in a coronal section (Fig. 21-4).

In the organization of the internal capsule these fibers cluster in order from front to back in fairly clear-cut bundles, as evidenced in local degenerative studies (Fig. 21-18, *C*). Most anterior of the projections are the *frontothalamic* fibers, which arise in the frontal cortex and pass to thalamic nuclei. Posteriorly adjacent are *frontopontine* fibers passing from the frontal cortex to pontine nuclei. Next are *pyramidal* fibers, which arise in area 4 and pass through the genu and adjacent capsule at the start of the posterior limb. The pyramidal pathway includes *corticobulbar* fibers, which arise in the lower half of area 4 and descend to the motor nuclei of the cranial nerves. These fibers locate in the genu. Immediately posterior to these are the *corticospinal* fibers from the upper part of the lateral surface of area 4. These fibers go to the motor nuclei in the ventral horn of the cervical enlargement for supply to the upper limbs. Next are the *corticospinal* fibers from the apex and medial surface of area 4 that pass to the lumbar enlargement for innervation of lower limb muscles. Posterior to the corticospinal bundles are the ascending radiations from the lateral nuclei of the thalamus to the *general somesthetic* area of the postcentral and neighboring gyri. Posteriorly adjacent are the *parieto-occipito-temporo-pontine* fibers, which pass from these cortical areas to the pontine nuclei (Fig. 22-13). In the adjacent retrolenticular part are the *geniculocalcarine* fibers of the visual radiations, which pass from the lateral geniculate body to the calcarine cortex (see Chapter 20). Mixed with these fibers in the retrolenticular part of the capsule are the reciprocal fibers interconnecting *pulvinar* and *parietal* cortex, and *corti-*

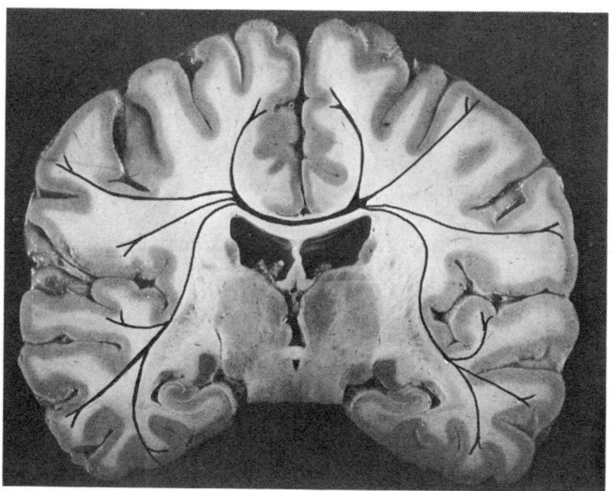

Fig. 21-19. Corpus callosum commissure.

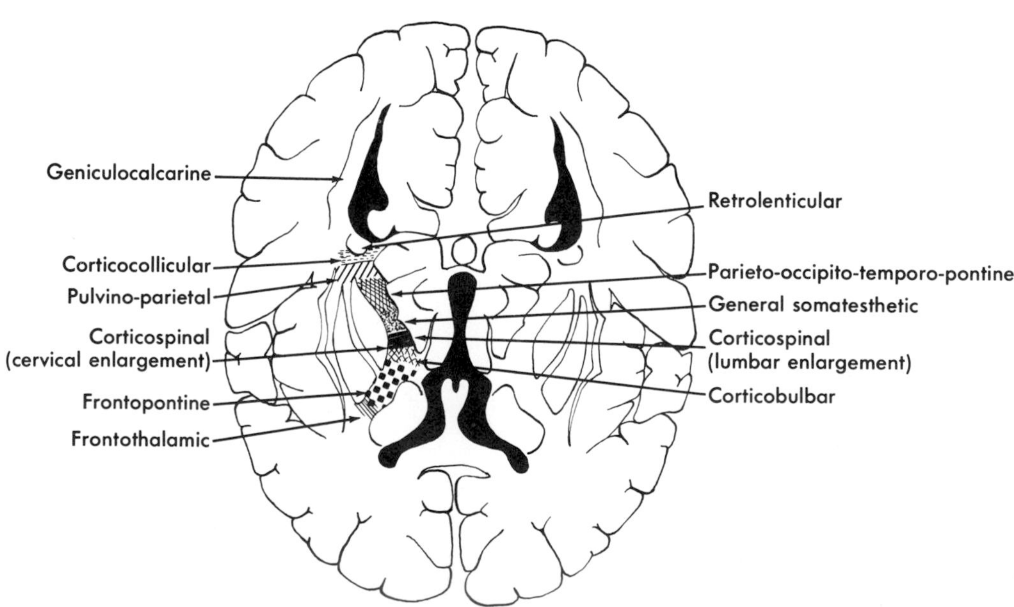

Fig. 21-20. Transverse diagram of internal capsule showing functional and regional topography.

cocollicular fibers most posteriorly. The *auditory radiations* occupy the sublenticular part of the capsule (see Chapter 19) in passing from the medial geniculate body to the transverse gyrus of Heschl.

Many diffuse fibers with known connections travel in the internal capsule without forming definitive bundles. These diffuse tracts include: (1) *cortico-thalamic* fibers, which are reciprocal paths of the thalamic radiations; (2) *thalamocortical* fibers, which include voluminous specific fiber connections without forming bundles (for example, anterior nucleus to cingulate gyrus); (3) *striocortical* and *corticostriate* fibers between precentral cortex and corpus striatum; (4) *corticorubral* and *rubrocortical* fibers, which interrelate cortex with red nucleus; and (5) *pulvinocortical* and *corticopulvinar* fibers, which tie the pulvinar to parietal and posterior superior temporal cortical areas. These components of the capsule form the major pathways of the extrapyramidal motor systems.

REFERENCES

1. Blinkov, S. M., and Glezer, I. I.: The human brain in figures and tables, New York, 1968, Plenum Publishing Corporation.
2. Campain, R., Jaeger, M., and Minckler, J.: The auditory cortex of man, Thesis, University of Denver, 1970.
3. Dekaban, A.: Neurology of infancy, Baltimore, 1959, The Williams & Wilkins Co.
4. Haymaker, W., Anderson, E., and Nauta, W. J. H.: The hypothalamus, Springfield, Illinois, 1958, Charles C Thomas, Publisher.
5. Hassler, R.: Anatomy of the thalamus. In Schaltenbrand, Z., and Bailey, P., editors: Introduction to sterotaxis with an atlas of the human brain, vol. I, Stuttgart, 1959, Georg Thieme Verlag.
6. Lorente de Nó, R.: Cerebral cortex. In Fulton, J., editor: Physiology of the nervous system, ed. 3, London, 1949, Oxford University Press.
7. McGoun, H. W.: The waking brain, Springfield, Illinois, 1958, Charles C Thomas, Publisher.
8. Minckler, J.: Communication disorders. In Minckler, J., editor: Pathology of the nervous system, vol. III, New York, 1971, McGraw-Hill Book Co.
9. Minckler, T., and Boyd, E.: Physical growth. In Minckler, J., editor: Pathology of the nervous system, vol. I, New York, 1968, McGraw-Hill Book Co.
10. Nielson, J. M.: Agnosias, apraxias, speech, and aphasia. In Baker, A. B., editor: Clinical neurology, ed. 2, vol. I, New York, 1962, Harper & Row, Publishers.
11. Noback, C. R.: The human nervous system, New York, 1967, McGraw-Hill Book Co.
12. Penfield, W., and Rasmussen, T.: The cerebral cortex of man, New York, 1950, The Macmillan Co.
13. Penfield, W., and Roberts, L.: Speech and brain mechanisms, Princeton, New Jersey, 1959, Princeton University Press.
14. Sperry, R. W.: Split-brain approach to learning. In Quarton, G. C., Melnechuk, T., and Schmitt, F. O., editors: The neurosciences, New York, 1967, The Rockefeller University Press.
15. von Bonin, G.: Essay on the cerebral cortex, Springfield, Illinois, 1950, Charles C Thomas, Publisher.

CHAPTER 22

MOTOR SYSTEMS

JEFF MINCKLER

The efferent and descending neural complexes in the human brain may be descriptively divided into nine groups. It should be noted that none can operate independently and that all of the complexes bear on most motor acts. (1) The *pyramidal system* is the voluntary motor pathway arising in the motor cortex of area 4. (2) The *extrapyramidal system* is an associated nonvolitional motor pathway arising mainly in the motor and premotor areas and relaying in the basal nuclei and parts of the thalamus and midbrain. (3) The *cortico-ponto-cerebellar system* arises in frontal, temporal, occipital, and parietal cortices and terminates in pontine nuclei, from which the pathway leads through cerebellum and midbrain nuclei to the final-common-path. (4) The *limbic system* figures in emotional responses and behavioral complexes closely related to autonomic activity and olfaction. It involves mainly the hippocampal complex, the thalamus, the cingulum, and the frontal lobes. (5) The *visceral efferent system* is closely related to visceral activity and is therefore less well established in its relationship to cerebral cortex. Although vital centers are controlled through this system, it operates largely without volition or conscious perception, and much of its activity is mediated through the hypothalmus. (6) The *neuroendocrine system* integrates hypothalamic and endocrine activities which are mediated through the pituitary gland. (7) *Other descending pathways* contribute to motor activity. These include many shorter-chain systems that bear eventually on final paths. (8) *Final-common-path cells* are those neurons that deliver the final volley to the effectors. (9) *Local neuromuscular units* and *servomechanisms* provide motor control to striated muscle. These structures are divorced from the other systems except when overcontrol is required.

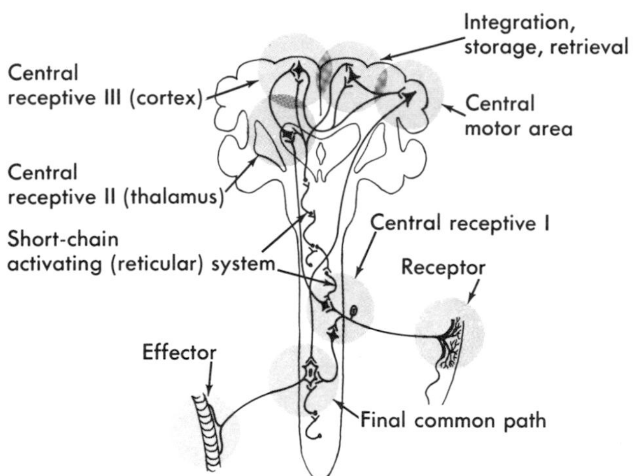

Fig. 22-1. Diagram of overall neural actions that culminate in motor effect.

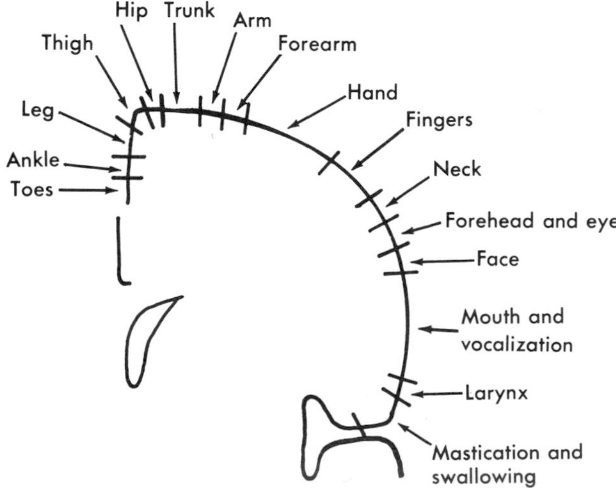

Fig. 22-2. Spatial representation in the motor cortex.

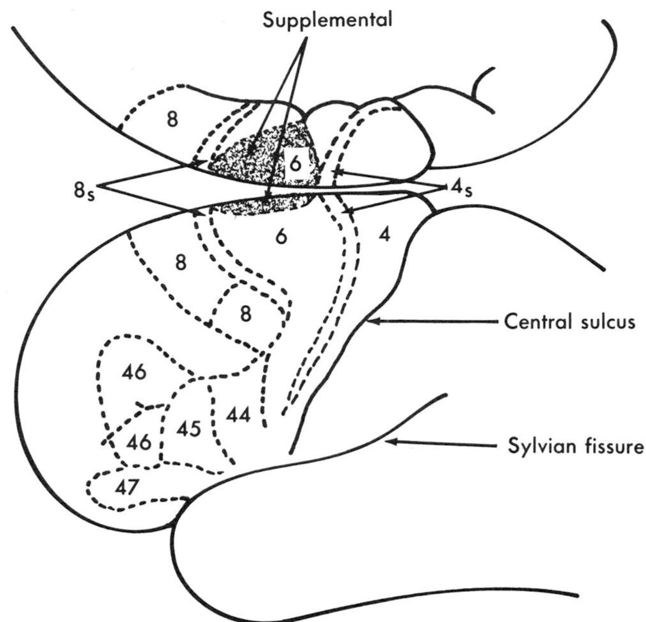

Fig. 22-3. Cerebral localization of motor fields, some of which are controversial or inconstant in human brain: area 4, volitional motor (see Fig. 22-2); area 4S, motor suppressor zone; areas 6 and 8, premotor areas; area 8S, suppressor zone; area 8, frontal eye fields, (controversial); areas 44, 45, 46, and 47 (of Broca), motor speech and writing symbols (controversial); cross-hatched supplemental area, motor related to speech (controversial).

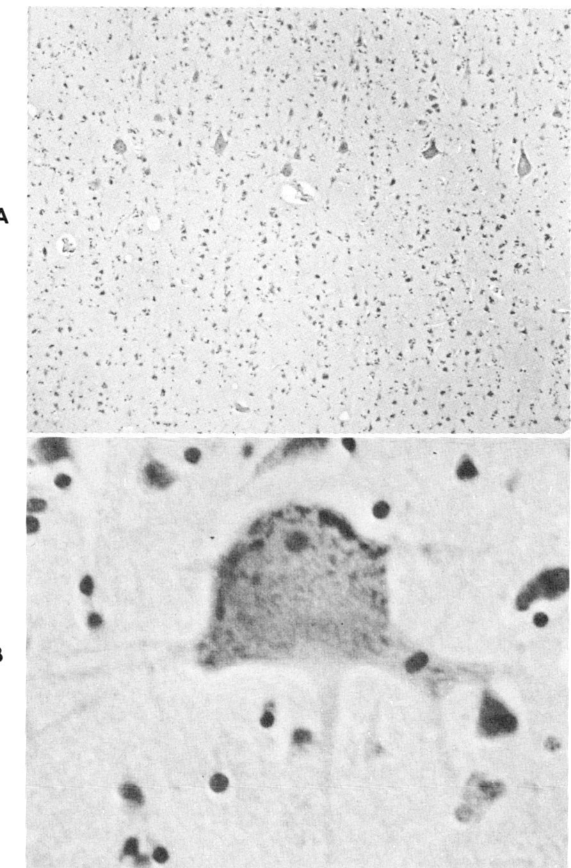

Fig. 22-4. A, Betz cell layer (H & E ×45.) **B,** Betz cell detail. Note clear axon hillock and directions taken by dendrites. (H & E ×500.)

PYRAMIDAL SYSTEM

Motor cortex

Efferent impulses arising in cortical area 4 are the products of interplay of all afferent systems, plus the reticular and associational activity bearing on the cortex (Fig. 22-1). This part of the motor fields represents volitional discharges. The spatial motor design representing body locations on the motor area 4 roughly parallels the sensory pattern (Fig. 22-2). Other closely related motor cortical efferent areas deserve special note (Fig. 22-3). A *suppression area, 4S,* represents a strip-zone immediately anterior to area 4; it causes cessation of existing muscle activity upon electrostimulation. *Frontal eye fields* occur in the posterior portion of the middle frontal gyrus and adjacent inferior frontal gyrus. These fields regulate eye movements, including associated movements of following. *Premotor (area 6)* cortex is regarded as supplementary motor cortex, but it has less specific localization correlated with movements. Ablation of area 6 produces degeneration of fibers admixed with the area 4 fibers (Fig. 22-7). *Area 8* (anterior to 6) is regarded as a contralateral suppressing field that permits correlated deviation movements of the eye rather than divergence. Of particular interest in speech and hearing are the opercular gyri of the frontal lobe *(44, 45, 46, and 47, Broca's area)*. These gyri secondarily regulate the ability to speak, although the motor cortex is uninvolved and no laryngeal paralysis exists. Regulation appears for the most part to be related to the left cerebral cortex (dominance), although emotional strain, singing, or rhythmic speech seems to have bilateral cortical representation in these areas of function. Somewhat more nebulous is the posterior fourth of the middle frontal gyrus, which is sometimes credited with regulation of *writing symbols.* A *supplemental motor area* exists at the vertex and medial aspect of areas 6 and 8.[10] This area plays a part in symbolic expression, and defects are ap-

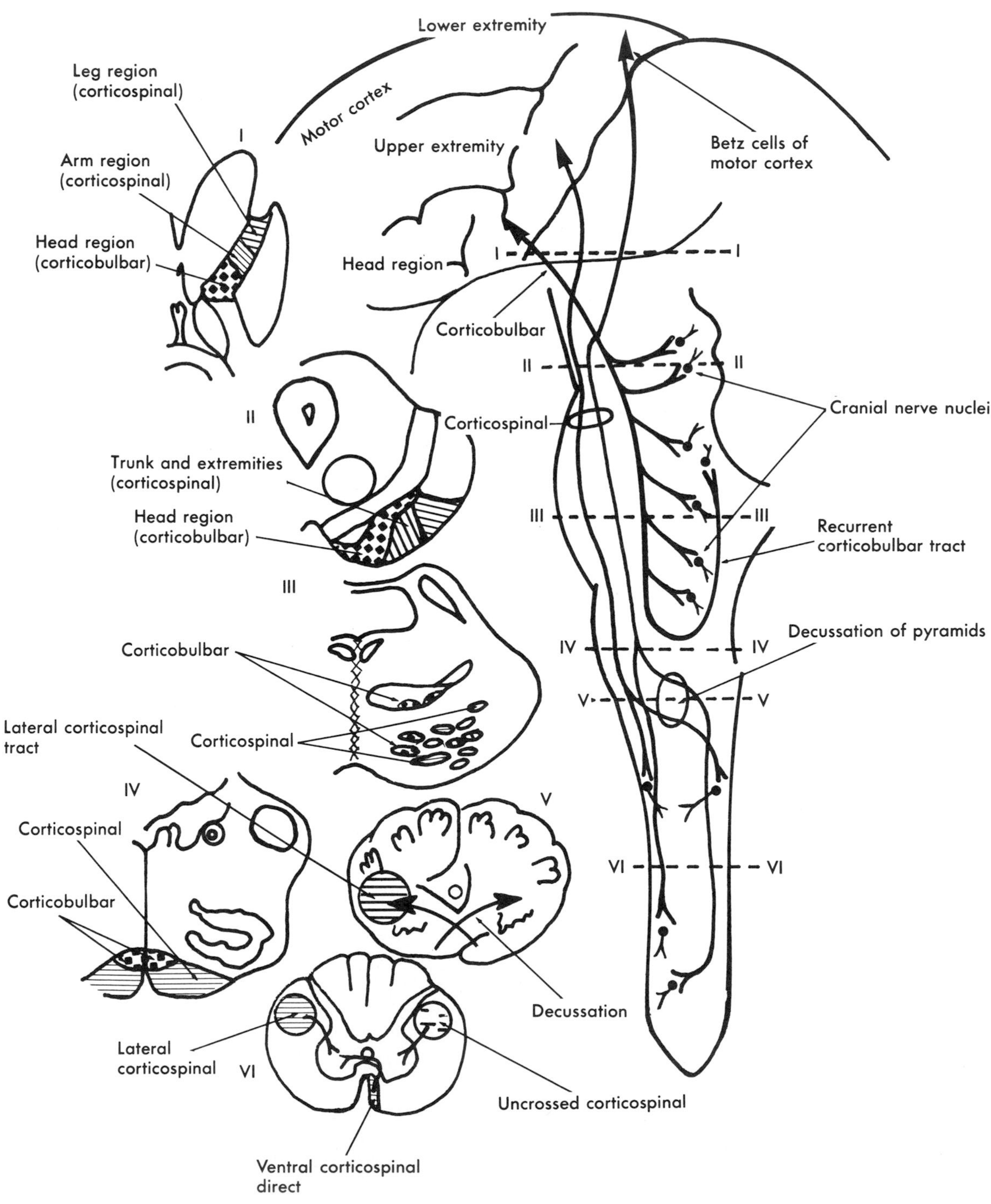

Fig. 22-5. Drawing of the course of the pyramidal tract.

parent in dysphasia. The exact mode of operation of these accessory motor fields is uncertain. While they are related to volitional acts, their connections are not as well established as those of the classical motor system, which presumably arise from the pyramidal cells of area 4.

Origin

The classical voluntary motor pathway, or pyramidal tract, arises in Betz cells and other pyramidal cells of area 4, which covers the precentral gyrus and the anterior gyrus of the paracentral lobule. The Betz cells are pyramidal in section and vary in diameter from 15 to 25 μ and in length from 35 to 70 μ (Fig. 22-4, *A*). The largest cells appear in the upper third of area 4, as might be expected from their distribution to the more distant parts of the spinal cord (Fig. 22-4, *B*). Betz cells number about 34,000 on each side; they account for a minor fraction (three percent) of the million or so fibers of a medullary pyramid. It seems unlikely that the Betz axons branch so remarkably. Other pyramidal cells of area 4 and probably of other allied motor fields (particularly area 6), and even the postcentral and association areas account for the fiber supply reaching the medulla and below (Fig. 22-7).[9]

Course

The corticobulbar fibers aggregate at the genu of the internal capsule (see Chapter 21). The corticospinal components occupy the anterior half of the posterior limb, with those to the upper limb (middle third of area 4) passing next to the corticobulbar fibers. The pyramidal fibers to the lower limbs (upper third of area 4) pass immediately posterior to those going to the upper limb (Fig. 22-5). In the midbrain, the pyramidal tract occupies the middle three-fifths of the basis pedunculi. In the pons the tract is broken into numerous linear strands by the transverse pontine fibers and by pontine nuclear masses (Fig. 22-6). These strands aggregate into the pyramids at the pontomedullary junction. The course of the fibers beyond the pyramids varies greatly. Approximately eighty-five percent of the fibers generally cross to the opposite side in the decussations of the pyramids (Fig. 22-7). These fibers enter the *lateral corticospinal tracts* of the spinal cord to provide the principal pyramidal route throughout the cord. A few fibers probably continue directly into the lateral corticospinal tracts. The main direct route for uncrossed fibers is via the *ventral corticospinal* pathway (about fifteen percent of the pyramidal fibers) (Fig. 22-5). In reaching the final paths (probably indirectly), both crossed and direct paths eventually relate to cells of the opposite side. The direct path crosses in the anterior commissure of the cord.

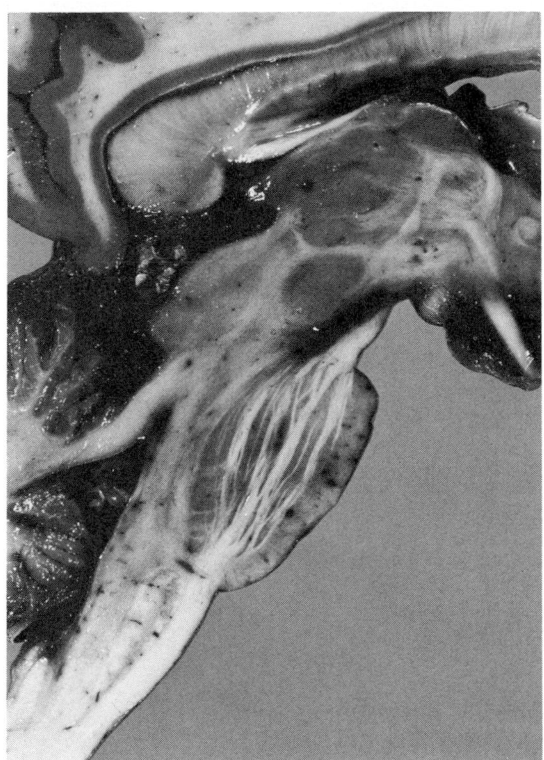

Fig. 22-6. Parasagittal section, unstained, showing linear strands of pyramidal tracts in pons. Note continuity with basis pedunculi above and with pyramid below.

The corticobulbar fibers travel as the *medial corticobulbar fasciculus* with the main pyramidal bundle to the regions of the cranial motor nuclei. Other corticobulbar fibers leave the main bundle (*aberrant*) high in the midbrain to reach the oculomotor areas. Some associate with the medial lemniscus (*lateral corticobulbar*) to reach the cranial nuclear area. The proportion of crossed and uncrossed fibers in the supply to cranial nuclei varies greatly. It has a profound effect on loss of function of nerve nuclei deprived of corticobulbar influence by unilateral tract destruction. Those nuclei receiving bilateral supply are not subject to the same extensive degree of paralysis that occurs in the muscle groups with unilateral supply (Fig. 22-8).

The spinal muscle groups most affected by unilateral pyramidal lesions are the muscles of the

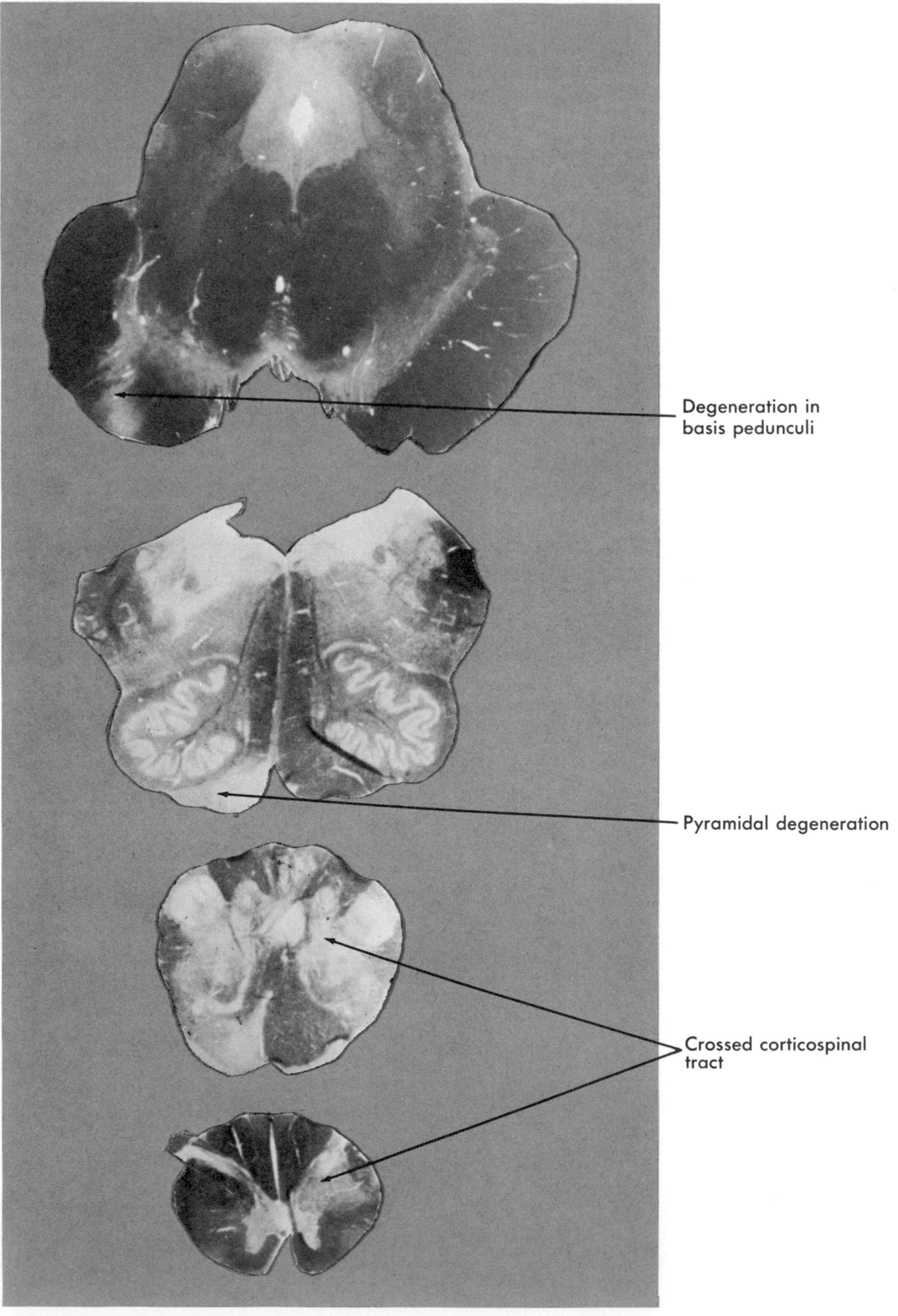

Fig. 22-7. Demyelination through brainstem following extirpation of area 6. Note concurrence with position of pyramidal tract throughout. Lowest figure shows crossed position of lateral corticospinal tract.

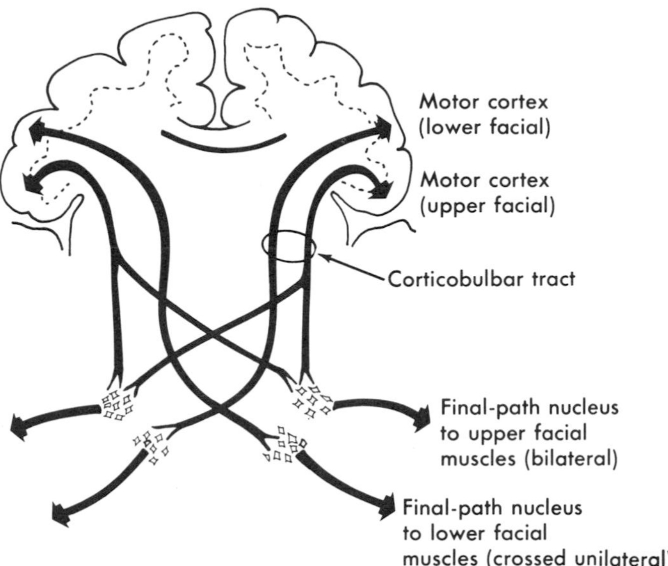

Fig. 22-8. Variation in degree of bilateral supply in corticobulbar fibers to nerve VII nuclei.

upper and lower extremities. In the cranial groups those exhibiting the most profound paralytic effects from high unilateral pyramidal interruption are the lower facial and trapezius muscles. An intermediate paralytic effect appears in the axial muscles of the trunk for the spinal group and in the muscles of the tongue for the cranial group. No paralytic effect occurs in the diaphragm from unilateral high corticospinal interruption, so bilateral supply of half crossing may be presumed. Of the cranial groups, bilateral corticobulbar supply is apparent for the ocular muscles, the upper facial muscles (frontalis and orbicularis oculi), the muscles of mastication, the muscles of deglutition (except the tongue), the muscles of the larynx, and the sternomastoid muscles.

Termination

The exact method of termination of the pyramidal fibers in man is not yet clear. Both the lateral and direct tracts reach the side opposite their origin. The route of the paths through the cord is shown at successive levels in Figs. 22-5 and 22-7. It is probable that neither the corticobulbar nor the corticospinal fibers terminate directly in relationship to final-path cells.[9] They probably end in relationship to internuncial cells, principally in the nucleus proprius or in the dorsal part of the ventral horn. No fibers relate to the intermediolateral column. The direct tract terminates in the upper thoracic region. Probably half the fibers terminate in the cervical cord, about thirty percent in the lumbosacral region, and twenty percent distributed throughout the thoracic segments. A diagram of a final-common-path cell and its probable receptive synaptic connections is shown in Fig. 15-3.

(For locations and characteristics of the motor nuclei and the distribution of the output from the nuclei see Chapters 6 and 7.)

EXTRAPYRAMIDAL SYSTEM

The extrapyramidal system represents an efferent cortical fiber complex that centers its activity in its relationship to the basal nuclei, particularly caudate, putamen, and globus pallidus (see Chapter 2). The claustrum and amygdala are excluded from the extrapyramidal system on functional grounds. The caudate head and the putamen, together with the intervening anterior limb of the internal capsule, constitute the corpus striatum (neostratum). Also, the combination of putamen with globus pallidus is called the lenticular (lens-shaped) nucleus. The globus pallidus alone is often called the pallidum, or paleostriatum. The total system also includes lower stem nuclei, which are thalamic, mesencephalic, and medullary in origin. The cerebellum is prominently tied into the system, as it is an accessory muscle regulatory device. The functions of the extrapyramidal system are motor-regulatory and operate apart from the direct motor system, although the influences are brought to bear on motor acts. The functions seem most closely tied to associated automatic activity, such as emotional expression or the extra movements occurring during walking (such as swinging arms). Deficiencies in the system are manifest in disabilities of muscular control without true paralysis (tremor at rest, rigidity, spasticity, stiffness, jerking movements, flailing, choreiform and athetoid movements, torsion). The system seems to be inhibitory to movements that are evoked experimentally in the corticospinal system. The caudate head seems to also relate to visceral motor functions.

Connections

The cerebral cortex connects to the basal nuclei either directly or by collaterals, and the nuclei interconnect in chain-like loops (for example, cortex to caudate to putamen to globus pallidus) (Fig. 22-9). The histologic details within the basal nuclei are not distinctive, except for abundant

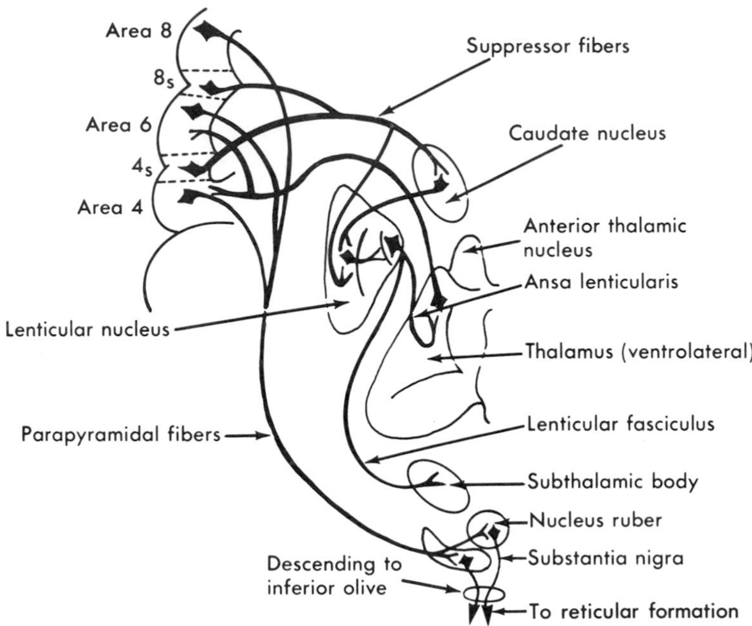

Fig. 22-9. Cortical connections with basal nuclei.

fibers in the pallidum. Both large and small nerve cells abound, and it is assumed that the large cells provide the long efferent fibers. The cortex also connects indirectly with the ganglia through the thalamus. Frontothalamic fibers reach the anterior and medial parts of the dorsal thalamus and the anterior part of the ventral nuclei. These thalamic nuclei project to both striatum and pallidum through the capsule as the thalamic fasciculus (field H1 of Forel). The head of the caudate and the adjacent putamen send fibers to the medial segment of the pallidum, while the bulk of the putamen relates to the lateral segment (Fig. 22-10).

Brainstem components

The efferent fibers from the basal nuclei downward arise both in the striatum and in the pallidum. The striatal fibers pass to the substantia nigra and are probably reciprocal (*strionigral* and *nigrostriatal*). These join direct *corticonigral* fibers and provide a continuing link to the lower extrapyramidal parts from relays in the striatum. The principal fiber mass descending from the nuclei arises from the large cells of the globus pallidus. These fibers form a floor for the pallidum and continue as the *ansa lenticularis* and *lenticular fasciculus.* The ansa curves around the anterior border of the internal capsule to terminate in the anterior part of the ventral nucleus of the thalamus. Some fibers pass through, as well as around, the capsule (Fig. 22-10). The lenticular fasciculus (bundle H2 of Forel) passes through the capsule and continues downward to multiple connections with brainstem nuclei of the extrapyramidal motor system. Much of this bundle probably synapses in the nucleus of the field of Forel and continues in a complex chain to lower nuclei. Fibers pass as the subthalamic fasciculus to the subthalamic body (of Luys); to the hypothalamus as the pallidohypothalamic tract; to the habenular nucleus; possibly to the nucleus of Darkschewitsch and to the nucleus of the medial longitudinal fasciculus of the opposite side via the posterior commissure; to the substantia nigra; to the reticular formation of the stem; to the motor nuclei of cranial nerves V and VII; and to the nucleus ruber. It is probably that some of these tracts are reciprocal, and some (possibly the connection with substantia nigra) are probably predominantly ascending.

Lower connections in the extrapyramidal chain are routed in three main ways to the final path. (1) Fibers from the substantia nigra descend in the reticulospinal tract. These reach the substantia nigra from the subthalamic body and the lenticular fasciculus, as do the longer descending tracts from the cortex and striatum. (2) From the subthalamic body some fibers pass directly to the nucleus ruber. Others pass with the thalamo-olivary bundle, tra-

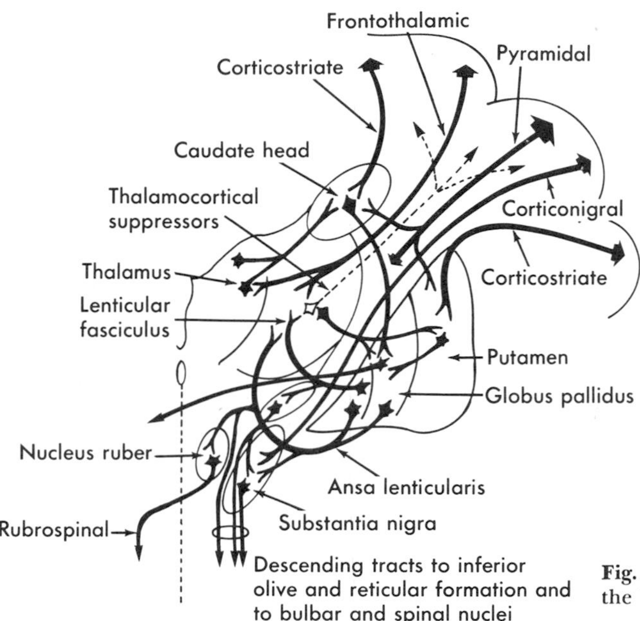

Fig. 22-10. Descending pathways relating to stem nuclei via the basal nuclei.

verse the cerebellar complex, and reach the ruber via the brachium conjunctivum. From the nucleus ruber they pass down the rubrospinal tract or reach the final paths via the reticular formation. (3) Some fibers enter the habenular complex and its descending continuum and the medial longitudinal fasciculus to descend in the sulcomarginal area. The *central tegmental bundle* (*thalamo-olivary fasciculus*) arises in the tegmentum of the midbrain and passes to the inferior olive (Fig. 22-11). The tract may be joined by fibers from the nucleus ruber, globus pallidus, and possibly the cortex. This connection of olive to cerebellum as a part of the extrapyramidal system is relatively massive, with olivocerebellar fibers providing con-

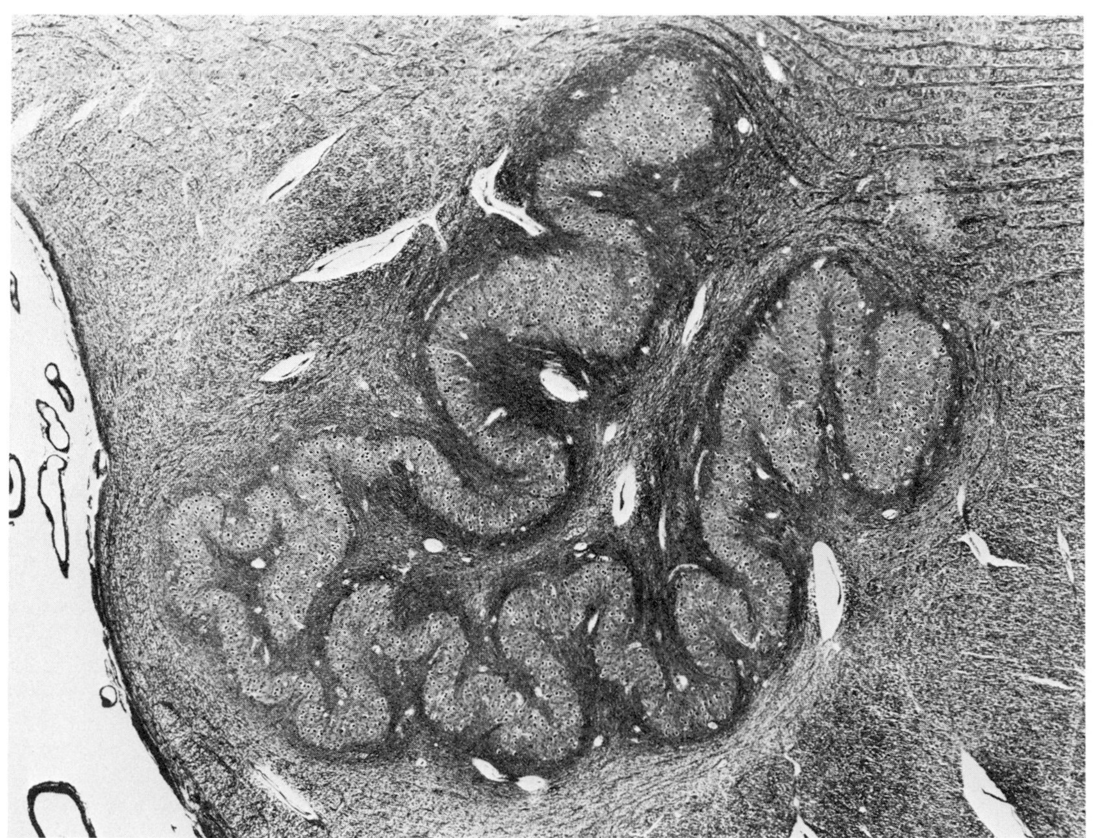

Fig. 22-11. Inferior olive.

siderable bulk of the corpus restiforme (Fig. 22-12). The olive relates the extrapyramidal system to the cerebellum much in the way that the pons relates the telencephalic cortex to the cerebellum. The inferior olive also discharges to the final-path areas via the olivospinal tract.

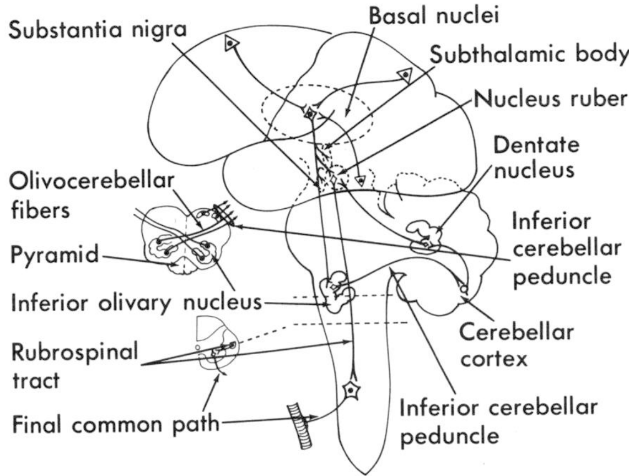

Fig. 22-12. Basal nuclei–inferior olivary complex relating to cerebellum and rubrospinal tract.

CORTICOPONTOCEREBELLAR SYSTEM

This efferent system from the cerebral cortex arises from frontal, parietal, occipital, and temporal cortices, and interrelates these areas intimately with the cerebellum. The function is directed to massive movements involving many muscles and is prominent in control of limb musculature. The *frontopontine* division runs in the internal capsule anterior to the pyramidal fibers at the genu and courses through the midbrain in the medial aspect of the basis pedunculi. In the radiations these fibers are mixed with frontothalamic fibers. *Parietopontine* fibers are mixed with the pyramidal elements. *Occipitotemporopontine* fibers course through the internal capsule posterior to the general sensory bundles and occupy a lateral position in the basis pedunculi. The corticopontine fibers terminate in relationship to pontine nuclei of the same side. *Pontocerebellar* fibers arise in the pontine nuclei, cross the midline in the pontine raphe, and terminate (via the *brachium pontis*) as *mossy fibers* adjacent to granular cells in the cerebellar cortex. Defects in this system contribute to disturbance in gait and unilateral transient torsion movements (Fig. 22-13).

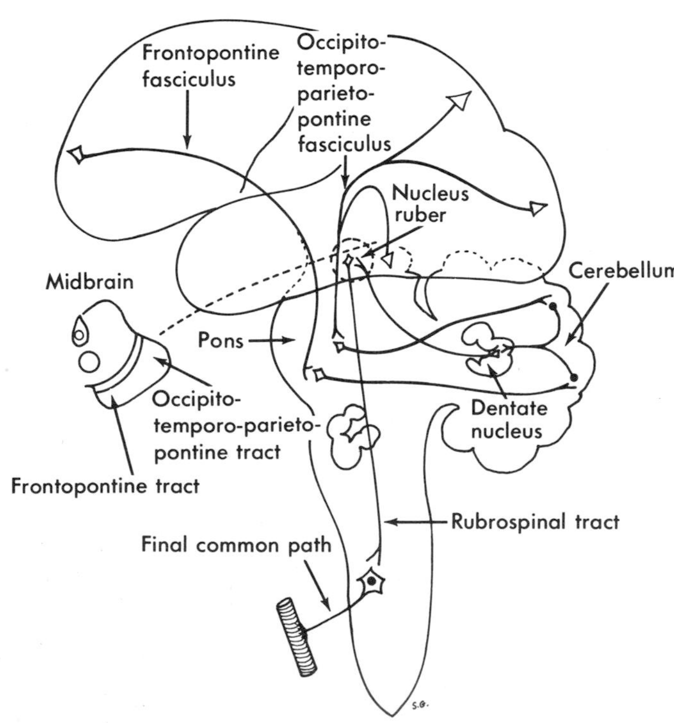

Fig. 22-13. Corticopontocerebellar system and relationship to rubrospinal tract.

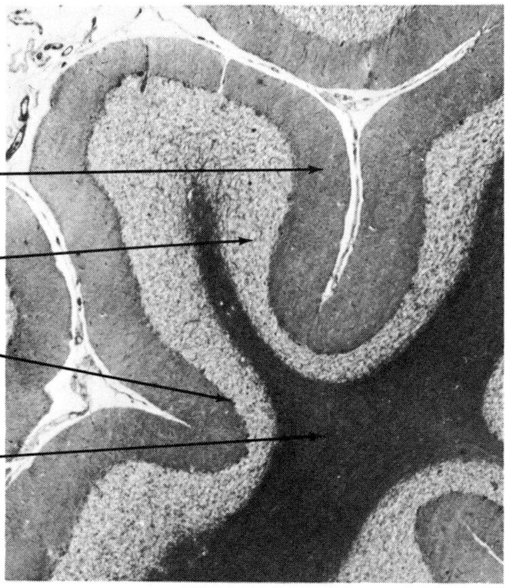

Cerebellum

The cerebellum has been represented as receiving fibers from all three peduncles and providing efferent fibers from the dentate and roof nuclei, which leave via the brachium conjunctivum and uncinate fasciculus. The largest afferent contributions by far arise in the two systems just described (corticopontocerebellar and basal nucleo-olivo-cerebellar). The connections are effected through the laminae of the cortex. These are arranged in *folia* (small longitudinal gyri) in the central vermis and both hemispheres (Fig. 22-14). The outermost cortical lamina is the *molecular layer*. Beneath this layer is a layer of *Purkinje* cells, and deep to this is a *granular layer*. The granular cells are distinguished by absence of Nissl substance and by little visible cytoplasm in routine stains. Deep to this are the fibers of the white matter.

Fig. 22-14. Layers of cerebellar cortex.

In summary, the afferent connections to the cerebellum include: (1) the *corpus restiforme,* conveying fibers from the nucleus dorsalis, nuclei gracilis and cuneatus, inferior olive, vestibular nuclei, and some direct from the dorsal funiculus and vestibular nerve; (2) *brachium pontis* from pontine nuclei of opposite side; and (3) *brachium conjunctivum,* carrying ventral spinocerebellar fibers. All afferent fibers reach the cortex through either *mossy fibers,* which terminate by glomerular tufts (eosin bodies) adjacent to many granular cells, or *climbing fibers,* which terminate prominently adjacent to the dendrites of Purkinje cells. The climbing fibers also terminate on *basket cells,* which run transversely across the folium to provide basket terminals around approximately twenty Purkinje cells. En route they give off bidirectional longitudinal collaterals to about six rows of Purkinje cells on either side. These climbing fibers also contact stellate cells (outer basket cells of disputed distribution) in the outer molecular layer and end on *Golgi cells,* which are bulky cells of the granular layer that interconnect granular and molecular layers. The *mossy fibers* arise outside the cerebellum and may represent the major type of ending for the tract sources just listed. The origin of the *climbing fibers* is disputed; they may represent either recurrent fibers from cerebellar sources or fibers from the inferior olivary nuclei. It should be noted that the orientation of the branching Purkinje cell is in the transverse plane of the folium (Fig. 22-15). Granule cell axons project into the maze of longitudinal parallel fibers of the molecular layer (Fig. 22-16).

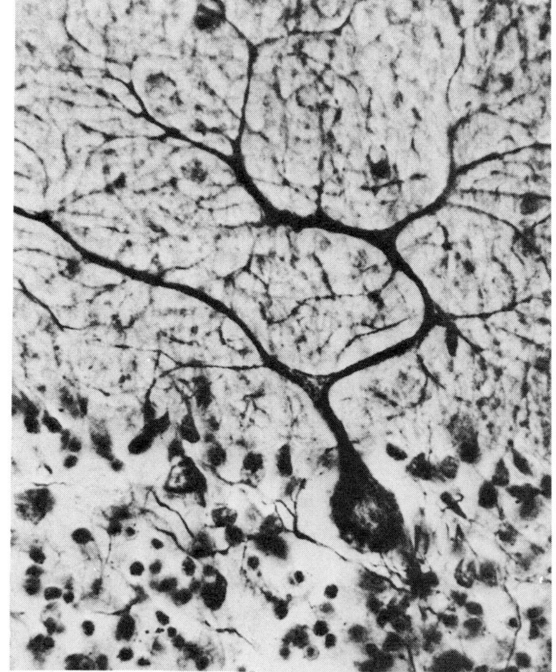

Fig. 22-15. Purkinje cells in cross section plane of folium.

The projections of white fibers from the cortex originate in Purkinje cells and terminate in the

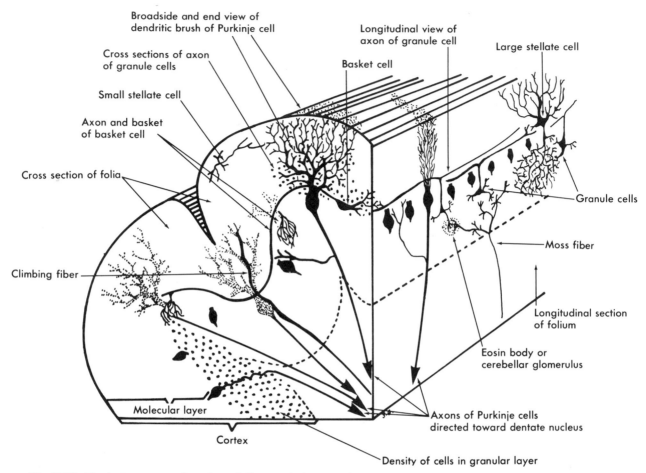

Fig. 22-16. Classical representation of cerebellar cortical connections centering on the Purkinje cell. (After Rasmussen.)

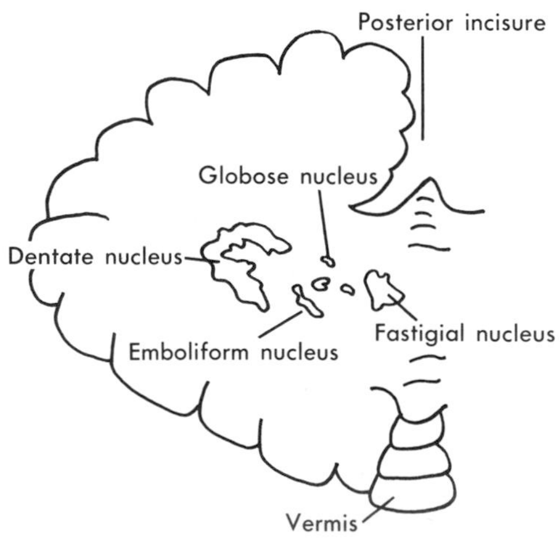

Fig. 22-17. Diagram of cerebellar nuclei.

dentate nuclei from lateral hemispheres and the *nucleus fastigius* from the vermis (Fig. 22-17). The *globose* and *emboliform* nuclei receive Purkinje axons from *paravermal* zones. Fibers from the *fastigial* nucleus are believed to form *cerebellomotor* tracts to the region of the cranial nerve nuclei and vestibular and spinal centers via the *uncinate fasciculus* and *juxtarestiform* body. Fibers from the *dentate nucleus* and the *emboliform and globose* nuclei form the brachium conjunctivum, which passes to the red nucleus (ruber) of the opposite side (via decussation of the brachium conjunctivum) and to the thalamus (dentatothalamic). In addition, there is fiber distribution to the oculomotor nucleus, to the inferior olive, and to the reticular formation. The flocculonodular lobe is the principal cerebellar vestibular area, and its efferent fibers are quickly directed to the oculo-

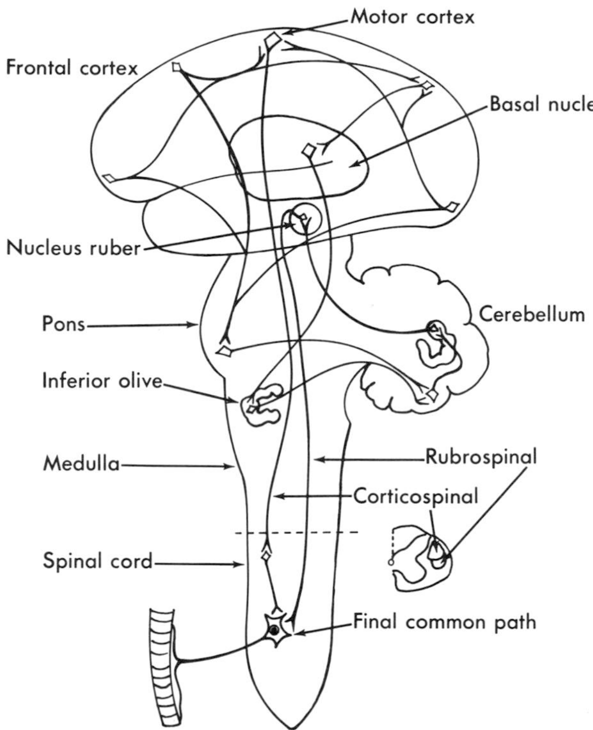

Fig. 22-18. Summary of major long descending pathways (pyramidal and rubrospinal) relating to voluntary motor, extrapyramidal, and corticopontocerebellar systems.

motor and related nuclei and the reticular formation (Figs. 18-12 to 18-14).

The efferent fibers from the cerebellum are brought into relationship with spinal final-common-path cells principally via the rubrospinal tract. The nucleus ruber is thus the main reflecting terminal for fibers passing from the cerebellum to the spinal cord. Through the rubrospinal, bulbospinal, and tectospinal tracts, cerebellar influences are added to other parapyramidal pathways to the lower centers (Fig. 22-18). The cerebellar hemisphere thus relates to the ipsilateral body musculature by virtue of the crossing of the rubrospinal tract. The flocculonodular lobe functionally relates principally to equilibration, and the remainder of the cerebellum to general proprioception.[5] As might be expected, cerebellar action potentials are evoked from stimulation of widely different areas (cortex, eye, ear, basal nuclei).

As previously mentioned, a loop feedback system exists from the thalamus, red nucleus, and tegmentum to the inferior olive, to the cerebellar cortex, and back via the brachium conjunctivum to the red nucleus and thalamus. It is possible that olivocerebellar connections relate to skilled movements, in contrast to the pathway from the accessory inferior olive, which relates to more primitive or unskilled movements (vermis). Thus, both extrapyramidal and corticopontocerebellar systems are tied into the motor activities.[5,6]

LIMBIC SYSTEM

Grossly defined, the limbic system includes the olfactory brain, the cingulum, the hippocampal formation and its outflow circuitry, the septal fields, and the hypothalamic outflow system to lower centers (Fig. 21-17). As the "visceral" brain, the limbic system interrelales visceral activity to emotional and behavioral activity; it thus becomes a part of the motor complex. It would appear that evolutionary considerations might permit removal of the viscerobehavioral motor complex from the human olfactory system. This liberty has been exercised in these pages.

The limbic system has adapted a combination of the neocortex and rhinencephalon to the efferent needs relating *affect* to general sensibility. While structurally manifest in the temporal lobe and hippocampal structures that discharge into hypothalamus via the fornices, the system is much more complex. The limbic outflow comingles in the thalamus with visceral influences arising from all sensory complexes as well as associative cortical areas and culminates in behavioral responses. A strong relationship exists with autonomic and neuroendocrine functions, although a separation of these three systems (limbic, neuroendocrine, and autonomic) does to some degree occur in the thalamus and its output.

The developmental importance of the olfactory contributions are apparent from the circuitry of olfactory origin into the limbic complex. The lateral olfactory stria sends fibers directly to the corticomedial segment of the amygdala, as well as to the adjacent piriform olfactory cortex. The intermediate stria terminates in the anterior perforated substance, and the medial stria in the parolfactory area (see Chapter 17). All these cortical areas project to the stria medullaris thalami and the habenular complex and to the descending olfactotegmental tract, which gives off collaterals to the hypothalamus (Figs. 17-8 and 17-14). The primary olfactory fields also reciprocally interrelate with the temporal lobe via the longitudinal striae over the corpus callosum, through the septum pellucidum, and via the stria terminalis. The basolateral amygdala indirectly connects to the hippocampal complex by relating to adjacent parahippocampal cortex and thence to the hippocampus itself.

The hippocampal formation is the start of the massive limbic efferent system to the hypothalamus. The structural features are shown in Figs. 21-17 and 22-19. The fibers originate in the hippocampal cortex, enter the fimbria and crus of the fornix, and continue through the body and column of the fornix to terminate in the mamillary body. Some collaterals terminate in intralaminar nuclei of the thalamus. At the underside of the corpus callosum some of the fibers cross to the opposite hippocampal formation via the hippocampal commissure (psalterium). The mamillary body sends fibers to the tegmentum (mamillotegmental tract). Reciprocal fibers come to the mamillary body from the tegmentum as the mamillary peduncle. A robust tract arises from the mamillary body and passes to the anterior nucleus of the thalamus (mamillothalamic tract of Vicq d' Azyr) (see Chapter 4). This brings the limbic output into the pathways emanating from the anterior nucleus. The limbic output continues to the habenular complex via the stria medullaris and to the cingulate cortex. The cingulate cortex interconnects widely with neocortex, particularly the frontal lobes. The intralaminar nuclei project to frontal cortex. The habenular complex projects to interpeduncular nuclei, and these in turn go to the dorsal longitudinal fasciculus for descent (Fig. 21-17).

Function

The diversity of connections of the limbic system and the closeness to visceral efferent activity makes the visceral brain impossible to define as a separate functional unit. It has already been stated that some measure of separation occurs in the hypothalamus among the limbic, autonomic, and neuroendocrine systems. These other systems localize to some degree in specific nuclear groups. The common functional product emanating from the action of each is represented in common in such events as heart rate, blood pressure, respiratory function, sweating, eating, pupillary changes, peristalsis, urinary bladder function, and sleep—all events commonly related to autonomic or endocrine reactions. The specific area in which the limbic system operates cannot be divorced from the activities just listed or even from more ordinary

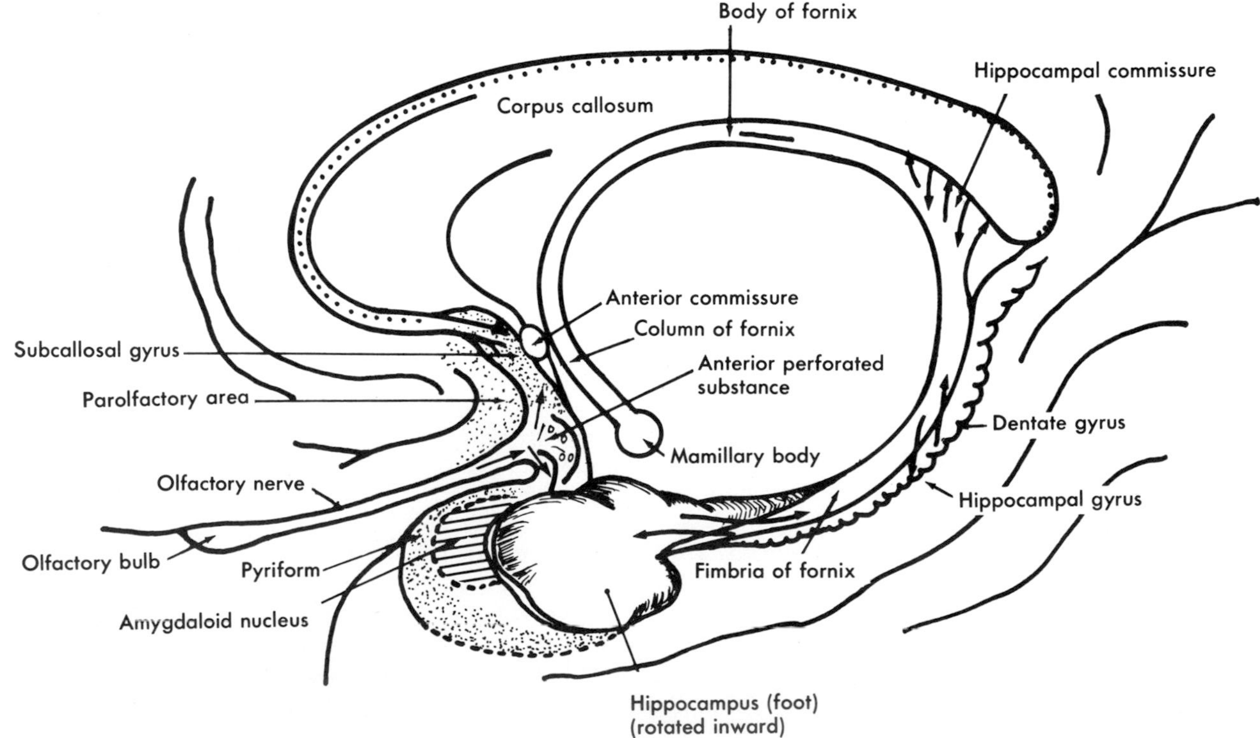

Fig. 22-19. The hippocampal complex as the way station and efferent system for the limbic lobe. Main pathway through fornix.

sensations that are somatically oriented. The special limbic feature added to these complexes seem to be *affect,* or sensory tone, which operates at levels recognized as emotional and as appended to the other reactions.

VISCERAL EFFERENT SYSTEM

The *general visceral efferent* (*autonomic*) *system* differs from the *somatic efferent* and *special visceral efferent* systems in several important respects. In general, the responses are autonomic and hence more dependent upon strictly reflex connections. The cerebrum and CNS in general are therefore less well defined in their relationship to the autonomic system than to the somatic efferent components. The final cells reach the effectors through cells in outlying ganglia, so at least one more neuron is interposed in the final-common-path delivery. There is anatomic distinctness in that central nuclei are separated and the peripheral nerves emanate from the CNS in two separate systems, *craniosacral* and *thoracolumbar,* each with its own ganglionic system. Physiologically the autonomic system often provides almost opposing functional patterns in the two anatomic groups. The structures innervated are smooth muscles, cardiac muscles, and glands rather than striated muscle. The craniosacral (parasympathetic) division is pharmacologically *cholinergic,* and the thoracolumbar (sympathetic) *adrenergic.* In the following pages the visceral efferent system will be subdivided for descriptive convenience into cerebral components, hypothalamus, descending pathways, special visceral efferent system, and autonomic system. (For general distribution patterns in the peripheral nerves that handle this system see Chapter 6.)

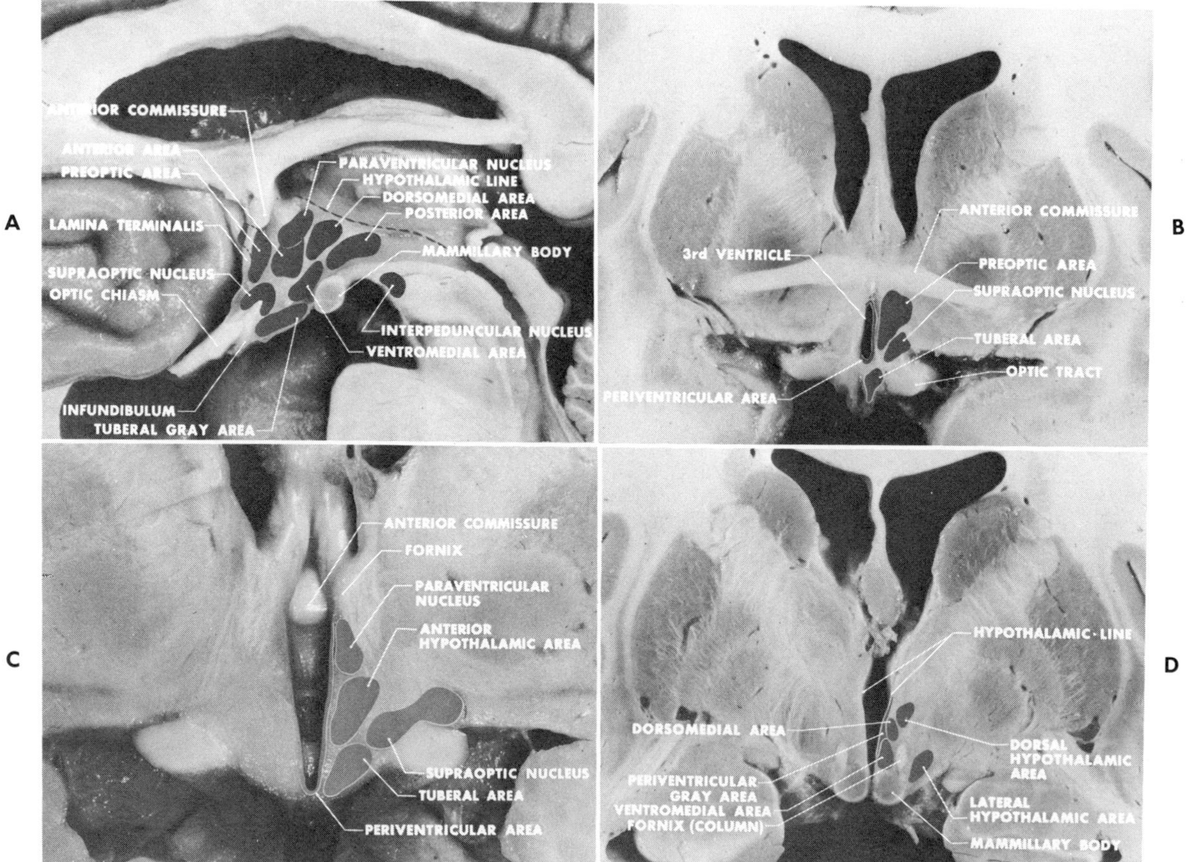

Fig. 22-20. Diagrams of hypothalamic nuclei superimposed on photo of sagittal section of brain; **B,** superimposed at coronal level of anterior commissure; **C,** superimposed at coronal level through tuber cinereum; **D,** superimposed at coronal level of mamillary bodies.

Cerebrum

Much of the evidence of cortical contributions to the visceral system is indirect and based upon autonomic disturbances in the presence of lesions. On this basis the temporal tip has been related to salivation, swallowing, and coughing. Similarly, the posterior insular area has also been related to salivation, and its anterior part to maintenance of blood pressure. Respiratory control relates to the precentral gyrus, and temperature regulation to the cingulum. In each instance it is presumed that the autonomic dysfunction is mediated through hypothalamic connections.

Hypothalamus

The behavioral ties of the hypothalamus have been reviewed in preceding paragraphs in connection with the limbic system. These relate to the outflow from the temporal lobe and the traffic pattern through the hypothalamus. The more specifically autonomic functions that localize in the hypothalamus include thermoregulation, water metabolism, feeding, sleep, chemical homeostasis, gastrointestinal function, cardiopulmonary regulation, and possibly vasomotor activity. These functions and others are included in the following outline, and the general locations are summarized in Fig. 22-20, *A* to *D*.[7]

HYPOTHALAMIC NUCLEI AND AREAS WITH FUNCTIONS

- I. *Nuclei*
  - A. *Supraoptic* (part of origin of hypothalamohypophyseal tract; water balance; thirst)
  - B. *Paraventricular* (part of origin of hypothalamohypophyseal tract)
  - C. *Mamillary* (suppression of gastric secretion; somnolence; catalepsy)
- II. *Area*
  - A. *Preoptic* (pulmonary edema and hemorrhage; bladder contraction; parasympathetic functions; heat regulation)
  - B. *Anterior* (sympathetic control; slowing heart; vasodilation; lowering blood pressure; gastrointestinal motility; heat regulation)
  - C. *Tuberal* (suppression of gastric secretions; feeding; hypothalamohypophyseal portal system to anterior lobe; gonadal failure; obesity; thirst; hunger; satiety)
  - D. *Dorsomedial* (parasympathetic functions)
  - E. *Ventromedial* (feeding; satiety; thirst; water intake; sympathetic functions)
  - F. *Posterior* (parasympathetic functions; some part in vasoconstriction; increased blood flow to heart and lungs; increased heart rate, blood pressure, gastrointestinal motility; temperature regulation)
  - G. *Periventricular* (none specific; possibly blood pressure control)
  - H. *Dorsal (lateral)* (cardiovascular adjustments to exercise)
  - I. *Lateral* (sleep; hypothermia; feeding; anorexia; pupil dilatation; peristalsis inhibition; loss of tone in stomach; polydipsia)

Descending pathways

The probable circuitry of descending outflow for limbic activities is shown in Fig. 21-18. The specific autonomic functions are probably mediated in part over the same outflow routes. It is presumed that a major responsibility in reaching final-common-path cells for viseral outflow from the hypothalamus falls to the reticular formation.

Special visceral efferent system

This system is branchial in origin, but it is similar to somatic efferent components in all other respects. No secondary postganglionic fibers exist, and the final paths of the CNS deliver directly to the effector organs. The visceral striated muscles involved are innervated as described in Chapter 6.

Autonomic system

The general features of the autonomic system (general visceral efferent vegetative, involuntary, visceral, splanchnic) have been described (p. 136). It supplies smooth and cardiac muscle and glands through inclusion of an intervening cell between the central final path and the end-organ effector. As mentioned, the system is involuntary and relates closely to hypothalamic functions. As the neural controlling device for viscera, the autonomic system plays the major role in vital functions (such as respiration, heart action, circulation). It is convenient to describe the autonomic system in terms of the pre- and postganglionic patterns for each of the two principal anatomic subdivisions, the craniosacral and thoracolumbar systems (Fig. 6-26).

Craniosacral system. This fiber system is parasympathetic. It is called cholinergic in function by virtue of the fact that its reactions generally parallel those arising from stimulation by acetylcholine. The distributions are summarized in Fig. 6-26.

The Edinger-Westphal nucleus is probably the

origin of the nerve III preganglionic fibers to the ciliary ganglion. These fibers synapse there with postganglionic fibers that supply the sphincter of the pupil and also the ciliary muscles (see Chapter 20). The *superior salivatory nucleus* gives rise to the preganglionic parasympathetic fibers that travel over nerve VII (nervus intermedius) to the sphenopalatine ganglion. Postganglionic fibers are both secretory and vasodilatory and supply the lacrimal glands and glands of the nose. Fibers of the same origin are routed over the chorda tympani as preganglionic fibers to the submandibular ganglion and to Langley's ganglion along the duct of the gland. Postganglionic fibers supply the submandibular and sublingual glands as well as the orolingual and buccal glands. The *inferior salivatory nucleus* is the source of preganglionic fibers that travel over nerve IX to the otic ganglion. The postganglionic cells are secretory and vasodilatory to the parotid gland. The *dorsal motor nucleus of the vagus nerve* gives rise to the long preganglionic fibers to parasympathetic ganglia in the walls of thoracic and abdominal viscera. The postganglionic fibers are very short and supply the glands and smooth muscles in the viscera. The vagus nerve is motor and secretory to the bowel, inhibitory to the heart, vasoconstrictor to the coronary arteries, and vasodilator to lung vessels. *Nucleus myoleioticus* (general visceral efferent sacral nucleus) gives rise to parasympathetic preganglionic outflow from S2, 3, and 4 to the ganglia in the left colon and pelvic viscera. Postganglionic fibers are short and extend the functions of the vagus to the organs supplied (see Chapter 6).

Thoracolumbar system. This division of the autonomic system is sympathetic. Functionally it is adrenergic, as it simulates in its actions the responses to adrenaline. The preganglionic fibers arise

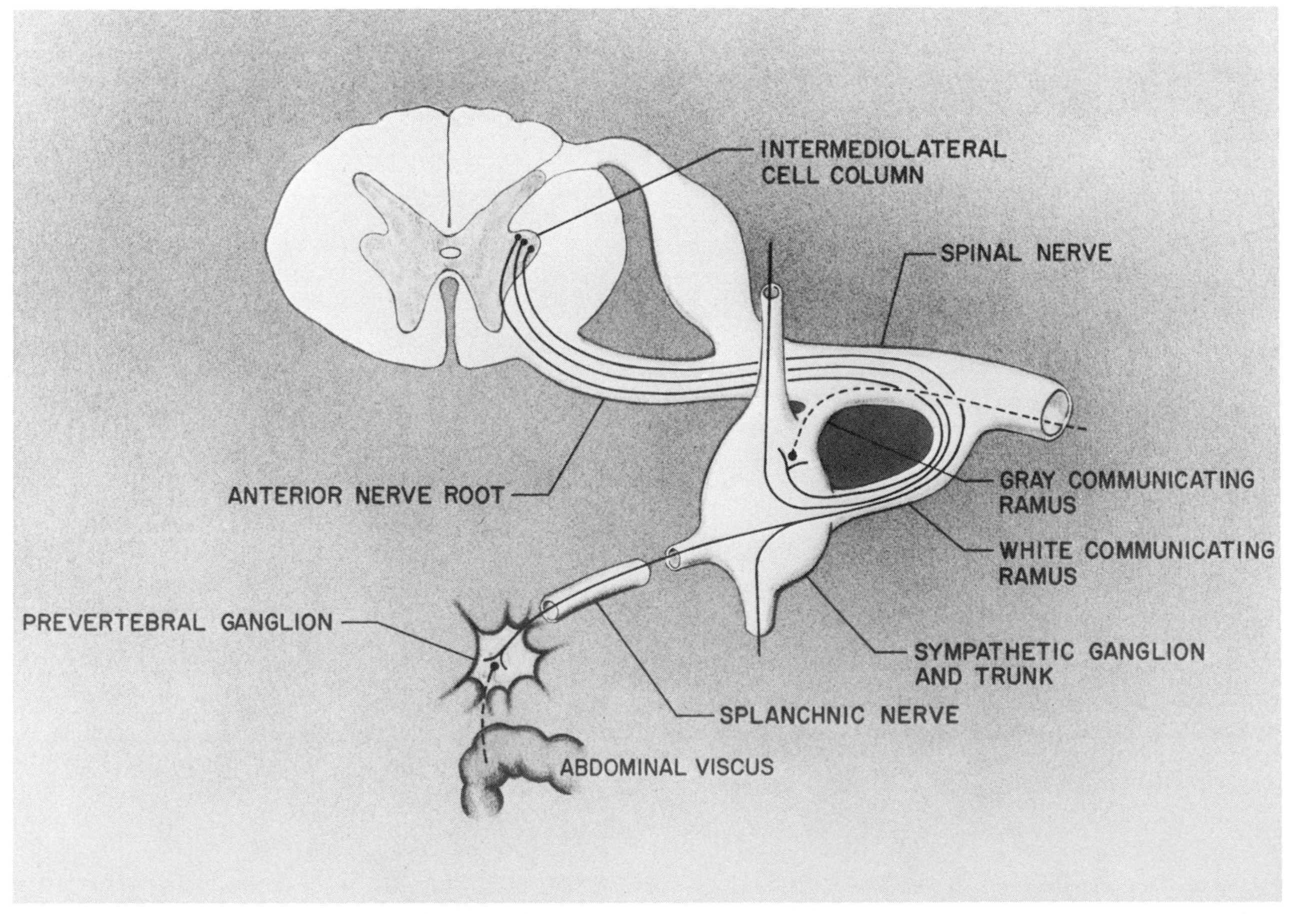

Fig. 22-21. Diagram of sympathetic ganglion connections.

in the *intermediolateral column* of cells of the ventral horn from segments T1 to L2 (Fig. 6-26). They exit with ventral roots of the same segments and reach the sympathetic ganglia via the white communicating rami (Fig. 22-21). Some bypass the first ganglia encountered and terminate in the more distant splanchnic ganglia. Postganglionic fibers pass from the sympathetic ganglia via vascular plexuses to the viscera. In general, sympathetic stimulation opposes in function that of parasympathetic stimulation. Sympathetic reactions include sudomotor, pilomotor, and vasomotor activity, pupillary dilatation, cardiac acceleration, bronchodilatation, and adrenal medullary secretion. The sympathetic outflow to the adrenal is direct and possesses no intervening postganglionic fiber. This adrenal supply pattern parallels that of special visceral efferent fibers. The functional effects of parasympathetic stimulation opposes the listed responses of the sympathetic effects. Segmental features of sympathetic supply are shown in Fig. 16-26 (see Chapter 6).

Histology

The central final cells of the autonomic system are fairly small, multipolar types without significant configuration differences in various nuclei (Fig. 22-22). They tend to have fewer dendritic processes than the final cells in somatic efferent groups. The fibers are for the most part myelinated and present no distinctive features until they reach the ganglia. Here the filaments come into relationship with *interstitial cells.* These cells probably are connective tissue and may be Schwannian in origin. The ganglion cells are structurally similar in both parasympathetic and sympathetic units. The terminals of preganglionic fibers are both axodendritic and axosomatic and form boutons and calyces. It is possible that these terminals physiologically change position. The ganglion cells themselves are predominantly mature elements with all the cytologic features of other nerve cells (Nissl substance, lipofuscin with age, large nucleus, and nucleolus) (Fig. 22-23). There is some evidence that young forms and growing forms of ganglion cells persist into adulthood and that these are replacement for normal attrition. There is no such cellular behavior in the CNS.

The postganglionic terminals in the effectors (smooth muscle, glands, cardiac muscle) are less well established than their counterparts in striated muscle. Most of the terminals occur as nerve nets or as free endings that apply to the wall of the effector cell.[1]

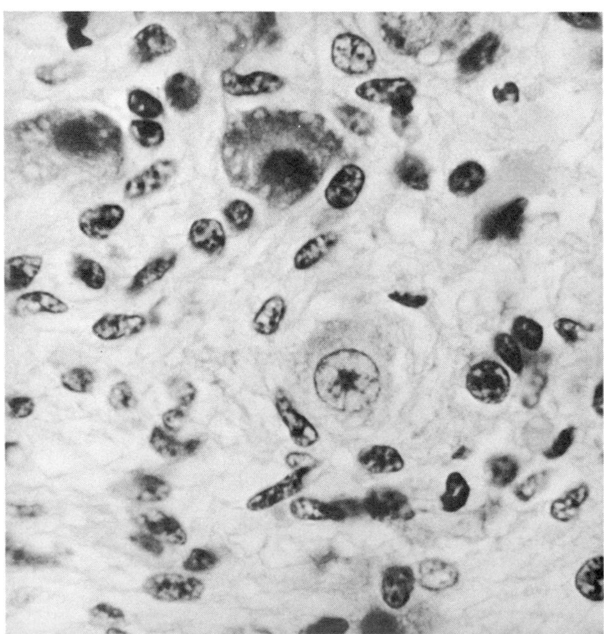

Fig. 22-22. Two common forms of sympathetic cells probably reflecting differences in metabolic state. (H & E ×1,250.)

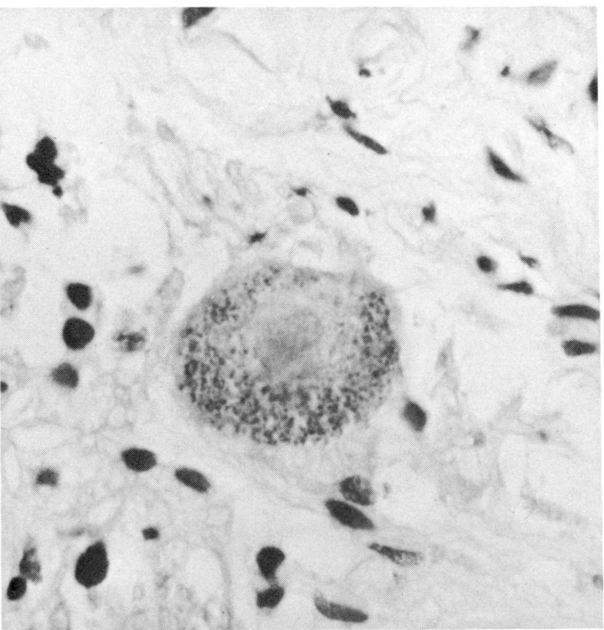

Fig. 22-23. Aging in sympathetic cell with deposits of lipofuscin in cytoplasm. (H & E ×1,250.)

NEUROENDOCRINE SYSTEM

Through the limbic and autonomic systems just outlined, it is apparent that cumulative sensory neural experience can be poured into emotional and visceral responses as a part of total human behavior. The hypothalamus appears to be the main mediating area in each complex. This part of the diencephalon also operates as a major central final path for regulating the pituitary gland and indirectly regulating its target organs.*

The neuroendocrine system in man is apparently dependent first upon the diverse afferent neural pathways that reach the hypothalamus. Based upon animal equivalents, it is believed that the system it also subject to a feedback of hormones from the involved target organs. These chemical substances in turn modify the thalamic output to the pituitary. Another item bearing on the thalamic integrative function in this system is the integrity of the homeostatic mechanisms for emotional and metabolic activity generated through limbic and autonomic systems. The hypothalamus appears to be involved in neuroendocrine function as the integrative field for neural, hormonal feedback, and metabolic homeostatic mechanisms (Fig. 22-24).†

In elaborating regulators for hormonal responses, thc hypothalamus functions through two separate hormonal systems. The first of these is represented in the *supraopticohypophyseal tract.* This tract originates in the supraoptic and paraventricular nuclei and projects to the posterior pituitary, or *neurohypophysis* (Fig. 22-25). The cells of these nuclei are specialized neurosecretory elements that form two hormones, vasopressin and oxytocin. Vasopressin, or antidiuretic hormone (ADH), is presumably formed in the supraoptic nucleus, and oxytocin in the paraventricular nucleus (Fig. 22-20, *C*). The neurohumoral substances travel down the neuraxes (axoplasmic flow) to be stored and released into the general circulation in the neurohypophysis. The course and storage in the tract can be detected by the massing of neurosecretory granules.[4] It is not known whether the posterior lobe cells themselves also produce hormone. Some hormone is possibly released into the circulation en route to the neurohypophysis. Vasopressin, which travels this route, acts on the kidney to conserve water. Oxytocin stimulates contraction of the smooth muscle of the uterus and the smooth muscle and myoepithelium of the breast in production of milk.

*See references 8, 11, 12, and 14.
†See references 7, 8, 11, and 14.

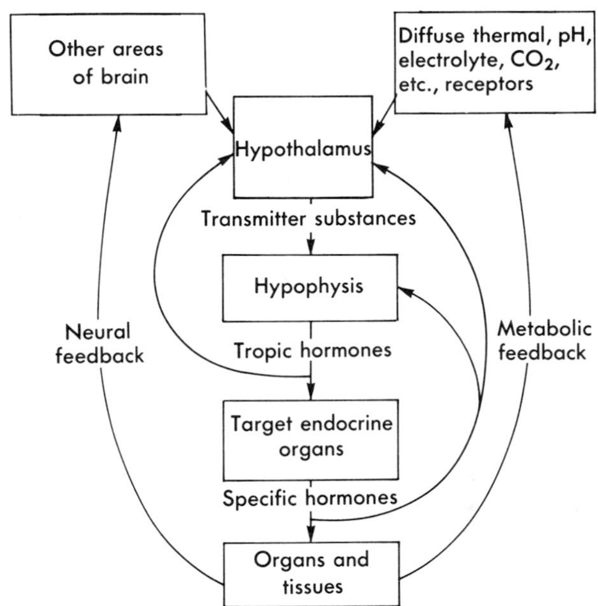

Fig. 22-24. Prototype of neuroendocrine function and feedback systems.

The second of the hormonal pathways from the hypothalamus provides for release of hormones in the central tuberal area (median eminence) (Fig. 22-20, *C*). The hormones possibly include those of the supraoptic and paraventricular nuclei, although this is by no means certain. The principal neurohumoral substances, which are as yet unidentified, are known as *releasing factors.* No nerve pathways are known to pass from the hypothalamus to the anterior lobe of the pituitary, which is the intermediate target organ in this system. The means by which these neurohumoral substances reach the anterior lobe must therefore vary from the pattern in the supraopticothypophyseal neural tract. The hormonal exchange is accomplished through a special vascular complex, the hypothalamoadenohypophyseal portal system (Fig. 22-26). This consists of a vascular network passing from the medial eminence to the anterior lobe. A primary vascular arterial plexus (Fig. 22-27) extends over the pars tuberalis and the median eminence. This plexus gives off a rich sinusoidal supply to the neurosecretory area within the median eminence. The arteries gather into portal vessels, which pass down the stalk and open into sinusoids that bathe the glandular cells of the anterior pituitary. The chemical nature of the hypothalamic releasing factors remain obscure. The following factors are suggested by experimental demonstration or by suppo-

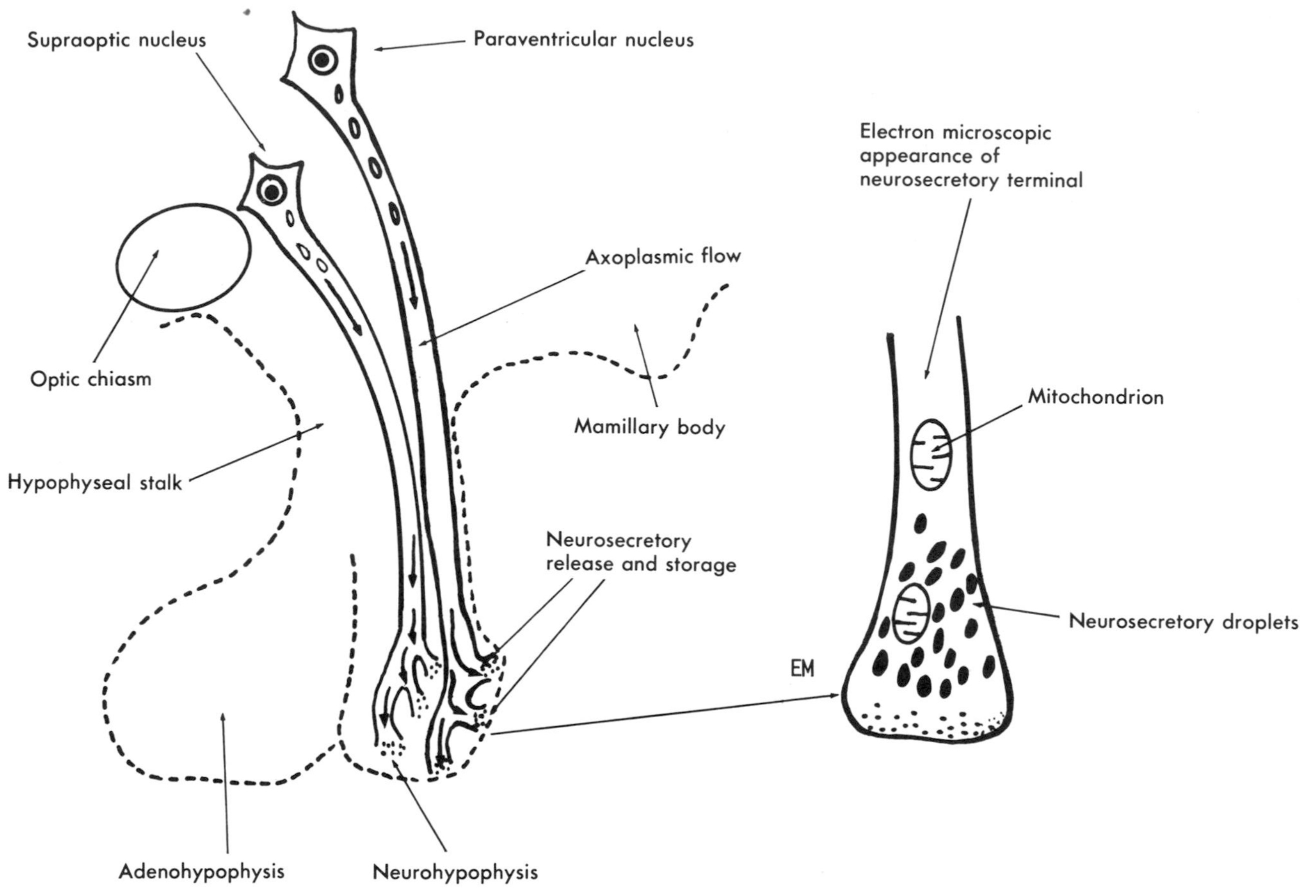

Fig. 22-25. Hypothalamus—neurohypophyseal tract.

sition: corticotropin releasing factors (CRF) for release of adrenocorticotropic hormone (ACTH); thyrotropic releasing factor for thyrotropic hormone; gonadotropin releasing factor; a factor causing synthesis and release of luteinizing hormone; one for follicle stimulation; and probably a factor for growth hormone.*

It should be emphasized that the neuroendocrine activity only adds an additional parameter to hypothalamic activity. The neuroendocrine system cannot be divorced from limbic and autonomic neural outflow. The final common paths of the latter systems generate responses that are productive of feedback systems, which in turn modify thalamic activity (Fig. 22-24).

OTHER DESCENDING PATHS

The motor complexes previously described are also influenced by additional descending fibers. These no doubt bear on the final-common-path cells and therefore contribute to the motor acts. These include the tectospinal tract, the vestibulospinal tracts, the premotor tract from area 6 and probably other cortical fibers that mix with the pyramidal bundles, the reticulospinal fibers, and the interstitiospinal fiber system.[9] Each of these systems has been mentioned in connection with some other neural complex, but it is important to recognize that they, too, are part of the overall motor system.

FINAL COMMON PATH

The final cells within the CNS that deliver the impulse to the effector represent the culmination of one or all the complex neural connections previously described (see Chapter 6). It would appear that firing any single final-common-path cell results in the same reaction regardless of the complexity of the neural pathways leading up to the firing. The physiologic effectiveness of the volley however becomes an aggregated effect of many final-com-

*See references 8, 11, 12, and 14.

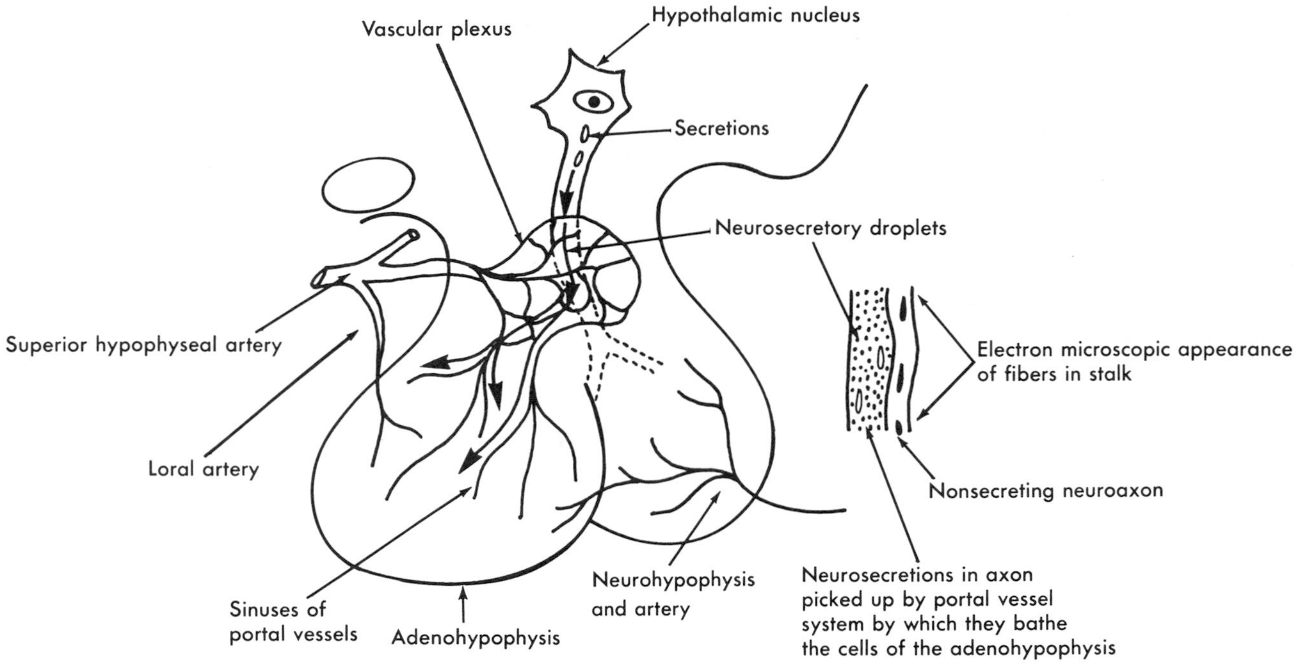

Fig. 22-26. Hypothalamoadenohypophyseal portal system.

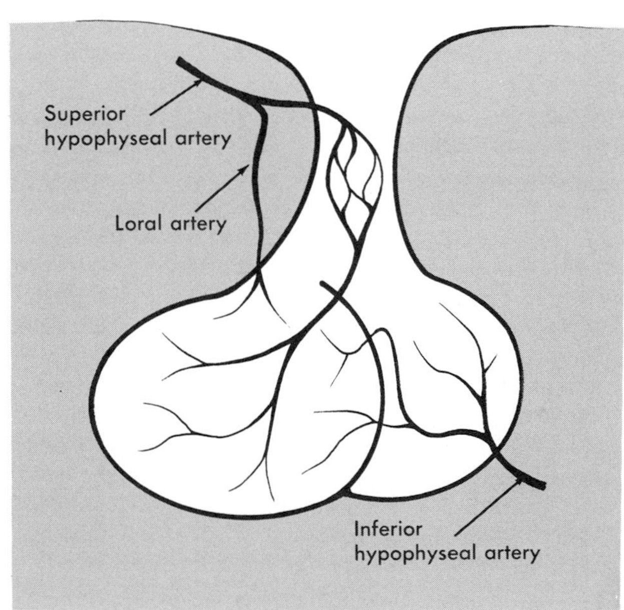

Fig. 22-27. Arterial supply to pituitary.

mon-path cells operating synchronously, in proper sequence, and synergistically. Most responsive acts that are purposeful or useful to an organism represent sequential events (movement of an arm, the rhythm of walking, the act of swallowing, the complex movements of writing or speaking, the sequential secretions as a bolus is passed along in the gastrointestinal tract, the turning toward a sound). These acts represent well-controlled (reflex, volitionally, or by habit) sequential firings of final-common-path cells. The synaptic connections involved are remarkably complex at any single cell. A large spinal final-common-path cell may have 4000 to 5000 synaptic terminals ending in relationship to it. Most of these are derived from internuncial cells or short-chain reticular formation fibers. Somewhat fewer are contributed from long ascending and descending tracts. Very few (or none) probably come directly from the corticospinal, or volitional, tracts, as these tracts operate through control of internuncial cells (Fig. 15-3). Those final-common-path cells mediating impulses to general somatic musculature deliver their signals directly to the muscles innervated. Those supplying smooth muscles and glands of the *autonomic* (general visceral efferent) system do so through distal connections (*ganglia*), which are outside the brain and spinal cord. The neural outflow that regulates the muscles of the special visceral efferent system arises in the brainstem and passes directly to the effectors. It can probably be presumed that different mechanisms operate in the control system for these various muscle groups. It should be noted that a feedback inhibitory arc is presumed to exist for final-path cells. This path is no doubt also mediated through internuncial cells (of Renshaw) (Fig. 15-3).

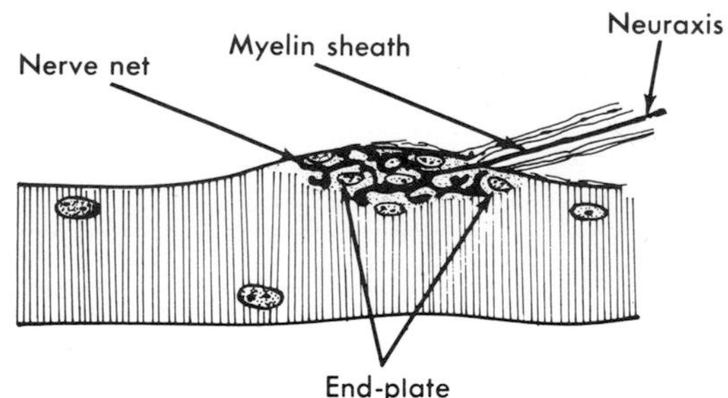

Fig. 22-28. Motor end-plate as seen under the light microscope.

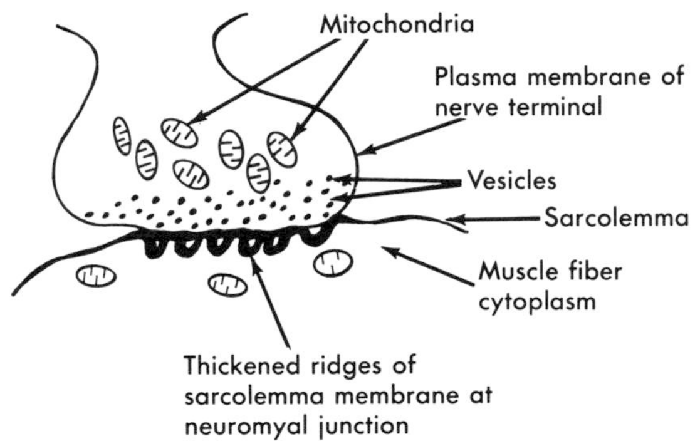

Fig. 22-29. Neuromyal junction diagrammed as seen in EM.

NEUROMUSCULAR UNIT

The delivery of an impulse to a striated muscle is accomplished through the *neuromuscular unit*. This applies to both somatic efferent and special visceral efferent systems, each of which terminates in striated muscle. Each axon involved may supply from one to more than 100 muscle fibers. The final-common-path cell and the muscle fibers it supplies are called the *motor unit*. The *neuromyal junction* is effected by a special end-organ (*end-plate*), which is applied to the sarcolemma of the muscle fiber and transmits the nerve impulse to the muscle. The end-plate arises by expansion of a single terminal filament (Fig. 22-28). In the healthy state the number of terminal end-plates almost matches the number of fibers innervated. In rare circumstances muscle fiber receives two end-plates, usually from the same terminals, so hyperneurotization, or multiple source innervation, of any single fiber probably does not occur.[13] The end-plates are located at the midpoint of a muscle fiber, the innervation band. Hence, the main mass of any fiber is aneural. Muscles that arise in metameres, such as abdominal muscles, possess an innervation band for each metamere.[3] The human end-plate is from 10 to 30 μ in cross section. It lies between the endomyseal cover and the sarcolemma and is not within the muscle fiber proper. Electron microscopy has clarified the structural details of the end-plate, which is diagrammed in Fig. 22-29.

The agent transmitting from nerve to muscle is probably a chemical mediator, *acetylcholine* (see Chapter 12). This chemical incites a change in the muscle fiber membrane potential, culminating in contraction. The acetylcholine is presumed to be inactivated by *acetylcholinesterase*, a specific destructive enzyme for the chemical transmitter. The change in membrane potential is thought to trigger the breakdown of adenosine triphosphate (ATP) to adenosine diphosphate (ADP). This reaction provides the energy for muscle contraction. This energy is probably expended in forming a loose chemical bonding between *myosin*, a protein making up the coarse myofibrils, and *actin*, a protein making up the fine myofibrils. The combination forms *actomyosin*, which is a contractile protein and is probably formed as interconnecting filaments between the coarse and fine myofibrils. The contractile process may be represented as a shortening of the helical actomyosin, producing overriding of the two sets of myofibrils. Another possible explanation for contraction is alternating attachment and detachment of the interconnecting filaments, myosin to actin, as the override progresses.

The physiologic status of skeletal muscle is also reflected in its isozyme pattern, which appears to be subject to epigenetic control. Thus, the physiologic demands of the muscle appear to be determinative for which isozyme of a given enzyme system is synthesized at any one time. In normal mammal and insect, the predominant isozyme of LDH (lactic dehydrogenase), for example, is the slow-moving electrophoretic fraction L_5. However, when the physiologic activity of the muscle alters (for example, to more closely resemble cardiac muscle in behavior, as in the sustained rhythmic beat of flight muscle in migrating birds or in sustained flight in insects; see Chapter 12) the isozyme pat-

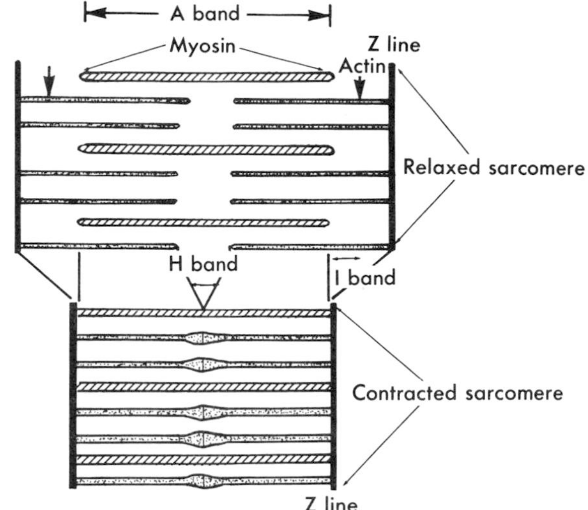

Fig. 22-30. Banding patterns of striated muscle. (After Huxley.)

tern changes, so that the electrophoretically fast-moving isozyme L_1, which normally predominates in cardiac muscle, becomes dominant in the flight muscles. Thus, the imposition of cardiac-type activity on skeletal muscle is compensated by the production of an isozyme better adapted kinetically to this pattern of activity.

In addition to shortening, the visible features in striated muscle that characterize the contraction process include alteration in the striate pattern of the fibers. Normally in the relaxed state the fiber is distinguished by transverse, dark, refractile bands (A-band, made up of coarse myofibrils) separated by intervening lighter bands (I-band) (Fig. 22-30). The A-band possesses a central, lighter, transverse zone (H-disk), and the I-band is divided centrally by a thin disk (Z-disk). The fiber is arbitrarily divided longitudinally into *sarcomeres* by the Z-disks. Fine myofibrils extend from the Z-disks at either end of the sarcomere to the H-disk at its center. The interconnecting filaments bridging between the coarse and fine myofibrils are are helical, permitting an overriding of the two sets of myofibrils. The slight overriding (interdigitating) of the myofibrils in the relaxed state produces the dark zones in the A-bands. In contraction the formation of contractile actomyocin in the interconnecting filaments between myofibrils pulls the Z-disks closer together. This obliterates the I-band; the H-band disappears, and the A-band remains the same length. These alterations in optical features characterize the contractile state and persist until relaxation.

Muscle spindles are regarded as principally receptor structures (Fig. 16-10), but they are known to receive numerous anterior root fibers as well (smaller efferent fibers). The spindle morphology has been reviewed (see p. 279) as a part of the deep sensibility sensory pick-up mechanisms together with *tendon spindles.* Each system participates in stretch responses. However, the tendon spindle is in "series" with the muscle and is stimulated directly as the muscle contracts. By contrast, the muscle spindles operate in "parallel" with regular or extrafusal muscle fibers. The spindle is made up of two to ten specialized intrafusal muscle fibers, which interconnect from perimysium or tendon to connective tissue elsewhere (Fig. 16-10). Extrafusal muscle contraction thus relaxes the intrafusal fibers.

Both ends of the spindles are striated and contractile and are innervated by motor units (fusimotor fibers) ending in motor end-plates or in nerve nets. The central region of the spindle however is noncontractile and contains nuclei, some of which are in clusters known as nuclear bags. These fibers relate to the afferent annulospiral endings. The flower spray endings (p. 279) relate to the myotubal areas, where the nuclei are in linear pattern as a central core (nuclear chains). The entire central field of the intrafusal filaments possesses a surrounding lymph space through which the nerve fibers pass.

The spindle thus has two main sets of afferent fibers (arising in annulospiral and flower spray endings) plus the fusimotor filaments to the contractile extremities. Other fine fibers in the neural complex of the spindle probably mediate pain and vascular control. The fusimotor fibers also display two patterns of terminals, which probably relate the nuclear bag filaments to the motor end-plates and the chain nuclear filaments to the nerve nets.[2] This complex arrangement provides an isolated reflex system of afferent to efferent fibers within the spindle itself. The spindle thus can respond to general extrafusal muscle stretch, and it can also operate independently and respond to the fusimotor system alone. The related afferent paths from both spindles and tendons are fed into the motor pool as significant influences on the reflex responses. These therefore must be added to the final-common-path complex of Fig. 15-3.

NEUROMUSCULAR SERVOMECHANISMS

As stated in previous chapters, there are numerous control systems that operate in the physiologic mechanics of the nervous system. Compensating mechanisms are brought into play in neural tissue in such processes as the respiratory act, maintaining chemical and pH levels in the related blood stream, gaseous exchanges, fluid retention, thermal excursions, and electrolyte balance. All these activities tend to maintain the body standards, which usually operate within rather narrow limits as a biologic system. Among control systems of particular interest in neurology are the *servomechanisms,* which indirectly regulate many complex neuromuscular acts. These are automatic, self-adjusting control devices that operate without requiring repetitive cerebral influence to sustain (for example) muscle position in the occurrence of changing load. For example, posture is maintained less by the standard neuromuscular units than by the servomechanism operating through small efferent fibers to muscle spindles. By control of the spindle, the length of the muscle (contraction versus stretch) is controlled without requiring total CNS participation for each adjustment. This sequence is presumed to be as follows: (1) A volitional impulse is transmitted to muscle with consequent contraction to meet the load. (2) A simultaneous efferent outflow (small fibers) reaches the spindle, which contracts and stimulates its receptor component. (3) The spindle receptor sends afferent impulses to its own CNS neuromuscular unit. (4) The same neuromuscular units respond with contraction until the receptor stimulus from the spindle ceases. In this manner a relatively minor neural expenditure occurs in sustained contractions of muscles that do not require higher center participation. The mechanisms afford a local means (without volition) for a muscle system to respond by added contraction to increased loading and by cessation of contraction when loading and stretch are balanced. While the neuromuscular servomechanism in posture is perhaps best understood, it seems clear that similar mechanisms must operate within the CNS to maintain the remarkable accommodating, adjusting, and sequential features so conspicuous in almost every neurophysiologic act. Important in these mechanisms is the *feedback.* Feedback refers to the returning impulse from a delivery area back to a control area that modifies the neural patterns to the delivery area.

REFERENCES

1. Botar, J.: The autonomic nervous system, Budapest, 1966, Akadémiai Kaidó.
2. Boyd, J. A.: The innervation of mammalian neuromuscular spindles, J. Physiol. **140**:14, 1958.
3. Coërs, C., and Woolf, A. L.: The innervation of muscle: a biopsy study, Springfield, Illinois, 1959, Charles C Thomas, Publisher.
4. De Robertis, E.: Histophysiology of synapses and neurosecretion, New York, 1964, The Macmillan Co.
5. Dow, R. S., and Moruzzi, G.: The physiology and pathology of the cerebellum, Minneapolis, 1958, The Universtiy of Minneapolis Press.
6. Eccles, J. C., Ito, M., and Szentágothai, J.: The cerebellum as a neuronal machine, New York, 1967, Springer-Verlag.
7. Haymaker, W., Anderson, E., and Nauta, W. J. H.: The hypothalamus, Springfield, Illinois, 1969, Charles C Thomas, Publisher.
8. Martini, L., and Ganong, W. F.: Neuroendocrinology, New York, 1967, The Academic Press, Inc.
9. Nyberg-Hansen, R.: Functional organization of descending supraspinal fibre systems to the spinal cord, Berlin, 1966, Springer-Verlag.
10. Penfield, W., and Roberts, L.: Speech and brain mechanisms, Princeton, New Jersey, 1959, Princeton University Press.
11. Scharrer, E., and Scharrer, B.: Neuroendocrinology, New York, 1963, Columbia University Press.
12. Segre, E. J., and Lloyd, C. W.: Neuroendocrine mechanisms. In Minckler, J., editor: Pathology of the nervous system, vol. I, New York, 1968, McGraw-Hill Book Co.
13. Stevens, C. F.: Neurophysiology, New York, 1966, John Wiley & Sons, Inc.
14. Szentágothai, J., and others: Hypothalamic control of the anterior pituitary, ed. 3, Budapest, 1968, Akadémiai Kiadó.

PART V Integrated functions

CHAPTER 23

PSYCHOBIOLOGY

DONALD SHEARN

Two avenues of vital concern to biologists and psychologists have provided the directions for this chapter—perception and behavioral plasticity. It it regretful that in following these avenues, others cannot be covered in this brief treatment of psychobiology.

PERCEPTION

Some psychophysical relations

One of the oldest formulations in psychophysics, the Weber-Fechner law, states that perceived stimulus intensity increases proportionally with the logarithm of stimulus intensity ($S = a \log I + b$, where S is perceived intensity, I is metered intensity, and a and b are constants). That is, to judge equal steps in the detection of increases in stimulus intensity, stimulus energy must be increased in logarithmic steps. The relationship between judgement of arithmetic steps and the corresponding logarithmic steps in stimulus intensity might be thought to reside in regions of great complexity of the nervous system, such as the cortex or the thalamus. However, data provided by Katz show that the logarithmic feature of the process enters at the very first stage of energy transduction by a receptor. When spike potential frequency is plotted as a function of logarithmic stimulus intensity (such as load on muscle), a proportional graph is drawn. When spike frequency is then plotted against the local or generator potential, which is scaled arithmetically rather than logarithmically, a proportional graph also follows. In short, it is in the coupling between the stimulation and generator potential of the receptor where the logarithmic relationship begins.[32]

However, it would be surprising if a single formulation such as the Weber-Fechner law could predict the behavior of all sensory modalities and conditions. Psychophysics had shown that while the law contained much fundamental truth about perception, it was often in error at the extremes of stimulus intensity. More recently, Stevens has argued for the use of a power function, $S = kI^n$ (where S is perceived intensity, I is stimulus intensity, and n varies with the sense modality).[71]

Contrast mechanisms in perception

Recently acquired evidence for lateral inhibition which works across the horizontal organization of sensory nerve cells, is considerably general and important. The psychologic principles that seem to share this characteristic with neurophysiology are color brightness and border contrast, Mach bands,[31] pitch discrimination, sound localization, and others.[59,77]

Microelectrode recordings from single nerve cells of the visual ganglia, lateral geniculate thalamus, or visual cortex made while various hues and patterns are presented to the retina have given rise to the concept of the *receptive field.* The pattern in the visual field and hence that playing on the retina that changes the spike activity of a particular cell defines the receptive field for that cell. Kuffler has observed that mammalian ganglion cells discharge with increasing frequency until the spot of light stimulating the retina reaches about 1 mm. in diameter; thereafter, larger spots of light produce decreasing responsitivity, suggesting that spatial summation of light on the retina has two processes.[45] The first process is facilitory, as the increasing spot activates more and more excitatory elements. This process is in line with the psychophysical principle known as Ricco's law.[31] The second is inhibitory and begins when the spot of light is large enough to encroach upon the surrounding negative synaptic connections. These neurologic perceptual processes have received considerable experimental attention. Hubel and Weisel's analyses of single units in the cat's striate cortex have provided important clues concerning how the geometry of the visual cortex relates to angular orientation of objects in the visual field.[39] Their data show that the circular receptive field with opponent center and periphery, found in ganglion regions and lateral geniculate bodies, gives way to a linear receptive field in the cortex (illustrated by drawing a row of overlapping circular fields). Each linear receptive field is tuned to a particular angular orientation of a line-shaped stimulus, and hence the spike frequency of the cell in question increases with increasing agreement between the stimulus angle and receptive field angle. Columnar organization of the cortex is such that cells of a given column appear to have the same receptive field axis orientation. More recently it has been learned that receptive fields are not always invariant networks, but may be more flexible circuits, changed by stimulation.[38]

Studies of color responses of cells in the primate lateral geniculate nucleus show not only a center-periphery antagonism, but also opposing hue responses involving red-green and yellow-blue pairs.[14] These opponent reactions recall the psychophysical phenomena of color contrast and negative after-images[31] and revitalize an old theory of color vision by Hering.[35]

Receptive field organization also plays a vital role in increasing visual acuity, as shown in research with the compound eye of *limulus*. This *limulus* preparation is more accessible than its mammalian counterpart, allowing direct measures of inhibition at the receptor as a light-dark edge stimulus is presented to the eye. Quantitative analysis has accounted for the enhancement of acuity by neural elements.[34] The method by which lateral inhibition proceeds to sharpen the edge response is illustrated in Fig. 23-1.

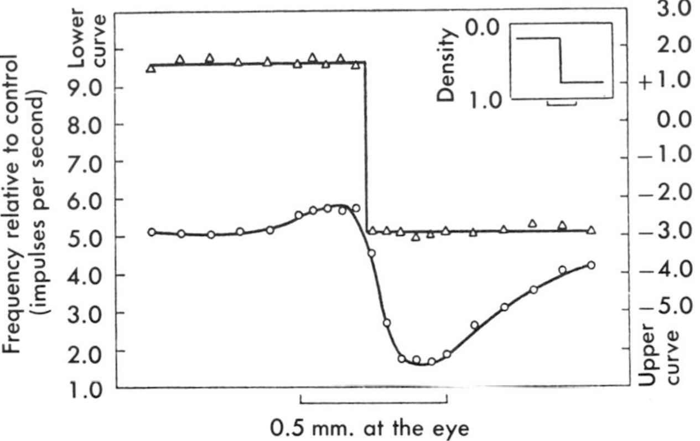

Fig. 23-1. Neural impulse response from a single photoreceptor of limulus. Upper right-hand insert shows the gradient of illumination that was moved across the retina in small steps. The top function shows response of the single unit when inhibition from neighboring units is removed by masking light from them. Bottom function shows response of normal situation without masking. (From Ratliff and Hartline: J. Gen. Physiol. **42:**1241, 1959.)

The somatotopic map of skin surface, determined by tactile stimulation and thalamic single-unit recording,[55] illustrates another kind of spatial isomorphism between the stimulus field and neural structure. Such relations differ from the tonotopic organization in hearing, where *frequency* of the sounding object is localized in various structures, such as the basilar membrane[77] or cortex.[79] The experimental analysis of the behavior of single cells in the acoustic system has given some interesting insights into tuning mechanisms. Katsuki has made unit recordings from nerve VIII, the inferior colliculus, trapezoid body, and medial geniculate nucleus, while varying both frequency and intensity of a pure tone stimulus. At these neural levels each cell is tuned to respond to one frequency at its threshold intensity. As intensity is increased, the bandwidth of frequencies that stimulates a cell widens, giving a *response area* for that cell. There is fairly good agreement between the psychophysical audibility curve (sensitivity as a function of frequency) and these electrophysiologic measures.[43] Recordings from cells in the primary auditory cortex have shown that the behavior is more complicated at that level. Some cells are tuned to more than one frequency, giving octave responses. Others shut off when the intensity becomes too loud.[37]

Thermally sensitive neurons react to spatial features of stimulation, as would be expected from the cutaneous surface, and to the stimulus temperature as well. The behavior of nerve fibers parallels a classic perceptual event known as *paradoxical cold,* in which further increases in skin temperature results in reporting by the subjects that the skin is colder.[81] The nerve fiber in question may respond to temperatures from 15° to 35° C. (cold), and then again above 45° C. (warm). The gap between 35° and 45° C. is handled by a second nerve fiber. Hence, the same neuron reacts to cold stimulation, turns off with intermediate stimulation, and

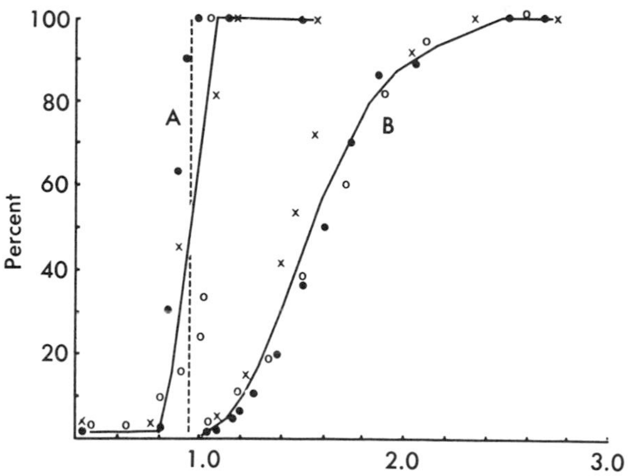

Fig. 23-2. Comparison of behavioral threshold, **A,** and evoked compound action potentials of brachial plexuses, **B,** in response to stimulation of the superficial radial nerve. The behavioral measure is the percent of maximum amplitude. Abscissa values are stimulus intensity values relative to neural threshold. Note sensitivity of behavioral measure. (From Bourassa & Swett: J. Neurophysiol. **30**:515, 1967.)

then reacts to warm stimulation, giving a paradoxical effect.

BEHAVIORAL PLASTICITY

Few extant organisms remain unchanged by environmental stimulation. The changes in behavior caused by stimulation, whether short-lived or enduring, are a form of memory. The range of such modifications is enormous when viewed across the species. The mollusk may demonstrate memory of prodding a few moments ago by simply withdrawing less noticeably on succeeding stimulations. A man may call out the name of a school chum not seen for twenty years upon viewing no more than the back of an aging head.

Role of proprioception

Cutaneous and muscular sensory systems offer excellent examples of sensitive interaction with mechanical aspects of the environment.[62] Experimental analysis using both behavioral data from trained cats responding to proprioceptive stimulation and action potentials evoked by the same stimulation has made it possible to relate the psychophysics and sensory physiology of proprioception. For example, Fig. 23-2 shows good correspondence between the behavioral and electrophysiologic responses plotted as a percentage of threshold, with the behavioral measure being only slightly more sensitive to cutaneous stimulation.[2] Only a very small number of cutaneous fibers must be activated to bring on both the appropriate learned response and evoked potentials at the brachial plexuses.

It seems easy to assume in view of such sensitivity that these receptor systems are necessary for all complex movement and learning. Experiments with deafferented monkeys have proven such an assumption untrue.[72] Following extensive dorsal rhizotomy these animals learned to avoid electric shocks with forelimb or finger responses in the absence of visual or auditory cues. The monkeys could run and climb with agility, even when blindfolded. Since theories of learning often use the assumption that proprioceptive feedback is critical in learning, these results are especially important.

Response habituation

Pavlov has observed that alerting reactions (*investigatory reflexes*) are greatly reduced with repeated presentation of the eliciting stimulus.[57] Clearly the cortical "inhibition" used by Pavlov to account for habituation is not the same as the "inhibition" designating certain synaptic events. As in many Pavlovian concepts using cortical terminology, the referents are actually behavioral rather than neural. However, it is of some importance that the term does imply an active process. In responding less and less to repetitive stimulation, the animal must have machinery that is busy registering the fact that the stimulation has already occurred. Later work, particularly the classic EEG investigations of Sharpless and Jasper, has provided more data on this point.[65] A brief tone at a frequency of 500 Hz. will initially evoke desynchronization of the suprasylvian EEG. With repetition of the 500 Hz. tone, this arousal response shortens and eventually ceases. If following this habituation some minutes or hours elapse without more stimulation, there will be spontaneous recovery of the desynchronized EEG with the next tone presentation, showing that the habituation is temporary. Additional presentations of the 500 Hz. tone will again produce habituation. If a tone at 1000 Hz. instead of 500 Hz. is introduced the desynchronized EEG pattern is elicited fully-blown (Pavlovian *disinhibition*). A tone of a pitch closer to the jaded 500 Hz. tone (such as 600 Hz.) evokes either a small EEG arousal response or none at all. Such gradations of response habituation as a function of similarity to the original habituating stimulus strongly suggest the phenomenon of stimulus generalization.

The experimental settings that produce response

habituation are the same ones that may produce response facilitation through the use of stimulation of higher intensities. For example, an occasional shock given haphazardly during a series of weak cutaneous stimulations is enough to sensitize a spinal reflex that otherwise would be negligible or rapidly habituated. (These shocks are not paired with the other stimulation as they would be in a conditioning experiment.) Thompson and Spencer view habituation and sensitization in spinal reflexes as independent processes that interact at the last stage of the limb flexion reflex.[73] They suggest that the interneurons contribute to the habituatory decrement, whereas motor neurons, including gamma motoneurons, which regulate muscle contraction, are most implicated in the increased magnitude reflex sensitization.

There is a considerable autonomic counterpart to these changes in EEG or striate motor reactions. Spontaneous recovery of the response with some change in stimulation, often as an orderly function of dissimilarity to the original habituating stimulus, are commonplace results with elicited changes in heart rate, vosomotor reactions, respiration, and the galvanic skin response. The processes of habituation and sensitization are recognized by Pavlov as *orienting reflexes* (reactions that habituate) and *defensive reflexes* (those reactions that do not habituate because of more intense stimulation).[69]

Pavlovian conditioning

One stimulus may be experimentally substituted for a second stimulus that already evokes a reaction or reflex under study. It is necessary to find a stimulus that naturally, or unconditionally, elicits the reaction, just as meat or acid in the mouth unconditionally elicits salivation.[57] When an unconditional stimulus for the reaction in question has been located, a stimulus that is neutral with respect to that reaction, such as a weak tone or light, is paired with it—first neutral stimulus, followed by the unconditional stimulus. Usually after a few pairings the neutral stimulus comes to elicit the reaction. The time between onset of the neutral stimulus (the conditional stimulus) and the unconditional stimulus is typically a few seconds. Two points are important in explaining this phenomenon. First, the stimulus that is imparting the effect, the unconditional stimulus, appears *last* in the conditioning sequence of conditional then unconditional stimulus. This procedure, which appears to work backwards in time, is opposite to neurophysiological conditioning, in which the conditioning shock appears first in order to impart its effect, followed by the testing shock. Second, the effective time scale of Pavlovian conditioning is in seconds rather than milliseconds, as in neurophysiology, this difference is of about one order of magnitude. Any conceptual scheme for memory that is used to relate neural behavior to Pavlovian conditioning must confront these differences.

When the conditional stimulus is presented alone to evoke its reaction (the conditional reflex or response), it will gradually lose its potency unless recharged by occasional pairings with the unconditional stimulus. The mere elapse of time however does not extinguish the response, and the response may survive for months or years in the absence of appropriate extinction or habituation procedures. It is necessary to repeatedly present the conditional stimulus alone in order to destroy its response-eliciting effect.

Considerable confusion still exists about the Pavlovian conditional stimulus, which evokes a reflex (frequently autonomic in nature), and other stimuli that cause more variable and often longer-lasting responses (usually of the striated musculature). The blue light in the monkey chamber, which occasions button pressing, is not a conditional stimulus any more than the moving baton of the symphony conductor. The type of stimulus that produces this second kind of behavior is discussed later under operant conditioning.*

Since Pavlov's early work with secretory conditional reflexes, the behavior studied in this manner has been extended to virtually every conceivable response system, including water balance and temperature regulation.[60] In the United States research has emphasized cardiovascular and other autonomic reactions and eyelid responses.[27,58,66]

Neural stimulation. In many experiments stimulation of neural structures has served as the conditional stimulus, and in a few such stimulation has also provided the unconditional stimulus. Using electrodes implanted in auditory cortex of dogs, Loucks has shown that stimulation of the brain can serve as conditional stimulation (CS).[39] He applied electric shock to the leg as unconditional stimulation (US). After a few pairings of cortical stimulation followed by shock to the leg, cortical stimulation alone elicited the same reaction that only shock had before. A control experiment in which the trigeminal nerve was sec-

*For discussion of the "pseudo reflex" and comparison of conditional and operant stimuli and responses see reference 68.

tioned has ruled out meningeal stimulation as the cause.[17] Brain stimulation as the US has been used successfully by Brogden and Gantt, who paired tone with cerebellar stimulation.[4] Further, both CS and US have taken the form of brain stimulation.[16] The loci of the CS in these studies might be occipital or suprasylvian cortex, while the US would be applied moments later to a site in the motor cortex.

Spinal conditioning. In view of these conditioning studies that make use of the cortex as loci both unconditional and conditional stimuli, it could be erroneously inferred that this structure is necessary for conditioning. Leg flexion responses have been conditioned in the decorticated dog using a tactile or auditory stimulus as the CS and electric shock as the US.[28] In other experiments the spinal cord has been surgically severed from the brain, and conditioning procedures have been carried on by tactile and electric shock stimulation to the legs. Recent successful experiments using cat subjects strongly suggest the possibility of spinal conditioning without the assistance of the brain.[18]

Unit conditioning. Yoshii and Ogura have conditioned single nerve cells using Pavlovian methods.[80] In these studies a tone or light that did not evoke spike potentials of a reticular formation cell was paired with shock to the sciatic nerve. After a few pairings the tone or light came to elicit spike activity. The phenomenon was transitory, disappearing with continued pairing. Bureš and Burešová have also conditioned single nerve cells in the hippocampus, thalamus, and neocortex as well as the reticular formation.[7] Their technique involved an auditory CS and direct chemical and/or electrical stimulation of the cells through the microelectrode. With this procedure twenty-six percent of the cells studied showed transitory reactions to the CS, and thirteen percent showed long-lasting conditioning effects (response to the tone as they had to the direct assault through the membrane).

EEG. Extensive Pavlovian conditioning of EEG has been done.[29,54] The desynchronized wave, the alpha block, is the common reaction naturally elicited by a light US. An auditory stimulus usually serves as the CS. As in all efforts to demonstrate Pavlovian conditioning, there is the possibility that one is simply sensitizing or dishabituating the subject with a strong stimulus so that a response is elicited to any subsequent stimulus.

Operant conditioning

The development of procedures that allow an investigator to supply a given response or a complex sequence of responses on demand is important in the study of relations between visible behavioral events and neural events. The limitations of Pavlovian conditioning become apparent in the difficulty of locating stimuli that naturally, or unconditionally, elicit certain complex behaviors in the animal or human subjects. It is difficult, for example, to obtain a replicable and intricate sequence of limb movements from the *Rhesus* monkey with Pavlovian conditioning. Since there is no stimulus that evokes such a sequence naturally, simple substitution of stimuli will not work. A better procedure for this purpose makes use of the *consequences* of responses to shape response patterns through *reinforcement* (reward) of desired responses and through nonreinforcement, or extinction, of undesirable responses. A response that can be strengthened by stimuli following quickly after its occurence is called an operant, and hence the term *operant conditioning*.[68] The strengthening of an operant may be demonstrated by increases in rate of responding.

Neural circuit analysis. The usefullness of operant techniques is illustrated by the work of Evarts, who examined the activity of the pyramidal tract during postural fixation.[21] In contrast to many classical studies of neural aspects of motor and sensory behavior in which the experimental animals have been heavily barbituated, Evarts made use of alert monkeys, trained with operant techniques to hold a particular limb position. Single-unit records obtained from chronically implanted electrodes showed that neuronal activity of the pyramidal tract is related to the muscular contraction around a joint rather than simple joint position or displacement.

A second illustration of the operant procedure in studying the nervous system is the work of Miller and Glickstein, who used highly-trained, awake monkeys in the traditional human reaction-time experiment.[51] Monkeys were trained with operant procedures to quickly release a telegraph key upon presentation of electrical stimulation to area 17. When the response latencies obtained with this interposed stimulation were compared with those obtained with normal visual stimulation, the former were found to be 30 msec. shorter, or about as much shorter as the time necessary to evoke potentials in area 17 with visual stimulation. The accountability of time segments in the neural circuit of the awake and behaving subject, from sensory input to motor output, may then proceed analytically. For example, Evarts has noted 70 msec. as the response latency from area 17 to the reaction of

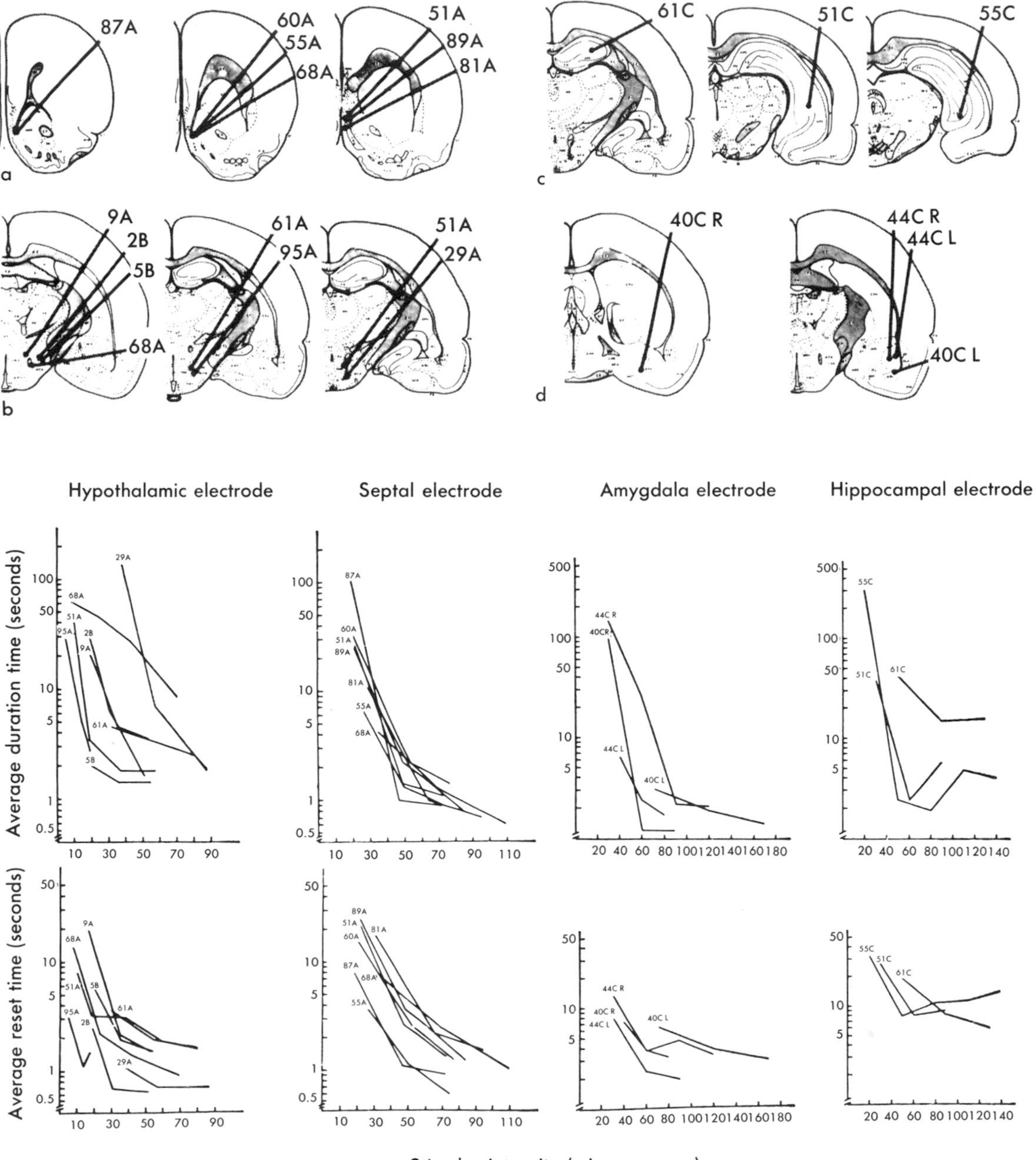

Fig. 23-3. Lever pressing rates of rats' turning brain stimulation on and off. Top shows electrode locations (*numbered*). Bottom shows response rates as a function of stimulus intensity for the various electrode locations (*numbered*). Average duration is the time brain stimulation is left on following response on the first lever before a second lever is depressed. Average reset duration is the amount of time stimulation is off between the second and the first lever sequence. Note that both on and off times shorten with increased intensity. (From Valenstein, E. S., and Valenstein, J. T.: Interaction of positive and negative reinforcing neural systems, Science 145:1456, 1969.)

pyramidal cells in motor cortex.[20] The response of motor cortex neurons has also been studied by playing the magnetic data tape backwards and summing the unit activity with respect to the key press response, which followed the neuronal response. The response of the unit might be a phasic burst of 200 to 300 msec. in some units or cessation of tonic activity in others.[48] Additional work has shown electromyographic reaction times in the biceps of about 80 msec. to auditory stimuli, and 125 msec. to visual stimuli. These reaction times are less variable and, of course, shorter than the key response itself.[49]

In addition to providing repeatable visible behavior for studying neural substrates, operant procedures have taken two additional directions.

Brain stimulation reinforcement. The first of these directions is brain self-stimulation as reinforcement for operant behavior.[56] In the most straight forward version of this procedure, a rat delivers a weak shock (such as 0.5 seconds of 100 ma. square or sine wave) through chronically implanted electrodes to his own brain (lateral hypothalamus or septum) each time he presses a small lever in his experimental chamber. Compulsive behavior is generated by this response-contingent stimulation, and rats may press their response keys thousands of times per hour, often without sign of satiation. Response-contingent brain stimulation becomes averse if continued for more than a second or so, depending upon the stimulus intensity. When provided with one lever to turn on brain stimulation and another to turn it off, rats will move back and forth from lever to lever, turning the current on and off.[75] As shown in Fig. 23-3, the animal shortens both on and off periods as the stimulation intensity is increased. This finding is consistent in a number of electrode sites. Although this paradigm raises some central questions regarding relations between brain mechanisms and learning and reinforcement, such questions remain unanswered for the most part.[30,56] There has been a change in emphasis in research from the anatomic loci of reinforcement to basic behaviors such as object carrying, eating and drinking elicited by hypothalamic stimulation, and in turn, the relations of these evoked behaviors to other behaviors that precede them and may be strengthened by them.[11,74] This shift in emphasis to motivation brings the analysis full circle to the classical work of Hess, in which autonomic and motor reactions elicited by hypothalamic stimulation were studied in the chronically implanted cat,[36] and to related work with intact rats, in which medial and lateral hypothalamic stimulation was shown to respectively inhibit and increase food intake.

Operant control of physiology. A second application of operant analysis concerns the reinforcement of responses heretofore thought to be beyond the pale of operant conditioning because of their involuntary or otherwise intractable nature. Response-contingent events have controlled cardiovascular reactions, glandular responses, neural gross potentials, and unit responses.[67] This application of operant procedures is well illustrated by the experiment of Fetz in which the behavior of single neurons of the motor cortex of Rhesus monkeys was conditioned with response-contingent reinforcement with banana pellets.[22] The results of this experiment are shown in Fig. 23-4. Each time the chronically implanted microelectrode detected a burst of spike activity well above baseline levels, the animal was automatically rewarded. These units were conditioned to fire actively only so long as reinforcement contingency was in effect. A control phase of the experiment, in which delivery of the reinforcer was uncorrelated with ongoing unit activity, ruled out any generalized activation due to evocation by the reinforcer.*

NEURAL ACCOUNTS OF BEHAVIORAL PLASTICITY

In addition to the kinds of conditioning and learning already discussed, experimentation is uncovering evidence of both a short- and long-term memory.[50] According to this dual-process view, electroconvulsive shock and retrograde amnesia disrupt short-term memory of events close in time to the trauma before permanent storage (long-term memory) is achieved. The neuronal contribution to short-term memory has been postulated to be electrical activity of reverbertory, or Renshaw, circuits during *consolidation* of the *memory trace.* Such delicate neural reverberation is easily breached by an electrical or pharmacologic stimulus directed at it. When the transmission from short- to long-term memory is complete and the memory trace has been consolidated, there are assumed permanent structural changes, e.g. enlarged presynaptic boutons.[19]

Anatomic factors in learning

The search for general mechanisms of memory that work across tracts of the brain has often been a discouraging and frustrating one.[46] The elusive *engram,* or neural encoding of an event, may not

*For discussion of experiments using operant procedures see reference 67.

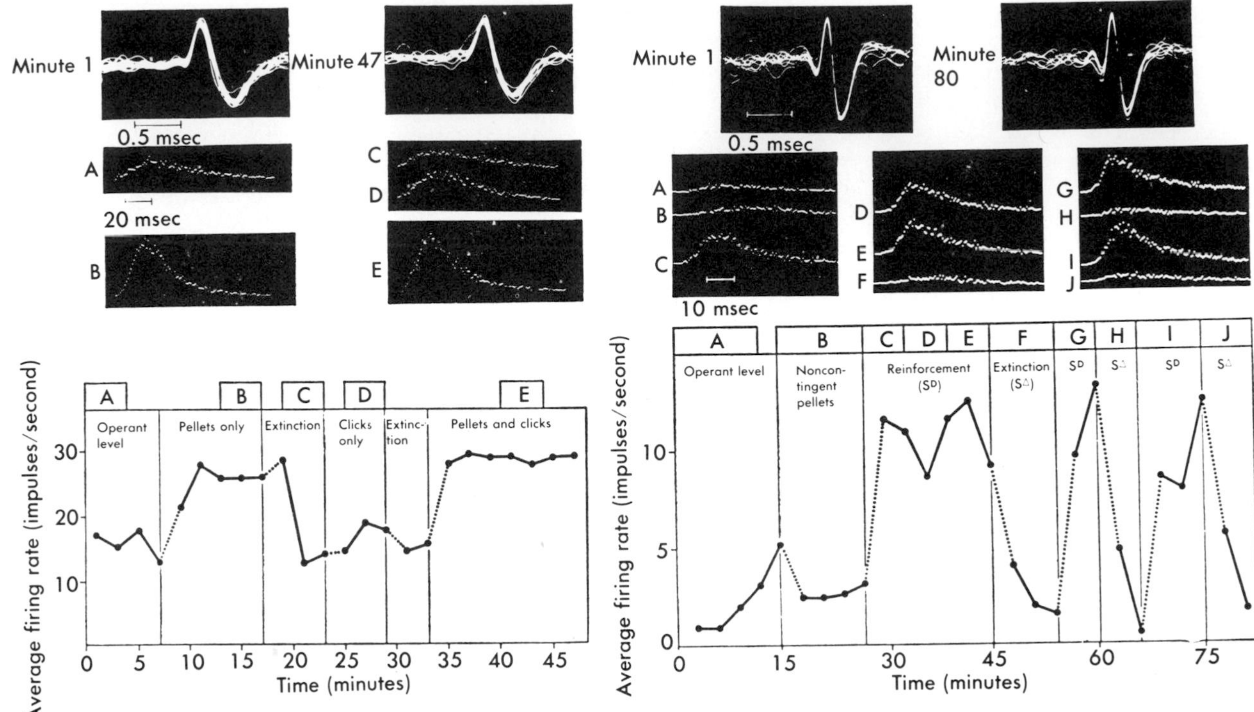

Fig. 23-4. Upper, Firing rate of precentral cortex cell as a function of reinforcement schedule. During operant level and extinction periods, neither food nor click feedback was presented. During pellets only period, the highest firing rates were reinforced with delivery of a food pellet, without click feedback. During clicks only period, a click was presented for each firing of the cell; finally, both pellets and clicks were provided. Interspike interval histograms above the graph show the relative number of intervals from 0 to 125 msec. occurring during the specified four-minute segments of the session. Several superimposed examples of the cell's action potential from the first and last minute of the session are illustrated at top. **Lower,** Firing rate of a precentral cell in a session with visual feedback and noncontingent reinforcement. Each point represents the average firing rate for the preceding three-minute interval. During operant level and extinction (S^{Δ}) periods, no food or feedback was provided. During the noncontingent pellets period, the meter was illuminated, and pellet delivery and meter deflection were determined by a tape recording of a previous session. The only change from noncontingent pellets to reinforcement (S^D) period was the correlation of pellet delivery and meter deflection with the activity of the monitored cell. In succeeding periods, reinforcement (S^D) alternated with extinction (S^{Δ}). Interspike interval histograms taken during the specified time segment show the number of intervals between 0 and 62.5 msec. all at the same vertical scale. Several superimposed action potentials from the first and last minute of the session are shown at top. (From Fetz, E. E.: Operant conditioning of cortical unit activity, Science **163:**955, 1969.)

be localized simply; loss of a learned habit does not typically follow from the destruction of a specific brain point. On the contrary, increases in the number of errors in rats executing a habit is a more or less a gradual function of the amount of cortical tissue ablated, a phenomenon widely known as *mass action* (Fig. 23-5). Judged by any criteria but memory for the correct response at the choice point, the performance of a rat with considerable sensorymotor destruction is shabby. However, his loss of memory appears to be a simple function of the amount of cortex removed. These data suggest that the "engram" concept suffers from the same inadequacies as that of the "brain center" in describing the true workings of the nervous system. Even when specific loci and pathways are implicated, as they have been in primate visual learning, the "engram" is still elusive.

Loss of learned visual discrimination is but one of the repercussions of bilateral temporal lobectomy known as the "Klüver-Bucy syndrome." Other modifications of behavior following the ablation include hypersexuality, docility, and mouthing of objects. Subsequent work has narrowed the critical area for impairment of visual memory to the inferior and middle temporal gyri and has implicated the posterior corpus callosum in a critical pathway between temporal gyrus and contralateral occipital

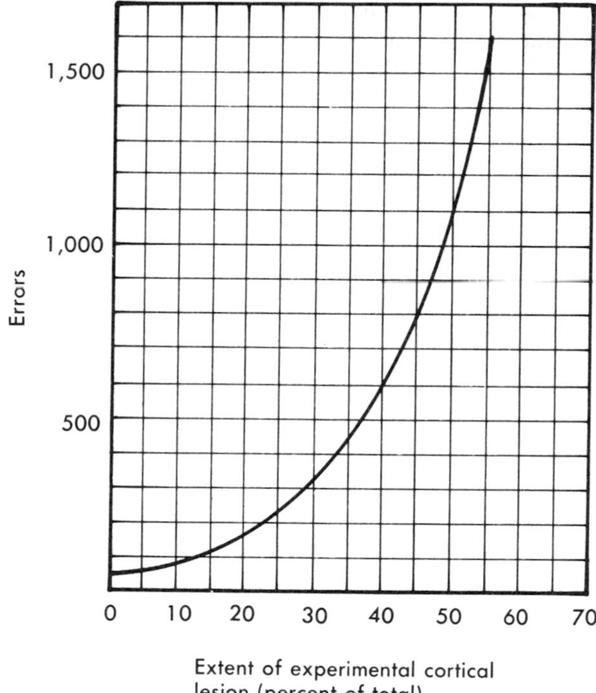

Fig. 23-5. Loss of a habit as a function of amount of cortical tissue ablated, demonstrating the mass action principle. (From The neuropsychology of Lashley by Beach and others, New York, 1950, McGraw-Hill Book Co. Used with permission of McGraw-Hill Book Co.)

lobe.[52] The loss of visual memory that ensues from these lesions is not the simple result of a sensory deficit, as would follow from ablation of a primary sensory area. The animal sees, but he may behave if he were viewing objects for the first time.*

Questions of distributed versus localized neural substrates in memory have been viewed by use of the *split-brain* preparation. The preparation may be surgical, involving transection of the optic chiasm, corpus callosum, and commissures,[70] or chemical, employing the temporary spreading depression hemidecortication brought about by application of KCl to one of the hemispheres.[6,63] Using the surgical split-brain preparation it is possible to condition responses occasioned by discriminative stimuli involving only one eye and one hemisphere. These responses are independent and even opposite to the stimulus-response patterns conditioned with the other eye-hemisphere combination. In essence, the subject has two brains for two sets of responses, which may be incompatible.

The results of these investigations underscore the role of commissural tracts in transferring information from one cerebral hemisphere to the other. The chemical split-brain procedure, while presently lacking histologic guarantees, enjoys the advantage of being temporary and reversible, allowing the investigator to return to conditions before spreading depression was employed or to depress the previously normal hemisphere while working with a recovered, previously depressed hemisphere. In one experiment rats that had learned to operate a lever when one hemisphere was depressed would not do so when it was recovered and the other hemisphere was depressed.[63] When both hemispheres were normal a single reinforced response on the lever was enough to cause "one-trial" or nearly instantaneous shift of information from one hemisphere to the other. Schneider however attributes these findings to forgetting caused by changes in stimulus conditions between training and test conditions.[64] He has conducted the one-trial transfer experiment, but with the added control of one reinforced trial with the hemisphere depressed that was previously intact during learning. The control subjects showed better subsequent performance than subjects given the single reinforcement with both hemispheres intact.

A procedure related to both the surgical and chemical split brain is one that makes use of organisms capable of regeneration of the CNS. This procedure has been used to show a transfer of learned information from one part of the visual system of the goldfish to another.[12] The fish learned a visual discrimination with one brachium intact and the other severed. These brachia respectively project from the dorsal or ventral retina to the ventral or dorsal tectum. Following neural regeneration, the previously untouched brachium was cut. Testing then showed that the visual discrimination had transferred intraretinally, employing neurons not active during the original conditioning.

Biochemical theories of memory

Optimism prevails for many in anticipating an adequate chemical account of learning and memory. Early theoretical sketches suggesting protein synthesis as a *template* mechanism for memory[44,53] have been augmented by considerable experimental and theoretical coverage following the implication of DNA in genetic function.[78] Hydén hypothesized that the RNA of a cell is modified by the electrical activity of the nerve impulse patterns reaching the

*For discussion of the problems introduced by the ablation method see reference 9.

cell, so that the same impulse patterns move readily across its synapse on subsequent occasions.[40] Each cell could conceivably react differentially to a large number of impulse patterns by creating a storehouse of various RNA templates. In well-known tests of this theory, Hydén and Egyhazi analyzed the RNA contents of various brain loci after rats had learned to walk on a wire or were exposed to rotation in a small centrifuge (to control for vestibular system activity).[41,42] The RNA content from Deiters cells of the vestibular nuclei in rats that learned the tight-rope task was 751 μm., as compared with 722 μm. for the centrifuge controls, and 683 μm. for untreated controls. An increased adenine-uracil ratio was observed in the animals that had learned the tight-rope problem. RNA changes were found in glial cells, underscoring the importance of these cells.[26] Increased base ratios of nuclear RNA disappeared soon after learning however if food was available afterwards. RNA changes were found in the vestibular system of the experimental rats, but not in the reticular formation of control rats. Why a comparison was made between a sensory system and the reticular formation and why any particular anatomic structure was analyzed are not clear. There is also the problem of meaningful comparison between the balancing and centrifugal animals with respect to RNA sampling in the vestibular system. RNA differences might be expected on the basis of activity differences of these very different tasks, aside from any presumed effect of the learning requirement. That is, the amount of neural activity elicited, apart from memory, may differ in different situations. One may also suggest that the correlation of RNA changes with learning possibly indicates that RNA is just one of several-by-products of cellular metabolism.[15]

Additional experiments designed to show the active role of RNA in learning have used two basic procedures—the ingestion or injection of RNA and the inhibition of RNA. After senile patients took yeast RNA orally, tests of short-term memory improved dramatically.[8] However, the mechanism for transporting ingested RNA across the bloodbrain barrier is unclear. In addition, effects of the large amounts of material consumed by the patients were not controlled. Intraperitoneal injection of RNA into young rats slightly improve their jumping performance in avoiding electric shock, but only when injection preceded the task for several days.[10] Nutritive and other side effects of the RNA were not ruled out.

Amnesia has been produced in a number of experiments in which protein synthesis is inhibited (typically by puromycin).[24] This amnesia may be attenuated by intracerebral saline injections at various times *after* learning and the injection of puromycin.*

Cholinergic agents. Another biochemical agent that may be implicated in memory is one that is active at the synapse. Acetylcholine (ACh) has been singled out by one group of investigators since it is known as a synaptic transmitter.[61] Because of the difficulties in evaluating ACh, experimenters have employed acetylcholine esterase (AChE), the ACh inactivator, to give an indirect estimate of the amount of ACh. In general, AChE levels were poorly or negatively related to maze learning, although a stronger relationship existed between these levels and rats bred for maze-learning ability. Later work by these investigators appears to upgrade the importance of early experiments (with emphasis being put upon its effect on cortex size) rather than AChE.[1] Recent efforts with synaptic chemicals have been reviewed by Deutsch, who has used anticholinesterases, such as diisopropyl fluorophosphate (DFP) and physostigmine, to produce loss of memory of a new habit by slowing the breakdown of ACh by AChE.[13] On the other hand, facilitation of a learned habit may be brought on with injections of DFP when the habit has almost been forgotten, showing that the time course of the behavior under study is critical in the effect of anticholinesterase agents.

*For discussions of puromycin and its effects and other issues related to protein synthesis and learning see references 3, 13, 25, and 32.

REFERENCES

1. Bennett, E. L., and others: Chemical and anatomical plasticity of brain, Science **146:**610, 1964.
2. Bourassa, C. M., and Swett, J. E.: Sensory discrimination thresholds with cutaneous nerve volleys in the cat, J. Neurophysiol. **Bu:**515, 1967.
3. Briggs, M. H., and Kitto, G. B.: The molecular basis of memory and learning, Psychol. Rev. **69:**537, 1962.
4. Brogden, W. J., and Gantt, W. H.: Intraneural conditioning—cerebellar conditioned reflexes, Arch. Neurol. Psychiat. **48:**437, 1942.
5. Bromiley, R. B.: Conditioned response in a dog after removal of neocortex, J. Comp. Physiol. Psychol. **41:**102, 1948.
6. Bureš, J.: Reversible decortication and behavior. In Brazier, M. A. B., editor: Central nervous system and behavior, New York, 1959, Josiah Macy, Jr., Foundation.
7. Bureš, J., and Burešová, O.: Plastic changes of unit activity based on reinforcing properties of extracellular stimulation of single neurons, J. Neurophysiol. **30:**98, 1967.
8. Cameron, D. E., and Solyom, L.: Effects of ribonucleic acid on memory, Geriatrics **16:**74, 1961.
9. Chow, K. L.: Effects of ablation. In Quarton, G. L.,

Melnechuk, T., and Schnutt, F. O., editors: The neurosciences, a study program, New York, 1967, The Rockefeller University Press.
10. Cook, L., and others: Ribonucleic acid: effect on conditioned behavior in rats, Science **141**:268, 1963.
11. Coons, E. E., and Cruce, J. A. F.: Lateral hypothalamus: Food current intensity in maintaining self-stimulation of hunger, Science **159**:1117, 1968.
12. Cronly-Dillon, J. R., Sutherland, N. S., and Wolf, J.: Intraretinal transfer of a learned shape discrimination in goldfish after section and regeneration of the optic nerve brachia, Exp. Neurol. **15**:455, 1966.
13. Deutsch, J. A.: The physiological basis of memory, Ann. Ren. Psychol. **20**:85, 1969.
14. De Valois, R. L.: Analysis and coding of color vision in the primate visual system. In Sensory receptors, Cold Spring Harbor, New York, 1965, Cold Spring Harbor Laboratory of Quantitative Biology.
15. Dingman, W., and Sporn, M. B.: Molecular theories of memory, Science **144**:26, 1965.
16. Doty, R. W., and Giurgea, C.: Conditioned reflexes established by coupling electrical excitations of two cortical areas. In Delafresnaye, J. F., editor: Brain mechanisms and learning, Oxford, 1961, Blackwell Scientific Publications Ltd.
17. Doty, R. W., Rutledge, L. T., Jr., and Larsen, R. M.: Conditioned reflexes established to electrical stimulation of cat cerebral cortex, J. Neuophysiol. **19**:401, 1956.
18. Dykman, R. A., and Shurrager, P. S.: Successive and maintained conditioning in spinal carnivores, J. Comp. Physiol. Psychol. **49**:27, 1956.
19. Eccles, J. C.: The physiology of nerve cells, Baltimore, 1957, The Johns Hopkins Press.
20. Evarts, E. V.: Pyramidal tract activity associated with a conditioned hand movement in the monkey, J. Neurophysiol. **29**:1011, 1966.
21. Evarts, E. V.: Activity of pyramidal tract neurons during postural fixation, J. Neurophysiol. **32**:375, 1969.
22. Fetz, E. E.: Operant conditioning of cortical unit activity, Science **163**:955, 1969.
23. Fitzgerald, L. A., and Thompson, R. F.: Classical conditioning of hindlimb flexion reflex in the acute spinal cat, Psychonomic Science **8**:213, 1967.
24. Flexner, L. B., Flexner, J. B., and Roberts, R.: Memory in mice analyzed with antibiotics, Science **155**:1377, 1967.
25. Gaito, J.: Macromolecules and brain. In Gaito, J., editor: Macromolecules and behavior, New York, 1966, Meredith Corporation.
26. Galambos, R.: A glia-neural theory of brain function, Proc. Nat. Acad. Sci., U.S.A. **47**:129, 1961.
27. Gantt, W. H.: Cardiovascular component of the conditional reflex to pain, food, and other stimuli, Physiol. Rev. **40**(4):266, 1960.
28. Girden, E., and others: Conditioned responses in a decorticate dog to acoustic, thermal and tactile stimulation, J. Comp. Psychol. **21**:367, 1936.
29. Glaser, G. H.: The normal electroencephalogram and its reactivity. In Glaser, G. H., editor, Electroencephalography and behavior, New York, 1963, Basic Books, Inc., Publishers.
30. Glickman, S. E., and Schiff, B. B.: A biological theory of reinforcement, Psychol. Rev. **74**:81, 1967.
31. Graham. C. H., editor: Vision and visual perception, New York, 1965, John Wiley & Sons, Inc.
32. Granit, R.: Receptors and sensory perception, New Haven, Connecticut, 1955, Yale University Press.
33. Grossman, S. P.: A textbook of physiological psychology, New York, 1967, John Wiley & Sons, Inc.
34. Hartline, H. K.: Visual receptors and retinal interaction Science **164**:270, 1969.
35. Hering, E.: Outlines of a theory of the light sense, Cambridge, Massachusetts, 1964, Harvard University Press. (Translated by L. M. Hurvich and D. Jameson.)
36. Hess, W. R.: The functional organization of the diencephalon, New York, 1957, Grune & Stratton, Inc.
37. Hind, J. E., and others: Unit activity in the auditory cortex. In Pasmussen, G. L., and Windle, W. F., editors: Neural mechanisms of the auditory and vestibular systems, Springfield, Illinois, 1960, Charles C Thomas, Publisher.
38. Hirsch, H. V. B., and Spinelli, D. N.: Visual experience modifies distribution of horizontally and vertically oriented receptive fields in cats, Science **168**:869, 1970.
39. Hubel, D. H., and Wiesel, T. N.: Receptive fields, binocular interaction and functional architecture in the cat's visual center, J. Physiol. **160**:106, 1962.
40. Hydén, H.: Biochemical changes in glial cells and nerve cells at varying activity. In Hoffman-Ostenhoff, O., editor: Biochemistry of the central nervous system, vol. III, London, 1959, Pergamon Press, Inc.
41. Hydén, H., and Egyhazi, E.: Nuclear RNA changes or nerve cells during a learning experiment in rats, Proc. Nat. Acad. Sci. U. S. A. **48**:1366, 1962.
42. Hydén, H., and Egyhazi, E.: Glial RNA changes during a learning experiment with rats, Proc. Nat. Acad. Sci. U. S. A. **49**:618, 1963.
43. Katsuki, Y.: Neural mechanisms of auditory sensation in cats. In Rosenblith, W. A., editor: Sensory communication, New York, 1961, John Wiley & Sons, Inc.
44. Katz, J. J., and Halstead, W. C.: Protein organization and mental function, Comp. Psychol. Monogr. **20 (103)**: 1, 1950.
45. Kuffler, S. W.: Discharge patterns and functional organization of mammalian retina, J. Neurophysiol. **16**:37, 1953.
46. Lashley, K. S.: In search of the engram. In Symposium of the Society of Experimental Biology, New York, 1950, Cambridge University Press.
47. Loucks, R. B.: Studies of neural structures essential for learning, II. The conditioning of salivary and striped muscle responses to faradization of cortical sensory elements, and the action of sleep upon such mechanisms, J. Comp. Psychol. **25**:315, 1938.
48. Luschei, E., Johnson, R., and Glickstein, M.: Response of neurons in the motor cortex during performance of a single repetitive arm movement (macaca, mulatta), Nature **217**:190, 1968.
49. Luschei, E., Saslow, G., and Glickstein, M.: Muscle potentials in reaction time, Exp. Neurol. **18**:429, 1967.
50. McGaugh, J. L.: Time-dependent processes in memory storage, Science **153**:1351, 1966.
51. Miller, J. M., and Glickstein, M.: Neural circuits involved in visumotor reaction time in monkeys, J. Neurophysiol. **30**:399, 1967.
52. Mishkin, M.: Visual mechanisms beyond the striate cortex. In Russell, R. W., editor: Frontiers in physiological psychology, New York, 1966, Academic Press, Inc.
53. Monne, L.: Functioning of the cytoplasm. In Nord, F. F., editor: Advances in enzymology, vol. VIII, New York, 1948, Interscience.

54. Morrell, F.: Electrophysiological contributions to the neural basis of learning, Physiol. Rev. **41**:443, 1961b.
55. Mountcastle, V. B., Powell, G. F., and Werner, G.: The relation of thalamic cells response to peripheral stimuli varied over an intensive continuum, J. Neurophysiol. **26**: 807, 1963.
56. Olds, J.: Hypothalamic substrates of reward, Physiol. Rev. **42**:554, 1962.
57. Pavlov, I.: Conditioned reflexes, New York, 1927, Oxford University Press.
58. Prokasy, W. F., editor: Classical conditioning, New York, 1965, Appleton-Century-Crofts.
59. Ratliff, F.: Match bands: quantitative studies on neural networks in the retina, San Francisco, 1965, Holden-Day, Inc.
60. Razran, G.: The observable unconscious and the inferable conscious in current Soviet psychophysiology: Interoceptive conditioning, sematic conditioning, and the orienting reflex, Psychol. Rev. **68**:81, 1961.
61. Rosenzweig, M. R., Krech, D., and Bennett, E. L.: A search for relations between brain chemistry and behavior, Psychol. Bull. **57**: 476, 1960.
62. Ruch, T. C., and Patton, H.: Psychology and biophysics, ed. 19, Philadelphia, 1965, W. B. Saunders Co.
63. Russell, I. S., and Ochs, S.: Localization of a memory trace in one cortical hemisphere and transfer to the other hemisphere, Brain **86**:37, 1963.
64. Schneider, A. M.: Control of memory by spreading cortical depression: a case for stimulus control, Psychol. Rev. **74**:201, 1967.
65. Sharpless, S., and Jasper, H. H.: Habituation of the arousal reaction, Brain **79**:655, 1956.
66. Shearn, D. W.: Does the heart learn, Psychol. Rev. **58**: 452, 1961.
67. Shearn, D. W.: Operant conditioning. In Greenberg, N. S., and Sternbach, R. A., editors: Handbook of psychophysiology, New York, In press, Holt, Rinehart & Winston, Inc.
68. Skinner, B. F.: The behavior of organisms: an experimental analysis, New York, 1938, Appleton-Century-Crofts.
69. Sokolov, E. N.: Neuronal models of the orienting reflex. In Brazier, M. A. B., editor: The central nervous systems and behavior, New York, 1960, Josiah Macy, Jr., Foundation.
70. Sperry, R. W.: Cerebral organization and behavior, Science **133**:1749, 1961.
71. Stevens, S. S.: To honor Fechner and repeal his law, Science **133**:80, 1961.
72. Taub, E., and Berman, A. J.: Movement and learning in the absence of sensory feedback. In Freedman, S. J., editor: The neuropsychology of spatially oriented behavior, Homewood, Illinois, 1968, Dorsey Press.
73. Thompson, R. F., and Spencer, W. A.: Habituation: a model phenomenon for the study of neuronal substrates of behavior, Psychol. Rev. **173**:16, 1966.
74. Valenstein, E. S., Cox, V. C., and Kakolewski, J. W.: Reexamination of the operant role of the hypothalamus in motivation, J. Comp. Physiol. Psychol. **77**:16, 1970.
75. Valenstein, E. S., and Valenstein, J. T.: Interaction of positive and negative reinforcing neural systems, Science **145**:1456, 1964.
76. von Békésy, G.: Experiments in hearing, New York, 1960, McGraw-Hill Book Co.
77. von Békésy, G.: Sensory inhibition, Princeton, New Jersey, 1967, Princeton University Press.
78. Watson, J. D., and Crick, F. H. C.: Molecular structure of nucleic acids, Nature (London) **171**:737, 1953
79. Woolsey, C. N.: Organization of cortical auditory system. In Rosenblith, W. A., editor: Sensory communication, New York, 1961, John Wiley & Sons, Inc.
80. Yoshii, N., and Ogura, H.: Studies on the unit discharge of brainstem reticular formation in the cat. I. Changes or reticular unit discharge following conditioning procedure, Med. J. Osaka Univ. **II**:1, 1960.
81. Zotterman, Y.: Thermal sensation. In Field, J., editor: Handbook of physiology, vol. I, Washington, 1959, American Physiological Society.

CHAPTER 24

MODELING AS A TOOL IN NEUROSCIENCE

TATE M. MINCKLER
THOMAS E. BAUER
LUANN M. RINGENBERG

Defined as a representation of reality condensed in structure, function, or time, the model becomes one of man's earliest recorded endeavors. It is therefore not a new tool, but a new application of an ancient tool that will be presented here.

There are many facets to the concept of modeling. Structural models include such everyday objects as toys, globes, portraits, representations of an atom, and architectural miniaturizations. Pure functional models are exemplified by computer programs, flow charts, circuit diagrams, and other abstract descriptions of reality. Combinations of structural and functional representations of the real world are recognized in flying airplane models, miniature road racing sets, etc. Models also may be discussed in terms of their descriptive or predictive function. Most of the structural models are descriptive, while most predictive models are mathematical or statistical in nature. The term simulation often appears in the context of predictive models. Simulation models usually mimic some real situation in reduced time frame allowing a prediction of the effect of various influences on the system in a fraction of real time. As an example of a predictive simulation model, consider a computer program which utilizes probability theory to optimize a marketing strategy.

Cybernetics is one aspect of modeling that deals with the principles of function shared by biologic and mechanical systems. Particular attention is given to the control, or feedback, mechanisms by which both men and machines execute complicated activities with a minimum of conscious judgmental participation.

The design of most types of models is based upon an understanding of the real world to be modeled. Unfortunately, not all of the real world is well enough understood to be copied. It is here that the conceptual modeling technique comes into play. The application to be described demonstrates how conceptual modeling can help to identify functional components and relationships in a complex subject. It can also be used to suggest possible mechanisms. The principal value of the technique is that it tends to force polarization of thinking and to pose organized questions about the real world.

METHOD OF DYNAMIC CONCEPT MODELING

The basic technique of model design is a cyclic pattern of testing and modifying. Specifically, the sequence of steps is as follows: (1) define the problem; (2) construct the simplest model possible that will accommodate the requirements that have been defined; (3) test the model with a real world situation; (4) redefine and/or modify the model based on the results of step 3; and (5) return to step 2 until the model allows the desired depth of understanding. When the tests have pointed out shortcomings in the original model, the design must be modified and new features must be introduced to handle these shortcomings.

Perhaps the most difficult step is the first one—defining the problem. If it is assumed that the objective of the model is to foster an understanding of the system, then the next step is to break the system down into its subsystems and to define the subfunctions as well as possible at this point. It may become apparent that certain of these subsystems are not really relevant to the problem under study, and, if so, these elements should be discarded. But, as will be seen later, during this first pass it is seldom known which components are really unimportant. At this stage, emphasis should be placed on identifying the known components of the system and the known attributes of these components. Also, since all systems can be regarded as subsystems of larger systems, it is important to recognize the position of each particular problem in this hierarchy in order to place it in proper perspective.

The next step is the construction of a model that will accommodate all of the features previously defined. The medium of construction becomes important here: out of what material will the model be built? The function that the model is expected to perform will help make this decision. Model airplanes or globes would be constructed of plastic, wood, or steel, while a model of a marketing strategy would be series of mathematical formulas. Later on in this chapter a memory model will be presented. If this model is intended to relate memory with specific anatomic areas, one might well produce a physical brain model out of an appropriate substance such as plastic. Since this model is intended to explain only functional relationships and not anatomic correlations, however, this type of medium is inappropriate; accordingly, the medium is of the flow diagram variety. To summarize this idea, a model has the overall function of representing reality; in accomplishing this it may take the form of a series of equations, a flow chart, or a hunk of plastic. Another feature that must be kept in mind during this step is simplicity. A cardinal rule of modeling is that the model should include only those components that are absolutely essential to accommodate whatever functions are performed by the system.

The model has now been defined and constructed using the best information available up to this point, and it is ready to be tested with a real world situation. This stage might be thought of as model validation. When attempting to validate the model, there are three types of criteria that must be tested for and kept in mind. These are reproduction of past data, tests of reasonableness, and checks for completeness. This step allows weak points or missing links in the model to be identified, and these will be used during the next step to suggest improvements.

At this point the level of understanding that the model has afforded must be evaluated. As long as the test phase continues to point out inadequacies, one must return to step 2 and repeat the cycle. When the model is able to satisfactorily handle all test situations presented to it and it is apparent that any further changes will not appreciably increase the level of understanding desired, the task is complete.

The application of these procedures to study of a system yields two results—a greater comprehension of the system and a model of the system. The first is a result of the fact that this is a dynamic learning process; the student is continually modifying his conception of the system in the light of new understanding and insight. The second product, the model itself, has intrinsic value in that it is now available as a teaching tool for others and may be used as a stepping stone toward even greater understanding.

CONCEPTUAL MODEL OF THE MEMORY FUNCTION OF THE BRAIN

In order to exemplify this technique of modeling, the function of memory should be considered. Because of obvious similarities between the functions of a computer and those of the brain, computer technology should be a suitable tool for this model.

For purposes of the present discussion, a simple description of a digital computer is sufficient. A computer consists of four main functional parts—a memory, a processor containing control, arithmetic and logical units, and input and output units. The memory unit gives the computer its ability to "remember" and can be used to store either programs (instructions to the computer) or data. The control unit interprets and executes the instructions. The arithmetic unit performs arithmetic, and the input/output units get raw data into and processed answers out of the computer.

A computer model of memory can be established by providing for input and output channels, at least one processor, and at least two kinds of memory units, one for short-term and one for long-term memory (Fig. 24-1).[2] For purposes of the functional model, the storage technique for each type of memory should be defined. It seems appropriate to use a

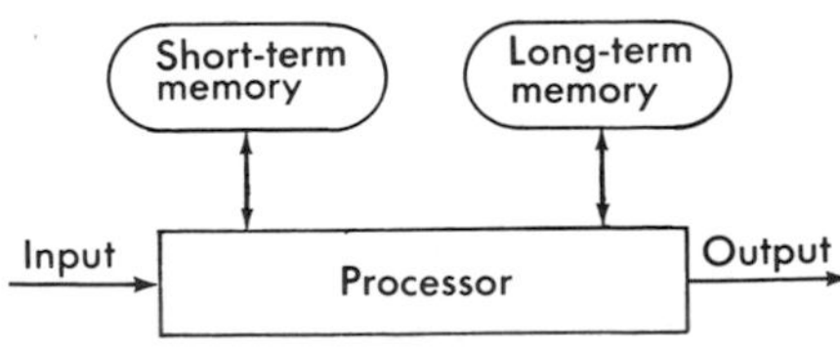

Fig. 24-1. First approximation of computer system to model the memory function of the brain.

serial data storage approach in short-term memory on a random-access disk of limited capacity, requiring only minimal processing between raw data input and temporary storage. The retrieval function therefore must randomly search the disk for recently input data, but so long as the amount of data so stored is limited in volume, reasonable retrieval times can be expected.

Long-term memory requires a far more sophisticated approach. Consideration of available computer storage methods suggests an inverted file storage approach. This technique, like an encyclopedia, stores both the data itself and extensive references to the data. As a simple example, all data in reference to individuals might be stored under a dictionary of names. Combination names, such as *Woodrow Wilson,* would appear under both *Woodrow* and *Wilson,* with cross references to the other associated name. Then when one asks for *Wilson,* the file for *Wilson* is found, and a list of associations are recovered—one for *Woodrow,* one for *Flip,* and one for each of the other *Wilson* associations. The inverted file computer is tremendously fast for retrieval of associations, but it is costly to establish and maintain, as every new block of data requires extensive rearrangement of the previous file of associations. These characteristics are similar to the observed delays (30 to 60 minutes) in learning by the brain as permanent or long-term memory; they are also consistent with the almost instantaneous recovery of association data. Most people can recall the formula for the circumference of a circle (πd) as fast or faster than they can recall what they ate for breakfast this morning (randomly stored in short-term memory).

The simple model of memory (Fig. 24-1) is ready to be tested against reality. One common area of memory behavior is traumatic amnesia, or temporary memory loss, following a blow to the head.

Amnesia for recent events

A common accompaniment of mild concussion is a progressive retrograde amnesia of temporary duration.[5] Up to 1 to 3 minutes after the accident, the patient can recall the events immediately preceding the accident. Then these events are lost, sometimes permanently, in spite of otherwise complete recovery. This type of amnesia is usually associated with some confusion in the immediate posttraumatic period, and memory of the first few minutes after the concussion usually is also lost. A case of permanent short-term memory deficit has also been recorded.[4] Following a motorcycle accident, a patient with intact long-term memory has continued to have difficulty with recent events. This pattern is also common in the elderly patient without specific traumatic cause.

Amnesia for past associations

A distinctly different type of amnesia occasionally occurs with concussion. Memory for past associations may be lost for minutes to months, or even forever. This is the classic, dramatic amnesia in which the patient cannot remember who he is or anything about himself. Memories for language concepts, music, and other things may be entirely intact. However, during temporary posttraumatic amnesia for past events, some information may be stored, since patients usually recover not only their complete memory for past associations, but also will remember at least some of the events that transpired during the amnesia phase. The computer model as constructed in Fig. 24-1 offers no means to produce these memory failures. The model must therefore be altered to accommodate these new functions.

At least several long-term memory units can be assumed on the simple observation that certain types of memory can be lost while others remain intact. To simulate the specific failure in amnesia, the model must have a store function and a retrieve function for each memory unit. Since memory for past personal associations can be lost and upon recovery made available again, the memory itself must have remained intact. Only the retrieval function needs to be damaged to produce the observed amnesia. In addition, since some recovered patients can recall events during the amnesia period, their store function must have been working.

These observations suggest separate store functions and retrieval functions for each of the long-term memory units. This is consistent with computer technology. Amnesia for long-term memory data is represented in the model by a retrieval function failure. The independent store function also may be damaged or intact.

In reviewing the progressive retrograde amnesia affecting short-term memory, several interesting features are apparent. In this case memory is *not* recovered after loss. Initially however there was certainly information in the file that was lost over a period of a few minutes. Therefore, one can assume separate storage and retrieval functions for short-term memory. Because of limited capacity, the data must be reviewed and refreshed periodically through the retrieval-storage loop. There is now a simple mechanism to accommodate retrograde amnesia. If the concussion temporarily dam-

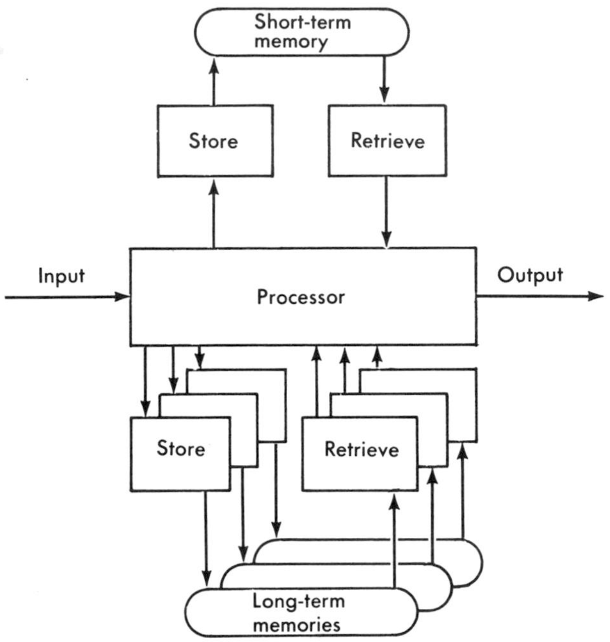

Fig. 24-2. Computer model of memory system, including separate Store and Retrieve functions for each memory unit.

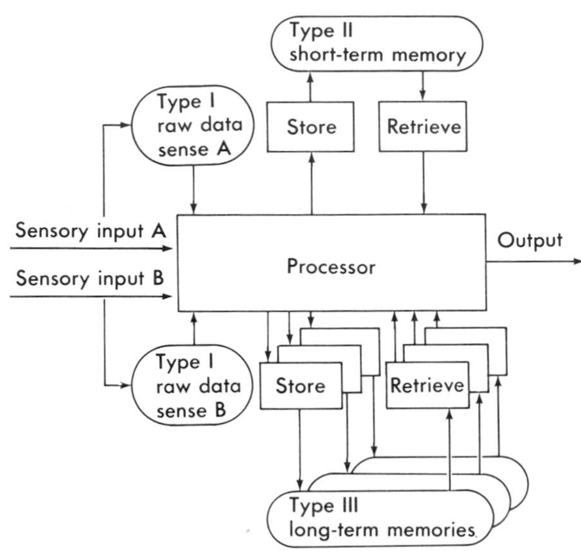

Fig. 24-3. Model of computer system to mimic basic memory functions. This model could be programmed to simulate normal memory processing, various amnesias, and eidetic behavior.

ages the store function, data already in the file can be retrieved, but it cannot be restored or refreshed. It is therefore lost progressively over a few minutes time. The new model (see Fig. 24-2), which can accommodate situations of traumatic amnesia, now handles memories of two distinct types and has functional components insuring that selective failure of these components will mimic at least one type of failure observed in nature.

Many reports attest to the existence of eidetic, or photographic, memory, which is rare in adults but as frequent as four percent in elementary aged children.[1] Eidetic images are apparently very much like a photograph, in that the content of the image can be recalled in great detail, whereas normal memory is in terms of interpreted content. The eidetic individual can look at a page of text and without awareness of its content memorize the image of the page. As long as years later, the page can be recalled and read from memory. Many people have degrees of this ability; some can, for example, remember the location on a page of text where an idea is presented. Common experience suggests that this type of memory may also exist for senses other than sight. One can frequently "replay" the last few phrases of a conversation and reinterpret the sounds into meaningful words.

As constructed, the model from Fig. 24-2 cannot accommodate any significant storage of unprocessed sensory data. The short-term memory is designed to handle interpreted data only. The model therefore must again be modified, this time by adding a third type of memory unit, designed as a buffer storage for raw incoming data. Since data are normally interpreted as they arrive but can be replayed if desired, there must be not only a new memory unit, but also a split path for incoming data. Duplicate messages can then be sent directly to the processor, which performs the interpretation, and can also be simultaneously sent to a raw data memory. Since the various senses have rather different incoming pathways and individual primary cortical areas, it seems reasonable to design the model with a separate raw data memory unit for each type of sensory data. For convenience in modeling, the raw data memory is called a type I memory unit, short-term memory a type II unit, and long-term memory a type III memory unit. The modified model appears as Fig. 24-3.

As a final test of this model of memory, it must include the functions of learning and forgetting. In terms of the computer model, learning is synonymous with storage, and the model has that capacity. Forgetting in computer terms requires either a failure to find, or intentional destruction of, stored data. Controlled destruction of data, or purging, is a common procedure in computer systems and can be modeled in several ways. The problem then is establishing the criteria and the mechanisms for purging or saving data.

Type II memory has been described as "serial" in structure. This means that items of data coming into the file are stored in the sequence of arrival. Since there is a finite limit to the amount of this storage available, means must be designed to save the data of value and eliminate that of lesser or no value. A value system is therefore proposed. For the computer model a special computer program can be written that evaluates each item of data on a scale of 0 through 9, with 0 the least and 9 the most valuable. This value is attached to the data as it is stored in type II memory. One means of purging the file is obvious; data of high value can be written on top of and therefore replace data of lowest value whenever the memory is full. Without some other technique however the file will soon be full of value 9 data. There must also be a means of transferring high value data to permanent (type III) memory. "Refreshment" of memory requiring periodic retrieval of data and restorage has been previously mentioned. If high value data is automatically transferred to the type III store program during refreshment, this should solve another part of the problem by continuously moving the more important data out of the type II file. The value-judgement program could then relook at medium value data at each refreshment pass. Depending on the passage of time, new information, or new relationships, medium value data could then be retained at the same value or rescaled upward or downward. These three mechanisms—replacement of low value data, transfer of high value data, and periodic reevaluation of medium value data—will accommodate the characteristics observed in learning and forgetting in type II memory.

This scheme also provides an introduction to understanding the initiation of learning in type III memory. The evaluation program provides the starting point for permanent learning. In the model then there must be a mechanism designed for storing a tremendous volume of data with many associations that can be recalled very rapidly. Fortunately, such a computer mechanism exists and has been briefly introduced as *inverted storage*.[3] Each data message coming into the type III store function is given a sequential number. The message is broken down into its contained concepts or words according to the preexisting organization of the file. The new message number is added to the existing list of message numbers already stored by each matching word or concept in the file. When a new word or concept is submitted, it is assigned to a new position in the organizational structure, and its message number is stored. In addition, the new message is compared with previous data in the file for other associations, and the new message number is stored against previous ideas. In this way new information is integrated with the old, and all data are interassociated. Although it may sound complicated, this inverted storage concept successfully operates in a number of current computer systems. Some of the characteristics of this type of file storage are of particular interest in terms of the memory model. The special advantage of this storage approach in computers is extremely rapid retrieval of associated data from files of very large volume. Its major disadvantage is the amount of processing required by the computer to reorganize the file after each new batch of data is added. The model system can therefore be programmed to add incoming data to the end of each file until the daily "housekeeping" run. "Housekeeping" in computer terms is the time each day when files are reorganized and cleaned up. This usually takes place overnight, when demands on the computer are at a minimum. The comparison to sleep and brain function is invitingly obvious, but not necessarily valid.

There have been outlined a series of mechanisms by which the model can simulate the function of acquiring permanent associations, or "learning." The mechanism of association in permanent memory (type III) was described as the attachment of numbers or pointers to each concept or word in various dictionaries. If it is assumed that during housekeeping the more recent associations get priority of placement in the string, and that there is some finite limit on the number of pointers recovered in a routine retrieval, a mechanism for the kind of forgetting commonly observed in type III memories is provided. For example, if over a period of years there are many other people named *Wilson* brought into the file, and *Flip Wilson* is not encountered during that time, then the pointer to *Flip* will be moved to the very end of the *Wilson* pointer list and will not be recalled when *Wilson* is asked for. However, the number of *Flips* encountered during those years is very small, and so the *Wilson* pointer in the *Flip* list is still recoverable. Very simply, if one hears the word *Wilson* he can name several *Wilsons* (but not *Flip*); however, if he hears *Flip*, he immediately remembers *Flip Wilson*. This explanation accounts for the frequently observed situation in which by asking certain questions one can recall specific associations, whereas other questions may not retrieve the desired data.

For the purposes of this treatise, the conceptual modeling of memory functions has been carried far enough (1) to illustrate the technique, (2) to suggest some ideas about how memory *could* function in the brain, and (3) to pose some interesting questions in the field of neuroscience. Is there an instant replay (type I) memory in man? Does the brain perform its housekeeping functions during sleep? Are dreams, for example, the occasional awareness of data routinely being reorganzed and reassociated?

It must be kept clearly in mind that however enticing the model may seem, it is simulating the function, not the mechanism, of memory. In so far as it performs parallel to the observed functions of the brain, it can be very useful, even to suggesting new avenues of research; it cannot however be accepted as the explanation of the real world without objective proof.

REFERENCES

1. Editorial: Photographic memory. The Sciences, vol. X, Oct. 1970, New York Academy of Sciences.
2. Editorial: The long and the short of memory. The sciences, vol. X, Dec. 1970, New York Academy of Sciences.
3. Lefkovitz, D.: File structures for on-line systems, Philadelphia, 1968, Computer Command and Control Co.
4. Warrington, E. K., and Shallice, T.: The selective impairment of auditory verbal short term memory, Brain **92**:885, 1969.
5. Yarnell, P. R., and Lynch, S.: Retrograde memory immediately after concussion, Lancet **1**:863, 1970.

SUGGESTED READINGS

Deutsch, S.: Models of the nervous system, New York, 1967, John Wiley & Sons, Inc.

Elliott, F. A.: Clinical neurology, Philadelphia, 1966, W. B. Saunders Co.

Hillier, F. S., and Lieberman, G. J.: Introduction to operations research, San Francisco, 1967, Holden-Day, Inc.

Quarton, G. C., Melnechuk, T., and Schmitt, F. O., editors: The neurosciences, New York, 1967, Rockefeller University Press.

von Neumann, J.: The computer and the brain, New Haven, Connecticut, 1958, Yale University Press.

Wiener, N.: Cybernetics or control and communication in the animal and the machine, Cambridge, Massachusetts, 1961, The M.I.T. Press.

Index

D

N

Q

R

T

U

V